PATHOLOGY OF BONE MARROW AND BLOOD CELLS

PATHOLOGY OF BONE MARROW AND BLOOD CELLS

DIANE C. FARHI, M.D.

Quest Diagnostics
Tucker, Georgia

with

CAROLYN CHILING CHAI, M.D.

Quest Diagnostics
San Juan Capistrano, California

ANDREW S. EDELMAN, M.D., PH.D.

Quest Diagnostics
Horsham, Pennsylvania

TALAT PARVEEN, M.D., M.S.

Quest Diagnostics
Tucker, Georgia

THUY-LIEU THI VO, M.D.

Quest Diagnostics
St. Louis, Missouri

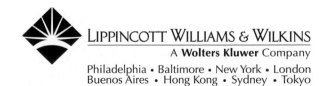

LIPPINCOTT WILLIAMS & WILKINS
A **Wolters Kluwer** Company

Philadelphia • Baltimore • New York • London
Buenos Aires • Hong Kong • Sydney • Tokyo

Acquisitions Editors: Ruth W. Weinberg/Jonathan Pine
Developmental Editor: Joanne Bersin
Production Editor: Elaine Verriest McClusky
Manufacturing Manager: Colin Warnock
Cover Designer: Armen Kojoyian
Compositor: TechBooks
Printer: Quebecor World Kingsport

© 2004 by LIPPINCOTT WILLIAMS & WILKINS
530 Walnut Street
Philadelphia, PA 19106 USA
LWW.com

Printed and bound in the United States of America

Library of Congress Cataloging-in-Publication Data

Farhi, Diane C.
    Pathology of bone marrow and blood cells/by Diane C. Farhi with Carolyn Chiling Chai . . . [et al.].
        p. ; cm.
    Includes bibliographical references and index.
    ISBN 0-397-51611-8
    1. Hematopoietic stem cell disorders—Histopathology.   2. Bone marrow—Histopathology.   I. Title.
    [DNLM: 1. Bone Marrow—pathology.   2. Blood Cells–pathology.   3. Bone Marrow
Examination—methods.   4. Hematologic Diseases—diagnosis.   5. Hematologic Tests—methods.
6. Lymphatic Diseases—diagnosis.   WH 380 F223p 2004]
    RC644.5.F37   2004
    616.4′1071—dc22

                                                                                                                2003069521

Care has been taken to confirm the accuracy of the information presented and to describe generally
accepted practices. However, the authors and publisher are not responsible for errors or omissions or for any
consequences from application of the information in this book and make no warranty, expressed or implied,
with respect to the currency, completeness, or accuracy of the contents of the publication. Application of this
information in a particular situation remains the professional responsibility of the practitioner.

The authors and publisher have exerted every effort to ensure that drug selection and dosage set forth in
this text are in accordance with current recommendations and practice at the time of publication. However,
in view of ongoing research, changes in government regulations, and the constant flow of information
relating to drug therapy and drug reactions, the reader is urged to check the package insert for each drug for
any change in indications and dosage and for added warnings and precautions. This is particularly important
when the recommended agent is a new or infrequently employed drug.

Some drugs and medical devices presented in this publication have Food and Drug Administration
(FDA) clearance for limited use in restricted research settings. It is the responsibility of the health care
provider to ascertain the FDA status of each drug or device planned for use in their clinical practice.

10 9 8 7 6 5 4 3 2 1

To patients and those who care for them.

CONTENTS

Jose
Costa

PREFACE

This book is intended to help physicians interpret peripheral blood and bone marrow specimens quickly, easily, and accurately. The recent and ongoing explosion of information in hematopathology has vastly complicated the diagnostician's task. We perceived a need for a synthetic treatment of the most important diagnostic points. We aimed to make the text accessible rather than encyclopedic, and have tried to avoid repetitive discussions of the same entity.

The discussions presented in the following pages are addressed primarily to those responsible for peripheral blood and bone marrow interpretation: general pathologists, hematopathologists, and hematologist/oncologists. We also kept in mind the needs of trainees in these fields and hope that this book helps them attain diagnostic proficiency.

We earnestly hope that we have succeeded in these goals. We regret any deficiencies or inaccuracies the reader may find and welcome suggestions for improvement.

ACKNOWLEDGMENTS

We gratefully acknowledge the assistance of many individuals, too numerous to mention individually, who made the publication of this volume possible. In particular, we thank Drs. Thomas E. Burgess, Raymond L. Kaplan, William M. Miller, and Ana K. Stankovic for valuable advice and critical review of portions of the manuscript. We thank Drs. Kaplan, Carlos R. Abramowsky, and Bahig M. Shebata for providing case material used to illustrate babesiosis and certain pediatric hematopoietic disorders.

We are indebted to Drs. Steven Silverberg and Pamela Murari for stimulating our interest in academic medicine and hematopathology, respectively.

On a more personal level, we thank our families and friends for their support and patience during the gestation of this book, which threatened at times to become interminable.

Above all, we express our gratitude to Providence for keeping us alive, sustaining us, and bringing us to the conclusion of this work.

1

BONE MARROW STRUCTURE, MORPHOLOGY, AND HEMATOPOIESIS

TALAT PARVEEN

BONE MARROW STRUCTURE

Bone marrow is a mesenchyme-derived, soft, semisolid, red gelatinous substance occupying the medullary cavities of the axial skeleton. In adults, bone marrow is the primary site of effective hematopoiesis and is composed of bony and vascular structures and hematopoietic tissue. The medullary cavity is encased by trabecular bone consisting of periosteum and cortical and subcortical bone (Fig. 1-1). It is supported by slender, curved, bony trabeculae or struts that interlace to form a delicate but strong network. The inner surface of the cortical bone and the outer surface of the bony trabeculae are lined by a single layer of thin, flat, elongated, endothelium-like cells or endosteal cells. Arterioles, sinusoids, and small peripheral nerves traverse the interstitial space (Fig. 1-2). The medullary cavity contains hematopoietic and stromal cells and extracellular matrix.

Bone marrow specimens from very young children show active bone remodeling. Plump osteoblasts on one side and active osteoclasts on the other line the trabecular bone, and the center often shows an irregular, basophilic cartilaginous core. With age, the cartilaginous core converts to bone, and osteoblastic and osteoclastic activity becomes less exuberant. In young to middle-aged adults, osteoblasts become patches of flattened cells and osteoclasts are rarely seen. In older adults, very little evidence of ongoing bone remodeling is present (1–5).

Blood vessels consist of the nutrient artery and the periosteal capillary network, which supply bone marrow with oxygenated blood to maintain hematopoiesis. The nutrient artery is the major source of blood supply and consists of ascending and descending branches, arterioles, and smaller branching vessels. These smaller branches of the nutrient artery further divide and ultimately form a sinusoidal network composed of ectatic, widely patent, and thin-walled channels. The return circulation occurs through the sinusoids. In humans, the sinusoids consist of an inner layer of endothelial cells with sparse subendothelial connective tissue and an outer incomplete layer of adventitial cells. The adventitial cells have long cytoplasmic processes that lie along the sinusoidal surface and project into the stroma to form the stromal framework. Cytoplasmic processes of macrophages also protrude through the endothelial cells into the sinusoidal lumen. The sinusoids may represent a major route of

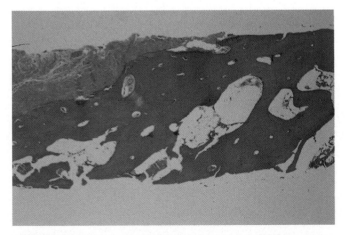

FIGURE 1-1. Bone marrow biopsy specimen: structure. Periosteum and cortical and subcortical bone.

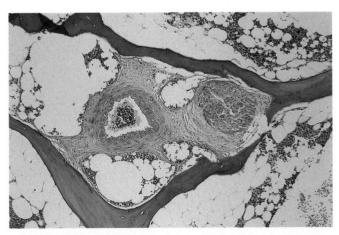

FIGURE 1-2. Bone marrow biopsy specimen: structure. Arteriole and nerve.

egress of hematopoietic cells from bone marrow. After maturation, hematopoietic cells migrate into the sinusoidal space to enter the blood circulation. The sinusoids are generally empty but sometimes contain actively dividing hematopoietic cells and megakaryocytes. True capillaries are difficult to identify, and lymphatic channels are not present in bone marrow. Enhanced stimulation of erythropoietic or granulopoietic activity leads to increased blood flow to bone marrow. The small arterioles appear thickened and more numerous in specimens from patients with chronic hypertension (6,7).

Peripheral nerves appear as short segments in core biopsy specimens. Although sensory and autonomic nerves apparently innervate bone marrow, relatively little is known of the relationship between the nervous system and hematopoiesis, blood flow, or other aspects of bone marrow biology (8,9).

BONE MARROW MORPHOLOGY AND HEMATOPOIESIS

The hematopoietic tissue is composed of hematopoietic and stromal cells and extracellular matrix. Hematopoietic cells and adipose tissue occupy the major portion of the bone marrow interstitial space, and the remaining stromal cells and extracellular matrix are present in a small amount.

In normal bone marrow, hematopoietic cells display an organized pattern. Immature myeloid precursors are lined up in rows adjacent to the bony trabeculae, away from the sinusoids. The maturing myeloid cells filter into the center of the bone marrow cavity and, when mature, pass directly through the cytoplasm of endothelial cells into the sinusoids and enter the circulation. The erythroid precursors form small, nonparatrabecular clusters or colonies that are composed of cells in varying stages of maturation. Occasionally, a central histiocyte (nurse cell) is present in the center of the erythroid cluster. These nests are located near the sinusoidal wall, and mature erythrocytes enter the sinusoids by directly passing through the cytoplasm of endothelial cells. In smears, the clusters may remain intact. Megakaryocytes reside adjacent to the sinusoidal wall in proximity to the erythroid islands. They extend their cytoplasmic processes through the cytoplasm of endothelial cells into the sinusoidal lumen and shed platelets directly into the circulation. Disorganization of this pattern or abnormal localization of the hematopoietic cells is a low-power clue to serious infections or clonal hematopoietic disorders (1,2).

General Features of Hematopoiesis

Hematopoiesis is a mechanism by which mature blood cells are formed from pluripotent hematopoietic stem cells. It is believed that multipotential hematopoietic stem cells and multipotential mesenchymal stem cells originate from common pluripotent stem cells that are capable of self-renewal and differentiation. In normal bone marrow, pluripotent

hematopoietic stem cells represent only a small proportion (approximately 0.05%) of the total hematopoietic cell mass and are intermixed with progenitor and more mature recognizable hematopoietic cells. Multipotential hematopoietic stem cells give rise to progenitor multilineage myeloid stem cells and progenitor lymphoid stem cells. Lymphoid stem cells differentiate into various subtypes of lymphocytes and plasma cells. Progenitor myeloid stem cell differentiation includes granulocytes (neutrophils, eosinophils, and basophils), mononuclear phagocytes (monocytes and macrophages), mast cells, erythroid cells, and megakaryocytes. This differentiation is achieved by progressive loss of proliferate activity and by gradually acquiring lineage-specific characteristics. Multipotential mesenchymal stem cells differentiate into a heterogeneous connective tissue lineage consisting of adipocytes, osteoblasts, osteoclasts, chondroblasts, endothelial cells, and fibroblasts such as reticular cells (3–13).

Development of Hematopoietic Tissue

Embryonic and Fetal Hematopoiesis

In humans, the yolk sac is the first site of blood cell production where hematopoiesis begins outside the embryo as blood islands during the third week of gestation. These hematopoietic cells are derived from mesoderm and predominantly consist of multipotential stem cells and primitive erythroblasts. The erythroblasts are large, nucleated, and megaloblastic. Identifiable mature neutrophils or megakaryocytes are not present during embryonic life.

At the 6th week of gestation, the hematopoietic tissue develops in the embryonic liver, which becomes the major site of hematopoiesis until the second trimester. During the early stages of fetal hepatic erythropoiesis, the hematopoietic tissue predominantly consists of hematopoietic stem cells and erythroid cells. Megakaryocytes appear during the 12th week and mature neutrophils after the 16th week of fetal development. More than half of the nucleated cells in the fetal liver are nucleated erythroid cells with a few megakaryocytes and granulocytes. Fetal hepatic erythropoiesis is normoblastic and results in nonnucleated red blood cells that are larger than adult red blood cells. The spleen does not normally function as an active site of hematopoiesis. In bone marrow, hematopoiesis starts during the 16th week of gestation and by the 26th week of intrauterine life, bone marrow becomes the primary site of hematopoiesis (14–22).

Neonatal and Childhood Hematopoiesis

After birth, hematopoiesis in the liver ceases, and bone marrow becomes the primary site of hematopoiesis. In neonates and young children, hematopoiesis occurs in most of the bone marrow cavities including the distal portion of long bones. Bone marrow cavities are filled with hematopoietic tissue (red marrow) with few fat cells (yellow marrow). Fat cells gradually appear between hematopoietic cells, beginning with the digits and advancing toward the axial skeleton (23,24).

Adult Hematopoiesis

In adults, hematopoiesis is confined to flat bones (skull, ribs, sternum, vertebrae, scapulae, clavicles, pelvis, and the upper half of the sacrum) and proximal portions of long bones (femur and humerus). The remaining bone marrow cavity is occupied by fat cells. The fat cell contents gradually increase with age, and in the elderly, most of the bone marrow cavity is filled with fatty tissue. Under conditions of stress, fat cells can be replaced by hematopoietic tissue. In mature adults, the subcortical region of trabecular bone is paucicellular, and in older adults, it is usually devoid of hematopoietic tissue. If this area is involved in hematopoiesis, it indicates abnormal hematopoiesis. The iliac crest is the standard biopsy site, in part because it retains some hematopoietic activity into the ninth decade and beyond, especially in the presence of a primary bone marrow disorder (23,24).

Regulation of Hematopoiesis

Hematopoiesis is a well-regulated but complex process in which the maturation of hematopoietic cells occurs in an orderly sequence. Regulation of hematopoiesis primarily occurs in the bone marrow microenvironment by cell-to-cell interaction and/or by the generation of specific hormones and various proteins called cytokines. This results in homing (recognition and adhesiveness of hematopoietic progenitor cells in their specific stromal microenvironment), proliferation, and differentiation of hematopoietic progenitor cells and egress of the developing hematopoietic cells (25–31).

Cytokines are a large family of proteoglycans produced primarily by stromal cells that act on receptor molecules to regulate hematopoiesis. The cytokines act on primitive stem cells and lineage-committed cells for their survival, renewal, proliferation, and differentiation and on mature cells for their functions. Cytokines may act locally at the site of their production or circulate in the blood. They usually affect more than one lineage and can exert a stimulatory (positive) or inhibitory (negative) influence on hematopoiesis (32–34).

The stimulatory (positive) cytokines or hematopoietic growth factors are glycoproteins that regulate the self-renewal of stem cells and the proliferation and differentiation of lineage-committed progenitor cells. They also affect the function of mature hematopoietic cells. Bone marrow stromal cells produce the majority of the stimulatory growth factors, except erythropoietin and thrombopoietin, which are primarily synthesized by peritubular cells of the kidney and liver, respectively. Stimulatory growth factors include stem cell factors (steel factor, kit ligand), granulocyte/monocyte colony-stimulating factor, granulocyte colony-stimulating

factor, monocyte colony-stimulating factor, erythropoietin, thrombopoietin, and various interleukins (interleukin-1 to interleukin-18) (35–45). Less significant regulatory hormones influencing the formation and proliferation of hematopoietic cells include growth hormone, insulin-like growth factor I, vascular endothelial growth factor, and platelet-derived growth factor (46–48).

The inhibitory (negative) cytokines inhibit the proliferation of normal hematopoietic progenitor cells in bone marrow and are produced by bone marrow stromal cells and macrophages. These inhibitory factors (cytokines) include transforming growth factor β, tumor necrosis factor α, macrophage inflammatory protein 1α, tetrapeptides, and pentapeptides. Some regulatory factors such as basic fibroblast growth factor and epidermal growth factor can exert their influence indirectly to inhibit hematopoiesis (49–52).

In addition to the cytokines, adhesion molecules are also essential for the regulation of hematopoiesis. The important adhesion molecules include adhesion molecules of the immunoglobulin supergene family, integrins, and selectin. The adhesion molecules (receptors) are present at the cell surface and bind with molecules (ligand) on the surface of target cells. These adhesion molecules mediate the attachment of various hematopoietic cells to each other, to stromal cells, and to extracellular matrix. They influence the induction, differentiation, and function of hematopoietic cells. Adhesion molecules also regulate the retention and release of hematopoietic cells in the bone marrow (53–55).

In recent years, numerous genes implicated as important regulators of hematopoietic stem cell growth, proliferation, differentiation, and fate have been identified, cloned, and sequenced. These genes include *SCL, GATA-2, HOX B4, c-mpl,* and *dlk* (56–60).

Hematopoietic Microenvironment

The hematopoietic microenvironment is a complex, highly organized structure composed of stromal cells (adipocytes, osteoblasts, osteoclasts, endothelial cells, and fibroblast-like reticular cells), accessory cells (T lymphocytes and monocytes), and their products (extracellular matrix and cytokines). The microenvironment provides support for hematopoietic tissue and regulates hematopoiesis by directly interacting with hematopoietic cells and/or by secreting various regulatory factors. The yolk sac in the embryo and the liver and bone marrow in the fetus provide the microenvironment for intrauterine hematopoiesis (51–68).

Stromal Cells

Bone marrow stromal cells consist of adipocytes, osteoblasts, osteoclasts, endothelial cells, and fibroblast-like reticular cells (Fig. 1-3). Although these cells are derived from multipotential stem cells, they do not develop into blood cells and are not found in normal peripheral blood. Stromal

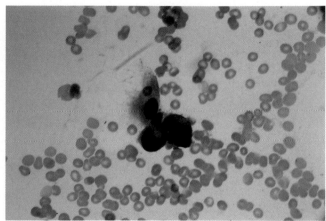

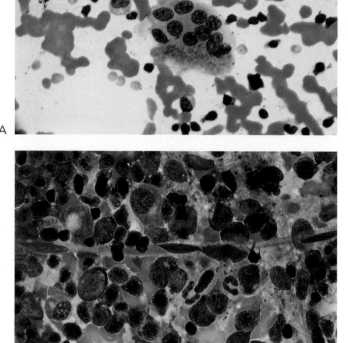

FIGURE 1-3. Bone marrow aspirate: stromal cells. **A:** An Osteoclast. **B:** Osteoblasts. **C:** Endothelial cells.

cells, together with extracellular matrix, provide a suitable microenvironment for the maturation and proliferation of hematopoietic cells (69,70).

Adipocytes (fat cells) are the largest cells in the bone marrow, measuring approximately 80 to 90 μm in diameter. They lie in close contact with hematopoietic cells and other stromal cells. In normal adults, fat cells are abundant and comprise 30% to 70% of bone marrow cells. Adipocytes are inversely proportional to hematopoietic cells. Whenever there is an increase or decrease in bone marrow hematopoietic cells, there is a corresponding decrease or increase in bone marrow adipocytes (fat cells). The mechanism of this inverse relationship between hematopoietic cells and fat cells is not well established (71–73).

Osteoblasts are large, ovoid or cuboid cells that measure 20 to 50 μm in diameter. The osteoblasts have a small eccentric nucleus and abundant basophilic cytoplasm with a clear Golgi zone located away from the nucleus. The osteoblast resembles a plasma cell but is much larger, and the Golgi zone is located away from the nucleus. They are derived from bone lining or endosteal cells. Osteoblasts are rarely seen in normal adult bone marrow (74,75).

Osteoclasts are large, multinucleated cells with abundant pale blue cytoplasm containing numerous azurophilic granules. They can measure 100 μm or greater in diameter. The individual nuclei are separate, uniform, and round. They

resemble megakaryocytes except that the nuclei do not overlap and the cytoplasm is agranular. In contrast to osteoblasts, osteoclasts originate from progenitor multilineage myeloid stem cells. Like osteoblasts, osteoclasts are infrequently found in bone marrow (76). Endothelial cells are elongated cells containing a flat nucleus with condensed chromatin and a moderate amount of cytoplasm. In bone marrow, adjacent endothelial cells overlap and completely line the inner surface of the sinusoids. The sinusoidal endothelial cells control trafficking and homing of hematopoietic stem cells, provide cellular contact, and regulate hematopoiesis by cytokine production (77–80).

Reticular cells resemble fibroblasts and produce reticulin fibers. They provide the support and regulatory factors essential for hematopoiesis. The reticular cells have long cytoplasmic processes that are in close contact with hematopoietic cells. The cytoplasmic processes of reticular cells extend in the marrow stroma between hematopoietic cells and are contigous with extracellular reticulin fibers. The delicate network formed by the cytoplasmic processes of reticular cells and reticulin fibers plays an important role in the bone marrow microenvironment. It supports hematopoietic tissue and contains various growth factors and cytokines essential for hematopoiesis. Most reticular cells are associated with sinusoids and other blood vessels. Ultrastructurally, there is no difference between reticular cells and perisinusoidal adventitial cells. Although reticular cells are normally non-phagocytic, they may contain phagocytized extruded erythroid nuclei in various pathologic conditions (81,82).

Extracellular Matrix

Extracellular matrix is a stromal cell product and an essential part of the bone marrow microenvironment. It is composed of reticulin fibers, glycoproteins, and a variety of proteoglycans (cytokines). Extracellular matrix is critical for compartmentalization of bone marrow and, in combination with stromal cells and growth factors, regulates hematopoiesis in bone marrow.

Reticulin fibers are composed of type III collagen. Stromal cells, especially reticular cells, produce them. Reticulin fibers form an incomplete, delicate network that provides a supportive framework for hematopoietic tissue. In human bone marrow, the normal level of reticulin fibers is low. Silver stain for reticulin shows a few fine reticulin fibers among hematopoietic cells adjacent to the trabecular bone and around the blood vessels. Reticulin fibers are increased in various hematologic and nonhematologic diseases and are considered an important factor in evaluating hematologic disorders.

Cytokines are regulatory growth factors of hematopoiesis and were discussed previously in reference to the regulation of hematopoiesis (83–87).

Hematopoietic Lineage

Hematopoietic lineage is composed of precursor and maturing myeloid cells, erythroid cells, monocytes, megakaryocytes, and lymphoid cells. Mast cells and macrophages, both derived directly from hematopoietic precursors, function as both hematopoietic cells and stromal elements of bone marrow. Under conditions of stress, there is an increase in one or more cell lineage, and immature forms may be seen in peripheral blood. However, in normal individuals, only mature cells are present in peripheral blood (88).

Granulocytes

Granulocytic lineage includes neutrophilic, eosinophilic, and basophilic cells and their precursors. It is regulated by granulocyte colony-stimulating factor. In bone marrow specimens from healthy individuals of all ages, granulocytic lineage predominates and constitutes approximately 50% to 70% of all nucleated cells. Most of these granulocytes are in neutrophils mature form (Fig. 1-4).

The earliest morphologically recognizable cell of the neutrophilic granulocyte is the myeloblast, which subsequently differentiates into the promyelocyte, myelocyte, metamyelocyte, band cell, and segmented neutrophil. This maturation occurs by a progressive decrease in the nuclear-to-cytoplasmic ratio, loss of nucleoli, condensation of chromatin material, nuclear segmentation, and simultaneous accumulation of primary (nonspecific azurophilic) and later secondary (specific) granules.

Myeloblasts measure 10–20 μm in diameter. They are characterized by a high nuclear-to-cytoplasmic ratio with a large, round, centrally located nucleus, finely dispersed chromatin, two to five prominent nucleoli, and scant to moderate pale blue cytoplasm. The blasts are divided into three subtypes based on the presence or absence of granules: type I, no cytoplasmic granules; type II, less than 20 azurophilic granules; and type III, more than 20 azurophilic granules.

Promyelocytes are the largest granulocytic cells and measure 10–20 μm in diameter. They have a large, eccentric, round to oval nucleus with a prominent nucleolus and a moderate amount of basophilic cytoplasm containing a few to many purple-red (primary nonspecific azurophilic) granules and a perinuclear pale area (Golgi zone). Promyelocytes and type III myeloblasts share some morphologic features, and sometimes it is difficult to differentiate between them.

Myelocytes are the last stage of granulocytic lineage capable of cell division and measure 10–18 μm in diameter. These cells have a relatively small, eccentric, round to oval or slightly indented nucleus with coarse, condensed chromatin and a moderate amount of cytoplasm containing purple-red (primary/azurophilic nonspecific) and light pink (secondary specific) granules.

Metamyelocytes are the next stage of maturation in the granulocyte series and measure 10–18 μm in diameter. They demonstrate indented nuclei and abundant acidophilic cytoplasm with a predominance of secondary granules.

Band cells measure 10–16 μm in diameter, have a horseshoe- or band-shaped nucleus (bilobed nucleus with no filaments) and abundant cytoplasm with secondary granules.

Segmented neutrophils are the last cells in this series. They measure 10–16 μm in diameter and are characterized by as many as five discrete nuclear segmentations connected to each other by filaments (89,104).

Eosinophils

Eosinophils demonstrate almost similar stages of proliferation and differentiation as neutrophils. The earliest morphologically recognizable cells are eosinophil promyelocytes. Eosinophil promyelocytes have round nuclei with dispersed chromatin and contain two types of granules: large, red-orange (eosinophilic) granules and large, bluish granules. Eosinophilic myelocytes and metamyelocytes contain only large, red-orange (eosinophilic) granules. Bilobed nuclei and numerous large eosinophilic cytoplasmic granules characterize the mature eosinophils, which are equal or slightly larger in size than neutrophils (89,90).

Basophils

Basophils, like eosinophils, demonstrate almost similar stages of proliferation, differentiation, and maturation as neutrophils. The earliest morphologically recognizable cells are

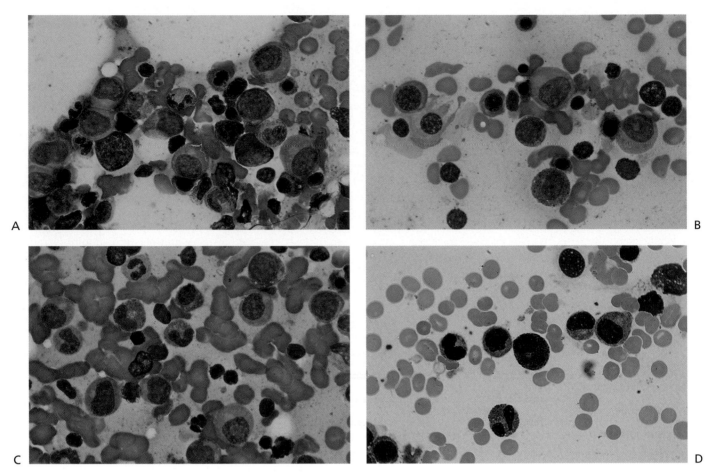

FIGURE 1-4. A–D: Bone marrow aspirate: morphology. Myeloid and erythroid cells in various stages of maturation.

basophil promyelocytes. Basophil promyelocytes, myelocytes, and metamyelocytes contain large, round, deeply basophilic granules. Mature basophils are usually bilobed and have numerous coarse, deeply basophilic granules that often overlie the nucleus. These granules stain metachromatically with toluidine blue stain (89).

Mast Cells

Mast cells are derived from multilineage myeloid stem cells and are closely related to basophils. They measure 12–25 μm in diameter. Mast cells are round, oval, or spindle-shaped and have round to oval nuclei with abundant cytoplasm containing numerous dark-purple to red-purple granules. In normal bone marrow, mast cells are inconspicuous and difficult to appreciate in biopsy specimens stained with hematoxylin and eosin. However, they are easily recognized in bone marrow biopsy specimens and aspirate smears stained with Wright-Giemsa stain (89).

Monocytes and Macrophages

Monocytes and macrophages are derived from the same progenitor cells as the granulocytic series. The proliferation and differentiation of these cells are controlled by monocyte/macrophage colony-stimulating factor. Gradual nuclear folding and acquisition of cytoplasmic granules characterize the morphologic stages of monocytic differentiation and maturation. These stages include monoblast, promonocyte, mature monocyte (bone marrow and blood), and macrophage.

Monoblasts are morphologically similar to myeloblasts except that they may have slightly lobulated or indented nuclei with scant agranular cytoplasm.

Promonocytes are the earliest recognizable cell in this series. Promonocytes measure 15–20 μm in diameter and are characterized by a large, round, lobulated or folded nucleus with fine chromatin and a moderate amount of cytoplasm containing a few azurophilic granules.

Mature monocytes have eccentric, oval, lobulated, folded, or indented nuclei with fine, lacy chromatin and abundant blue-gray, vacuolated cytoplasm. They measure 15–18 μm in diameter. Monocytes are released from bone marrow into the blood circulation and then migrate to different body sites where they transform into tissue macrophages or histiocytes.

Macrophages are derived from monocytes and function as phagocytic cells in the bone marrow and other tissue sites. Macrophages are larger than monocytes and measure

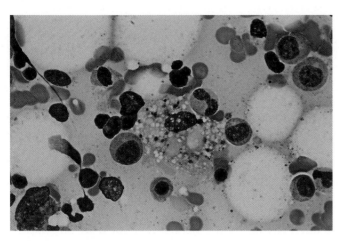

FIGURE 1-5. Bone marrow aspirate: morphology. A macrophage, myeloid cells, and erythroid cells.

20–30 μm in diameter. A large, round to oval nucleus with lacelike chromatin and abundant pale blue vacuolated cytoplasm containing azurophilic granules and intracytoplasmic inclusions characterizes them. These inclusions vary in size and shape and contain phagocytized debris (Fig. 1-5). In bone marrow, macrophages are usually present in the center of erythroid islands, plasma cell islands, and lymphoid aggregates and adjacent to the endothelial cells. They are also randomly scattered among hematopoietic cells (91,92).

Erythroid Cells

Erythroid cells constitute approximately 10% to 40% of bone marrow nucleated cells. Erythropoietin is responsible for the stimulation, proliferation, and differentiation of erythroid precursors. Erythroid cells, in order of maturation, include pronormoblasts (proerythroblasts), basophilic normoblasts, polychromatophilic normoblasts, orthochromic normoblasts, reticulocytes, and erythrocytes. The cytoplasm changes from deep blue to pink as RNA is lost and hemoglobin accumulates (Fig. 1-6). In normal bone mar-

row, normoblasts are low in number and more mature forms predominate.

Pronormoblasts are the largest and earliest recognizable erythroid precursor and measure 14–19 μm in diameter. Pronormoblasts are characterized by a large, round nucleus with dispersed chromatin and a single, centrally located nucleolus surrounded by an even rim of deeply basophilic agranular cytoplasm.

Basophilic erythroblasts measure 12–17 μm in diameter. They are smaller than pronormoblasts with more condensed chromatin, no nucleolus, and medium-blue cytoplasm; binuclear forms are occasionally found.

Polychromatophilic normoblasts are smaller than basophilic normoblasts and measure 12–15 μm in diameter. They have smaller nuclei with more condensed chromatin, blue-pink cytoplasm, and a low nuclear-to-cytoplasmic ratio. Polychromasia is owing to cytoplasmic RNA, which stains blue, and cytoplasmic hemoglobin, which stains red. The polychromatic normoblast is the last cell in normoblastic maturation capable of cell division.

Orthochromic normoblasts are smaller than polychromatophilic normoblasts, measure 8–12 μm in diameter and are characterized by pyknotic nuclei and pink-blue cytoplasm. The cytoplasm contains abundant hemoglobin and a small amount of RNA.

Reticulocytes are similar to orthochromatic normoblasts except that they are anucleate. They measure 7–10 μm in diameter. The reticulocytes are formed by extrusion of orthochromatic normoblast nuclei. Bone marrow erythrocytes are motile and first migrate to the sinusoids and then into the blood circulation. The supravital stains such as brilliant cresyl blue show a skein of ribosomal RNA material in the cytoplasm, termed reticulin, with Wright-Giemsa stain; such cells are termed polychromatophilic red blood cells. Reticulocytes circulate in the blood for 1 to 2 days before becoming mature erythrocytes.

Mature erythrocytes are slightly smaller and acidophilic and show no basophilia with Wright-Giemsa or similar

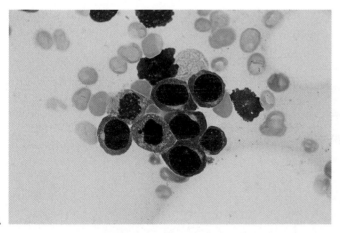

A

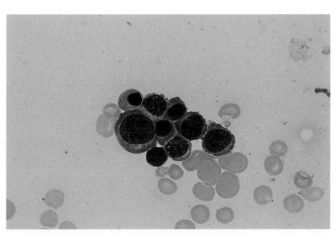

B

FIGURE 1-6. Bone marrow aspirate: morphology. **A, B:** Erythroid cells in various stages of maturation.

stains. They measure 7–8 μm in diameter and have a circular or biconcave shape. The life span of a mature erythrocyte is approximately 120 days. During this period, they gradually lose some enzymatic activity and are finally destroyed by phagocytic reticuloendothelial cells (93,94,104).

Megakaryocytes

Megakaryocytes are derived from multipotential hematopoietic stem cells. Thrombopoietin is the growth factor that primarily regulates megakaryocytopoiesis. It stimulates proliferation and differentiation of megakaryocytic progenitor cells and enhances the production of platelets. The committed progenitor cells are morphologically indistinguishable from progenitor lymphoid cells. The cells in the megakaryocytic series are least in number (less than 1% of nucleated cells) but the largest of all hematopoietic cells. The normal range is three to four megakaryocytes per high-power field; clustering indicates a pathologic process. Megakaryocytic maturation is unique and characterized by endomitosis (nuclear division without cytoplasmic division), resulting in a gradual increase in nuclear segmentation and DNA content (hyperdiploid). The DNA content may vary from 2 to 64 N; most cells contain 8 to 16 N. The stages of maturation are megakaryoblast, promegakaryocyte, granular megakaryocyte, mature megakaryocyte, and platelets.

Megakaryoblasts are the earliest morphologically recognizable cells and have a single, large, oval, lobate, or kidney-shaped nucleus with multiple small nucleoli and a narrow rim of deeply basophilic agranular cytoplasm. Megakaryoblasts measure 20–45 μm in diameter.

Promegakaryocytes are larger than megakaryoblasts and measure 20–80 μm in diameter. They have a single, multilobed, horseshoe-shaped, nucleus and a moderate amount of basophilic cytoplasm containing a few azurophilic granules.

Granular megakaryocytes are the next stage of development and are characterized by a single, overlapping, multi-lobed nucleus and abundant cytoplasm containing numerous azurophilic granules.

Mature megakaryocytes measure 30–100 μm in diameter. They have a single, tightly packed, multilobed nucleus with abundant eosinophilic cytoplasm containing numerous azurophilic granules, forming small aggregates (Fig. 1-7). In bone marrow, megakaryocytes lie adjacent to the sinusoids and shed platelets directly into the circulation by extending their cytoplasmic processes into the sinusoidal lumen.

Mature platelets are small, measure 2–4 μm in diameter and have an irregular outline. The cytoplasm is pale blue and contains numerous azurophilic granules. These platelets are formed by cytoplasmic fragmentation of mature granular megakaryocytes (95–97,104).

Lymphocytes and Plasma Cells

Lymphoid cells are also derived from multipotential stem cells and are primarily regulated by interleukins. Lymphoblasts are the earliest morphologically recognizable cells. They are characterized by a high nuclear-to-cytoplasmic ratio, round to oval nuclei with fine chromatin, one or two nucleoli, and a small amount of basophilic agranular cytoplasm. Lymphoblasts are sometimes difficult to differentiate from other blasts. The lymphoid maturation results in two major groups of cells: T and B lymphocytes. B-cell maturation occurs in bone marrow, whereas T-cell maturation and differentiation are completed in the thymus. Stages of lymphoid cell maturation are difficult to appreciate in bone marrow. Morphologically, B and T lymphocytes are indistinguishable and can only be differentiated by surface antigens identified by immunophenotyping. The mature lymphocytes are slightly larger than erythrocytes and measure 7–10 μm in diameter. They are characterized by a round nucleus with coarse, condensed chromatin, inconspicuous nucleoli, and scanty deep blue cytoplasm.

In adults, lymphocytes constitute less than 20% of the total nucleated cells of bone marrow. However, in children, especially in very young children, B-cell precursors (hematogones) may account for as many as 40% of nucleated cells and may be increased in some conditions. After 6 years of age, hematogones decrease until middle age and after, when they comprise approximately 1% to 2% of total nucleated cells of bone marrow. Benign lymphoid aggregates occasionally occur in adults, especially in women and the elderly. They are associated with a variety of disorders and when present are commonly found adjacent to the sinusoidal walls.

Plasma cells measure 10–18 μm in diameter and are the last stage of maturation in B-cell lineage. In bone marrow, they are present in low numbers (estimated range, 0.5%–1.5%). The plasma cells are characterized by an eccentric nucleus with coarse chromatin and ample deeply basophilic cytoplasm containing a perinuclear area (Golgi zone) (98–104).

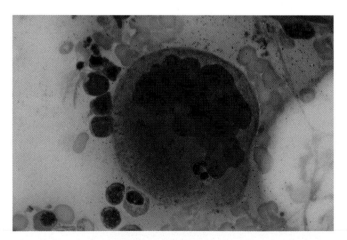

FIGURE 1-7. Bone marrow aspirate: morphology. A megakaryocyte, myeloid cells, and erythroid cells.

REFERENCES

Bone Marrow Structure

1. Compston JE. Bone marrow and bone: a functional unit. *J Endocrinol* 2002;173:387–394.
2. Wickramasinghe SN. Bone marrow. In: Stenberg SS, ed. *Histopathology for pathologists,* 2nd ed. Philadelphia: Lippincott–Raven Publishers, 1997:707–742.
3. Peterson P, Ellis JT. The development, morphology, and function of normal bone marrow: a review. In: Wasserman LR, Berk PD, Berlin NI, eds. *Polycythemia vera and the myeloproliferative disorders.* Philadelphia: WB Saunders, 1995:1630–1639.
4. Gulati GL, Ashton JK, Hyun BH. Structure and function of bone marrow and hematopoiesis. *Hematol Oncol Clin North Am* 1988;2:495–511.
5. Burkhardt R. Bone marrow histology. In: Catovsky D, ed. *Methods in hematology. The leukaemic cell.* Edinburgh: Churchill Livingstone, 1981:49–86.
6. Iversen PO. Blood flow to the haemopoietic bone marrow. *Acta Physiol Scand* 1997;159:269–276.
7. Wickramasinghe SN. Observations on the ultrastructure of sinusoids and reticular cells in human bone marrow. *Clin Lab Haematol* 1991;13:263–278.
8. Reimann I, Christensen SB. A histological demonstration of nerves in subchondral bone. *Acta Orthop Scand* 1977;48:345–352.
9. Artico M, Bosco S, Cavallotti C, et al. Noradrenergic and cholinergic innervation of the bone marrow. *Int J Mol Med* 2002;10:77–80.

Bone Marrow Morphology and Hematopoiesis

1. Foucar K. Hematopoiesis and morphologic review of bone marrow. In: Foucar K, ed. *Bone marrow pathology,* 2nd ed. Chicago: ASCP Press, 2000:1–29.
2. Brunning RD. Normal bone marrow. In: Brunning RD, Mckenna RW, eds. *Tumors of the bone marrow. Atlas of tumor pathology,* 3rd fascicle. Washington, DC: Armed Forces Institutes of Pathology, 1994:2–18.
3. Weissman IL, Anderson DJ, Gage F. Stem and progenitor cells: origins, phenotypes, lineage commitments, and transdifferentiations. *Annu Rev Cell Dev Biol* 2001;17:387–403.
4. Ziegler BL, Kanz L. Expansion of stem and progenitor cells. *Curr Opin Hematol* 1998;5:434.
5. Ogawa M. Differentiation and proliferation of hematopoietic stem cells. *Blood* 1993;81:284.
6. Ogawa M, Porter PN, Nakahata T. Renewal and commitment to differentiation of hematopoietic stem cells (an interpretive review). *Blood* 1983;61:823–829.
7. Scott MA, Gordon MY. In search of the haematopoietic stem cell. *Br J Haematol* 1995;90:738–743.
8. Morrison SJ, Uchida N, Weissman IL. The biology of hematopoietic stem cells. *Annu Rev Cell Dev Biol* 1995;11:35–71.
9. Quensbury PJ, Colvin GA. Hematopoietic stem cells, progenitor cells, and cytokines. In: Beutler E, Erslev AJ, Lichtman M, et al., eds. *Williams hematology,* 6th ed. New York: McGraw-Hill, 2000:153–174.
10. Hoffbrand AV, Pettit JE. Normal haematopoiesis and blood cells. In: Hoffbrand AV, Pettit JV, eds. *Color atlas of clinical hematology,* 3rd ed. London: Mosby, 2000:1–40.
11. Trinchieri G. The hematopoietic system and hematopoiesis. In: Knowles DM, ed. *Neoplastic hematopathology,* 2nd ed. Baltimore: Williams & Wilkins, 2000:1–19.
12. Evans T. Developmental biology of hematopoiesis. *Hematol Oncol Clin North Am* 1997;11:1115–1147.
13. Sieff CA, Nathan DG, Clark SC. The anatomy and physiology of hematopoiesis. In: Nathan DG, Orkin SH, eds. *Hematology of infancy and childhood, volume 1,* 5th ed. Philadelphia: WB Saunders, 1998:161–236.
14. Palis J, Yoder MC. Yolk-sac hematopoiesis: the first blood cells of mouse and man. *Exp Hematol* 2001;29:927–936.
15. Huyhn A, Dommergues M, Izac B, et al. Characterization of hematopoietic progenitors from human yolk sacs and embryos. *Blood* 1995;86:4474–4485.
16. Tavassoli M. Embryonic and fetal hemopoiesis: an overview. *Blood Cells* 1991;17:269–281, 282–286.
17. Timens W, Kamps WA. Hemopoiesis in human fetal and embryonic liver. *Microsc Res Tech* 1997;39:387–397.
18. Calhoun DA, Li Y, Braylan RC, et al. Assessment of the contribution of the spleen to granulocytopoiesis and erythropoiesis of the mid-gestation human fetus. *Early Hum Dev* 1996;46:217–227.
19. Peault B. Hematopoietic stem cell emergence in embryonic life: developmental hematology revisited. *J Hematother* 1996;5:369–378.
20. Slayton WB, Li Y, Calhoun DA, et al. The first-appearance of neutrophils in the human fetal bone marrow cavity. *Early Hum Dev* 1998;53:129–144.
21. Slayton WB, Juul SE, Calhoun DA, et al. Hematopoiesis in the liver and marrow of human fetuses at 5 to 16 weeks postconception: quantitative assessment of macrophages and neutrophil populations. *Pediatr Res* 1998;43:774–782.
22. Pahal GS, Jauniaux E, Kinnon C, et al. Normal development of human fetal hematopoiesis between eight and seventeen weeks' gestation. *Am J Obstet Gynecol* 2000;183:1029–1034.
23. Goyette RE. *Hematopoiesis. Hematology, a comprehensive guide to the diagnosis & treatment of blood disorders.* Los Angeles: PMIC, 1997:1–25.
24. Davey FR, Hutchison. Hematopoiesis. In: Henry JB, ed. *Clinical diagnosis and management by laboratory methods,* 20th ed. Philadelphia: WB Saunders, 2001:520–541.
25. Smith BR. Regulation of hematopoiesis. *Yale J Biol Med* 1990;63:371–380.
26. Hardy CL, Minguell JJ. Cellular interactions in hemopoietic progenitor cell homing: a review. *Scanning Microsc* 1993;7:333–341.
27. Hardy CL, Megason GC. Specificity of hematopoietic stem cell homing. *Hematol Oncol* 1996;14:17–27.
28. Hardy CL. The homing of hematopoietic stem cells to the bone marrow. *Am J Med Sci* 1995;309:260–266.
29. Whetton AD, Graham GJ. Homing and mobilization in the stem cell niche. *Trends Cell Biol* 1999;9:233–238.
30. Papayannopoulou T, Craddock C. Homing and trafficking of hemopoietic progenitor cells. *Acta Haematol* 1997;97:97–104.
31. Mazo IB, von Andrian UH. Adhesion and homing of blood-borne cells in bone marrow microvessels. *J Leukoc Biol* 1999;66:25–32.
32. Majka M, Janowska-Wieczorek A, Ratajczak J, et al. Numerous growth factors, cytokines, and chemokines are secreted by human CD34 (+) cells, myeloblasts, erythroblasts, and megakaryoblasts and regulate normal hematopoiesis in an autocrine/paracrine manner. *Blood* 2001;97:3075–3085.
33. Moore MA. Cytokine and chemokine networks influencing stem cell proliferation, differentiation, and marrow homing. *J Cell Biochem Suppl* 2002;38:29–38.
34. Whetton AD, Spooncer E. Role of cytokines and extracellular matrix in the regulation of hemopoietic stem cells. *Curr Opin Cell Biol* 1998;10:721–726.
35. Broudy VC. Stem cell factor and hematopoiesis. *Blood* 1997;90:1345.

36. Lorentz A, Schuppan D, Gebert A, et al. Regulatory effects of stem cell factor and interleukin-4 on adhesion of human mast cells to extracellular matrix proteins. *Blood* 2002;99:966–972.

37. Lemoli RM, Fortuna A, Fogli M, et al. Stem cell factor (c-kit ligand) enhances the interleukin-9-dependent proliferation of human CD34+ and CD34+CD33−DR− cells. *Exp Hematol* 1994;22:919–923.

38. Bruno E, Luikart SD, Long MW, et al. Marrow-derived heparan sulfate proteoglycan mediates the adhesion of hematopoietic progenitor cells to cytokines. *Exp Hematol* 1995;23:1212–1217.

39. Bunting KD. ABC transporters as phenotypic markers and functional regulators of stem cells. *Stem Cells* 2002;20:11–20.

40. Messner HA. The role of CFU-GEMM in human hemopoiesis. *Blut* 1986;53:269–277.

41. Kondo M, Scherer DC, Miyamoto T, et al. Cell-fate conversion of lymphoid-committed progenitors by instructive actions of cytokines. *Nature* 2000;407:383–386.

42. Jelkmann W, Metzen E. Erythropoietin in the control of red cell production. *Anat Anz* 1996;178:391–403.

43. Kato T, Matsumoto A, Ogami K, et al. Native thrombopoietin: structure and function. *Stem Cells* 1998;16[Suppl 2]:11–19.

44. Wendling F. Thrombopoietin: its role from early hematopoiesis to platelet production. *Haematologica* 1999;84:158–166.

45. Caen JP, Han ZC, Bellucci S, et al. Regulation of megakaryocytopoiesis. *Haemostasis* 1999;29:27–40.

46. Bruno E, Cooper RJ, Wilson EL, et al. Basic fibroblast growth factor promotes the proliferation of human megakaryocyte progenitor cells. *Blood* 1993;82:430–435.

47. Merchav S. The haematopoietic effects of growth hormone and insulin-like growth factor 1. *J Pediatr Endocrinol Metab* 1998;11:677–685.

48. Duhrsen U, Martinez T, Vohwinkel G, et al. Effects of vascular endothelial and platelet-derived growth factor receptor inhibitors on long-term cultures from normal human bone marrow. *Growth Factors* 2001;19:1–17.

49. Parker AN, Pragnell IB. Inhibitors of haemopoiesis and their potential clinical relevance. *Blood Rev* 1995;9:226–233.

50. Sato T, Selleri C, Anderson S, et al. Expression and modulation of cellular receptors for interferon-gamma, tumour necrosis factor, and Fas on human bone marrow CD34+ cells. *Br J Haematol* 1997;97:356–365.

51. Zermati Y, Fichelson S, Valensi F, et al. Transforming growth factor inhibits erythropoiesis by blocking proliferation and accelerating differentiation of erythroid progenitors. *Exp Hematol* 2000;28:885–894.

52. Dooley DC, Oppenlander BK, Spurgin P, et al. Basic fibroblast growth factor and epidermal growth factor downmodulate the growth of hematopoietic cells in long-term stromal cultures. *J Cell Physiol* 1995;165:386–397.

53. Prosper F, Verfaillie CM. Regulation of hematopoiesis through adhesion receptors. *J Leukoc Biol* 2001;69:307–316.

54. Schmitz B, Park IA, Kaufmann R, et al. Influence of cytokine stimulation (granulocyte macrophage-colony stimulating factor, interleukin-3 and transforming growth factor-beta-1) on adhesion molecule expression in normal human bone marrow fibroblasts. *Acta Haematol* 1995;94:173–181.

55. Ryan DH, Tang J. Regulation of human B cell lymphopoiesis by adhesion molecules and cytokines. *Leuk Lymphoma* 1995;17:375–389.

56. Calabretta B, Skorski T. Gene regulatory mechanisms operative on hematopoietic cells: proliferation, differentiation, and neoplasia. *Crit Rev Eukaryot Gene Expr* 1997;7:117–124.

57. Sensebe L, Deschaseaux M, Li J, et al. The broad spectrum of cytokine gene expression by myoid cells from the human marrow microenvironment. *Stem Cells* 1997;15:133–143.

58. Jordan CT, Van Zant G. Recent progress in identifying genes regulating hematopoietic stem cell function and fate. *Curr Opin Cell Biol* 1998;10:716–720.

59. Chichester CO, Fernandez M, Minguell JJ. Extracellular matrix gene expression by human bone marrow stroma and by marrow fibroblasts. *Cell Adhes Commun* 1993;1:93–99.

60. Barry F, Boynton RE, Liu B, et al. Chondrogenic differentiation of mesenchymal stem cells from bone marrow: differentiation-dependent gene expression of matrix components. *Exp Cell Res* 2001;268:189–200.

61. Bianco P, Riminucci M, Gronthos S, et al. Bone marrow stromal stem cells: nature, biology, and potential applications. *Stem Cells* 2001;19:180–192.

62. Majumdar MK, Banks V, Peluso DP, et al. Isolation, characterization, and chondrogenic potential of human bone marrow-derived multipotential stromal cells. *Cell Physiol* 2000;185:98–106.

63. Peled A, Kalai M, Toledo J, et al. Stroma-cell dependent hematopoiesis. *Semin Hematol* 1991;28:132.

64. Dennis JE, Charbord P. Origin and differentiation of human and murine stroma. *Stem Cells* 2002;20:205–214.

65. Seshi B, Kumar S, Sellers D. Human bone marrow stromal cell: coexpression of markers specific for multiple mesenchymal cell lineages. *Blood Cells Mol Dis* 2000;26:234–246.

66. Turner ML, Masek LC, Hardy CL, et al. Comparative adhesion of human haemopoietic cell lines to extracellular matrix components, bone marrow stromal and endothelial cultures. *Br J Haematol* 1998;100:112–122.

67. Linenberger ML, Jacobson FW, Bennett LG, et al. Stem cell factor production by human marrow stromal fibroblasts. *Exp Hematol* 1995;23:1104–1114.

68. Simmons PJ, Zannettino A, Gronthos S, et al. Potential adhesion mechanisms for localisation of haematopoietic progenitors to bone marrow stroma. *Leuk Lymphoma* 1994;12:353–363.

69. Dexter TM, Coutinho LH, Spooncer E, et al. Stromal cells in haemopoiesis. *Ciba Found Symp* 1990;148:76–86, 86–95.

70. Pittenger MF, Mackay AM, Beck SC, et al. Multilineage potential of adult human mesenchymal stem cells. *Science* 1999;284:143–147.

71. Tavassoli M. Marrow adipose cells and hemopoiesis: an interpretative review. *Exp Hematol* 1984;12:139–146.

72. Gimble JM. The function of adipocytes in the bone marrow stroma. *New Biol* 1990;2:304–312.

73. Zuk PA, Zhu M, Mizuno H, et al. Multilineage cells from human adipose tissue: implications for cell-based therapie. *Tissue Eng* 2001;7:211–228.

74. Chen JL, Hunt P, McElvain M, et al. Osteoblast precursor cells are found in CD34+ cells from human bone marrow. *Stem Cells* 1997;15:368–377.

75. Taichman RS, Emerson SG. Human osteoblasts support hematopoiesis through the production of granulocyte colony stimulating factor. *Exp Med* 1994;179:1677–1682.

76. Hayase Y, Muguruma Y, Lee MY. Osteoclast development from hematopoietic stem cells: apparent divergence of the osteoclast lineage prior to macrophage commitment. *Exp Hematol* 1997;25:19–25.

77. Reyes M, Dudek A, Jahagirdar B, et al. Origin of endothelial progenitors in human postnatal bone marrow. *J Clin Invest* 2002;109:337–346.

78. Oberlin E, Tavian M, Blazsek I, et al. Blood-forming potential of vascular endothelium in the human embryo. *Development* 2002;129:4147–4157.

79. Rafii S, Mohle R, Shapiro F, et al. Regulation of hematopoiesis by microvascular endothelium. *Leuk Lymphoma* 1997;27:375–386.

80. Rafi S, Shapiro F, Pettengell R, et al. Human bone marrow microvascular endothelial cells support long term proliferation and differentiation of myeloid and megakaryocytic progenitors. *Blood* 1995;86:3353–3363.

81. Nagao T. Characteristics of bone marrow fibroblasts and their significance in hematopoiesis. *Tokai J Exp Clin Med* 1987;12:1–6.

82. Wickramasinghe SN. Bone marrow. In: Stenberg SS, ed. *Histopathology for pathologists,* 2nd ed. Philadelphia: Lippincott–Raven Publishers, 1997:707–742.

83. Klein G. The extracellular matrix of the hematopoietic microenvironment. *Experientia* 1995;51:914–926.

84. Gordon MY. Extracellular matrix of the marrow microenvironment. *Br J Haematol* 1988;70:1.

85. Armstrong JW, Chapes SK. Effects of extracellular matrix proteins on macrophage differentiation, growth, and function: comparison of liquid and agar culture systems. *J Exp Zool* 1994;269:178–187.

86. Turner ML, Masek LC, Hardy CL, et al. Comparative adhesions of human haematopoietic cell lines to extracellular matrix components, bone marrow stromal and endothelial cultures. *Br J Haematol* 1998;100:112–122.

87. Beckman EN, Brown AW Jr. Normal reticulin level in iliac bone marrow. *Arch Pathol Lab Med* 1990;114:1241–1243.

88. Manz MG, Miyamoto T, Akashi K, et al. Isolation of human clonogenic common myeloid progenitors. *Proc Natl Acad Sci U S A* 2002;99:11872–11877.

89. Bedi A, Sharkis SJ. Mechanisms of cell commitment in myeloid cell differentiation. *Curr Opin Hematol* 1995;2:12–21.

90. Walsh GM. Human eosinophils: their accumulation, activation and fate. *Br J Haematol* 1997;97:701–709.

91. Cavanagh LL, Saal RJ, Grimmett KL, et al. Progenitor cells capable of myeloid differentiation cause proliferation in monocyte-derived dendritic cell cultures. *Blood* 1998;92:1598–1607.

92. Reid CD. The dendritic cell lineage in hematopoiesis. *Br J Haematol* 1997;96:217–223.

93. Moritz KM, Lim GB, Wintour EM. Developmental regulation of erythropoietin and erythropoiesis. *Am J Physiol* 1997;273:1829–1844.

94. Howen B. Reticulocyte maturation. *Blood Cells* 1992;18:167.

95. Dolzhanskiy A, Basch RS, Karpatkin S. Development of human megakaryocytes. *Blood* 1996;87:1353–1360.

96. Long MW. Megakaryocyte differentiation events. *Semin Hematol* 1998;35:192–199.

97. Gewirtz AM. Megakaryocytopoiesis, the state of the art. *Thromb Haemost* 1995;74:204.

98. Akashi K, Reya T, Dalma-Weiszhausz D, et al. Lymphoid precursors. *Curr Opin Immunol* 2000;12:144–150.

99. Duchosal MA. B-cell development and differentiation. *Semin Haemotol* 1997;34:2–12.

100. Hardy RR, Hayakawa K. B cell development pathways. *Annu Rev Immunol* 2001;19:595–621.

101. Spits H, Lanier LL, Phillips JH. Development of human T and natural killer cells. *Blood* 1995;85:2654–2670.

102. Denny T, Yogev R, Gelman R, et al. Lymphocyte subsets in healthy children during the first 5 years of life. *JAMA* 1992;1484–1488.

103. Erkeller-Yuksel FM, Deneys V, Yuksel B, et al. Age-related changes in human blood lymphocyte subpopulations. *J Pediatr* 1992;120:216–222.

104. Bell A. Morphology of human blood and marrow cells; hematopoiesis. In: Harmening DM ed. *Clinical histology and fundamentals of hemostasis.* Philadelphia: F A Davis, 2002:1–38.

BONE MARROW PROCEDURE, EXAMINATION, AND REPORTING

TALAT PARVEEN

BONE MARROW PROCEDURE

Indications and Contraindications

Bone marrow examination is an important and effective way to diagnose hematologic and nonhematologic disorders, determine staging of Hodgkin disease, malignant non-Hodgkin lymphoma and solid tumors, detect micrometastasis in patients with carcinoma, evaluate postchemotherapy patients and post–bone marrow transplant recipients, assess bone marrow iron stores, and culture the organisms, particularly in patients infected with human immunodeficiency virus (Table 2-1). Diagnosis of leukemia and staging of lymphoma are among the most important indications of bone marrow examination (1–20). In rare instances, in the absence of peripheral blood abnormality, the diagnosis of leukemia has been made primarily based on bone marrow evaluation (21).

The bone marrow examination should be performed only when it is necessary. There is no absolute contraindication except if the patient does not meet the specific criteria for bone marrow biopsy (22–25).

Bone Marrow Biopsy and Aspiration Sites and Technique

The technical steps used in obtaining the bone marrow sample are simple and fairly well standardized. An accurate procedure performed by an experienced physician or physician assistant provides optimal information and minimizes the need to repeat a biopsy for morphologic evaluation and special studies (26–29).

Although several sites have been used for bone marrow biopsy and aspiration, for safety reasons, convenience, and better sampling, the posterior superior iliac crest is the preferred site in adults and children. In infants, because active hematopoiesis occurs in long bones, aspiration from the anterior aspect of the tibial tuberosity is the recommended site. Patients who cannot lie on their stomach can be approached through the anterior superior iliac crest or

sternum. Sternal aspiration is recommended for obese patients because the sternum can be relatively easily accessible, for the elderly because it may be more representative of hematopoiesis, and for patients with lesions of the sternum and/or rib. However, because of the structure and anatomy of the sternum, bone marrow biopsy cannot be performed at this site. In esophageal cancer and non–small cell lung cancer, rib segment resection during surgery has been recommended to detect isolated tumor cells in the bone marrow (30–35).

TABLE 2-1. INDICATIONS FOR BONE MARROW EXAMINATION

Evaluation of hematologic disorders
  Unexplained anemia
  Unexplained leukopenia and leukocytosis
  Unexplained thrombocytopenia and thrombocytosis
  Pancytopenia
  Leukemia
  Myelodysplasic syndromes
  Myeloproliferative disorders
  Lymphoproliferative disorders
  Plasma cell dyscrasia
  Staging of Hodgkin disease and non-Hodgkin lymphoma
  Unexplained splenomegaly, hepatomegaly, lymphadenopathy

Evaluation of nonhematologic disorders
  Staging of carcinoma and solid tumors prone to metastasize to bone
  Fever of unknown origin
  Infectious diseases
  Unexplained hypercalcemia
  Diagnosis of febrile illnesses in patients with human immunodeficiency virus infection
  Rare diseases such as systemic mast cell disease, metabolic bone disease, lipid storage diseases, and hemophagocytic syndrome

Miscellaneous conditions
  Bone marrow assessment before bone marrow transplantation
  Monitoring of chemotherapy effect
  Evaluation of trabecular bone in metabolic disease

Because both bone marrow biopsy and aspiration are required for bone marrow evaluation, both should be performed as part of the same procedure. Therefore, this discussion includes both procedures. Before starting the procedure, the technique, complications, and alternative diagnostic methods are explained to the patient and an informed consent is obtained from the patient or guardian. The patient should be reassured about the safety of the procedure, and if he or she is overanxious, a mild sedative may be required. All supplies including extra syringes and transport media or appropriate anticoagulant tubes for special studies such as flow cytometry, chromosomal analysis, and molecular genetics should be checked. The patient is instructed to lie comfortably on one side (lateral decubitus position) with his or her back facing toward the operator (physician/physician assistant). It is extremely important to locate the posterior superior iliac spine correctly. The posterior superior iliac spine is located lateral to the sacral prominence and is identified by a dimple in the skin forming one of the lateral points of the rhomboid. The skin overlying the iliac crest is marked. Using standard antiseptic techniques, the area is sterilized. Bone marrow trays containing all necessary sterile items for the procedure are commercially available. After opening the tray, all the items should be checked quickly to ensure that they are intact and the stylet is working properly. A local anesthetic such as 2% lidocaine is used to anesthetize the overlying skin and subsequently the periosteum of the posterior superior iliac spine. Usually approximately 5 to 10 mL of a local anesthetic is required to anesthetize the skin and the periosteum adequately. After approximately 5 minutes, a small skin incision is made with a knife blade. The sequence of performing bone marrow aspiration and biopsy has not been standarized and depends on the personal preference of the operator. Usually, the aspiration is performed first so that touch imprints can be made if dry tap (no aspiration) is obtained. The aspiration artifact (discussed below) can be avoided if the biopsy is performed from a slightly different site.

If the aspiration is performed first, the bone marrow aspiration needle is introduced through the skin and periosteum into the cortical bone. The needle is pushed with a firm, twisting, clockwise and counterclockwise motion until it penetrates the cortical bone into the medullary cavity. Usually when the cortex is penetrated, the operator feels a subtle decrease in resistance. After achieving a firm fixation of the needle shaft in the bone marrow cavity, the central stylet is unlocked and removed immediately. A large, sterile, heparinized syringe is then attached. The patient should be warned that he or she might experience an unpleasant sensation or a significant amount of pain during the aspiration. Approximately, 1 to 2 mL of bone marrow is aspirated quickly in the syringe. The initial aspirate should be used for morphologic evaluation. Additional aspirate can be obtained for special studies such as flow cytometry, chromosomal analysis, molecular genetics, and culture.

After the bone marrow aspirate is obtained, the biopsy needle is advanced in a slightly different direction for another 1 to 2 cm. The needle is rotated in a circular, back-and-forth motion several times to dislodge the core from its surroundings and then the needle is gently withdrawn. The core biopsy is recovered from the needle by inserting another stylet or probe through the pointed end of the needle. When the procedure is finished, pressure is applied at the biopsy site for approximately 5 minutes (10 to 15 minutes in thrombocytopenic patients), and the site is covered with a small bandage (26–29).

Bilateral bone marrow (from both the right and left iliac crests) examination is useful for staging of non-Hodgkin lymphoma, Hodgkin disease, carcinoma, and sarcoma. However, it is not indicated in acute leukemia, chronic leukemia, myeloproliferative disorder, myelodysplastic syndrome, multiple myeloma, and other primary bone marrow diseases. These biopsy specimens should be labeled as such and processed separately (36,37).

Complications

In general, bone marrow aspiration and biopsy are invasive but fairly safe and well-tolerated procedures with low risk of morbidity and mortality. The complications of biopsy are rare, and usually not serious and primarily consist of residual pain lasting for a few hours, hemorrhage, small hematoma, wound infection at the biopsy site and needle related incidence. The risk of bleeding may be higher in patients with thrombocytopenia and abnormal platelet function. Serious and untoward events may rarely occur, such as uncontrollable bleeding, neuropathy, osteomyelitis, tumor seeding along the needle track, pericardial ramponade, cardiac arrest, and death. Bone marrow transplant donors have a relatively higher rate of local complications because of repeated iliac crest aspiration. In patients with severe bleeding disorders owing to congenital or acquired coagulation factor deficiency disorders, replacement therapy and close observation in the hospital for 24 hours after the procedure is recommended (38–41).

BONE MARROW EXAMINATION

In recent years, advances in the treatment of hematologic malignancies and in bone marrow transplantation has renewed interest among pathologists and hematologists in methods to obtain and prepare bone marrow for diagnostic purposes. Although new methodologies have enhanced and refined the diagnostic abilities of bone marrow examination, the morphologic examination of bone marrow remains the most important diagnostic tool. A thorough and satisfactory evaluation of a bone marrow sample for diagnostic studies includes examination of peripheral blood smears, bone marrow aspirate smears, bone marrow aspirate clot sections, bone marrow touch imprints, and bone marrow biopsy sections. Ideally, bone marrow examination should be performed by a trained hematopathologist who is competent in both histopathology and hematology and is capable of evaluating a bone marrow biopsy specimen as well as bone marrow aspirates. The semisolid nature of bone marrow permits morphologic evaluation as a liquid (smear preparation) and a solid (clot material and core biopsy). The examiner thus gains both cytologic and histologic information. The importance of bringing these two morphologic forms together to be examined by a single observer cannot be overemphasized. A general approach to the morphologic examination of bone marrow and the ways in which different types of examination complement one another in establishing a diagnosis are discussed in the following sections (1–4).

Peripheral Blood Smear

The initial diagnosis of hematopoietic disorders is usually made based on a peripheral blood smear and complete blood count examination. Whenever possible, a blood smear from a capillary puncture should be prepared before the bone marrow is obtained. Although anticoagulated blood is not recommended because it may alter the cellular morphology, the peripheral blood smear can be prepared from anticoagulated blood, preferably within 3 hours of withdrawal [ethylenediaminetetraacetic acid (EDTA) is a better anticoagulant for morphologic examination].

The blood films are prepared by placing a drop of blood in the middle of a slide, 1 to 2 cm from the frosted end. A spreader slide is held at a 30- to 45-degree angle and moved backward until it just comes in contact with the drop of blood. The spreader slide is then moved forward quickly but gently and smoothly. The smear should be thin, evenly distributed, and free of holes. The slide should be labeled and air-dried. A peripheral blood smear is usually stained with Wright-Giemsa or other Romanowsky blood stains.

The morphologic evaluation of a peripheral blood smear includes examination of white blood cells (granulocytes, monocytes, and lymphoid cells), red blood cells, and platelets.

The granulocytic series includes neutrophils, neutrophilic bands, eosinophils, and basophils. Neutrophils are characterized by nuclear lobulation, the presence of secondary granules, and as many as five distinct nuclear lobules. Neutrophilic bands have a bilobed nucleus with no filaments. The morphologic difference between a neutrophil and a band is arbitrary. Eosinophils are bilobed and contain abundant eosinophilic granules. Basophils are usually bilobed and contain numerous coarse basophilic granules.

Lymphocytes are slightly larger than erythrocytes and have a round nucleus with coarse chromatin and scanty basophilic cytoplasm. A small number of lymphocytes are larger and contain abundant cytoplasm with azurophilic granules. These are called large granular lymphocytes.

Monocytes are large cells with a folded nucleus and abundant cytoplasm. They vary in size and shape and may exhibit cytoplasmic vacuoles and/or cytoplasmic projections (pseudopods).

Red blood cells (erythrocytes) are relatively uniform in size and shape and appear as circular, homogeneous disks with a central pale area. These red blood cells are approximately the size of a lymphocyte and range from 6 to 8 mm in diameter. Nucleated red blood cells are not normally present in the peripheral blood except in newborns.

Platelets are the smallest hematopoietic cells. They are round to oval in shape, measure 2 to 4 mm in diameter, and contain cytoplasmic granules (4,5).

Bone Marrow Aspirate Smear

Bone marrow aspirate smears are primarily used for the assessment of differential count, maturational stage, morphologic details, myeloid-to-erythroid (M:E) ratio (normal range, 3:1) and to evaluate bone marrow iron stores. The morphology of normal bone marrow cells was discussed in Chapter 1 in the sections on bone marrow morphology and hematopoiesis. Bone marrow aspirates are more sensitive in detecting bone marrow involvement by lymphoblastic lymphoma and small, noncleaved cell lymphoma than is bone marrow trephine biopsy. They are also useful to perform cytochemical stains, immunophenotypic analysis, cytogenetics, molecular genetics, and other specialized studies (5–8).

Bone marrow aspirate smears may be made by ejecting fresh material and preparing at the bedside or by promptly discharging the syringe contents into a tube containing EDTA and quickly but gently mixing to achieve anticoagulation (heparin is unsatisfactory for morphologic evaluation). The anticoagulated specimen is then poured into a clean watch glass or other suitable surface. The gray particles of marrow are visible with the naked eye and can be gently picked up with a clean forceps, placed in the center of a clean glass slide, and a drop or two of marrow blood is added. A clean glass slide or coverslip is carefully placed on top of the blood and marrow drop. While keeping them in close apposition, the upper and lower slides are quickly and gently pulled in opposite directions. The upper slide is discarded. The lower slide is used for morphologic evaluation or special studies.

There has been much discussion of the relative merits of smears made without versus with anticoagulation; both seem adequate. Many other methods have been devised for separating marrow samples into fractions, each with its own purpose. Although these methods are valuable for demonstrating some marrow features, they have generally proved too cumbersome or labor intensive to be widely adopted.

After the smears are prepared and well-dried, it is sufficient to stain two smear slides with Wright-Giemsa or other Romanowsky blood stains and one smear slide for iron with Prussian blue stain. Using the Wright-Giemsa stain requires skill, and it is difficult to achieve optimal results. Careful adjustment of an automatic stainer or, alternatively, of the manual method is required to produce the right balance of acidophilic and basophilic staining. The best particle preparations should be used, keeping four to six unstained smears in reserve for special studies, if needed.

In the aspirate preparation, the particle is usually arranged in a distinct zonal pattern consisting of a central zone of fatty tissue, a middle zone of abundant hematopoietic cells, and a peripheral hemodiluted area predominantly composed of blood. The middle hematopoietic zone is also arranged in a distinct pattern consisting of an inner layer of mast cells, plasma cells, histiocytes, and megakaryocytes and an outer layer composed of sheets of hematopoietic precursors. If mast cells and plasma cells are found here, it indicates that they are increased in number. The M:E ratio and hematopoietic maturation are judged in the middle zone. In the absence of a clear middle zone, the M:E ratio may not be interpretable, but determinations can still be made regarding maturation, dysplastic and megaloblastic changes and the presence or absence of ring sideroblasts, blasts, Auer rods, etc. Occasionally, a single particle represents a lymphoid aggregate rather than fatty tissue or hematopoietic cells; these must be recognized as focal lesions and should not be given undue weight.

Bone Marrow Aspirate Clot Sections

Preparation of aspirate clot sections plays an important role in bone marrow evaluation and should be included in the routine examination of bone marrow. Clot sections substantially increase the chances of finding a focal lesion, such as a granuloma, or metastatic disease. They are especially helpful in diagnosing lymphoproliferative disorders (9).

The aspirate clot section is made by allowing a semisolid clot to drain on an absorbent filter paper or other suitable substance; it is then scraped together, lifted on a scalpel blade, and gently immersed in formalin where it will solidify. Alternatively, the technician may squirt some sample directly into formalin. Histologic sections are obtained from paraffin-embedded clot material and routinely stained with hematoxylin and eosin (H&E).

Bone Marrow Touch Imprints

A poor aspirate return is a sign of the needle not being in the medullary space or needle being in the medullary space, but aspiration is impeded by fibrosis, fat, infiltration tumor, or marrow necrosis. In such cases, a touch imprint of the core biopsy specimen is especially helpful in permitting cytologic examination of the bone marrow elements. Touch imprints are often made by gently rolling the freshly obtained core biopsy specimen between two glass slides or by gently pressing the glass slides over the specimen before fixation. They are air-dried and usually stained with Wright-Giemsa stain. The touch imprints are reliable tools for independent rou-

tine use to determine the cellular composition of normal bone marrow and to evaluate bone marrow diseases. They are particularly useful when a bone marrow biopsy fails to yield an aspirate specimen (dry tap) or the biopsy specimen is inadequate. In these instances, touch imprints can be used to evaluate for neoplastic hematologic disorders and to identify nonhematologic malignancies, especially solid tumors. They can also be used for molecular diagnosis in leukemia. There are advantages to using touch imprints: Multiple touch imprints can be easily prepared, they correlate better with the core biopsy than the aspirate smear, and there is minimal hemodilution error (10–13).

Bone Marrow Core Biopsy

A bone marrow core biopsy specimen in adults should measure at least 1.6 cm or more and, after processing, 1.2 cm in section. If the biopsy is smaller than 1.6 cm, a repeat biopsy, preferably on the contralateral side, should be considered. In children, 0.5-cm bone marrow biopsy sections (after processing) have been reported to be adequate. If no aspiration (dry tap) is obtained, touch imprints should be made; otherwise, the biopsy specimen should be immediately placed in an appropriate fixative. Although various types of fixative are commercially available, those containing mercury salts, such as Zenker or B5 fixative (prepared by mixing 1 mL of 10% formaldehyde and 9 mL of B5 solution immediately before use) provide the best preservation of nuclear and cytoplasmic detail with minimal shrinkage. Proper environmental safety precautions must be observed if mercury-containing fixatives are used. However, excellent results can also be obtained with buffered formalin, with care and attention to fixation times. The bone marrow biopsy should be fixed for at least 2 hours; the fixative is then decanted and the decalcified solution is added. The biopsy specimen should be decalcified for 1 hour. Histologic sections are obtained from the paraffin-embedded core biopsy specimen and routinely stained with H&E.

Bone marrow core biopsy sections provide a better and more detailed estimate of bone marrow cellularity, cellular relationships, architecture, and morphology. They are particularly useful for patients with marrow fibrosis caused by hematologic and nonhematologic malignancies resulting in dry tap (no aspiration). The core biopsies are essential for identification of metastatic malignancies and pathologic processes such as granulomas, amyloidosis necrosis, and abscess. They are also important for studying the distribution and quantity of reticulin and collagen fibers. Core biopsies may be helpful in diagnosing some vascular lesions (thrombotic thrombocytopenic purpura and polyarteritis nodosa). Additionally, the core biopsies can be used to perform immunohistochemical stains and molecular studies (14–19).

Bone marrow biopsy specimens are also helpful in identifying the structural abnormalities of bone, which include thickening, thinning, irregular margins, uncalcified rims of osteoid, active osteoblasts and osteoclasts (in a patient older than 21 years of age), prominent cement lines, and widely spaced cross-sections of bone.

The M:E ratio is often lower in core biopsies than it appears in aspirate smears, at approximately 2:1. Megakaryocytes are evenly distributed throughout the marrow space at the rate of approximately one per 40× field. Myeloid precursors are arranged along the trabecular margin and then filter out in an irregular pattern into the center of the interstitial space. Erythroid colonies are more cohesive, forming groups of small, dark, round nuclei surrounded by scant cytoplasm. Marrow sinusoids wend through the central marrow space and may be either collapsed or dilated. Megakaryocytes and other hematopoietic cells may be found within the sinusoids.

Three H&E-stained levels properly fixed, embedded, and sectioned are sufficient for evaluation. Although periodic acid–Schiff and Giemsa stains are still widely used, they contribute little additional information to well-executed H&E-stained sections. Histochemical and immunoperoxidase stains can also be performed, if needed.

Bone Marrow Cellularity

Accurate assessment of bone marrow cellularity or hematopoietic-to-adipose tissue ratio is necessary to establish the diagnosis of malignant and nonmalignant hematopoietic disorders, to monitor the effect of cytotoxic therapeutic agents, and to evaluate donors for bone marrow transplantation.

It is easier and more accurate to estimate bone marrow cellularity from a bone marrow core biopsy section compared with an aspirate smear. The medullary cavity is examined to evaluate bone marrow cellularity. The biopsy site and patient age are critical for the evaluation of marrow cellularity; the cellularity of the bone marrow depends on the location of the sample and age of the person. The bone marrow cellularity declines approximately 10% with each decade of life. Bone marrow cellularity is approximately 100% at birth; in young children, the ratio is more than 9:1; in young adults, the ratio is 2:1; in middle age, the ratio decreases to 1:1; and in older adults, the ratio gradually decreases to 1:9 (Fig. 2-1). Biopsy sites distal to the iliac crest show earlier and more complete fatty replacement; more proximal sites (ribs, spine, and skull) retain active hematopoietic marrow throughout life (20–22).

Bone marrow cellularity may vary in a single specimen. The overall cellularity should be estimated to judge the bone marrow as normocellular, hypocellular, or hypercellular. Depending on the age of individual, normocellular bone marrow contains a varying proportion of fatty tissue, as discussed above. In adults, hypocellular bone marrow predominantly consists of mature fat cells (usually 75%) with an increased number of fibroblasts and collagen fibers. Granulocytic, ery-

throcytic, and megakaryocytic lineage is usually decreased, and lymphocytes, plasma cells, and mast cells are relatively or absolutely increased in number. However, different cell lines may not be affected to the same degree. Care should be taken not to misinterpret artifacts (procedural or processing) as hypocellularity. Hypercellular bone marrow contains few or no fat cells and largely consists of cellular elements (>75%). The increased cellularity may be owing to proliferation of one cell line or all cell lines. If all cell lines are affected, the marrow cells may show a normal distribution with a normal ratio or they may show a normal distribution with a predominance of either mature cells or immature cells.

Common causes of hypocellular and hypercellular bone marrow are listed in Table 2-2.

Bone Marrow Iron

Assessment of bone marrow iron stores is valuable in determining the adequacy of iron stores and in the differential diagnosis of anemias. It is decreased or absent in iron deficiency anemia and normal or increased in most other anemias. However, if iron storage function is impaired, such as in myeloproliferative disorders, iron stores may be absent without iron deficiency. Iron assessment from marrow was common for the diagnosis of iron deficiency anemia but has now been supplanted by serum iron, serum ferritin, and serum transferrin receptor studies. Assessment of bone marrow iron may be helpful to confirm the diagnosis of iron deficiency anemia if serum iron and iron binding capacity is unable to provide a definite answer (23–28).

In bone marrow, iron granules are formed in red blood cell precursors and stored in reticuloendothelial cells. Special stains such as Prussian blue are necessary to adequately demonstrate the presence of iron stores. Nucleated red blood cells containing punctate intracytoplasmic iron granules are known as sideroblasts. In normal bone marrow, sideroblasts constitute approximately 20% to 40% of red blood cell precursors. Sideroblasts are decreased in iron deficiency anemia, anemia of chronic diseases, and after acute blood loss. They are increased in conditions with accelerated red blood cell turnover such as hemolytic anemia. The pattern and amount of iron deposit in sideroblasts have a diagnostic significance. Nucleated red blood cells containing five or more granules encircling at least two-thirds of the nucleus are called ring sideroblasts. Ring sideroblasts are pathologic and seen in congenital and acquired sideroblastic anemias, after toxin and drug exposure, and in some infections.

Bone marrow iron stores are identified in the cytoplasm of reticuloendothelial cells, which are characterized by a small nucleus, no nucleolus, and abundant cytoplasm, often with long cytoplasmic processes. The reticuloendothelial cells acquire most of their iron by erythrophagocytosis. Iron in reticuloendothelial cells is stored in the form of hemosiderin (ferric hydroxide and denatured ferritin aggregates) and ferritin (ferric hydroxide and apoferritin complex). Hemosiderin is

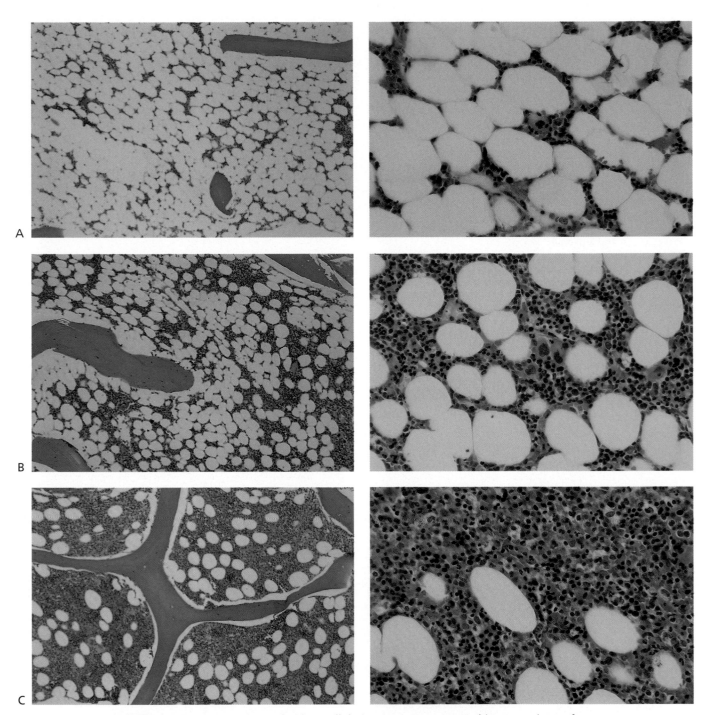

FIGURE 2-1. Bone marrow examination: cellularity. Bone marrow core biopsy specimens from adult men (30–35 years of age). Hypocellular bone marrow (**A**). Normal cellular bone marrow (**B**). Hypercellular bone marrow (**C**).

a more stable and less available form of storage iron than ferritin. The hemosiderin granules vary in size and are water insoluble. They appear as yellow to brown granules on H&E stain and greenish blue with Prussian blue stain. Ferritin is water soluble and not visible on H&E or Prussian blue stain. In normal bone marrow, reticuloendothelial cells containing hemosiderin granules are seen in every third or fourth oil immersion field. If iron stores are increased, hemosiderin gran-

ules are seen in every oil immersion field. With decreased iron stores, very few or no hemosiderin-containing reticuloendothelial cells are noted.

Iron stain (Prussian blue) can be performed on bone marrow aspirate smears and on histologic sections. They are more accurate and reliable when performed on aspirate smears. Iron stains performed on clot sections are less sensitive because some iron is lost during processing. Iron stores may

TABLE 2-2. BONE MARROW CELLULARITY

Hypocellular bone marrow
  Physiologic state (e.g., normal aging process)
  Exposure to various toxins (e.g., drugs, chemotherapeutic
    agents, organic solvents, and ionizing radiation)
  Infections (e.g., viral, mycobacteriosis)
  Idiopathic
  Congenital (Fanconi anemia or constitutional hypoplastic
    anemia)
  Preleukemic state (e.g., idiopathic acquired aplastic
    anemia, refractory anemia, and paroxysmal nocturnal
    hemoglobinuria)

Hypercellular bone marrow
  Physiologic state (e.g., newborn)
  Leukemoid reactions (e.g., infections, tumors, other)
  Preleukemia and leukemia
  Myeloproliferative disorders
  Lymphoproliferative disorders
  Anemia (e.g., pernicious anemia, hemolytic anemia, and
    some refractory anemias)
  Miscellaneous conditions (e.g., hypersplenism)

be evaluated in bone marrow core biopsy sections but are unreliable because of decalcification, which leaches out iron and calcium (29–31). If iron remains after this process, it is safe to assume that iron stores are increased. Lipofuscin looks like iron on H&E stain, and a special stain for iron (Prussian blue) may be necessary to differentiate between them.

No exact data are available for the quantitative assessment of iron stores. Iron stores are usually reported as negative or 1+ to 5+. In adults, 2+ is considered to be normal, 3+ slightly increased, 4+ moderately increased, and 5+ markedly increased. We recommended reporting iron stores as absent, decreased, adequate, and increased (Fig. 2-2). This classification provides the clinicians an adequate and better understanding of a patient's iron stores.

Common causes of increased and decreased iron stores are listed in Table 2-3.

Bone Marrow Artifacts

A variety of artifacts may be observed in bone marrow aspirate smears and histologic sections secondary to poor technique, sampling error, and preparation artifacts (Table 2-4) (Fig. 2-3A–C). It has been claimed that if bone marrow aspiration is followed by bone marrow biopsy at the same site, it causes artifactual depletion of bone marrow cellularity and hemorrhage, so-called aspiration artifact. This artifact usually occupies a relatively small area and can be avoided by further advancing the biopsy needle and performing the core

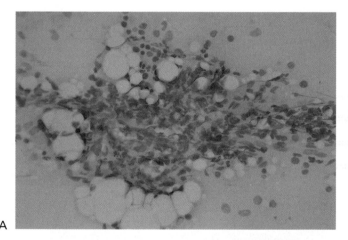

A

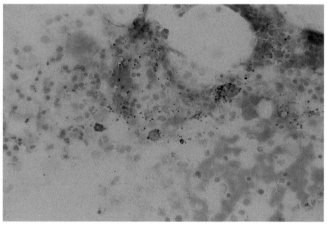

B

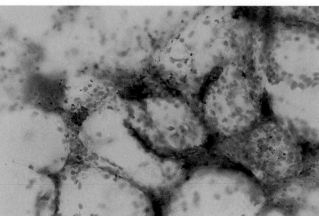

C

FIGURE 2-2. Bone marrow examination: iron stores. Bone marrow aspirate smears (Prussian blue). **A:** Decreased iron stores. **B:** Adequate iron stores. **C:** Increased iron stores.

TABLE 2-3. BONE MARROW IRON STORES

Increased iron stores
  Anemia of chronic disease
  Anemias associated with ineffective erythropoiesis or
    extravascular hemolysis
  Hemosiderosis
  Hemochromatosis
  Sideroblastic anemia
  Pernicious anemia in relapse
  After repeated transfusions
  Anemia associated with infections, hepatic cirrhosis, uremia,
    rheumatoid arthritis, and neoplastic diseases
  Rare conditions such as Gaucher disease

Decreased/absent iron stores
  Iron deficiency anemia
  Myeloproliferative disorders
  Congenital atransferrinemia
  Idiopathic pulmonary hemosiderosis
  Paroxysmal nocturnal hemoglobinuria
  Intravascular hemolysis (intracardiac prosthesis)
  Newborn

TABLE 2-4. BONE MARROW ARTIFACTS

Technical artifacts
  Crushed core biopsy specimen
  Crushed aspirate particles
  Small, inadequate sample
  Core biopsy consisting of cortical bone or hypocellular
    subcortical region

Sampling error
  Aspiration artifact (aspiration of marrow from core biopsy site)
  Core biopsy from previous biopsy site
  Artifactually embedded nonneoplastic glands (sweat or
    sebaceous gland)
  Fragments of skin, fibrocartilage, skeletal muscle
  Foreign bodies

Preparation artifacts
  Aspirate smears too thick
  Drying artifact of aspirate smears
  Overstaining or understaining of aspirate smears
  Inadequate fixation of biopsy and clot specimens
  Overfixation of biopsy and clot specimens in B5 fixative
  Inadequate washing of B5-fixed specimens
  Excessive decalcification of core biopsy
  Overstaining or understaining of biopsy and clot sections
  Biopsy and clot sections too thick
  Water contamination of staining solutions
  Staining contaminated by fungal/bacterial overgrowth

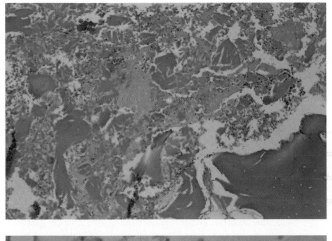
A

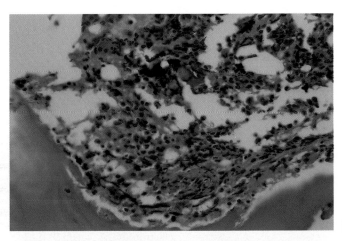
B

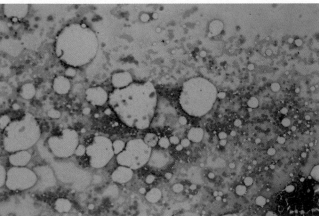
C

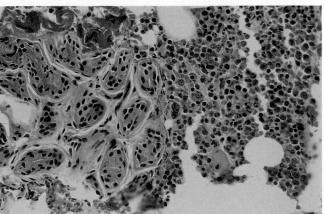
D

FIGURE 2-3. Bone marrow examination: artifacts. **A:** Bone marrow core biopsy, predominantly crushed cortical bone. **B:** Bone marrow core biopsy, crushed bone marrow. **C:** Bone marrow aspirate, poorly stained aspirate. **D:** Bone marrow core biopsy, glandular structures (sweat glands).

biopsy in a slightly different direction away from the aspiration site (32,33).

A nonneoplastic glandular structure such as a dermal sweat gland, owing to technical artifact, may become embedded in the center of a core biopsy and may be misinterpreted as adenocarcinoma (34) (Fig. 2-3D).

Different types of pigments such as hemosiderin pigments, melanin pigments, formalin pigments, ceroid pigments, and malarial pigments may be noted in the bone marrow. Anthracotic pigment and thorotrast pigment have also been reported. Sometimes numerous naked nuclei appear in the smears; it is important not to mistake these for the smudged nuclei of tumor cells. In most cases, when the smears are compared with sections, they correspond to erythroid precursors, and iron stain demonstrates both intracellular iron stores and ring sideroblasts.

BONE MARROW REPORT

The final bone marrow report is an important method in which the results of a complex study are relayed to the clinicians. It requires a multiparameter, multidisciplinary, and collaborative diagnostic approach. The clinician and the pathologist are partners in this endeavor (1).

TABLE 2-5. STEPS IN BONE MARROW EXAMINATION AND REPORTING

Preliminary review of data	
Demographic data	Age, gender, ethnic group
Clinical impression	History, clinical assessment, or diagnostic query
Laboratory studies	Complete blood count with white blood cell differential count; other pertinent studies may include Coombs test, hemoglobinopathy evaluation, serologic studies for infectious agents, serum protein electrophoresis
Pathologic examination	
Peripheral blood smears	1 Wright-Giemsa
Aspirate smears	2 Wright-Giemsa, 1 iron stain
Aspirate clot	3 H&E levels, 1 iron stain
Touch imprints	1 Wright-Giemsa
Core biopsy	3 H&E levels, 1 iron stain
Summary of findings	
Diagnosis	Site and procedure, followed by brief, clearly worded diagnosis
Comment (optional)	Reconcile clinical and pathologic findings, address unusual findings, offer differential diagnosis, recommend further testing, suggest management options, record clinician contacts

H&E, hematoxylin and eosin.

The bone marrow report should be thorough, concise, and systematic. It should include a brief clinical history, pertinent laboratory data including complete blood count, and morphologic examination of peripheral blood smears, bone marrow aspirate smears, clot sections, core biopsy sections, and touch imprints. All significant positive and negative findings and general information such as anatomic site and number of biopsies (unilateral or bilateral) should be described. Immunophenotypic analysis, cytogenetic studies, and molecular data, often derived in separate laboratories, must be integrated with the morphologic findings to establish an accurate and clinically useful diagnosis. A brief comment may be added after the diagnosis, especially if a definite diagnosis could not be established or a differential diagnosis is entertained. Also, additional studies or confirmatory tests may be recommended (2,3).

In recent years, numerous computer-based interpretative bone marrow reporting systems have also been developed (4–7).

The steps of a bone marrow examination and the final report are summarized in Table 2-5.

REFERENCES
Bone Marrow Procedure

1. Sills RH. Indications for bone marrow examination. *Pediatr Rev* 1995;16:226–228.
2. Mark HF, Gray Y, Mark Y, et al. A multimodality approach in the diagnosis of patients with hematopoietic disorders. *Cancer Genet Cytogenet* 1999;109:14–20.
3. Nigam S, Rani S, Singh T, et al. Clinical, hematological and histomorphological profile of myelodysplastic syndrome. *J Assoc Physicians India* 2001;49:430–434.
4. Annaloro C, Lambertenghi DG, Oriani A, et al. Prognostic significance of bone marrow biopsy in essential thrombocythemia. *Haematologica* 1999;84:17–21.
5. Bartl R, Frisch B. Clinical significance of bone marrow biopsy and plasma cell morphology in MM and MGUS. *Pathol Biol (Paris)* 1999;47:158–168.
6. Florena AM, Iannitto E, Quintini G, et al. Bone marrow biopsy in hemophagocytic syndrome. *Virchows Arch* 2002;441:335–344.
7. La Civita L, Mariani G, Porciello G. Bone involvement in Gaucher's disease: "bone crisis" or disease complication? *Clin Exp Rheumatol* 1996;14:195–198.
8. Buhr T, Langer F, Schlue J, et al. Histopathology of leukaemic non-Hodgkin's lymphoma in bone marrow. *Pathologe* 2002;23:438–447.
9. Pittaluga S, Tierens A, Dodoo YL, et al. How reliable is histologic examination of bone marrow trephine biopsy specimens for the staging of non-Hodgkin lymphoma? A study of hairy cell leukemia and mantle cell lymphoma involvement of the bone marrow trephine specimen by histologic, immunohistochemical, and polymerase chain reaction techniques. *Am J Clin Pathol* 1999;111:179–184.
10. Howell SJ, Grey M, Chang J, et al. The value of bone marrow examination in the staging of Hodgkin's lymphoma: a review of 955 cases seen in a regional cancer centre. *Br J Haematol* 2002;119:408–411.
11. Mahoney DH Jr, Schreuders LC, Gresik MV, et al. Role of staging

bone marrow examination in children with Hodgkin disease. *Med Pediatr Oncol* 1998;30:175–177.

12. Bunin N, Johnstone DA, Roberts WM, et al. Residual leukemia after bone marrow transplant in children with acute lymphoblastic leukemia after first haematological relapse or with poor initial presenting features. *Br J Haematol* 2003;120:711–715.

13. Simmons R, Hoda S, Osborne M. Bone marrow micrometastases in breast cancer patients. *Am J Surg* 2000;180:309–312.

14. Weckermann D, Muller P, Wawroschek F, et al. Micrometastases of bone marrow in localized prostate cancer: correlation with established risk factors. *J Clin Oncol* 1999;17:3438–3443.

15. Kjurkchiev G, Valkov I. Role of touch imprint and core biopsy for detection of tumor metastases in bone marrow. *Diagn Cytopathol* 1998;18:323–324.

16. Reddy VV. Topics in bone marrow biopsy pathology: role of marrow topography in myelodysplastic syndromes and evaluation of post-treatment and post-bone marrow transplant biopsies. *Ann Diagn Pathol* 2001;5:110–120.

17. Perkins S. Diagnosis of anemias. In: Kjeldsberg C, Elenitoba-Johnson K, Foucar C, et al., eds. *Practical diagnosis of hematologic disorders,* 3rd ed. Chicago: ASCP Press, 2000:19–20.

18. Luther JM, Lakey DL, Larson RS, et al. Utility of bone marrow biopsy for rapid diagnosis of febrile illnesses in patients with human immunodeficiency virus infection. *South Med J* 2000;93:692–697.

19. Hussong J, Peterson LR, Warren JR, et al. Detecting disseminated *Mycobacterium avium* complex infections in HIV-positive patients. The usefulness of bone marrow trephine biopsy specimens, aspirate cultures, and blood cultures. *Am J Clin Pathol* 1998;110:806–809.

20. Kilby JM, Marques MB, Jaye DL, et al. The yield of bone marrow biopsy and culture compared with blood culture in the evaluation of HIV-infected patients for mycobacterial and fungal infections. *Am J Med* 1998;104:123–128.

21. Shanks D, Linke R, Saxon B. Bones, groans and blasts. *J Paediatr Child Health* 2001;37:504–506.

22. Jubelirer SJ, Harpold R. The role of the bone marrow examination in the diagnosis of immune thrombocytopenic purpura: case series and literature review. *Clin Appl Thromb Hemost* 2002;8:73–76.

23. George JN, Woolf SH, Raskob GE, et al. Idiopathic thrombocytopenic purpura: a practical guideline developed by explicit methods for the American Society of Hematology. *Blood* 1996;88:3–40.

24. Cheung NK, Heller G, Kushner BH, et al. Detection of metastatic neuroblastoma in bone marrow: when is routine marrow histology insensitive? *J Clin Oncol* 1997;15:2807–2817.

25. Westerman DA, Grigg AP. The diagnosis of idiopathic thrombocytopenic purpura in adults: does bone marrow biopsy have a place? *Med J Aust* 1999;170:216–217.

26. Foucar K. Bone marrow examination: indications and techniques. In: Foucar K, ed. *Bone marrow pathology,* 2nd ed. Chicago: ASCP Press, 2000:31–49.

27. Bain BJ. Bone marrow trephine biopsy. *J Clin Pathol* 2001;54:737–742.

28. Bain BJ. Bone marrow aspiration. *J Clin Pathol* 2001;54:657–663.

29. Hodges A, Koury MJ. Needle aspiration and biopsy in the diagnosis and monitoring of bone marrow diseases. *Clin Lab Sci* 1996;9:349–353.

30. Hernandez-Garcia MT, Hernandez-Nieto L, Perez-Gonzalez E, et al. Bone marrow trephine biopsy: anterior superior iliac spine versus posterior superior iliac spine. *Clin Lab Haematol* 1993;15:15–19.

31. Reid MM, Roald B. Adequacy of bone marrow trephine biopsy specimens in children. *J Clin Pathol* 1996;49:226–229.

32. Reid MM, Roald B. Bone marrow trephine biopsy in infants.

European Neuroblastoma Study Group. *Arch Dis Child* 1997;77:60–61.

33. Sola MC, Rimsza LM, Christensen RD. A bone marrow biopsy technique suitable for use in neonates. *Br J Haematol* 1999;107:458–460.

34. Mattioli S, D'Ovidio F, Tazzari P, et al. Iliac crest biopsy versus rib segment resection for the detection of bone marrow isolated tumor cells from lung and esophageal cancer. *Eur J Cardiothorac Surg* 2001;19:576–579.

35. Bonavina L, Soligo D, Quirici N, et al. Bone marrow-disseminated tumor cells in patients with carcinoma of the esophagus or cardia. *Surgery* 2001;129:15–22.

36. Wang J, Weiss LM, Chang KL, et al. Diagnostic utility of bilateral bone marrow examination: significance of morphologic and ancillary technique study in malignant. *Cancer* 2002;4:1522–1531.

37. Valdes-Sanchez M, Nava-Ocampo AA, Palacios-Gonzalez RV, et al. Diagnosis of bone marrow metastases in children with solid tumors and lymphomas. Aspiration, or unilateral or bilateral biopsy? *Arch Med Res* 2000;31:58–61.

38. Bain BJ. Bone marrow biopsy morbidity and mortality. *Br J Haematol* 2003;121:949–951.

39. Dieu RL, Luckit J, Sundarasun M. Complications of trephine biopsy. *Br J Haematol* 2003;121:822.

40. Salem P, Wolversons MK, Reimers HJ, et al. Complications of bone marrow biopsy. *Br J Haematol* 2003;121:821.

41. Citron ML, Krasnow SH, Grant C, et al. Tumor seeding associated with bone marrow aspiration and biopsy. *Arch Intern Med* 1984;144:177.

Bone Marrow Examination

1. Barekman CL, Fair KP, Cotelingam JD. Comparative utility of diagnostic bone-marrow components: a 10-year study. *Am J Hematol* 1997;56:37–41.

2. Bain BJ. The normal bone marrow. In: Bain BJ, Clark DM, Lampert IA, eds. *Bone marrow pathology,* 3rd ed. Oxford: Blackwell Science, 2001.

3. Sabharwal BD, Malhotra V, Aruna S, et al. Comparative evaluation of bone marrow aspirate particle smears, imprints and biopsy sections. *J Postgrad Med* 1990;36:194–198.

4. Naeim F. Normal bone marrow structure and blood cells. In: Naeim F, ed. *Atlas of bone marrow and blood pathology.* Philadelphia: WB Saunders, 2001:1–12.

5. Davey FR, Hutchison RE. Hematopoiesis. In: Henry JB, ed. *Clinical diagnosis and management by laboratory methods,* 20th ed. Philadelphia: WB Saunders, 2001:520–540.

6. Bain BJ. The bone marrow aspirate of healthy subjects. *Br J Haematol* 1996;94:206–209.

7. Subira M, Domingo A, Santamaria A, et al. Bone marrow involvement in lymphoblastic lymphoma and small non-cleaved cell lymphoma: the role of trephine biopsy. *Haematologica* 1997;82:594–595.

8. Cetto GL, Iannucci A, Perini A, et al. Bone marrow evaluation: the relative merits of particle sections and smear preparations. *Appl Pathol* 1983;1:181–193.

9. Aboul-Nasr R, Estey EH, Kantarjian HM, et al. Comparison of touch imprints with aspirate smears for evaluating bone marrow specimens. *Am J Clin Pathol* 1999;111:753–758.

10. Navone R, Colombano MT. Histopathological trephine biopsy findings in cases of "dry tap" bone marrow aspirations. *Appl Pathol* 1984;2:264–271.

11. James LP, Stass SA, Schumacher HR. Value of imprint preparations of bone marrow biopsies in hematologic diagnosis. *Cancer* 1980;46:173–177.

12. Kjurkchiev G, Valkov I. Role of touch imprint and core biopsy for detection of tumor metastases in bone marrow. *Diagn Cytopathol* 1998;18:323–324.
13. Crisan D, Farkas DH. Bone marrow biopsy imprint preparations: use for molecular diagnostics in leukemias. *Ann Clin Lab Sci* 1993;23:407–422.
14. Brown DC, Gatter KC. The bone marrow trephine biopsy: a review of normal histology. *Histopathology* 1993;2:411–422.
15. Bishop PW, McNally K, Harris M. Audit of bone marrow trephines. *J Clin Pathol* 1992;45:1105–1108.
16. Aronica PA, Pirrotta VT, Yunis EJ, et al. Detection of neuroblastoma in the bone marrow: biopsy versus aspiration. *J Pediatr Hematol Oncol* 1998;20:330–334.
17. Jatoi A, Dallal GE, Nguyen PL. False-negative rates of tumor metastases in the histologic examination of bone marrow. *Mod Pathol* 1999;12:29–32.
18. Bird AR, Jacobs P. Trephine biopsy of the bone marrow. *S Afr Med J* 1983;64:271–276.
19. Dunphy CH, Dunphy FR, Visconti JL. Flow cytometric immunophenotyping of bone marrow core biopsies: report of 8 patients with previously undiagnosed hematologic malignancy and failed bone marrow aspiration. *Arch Pathol Lab Med* 1999;123:206–212.
20. Justesen J, Stenderup K, Ebbesen EN, et al. Adipocyte tissue volume in bone marrow is increased with aging and in patients with osteoporosis. *Biogerontology* 2001;2:165–171.
21. Muschler GF, Nitto H, Boehm CA, et al. Age- and gender-related changes in the cellularity of human bone marrow and the prevalence of osteoblastic progenitors. *J Orthop Res* 2001;19:117–125.
22. Friebert S, Shepardson L, Shurin SB, et al. Pediatric bone marrow cellularity: are we expecting too much? *J Pediatr Hematol Oncol* 1998;20:439–443.
23. Cetin M, Gonul A, Kara A, et al. Profile of bone marrow iron stores in childhood iron deficiency anemia. *Turk J Pediatr* 1999;41:329–334.
24. Barron BA, Hoyer JD, Tefferi A. A bone marrow report of absent stainable iron is not diagnostic of iron deficiency. *Ann Hematol* 2001;80:166–169.
25. Spivak JL. Iron and the anemia of chronic disease. *Oncology (Huntingt)* 2002;16[Suppl 10]:25–33.
26. Punnonen K, Irjala K, Rajamaki A. Serum transferrin receptor and its ratio to serum ferritin in the diagnosis of iron deficiency. *Blood* 1997;89:1052–1057.
27. Joosten E, Van Loon R, Billen J, et al. Serum transferrin receptor in the evaluation of the iron status in elderly hospitalized patients with anemia. *Am J Hematol* 2002;69:1–6.
28. Song JS, Park W, Bae SK, et al. The usefulness of serum transferrin receptor and ferritin for assessing anemia in rheumatoid arthritis: comparison with bone marrow iron study. *Rheumatol Int* 2001;21:24–29.
29. Fong TP, Okafor LA, Thomas W Jr, et al. Stainable iron in aspirated and needle-biopsy specimens of marrow: a source of error. *Am J Hematol* 1977;2:47–51.
30. DePalma L. The effect of decalcification and choice of fixative on histiocytic iron in bone marrow core biopsies. *Biotech Histochem* 1996;71:57–60.
31. Meredith JT, Cerezo LA. Comparison of stainable iron in thick bone marrow aspirate smears and decalcified biopsy specimens. *Lab Med* 1988;19:493–496.
32. Douglas DD, Risdall RJ. Bone marrow biopsy technic. Artifact induced by aspiration. *Am J Clin Pathol* 1984;82:92–94.
33. Wolff SN, Katzenstein AL, Phillips GL, et al. Aspiration does not influence interpretation of bone marrow biopsy cellularity. *Am J Clin Pathol* 1983;80:60–62.
34. McCluggage WG, Clarke R, Bharucha H. Non-neoplastic glandular structures in bone marrow: a technical artefact. *J Clin Pathol* 1995;48:1141–1142.

Bone Marrow Report

1. Hyun BH, Stevenson AJ, Hanau CA. Fundamentals of bone marrow examination. *Hematol Oncol Clin North Am* 1994;8:651–663.
2. Foucar K. Bone marrow examination: indications and techniques. In: Foucar K, ed. *Bone marrow pathology,* 2nd ed. Chicago: ASCP Press, 2000:31–49.
3. Cotelingam JD. Bone marrow biopsy: interpretive guidelines for the surgical pathologist. *Adv Anat Pathol* 2003;10:8–26.
4. Asare AL, Caldwell CW. An information system for improving clinical laboratory outcomes. Proc American Medical Informatics Association Symposium, 2000:22–26.
5. Nguyen DT, Diamond LW, Cavenagh JD et al. Haematological validation of a computer-based bone marrow reporting system. *J Clin Pathol* 1997;50:375–378.
6. Diamond LW, Tamino PB, Seal AH, et al. Multiparameter case studies using knowledge-based systems in hematology. *Comput Methods Programs Biomed* 1995;48:59–64.
7. Diamond LW, Mishka VG, Seal AH, et al. multiparameter interpretative reporting in diagnostic laboratory hematology. *Int J Biomed Comput* 1994;37:211–224.

3

ANCILLARY STUDIES

CAROLYN CHILING CHAI

Ancillary studies offer valuable information, in addition to that provided by Romanowsky and hematoxylin and eosin staining, for the differential diagnosis of hematologic disorders. With the advances in lineage testing, prognostic evaluation, and treatment, ancillary studies including immunohistochemistry, flow cytometry, and cytogenetic analyses have become increasingly important for patient care. Despite new techniques, however, morphologic examination remains the crucial first step in arriving at a correct diagnosis. The principles and general applications of the ancillary studies are discussed here. Please refer to special textbooks for technical details.

CYTOCHEMISTRY AND HISTOCHEMISTRY

Cytochemistry and histochemistry are the study of chemical elements in the cells, which may be enzymes or nonenzymes. With the development of other techniques, cytochemistry and histochemistry are used mostly in conjunction with them and not as a sole diagnostic tool (1).

In cytochemistry, smears from bone marrow, lymph node, spleen, or peripheral blood are the preferred specimens. Fresh smears should be used whenever possible to ensure optimal enzyme activity. Smears for nonenzymatic stains, such as periodic acid–Schiff (PAS) or Sudan black B, may remain stable for months or years at room temperature.

Acid Phosphatase

A lysosomal enzyme, acid phosphatase hydrolyzes naphthol AS-BI phosphoric acid in most hematopoietic cells. Almost all blood cells contain seven nonerythroid isoenzymes (0, 1, 2, 3, 3b, 4, and 5), but their isoenzyme 5 is minimal. Hairy cells, histiocytes, Gaucher cells, and osteoclasts produce abundant isoenzyme 5. With L(+) tartrate treatment, all isoenzyme activity is abolished except isoenzyme 5. Although not entirely specific, tartrate-resistant acid phosphatase is useful in the diagnosis of hairy cell leukemia (2–5) (Fig. 3-1).

Esterases

Esterases split naphthol and naphthol derivatives from their esters in hematopoietic cells and include chloracetate esterase for granulocytes, α-naphthyl acetate esterase for T cells, α-naphthyl butyrate esterase for monocytes, and aminocaproate esterase for mast cells.

Chloracetate esterase, also called specific esterase, is found in primary granules in myeloid and mast cells and gives a red color to cytoplasm. It hydrolyzes naphthol AS-D chloroacetate and is resistant to sodium fluoride. It parallels the myeloperoxidase and Sudan black B reactions but has the advantage of applying on paraffin-embedded sections and therefore can be used to diagnose granulocytic sarcoma (6). Mast cells and myeloid cells including myeloblasts are positive for chloracetate esterase. The chloracetate esterase reaction does not occur in decalcified tissue.

α-Naphthyl acetate esterase is present in monocytes, macrophages, megakaryocytes, plasma cells, and lymphocytes. Dotlike activity correlates with T helper cells. Megakaryocytes and plasma cells generally show diffuse cytoplasmic staining. The enzymes of the monocytes and

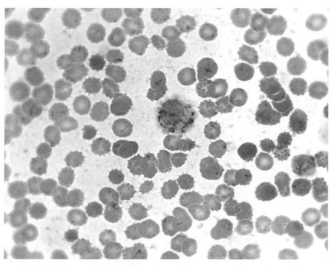

FIGURE 3-1. Cytochemical stain using tartrate-resistant acid phosphatase in hairy cell leukemia.

histiocytes are inhibited by sodium fluoride, whereas those of megakaryoblasts are not. A positive α-naphthyl acetate esterase with negative α-naphthyl butyrate esterase activity is characteristic of acute megakaryocytic leukemia (AML-M7).

α-Naphthyl butyrate esterase, also called nonspecific esterase, is positive in monocytes and histiocytes and shows diffuse cytoplasmic staining. T helper cells exhibit a dotlike staining pattern. It is commonly used in the diagnosis of acute monocytic leukemias (AML-M4 and M5) (2,3).

Aminocaproate esterase uses naphthol AS ε-aminocaproate as substrate. Mast cells show diffuse cytoplasmic positivity (3); other cells are usually negative. It is useful in the diagnosis of mast cell diseases.

Leukocyte Alkaline Phosphatase

Leukocyte alkaline phosphatase is an enzyme in secondary granules in neutrophils, band forms, and metamyelocytes. The enzymatic activity increases with cellular maturation. One hundred neutrophils and band forms are counted on the peripheral blood smear and scored. The activity score ranges from 0 to 4+. The normal score is 20 to 100 (4). Eosinophils are negative for leukocyte alkaline phosphatase and should not be mistaken for neutrophils during scoring.

A decreased leukocyte alkaline phosphatase score is seen in chronic myelogenous leukemia, paroxysmal nocturnal hemoglobinuria, sickle cell anemia, and sideroblastic anemia. An elevated score may be seen in leukemoid reaction, polycythemia vera, and third-trimester pregnancy.

Myeloperoxidase

Myeloperoxidase is an enzyme in the primary granules of myeloid lineage from the promyelocyte to neutrophil stages including eosinophils. Monocytes may be weakly positive. Blue-black granules indicate positive myeloperoxidase. Blasts with positive myeloperoxidase staining indicate myeloid lineage and distinguish acute myelogenous leukemia from acute lymphoblastic leukemia. Myeloperoxidase in eosinophils resists cyanide inhibition and identifies acute myelogenous leukemia with eosinophilic differentiation (7). Auer rods also demonstrate myeloperoxidase positivity (2,8,9).

Periodic Acid–Schiff

PAS stains cytoplasmic glycogen in many cell lines including lymphocytes, granulocytes, monocytes, and megakaryocytes. It distinguishes normal red cells and precursors (PAS negative) from leukemic cells of erythroid lineage (PAS positive) and therefore is important in the diagnosis of acute erythroid leukemia (AML-M6). It also distinguishes B-precursor lymphoblastic leukemia/lymphoma from B-cell type (Burkitt lymphoma). The former is positive for PAS (4,10–12).

Adding diastase removes glycogen and identifies the carbohydrate portion of the intracellular immunoglobulin (Ig) in plasma cells and plasmacytoid lymphocytes. Russell bodies and Dutcher bodies are positive. PAS with diastase is also useful for distinguishing the intensely red-staining megakaryocytes from the negative-staining Reed-Sternberg cells.

Perls Prussian Blue

Perls Prussian blue stain detects storage iron (ferritin and hemosiderin) in macrophages and erythroblasts and is most useful in aspirate smears when sufficient particles are present (13,14). Ferritin produces blue haze or streaks but may not be detected at normal levels. Hemosiderin is formed as granules or droplets (15). Bone marrow contains both intracellular and extracellular iron, the former in erythroblasts and the latter from crushed macrophages. Iron assessment is based mainly on intracellular iron because artifactual deposit may sometimes resemble extracellular iron. Iron store is graded as 1+ to 6+, with grades 1+ to 3+ considered within the normal range (13,16,17). Bone marrow of hematologically normal individuals typically contains 20% to 50% sideroblasts (18–20) (Table 3-1).

Reticulin

Histologic sections, either from trephine biopsy or particle section, can be stained with reticulin using the silver-impregnation technique. Hematologically normal bone marrow has a minimal reticulin deposit, although reticulin may be present around blood vessels or bony trabeculae. Increased reticulin fibers provide nonspecific evidence of abnormal marrow and a focal increase in the reticulin deposit helps to detect abnormalities that might be overlooked by routine hematoxylin and eosin stain (21) (Table 3-2).

Sudan Black B

Sudan black B is a fat-soluble dye. It stains lipids in primary and secondary granules of the myeloid series and lysosomal granules in monocytes. The staining pattern correlates with that of myeloperoxidase and is slightly more sensitive for early myeloid precursors. The staining intensity and

TABLE 3-1. BONE MARROW STORAGE IRON

0	No stainable iron (negative)
1	Small iron particles visible under oil objective
2	Small iron particles visible under low objective
3	Numerous small iron particles throughout marrow particles
4	Large iron particles throughout marrow; tend to aggregate
5	Dense large iron clumps throughout marrow
6	Very large iron clumps that obscure cellular details

From Gale E, Torrance J, Bothrell T. The quantitative estimation of total iron stores in human bone marrow. *J Clin Invest* 1963;42: 1076–1082.

TABLE 3-2. RETICULIN QUANTITATION IN BONE MARROW

0	No reticulin fibers
1	Occasional fine reticulin fibers
2	Fine reticulin fiber network throughout most sections with no coarse fibers
3	Diffuse fiber network with scattered thick fibers but no mature collagen
4	Diffuse thick fiber network with areas of collagenization

From Bauermeister DE. Quantification of bone marrow reticulin—a normal range. *Am J Clin Pathol* 1971;56:24–31.

TABLE 3-3. COMMONLY USED ANTIGENS IN BONE MARROW BIOPSY (FOR PARAFFIN TISSUE)

B cells	CD20, CD79a
T cells	CD2, CD3, CD4, CD5, CD7, CD8, UCHL-1
B precursors	CD10, CD79a, TdT
Natural killer/cytotoxic T cells	CD56, TIA-1, granzyme B, perforin
Myeloid cells	Myeloperoxidase, lysozyme
Immature cells	CD1a, CD34, TdT

TdT, terminal deoxynucleotidyltransferase.

coarseness increase with myeloid maturation. Positive cells have brown-black cytoplasmic granules (9,22). Because of its fat solubility, Sudan black B may stain lymphoblasts containing fat granules such as in B-cell lymphoblastic leukemia/small noncleaved cell lymphoma.

Compared with myeloperoxidase, Sudan black B stain is preferred in specimens that are older than 2 weeks.

Terminal Deoxynucleotidyltransferase

Terminal deoxynucleotidyltransferase is a DNA polymerase in T- and B-cell precursors and is used to identify lymphoblasts in acute lymphoblastic leukemia/lymphoma. However, it is not specific and has been noted in 5% to 10% of patients with acute myelogenous leukemia, as many as 30% of patients with chronic myelogenous leukemia in blast crisis, and as many as 50% of patients with acute undifferentiated leukemia. It is present in 2% to 7% of hematopoietic cells in children younger than 5 years old, in 1% to 2% in adult bone marrow, and in as many as 20% in regenerating bone marrow (8).

IMMUNOHISTOCHEMISTRY

With the growing number of antibodies for paraffin-embedded tissue and the ease of performing paraffin staining, immunohistochemistry has achieved widespread use in hematopathology (1–3). It can be used with acid- or ethylenediaminetetraacetic acid–decalcified trephine biopsy or nondecalcified samples (4). Antigen retrieval by the wet-heat method or by minimization of nonspecific staining owing to endogenous enzyme activity has greatly improved the staining results. Immunohistochemistry can detect membrane, cytoplasmic, and nuclear antigens and may provide specific genetic information such as ALK-1, Bcl-1, and Bcl-2 in anaplastic large cell lymphoma, mantle cell lymphoma, and follicular center cell lymphoma, respectively.

Immunohistochemical staining of the trephine biopsy and particle section is ideal for assessment of focal lesions to determine lineage differentiation or stage of maturation that may not be detected by flow cytometry analysis in patients with a dry tap (5–7). This is often seen when significant reticulin fibrosis is associated with an infiltrate that hinders aspiration of the abnormal cells, such as in bone marrow involvement by follicular center cell lymphoma, Hodgkin lymphoma, carcinoma, or small round cell tumors. In the evaluation of acute leukemia and lymphoproliferative disorders, flow cytometry is preferred because of the limitations in the detection of some antigens by immunohistochemistry. Like all immunophenotypic analyses, a panel of antibodies should be applied to increase the detection sensitivity and specificity. For example, T-cell antigen CD5 is also present in B-cell chronic lymphocytic leukemia/small lymphocytic lymphoma and mantle cell lymphoma. Commonly used B- and T-cell markers in immunohistochemistry are listed in Table 3-3.

Compared with flow cytometry, which is able to assess multiple antigens on a single cell and several thousand cells simultaneously, immunohistochemistry is limited by the number of slides available for staining. However, it detects focal lesions and provides morphologic evaluation of the cell distribution pattern. The number of antibodies and, therefore the detection spectrum in immunohistochemistry, are also becoming increasingly extensive.

FLOW CYTOMETRY

Flow cytometry analysis has a broad range of applications in the evaluation of hematologic diseases. The most common is immunophenotyping of peripheral blood, bone marrow, and lymph node to identify clonality or leukemias. Other applications include determining CD4/CD8 ratio and absolute lymphocyte count, establishing the presence of congenital immunodeficiency, determining ploidy and S phase of the tumors, and evaluating red blood cells with specific defects (CD55, CD59) associated with paroxysmal nocturnal hemoglobinuria. Multicolor flow cytometry can detect minimal residual disease or nonhematopoietic lesions (1). Useful guidelines are listed in several consensus reports (2–10).

The principle of flow cytometry is that cells bearing a specific antigen are detected by monoclonal antibody labeled with a fluorochrome. This allows classification of cells by light scatter and fluorescent intensity. Multiple fluorochromes can be used so that simultaneous expression of multiple antigens can be studied. Although flow cytometry analysis primarily detects surface antigens, when permeabilized, cytoplasmic and nuclear antigens can also be studied. It is convenient for detecting a large number of cells in peripheral blood, bone marrow aspirate, cerebrospinal fluid, body fluids, or lymph node and tissue suspensions. The gating strategies with increased detection sensitivity also increase the ability to detect minimal residual disease (11). When peripheral blood is used, immunophenotyping can be applied either to a mononuclear cell preparation or to whole blood in which the red cells are lysed (12).

Leukemic blasts express dim CD45, whereas non-hematopoietic tumors and some blasts in acute lymphoblastic leukemia lack CD45 expression. To maximize sensitivity and specificity, an ideal leukemia panel should contain at least two antibodies per cell lineage. Gating is essential for an accurate immunophenotyping, especially when cells are heterogeneous or when target cells are few. Sclerotic bone marrow may yield too few cells for adequate analysis; therefore, correlating light scatter and immunophenotypic pattern with cellular morphology may help to detect some cells of interest when standard gating protocols fail to detect them. This is also true when benign lymphocytes outnumber malignant cells (e.g., in Hodgkin lymphoma) or when aspirate is taken from a benign area in partially involved marrow. Immunohistochemical stains should be applied in these circumstances for morphologic correlation (1,13,14). The choice of the diagnostic antibodies is based on differential diagnosis. Reactive lymphocytosis requires both B- and T-cell antigens, whereas in lymphoproliferative disorders, B-cell antigens and light chain clonality should be focused. Some acute leukemias or lymphomas show aberrant antigen expression (Fig. 3-2). The ultimate results of flow cytometry should correlate with the clinical history, automated hematology panel, morphologic review, and other laboratory data.

CYTOGENETICS

Cytogenetic analysis provides valuable information on the karyotypic change and prognostic significance of leukemias and lymphomas. It helps to distinguish neoplastic processes from reactive ones, such as distinguishing reactive eosinophilia from eosinophilic leukemia and reactive lymphocytosis from B-cell lymphoproliferative disorders.

Conventional cytogenetic analysis involves examining metaphase spreads and can be performed with peripheral blood, bone marrow, or lymph node aspirate, either as direct preparation or after culturing. It can be performed only on viable cells (1). Cells are arrested in metaphase, lysed, and then visualized with stains or a fluorescent agent. Each chromosome is identified by size, banding pattern, and the centromere location and then either illustrated by a karyogram or expressed as a karyotype. Common cytogenetic abnormalities associated with hematopoietic neoplasms are those with tyrosine kinase translocations, those with retinoic acid translocations, those that disrupt transcription factors, and those with 11q23 abnormality (2).

Common examples of translocation with resultant tyrosine kinase fusion proteins are BCR/abl of t(9;22)(q32;q11) in chronic myelogenous leukemia and some acute myelogenous leukemia, TEL/ABL of t(9;12)(q32;p13) in some acute and chronic leukemias, and TEL/PDGFRβ of t(5;12)(q33;p13) in some chronic myelomonocytic leukemia. A classic example of retinoic acid translocation is t(15;17)(q22;q11.2), unique to acute promyelocytic leukemia and resulting in PML/RARα fusion protein. All-trans retinoic acid counteracts this leukemic fusion protein and is unique in the treatment of acute promyelocytic leukemia (Fig. 3-3). Translocations involving transcription factor genes are common in acute leukemia, with the best known being the core binding factor in normal hematopoiesis. AML1 and CBFβ proteins, encoded on chromosomes 21q22 and 16q22, respectively, are important components of core binding factor. Disruption of these chromosome regions, such as in t(3;21), t(8;21), t(12;21), inv(16), and t(16;16), disrupts normal hematopoiesis and results in the development of acute leukemia. The leukemia types vary; the AML1/ETO fusion product of t(8;21)(q22;q22) results in acute myelogenous leukemia with maturation (AML-M2). The CBFβ/MYH11 fusion product of inv(16)(p13;q22) or t(16;16)(p13;q22) is

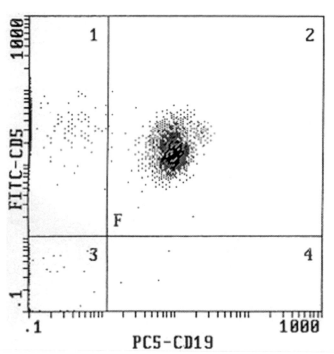

FIGURE 3-2. Flow cytometry analysis demonstrates B-cell chronic lymphocytic leukemia with aberrant CD5 expression.

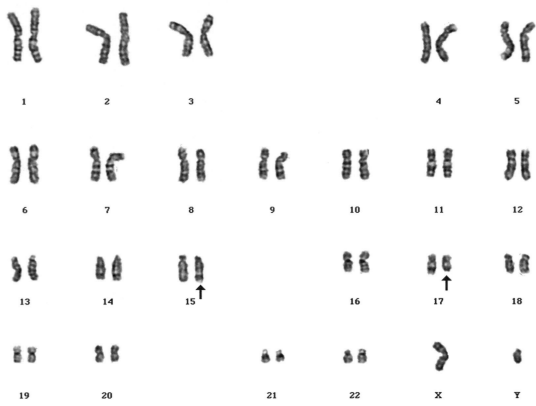

FIGURE 3-3. Conventional cytogenetic analysis demonstrates t(15;17) in a patient with acute promyelocytic leukemia.

seen in acute myelomonocytic leukemia with abnormal eosinophils (AML-M4eo). AML1/EVI1, AML1/EAP, and the AML1/MDS1 fusion products of t(3;21)(q26;q22) result in myelodysplastic syndrome–associated processes and the TEL/AML1 fusion product of t(12;21)(p13;q22) results in pediatric acute lymphoblastic leukemia. Abnormalities of chromosome 11q23 involving the MLL gene are seen in many translocations and different leukemias (3). The t(4;11)(q21;q23) is associated with precursor B-cell acute lymphoblastic leukemia in infants with aberrant CD15 expression. The t(9;11)(p22;q23) is associated with adult acute myelogenous leukemia with monocytic differentiation. Secondary acute myelogenous leukemia after topoisomerase II inhibitor treatment also exhibits the 11q23 abnormality, usually with monocytic differentiation.

In newly diagnosed leukemia or suspected myelodysplastic syndrome, traditional karyotypic analysis is the first line because of the high likelihood of multiple acquired genetic anomalies. It can detect a chromosome abnormality that carries a specific prognosis that affects the treatment choice. It may distinguish malignant from reactive conditions (e.g., large granular lymphocytosis from large granular cell lymphoma leukemia and hypereosinophilia from eosinophilic leukemia), monitor treatment in chronic myelogenous leukemia, detect treatment-related myelodysplasia, and monitor minimal residual disease. However, some leukemias yield insufficient metaphase for examination and may produce a false-negative result. Probes are not available for many recurring abnormalities at present.

MOLECULAR GENETICS

In recent years, Southern blotting and polymerase chain reaction (PCR) have allowed confirmation of abnormalities detected by conventional cytogenetics and have detected additional genetic abnormalities, including point mutation and gene rearrangements. They are being used increasingly to establish clonality and for diagnosis and follow-up of hematologic neoplasms. They also detect chromosome translocation, mutation, amplification, and viral DNA and RNA. However, Southern blotting requires radioactive material and a large quantity of DNA, which limits the detection sensitivity. It also has a long turnaround time (1).

Both Southern blot analysis and PCR detect tumor clonality (2–4) by identifying their antigen receptor gene rearrangement [Ig and T-cell receptor (TCR)] and establish tumor lineage. They differ slightly in that the probes in Southern blot analysis detect IgH J region or TCR β and γ chains, whereas in PCR, the primers are complementary to IgH V and J regions or TCR β and γ chains. In the polyclonal lymphoid population, the rearrangement is random and no single band is present. In a monoclonal population, all lymphocytes share the same rearrangement and produce a single discrete band on electrophoresis. Molecular technique is especially valuable in detecting somatic hypermutation in B-cell lymphoproliferative disorders. Much more is known about the B-cell maturation than that of T cells, mainly the maturation of the Ig molecule within germinal centers. Lymphomas derived from a pregerminal center (nonmutated), germinal center (hypermutated with evidence of ongoing mutation), and postgerminal center (hypermutated with no ongoing mutation) lymphoid cells have different mutation patterns (5). A chronic lymphocytic leukemia has been described to differ by showing pregerminal center and postgerminal center patterns of IgH hypermutation.

PCR has a higher sensitivity for detecting small clonal populations, but it detects only 80% of B-cell neoplasms using a primer for the IgH V region (6). Most of the remaining 20% are detectable by Southern blot analysis. Negative PCR results are usually followed by a Southern blot. The sensitivity varies among lymphoma types, with follicular lymphoma having the lowest sensitivity, likely owing to its high rate of somatic hypermutation and subsequent failure to respond to consensus primers for the V region (1,2). Mantle cell lymphoma and small lymphocytic lymphoma, conversely, have a higher detection rate by PCR. In cases in which translocation cannot be detected by PCR, reverse transcriptase PCR may be used.

IgH and TCR gene rearrangement is not lineage specific and may be seen in acute lymphoblastic leukemia and acute myelogenous leukemia. Moreover, it has been detected in reactive conditions. Therefore, the results should be interpreted with caution and correlated with histology and clinical findings. For a B-cell lineage study, κ and λ light chain gene rearrangements are much more specific than the IgH gene (Fig. 3-4). Some nonneoplastic conditions, including acquired immunodeficiency syndrome, autoimmune disorders, and Castleman disease, may also show clonal gene rearrangement of antigen receptors. Classic stimulated germinal centers and disorganized progressive transformation of germinal centers have recently been reported to show somatic hypermutation (7,8). In addition, the lack of a clonal band does not exclude malignancy.

Some fusion genes can be detected by PCR or reverse transcriptase PCR by employing specific primers that flank the chromosome breakpoints. It is rapid and highly sensitive and does not require viable cells as does conventional cytogenetics. However, it detects only the abnormalities that are

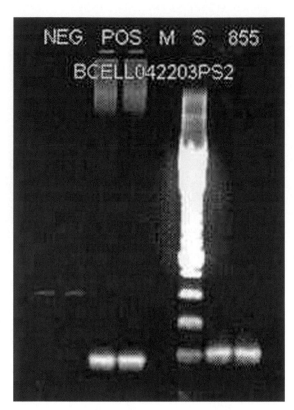

FIGURE 3-4. Molecular study using polymerase chain reaction to detect monoclonal immunoglobulin H in a patient with B-cell lymphoma.

being specifically sought. Commonly detected translocations include t(9;22)(q34;q11) in chronic myelogenous leukemia and some acute lymphoblastic leukemias, t(2;5)(p23;q25) in anaplastic large cell lymphoma, and t(8;21)(q22;q22), t(15;17)(q22;q21), and inv(16)(p13;q22) in acute myelogenous leukemia (6). Some translocations may persist in low numbers after treatment. Their detection by PCR does not necessarily predict relapse. For this reason, quantitative PCR may be more valuable for the detection of minimal residual disease (2,9–11).

FLUORESCENCE *IN SITU* HYBRIDIZATION

Fluorescence *in situ* hybridization (FISH) is a molecular genetic technique using a labeled probe to interphase nuclei or metaphase spreads and visualization under a fluorescence microscope (1–4). By using different fluorochromes, it is possible to identify multiple DNA sequences in a single preparation simultaneously. Chromosome abnormalities can be detected in tumor cells without entering mitosis (such as in chronic lymphocytic leukemia) and in peripheral blood or bone marrow films previously stained with Romanowsky or immunohistochemical stain, allowing cytologic and karyotypic correlation. It can be used to detect numeric abnormalities (e.g., trisomy 21, monosomy 7), translocations

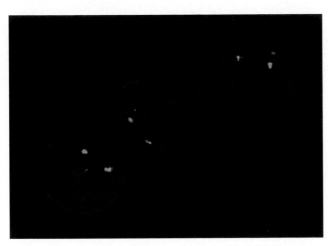

FIGURE 3-5. Fluorescence *in situ* hybridization demonstrates t(9;22) in a patient with chronic myelogenous leukemia.

(e.g., MLL gene), and isochromosome formation, and deletion or amplification of chromosome material (e.g., p53). Other advantages of FISH include the ability to confirm a suspected abnormality when chromosome morphology is poor and to scan a large number of cells to catch a low number of abnormality (e.g., detecting minimal residual disease). Interphase FISH analysis is much faster than G-banding metaphase analysis because the cells do not need to grow in the culture. However, only part of the chromosome is analyzed, and some important information may be missed. Spectral karyotyping uses a complex panel of probes simultaneously and identifies all chromosomes in a metaphase preparation. It is particularly useful in detecting complex chromosome abnormalities (5).

Assessing chromosome translocation requires two separate probes of different colors. Each probe is complementary to the DNA sequence near the translocation site. The sample is then visualized using a fluorescence microscope. In nontranslocated chromosomes, two separate colored signals are detected. If a translocation is present, a third single fusion signal is also detected. A good example is t(9;22) (Fig. 3-5).

FISH is limited by its detection of only the abnormalities for which the probes are used [e.g., a probe for t(9;22) does not detect inv(16)]. Secondary abnormalities are not recognized (e.g., those detecting Ph$^+$ miss 11q23). False positivity or negativity is present in screening trisomy or monosomy, so the low frequency of the abnormalities is not reliably detected (6). In bone marrow fibrosis, an abnormality may not be detected because of inadequate sampling. The application of FISH in bone marrow trephine biopsy is more limited at present.

ACKNOWLEDGMENTS

The author gives sincere thanks to Dr. Diane Farhi for reviewing this chapter.

REFERENCES

Cytochemistry and Histochemistry

1. Scott CS, Den Ottolander GJ, Swirsky D, et al. Recommended procedures for the classification of acute leukemias. *Leuk Lymphoma* 1993;11:37–49.
2. Brunning RD, Mckenna RW. *Tumor of the bone marrow, Atlas of Tumor Pathology,* 3rd series, fascicle 9. Washington, DC: AFIP, 1994:19–142.
3. Foucar K. *Bone marrow pathology,* 2nd ed. Chicago: ASCP Press, 2001.
4. Steine-Martin EA, Lotspeich-Steininger CA, Keopke JA. *Clinical hematology, principles, procedures, correlations,* 2nd ed. Philadelphia: Lippincott–Raven Publishers, 1998.
5. Yam LT, Li CY, Crosby WH. Cytoplasmic identification of monocytes and granulocytes. *Am J Clin Pathol* 1971;55:283–290.
6. Traweek ST, Arber DA, Rappapot H, et al. Extramedullary myeloid cell tumors. An immunohistochemical and morphologic study of 28 cases. *Am J Surg Pathol* 1993;17:1011–1019.
7. Gabbas AG, Li CY. A non-lymphoblastic leukemia with eosinophilic differentiation. *Am J Hematol* 1986;21:29–38.
8. Li CY, Yam LT. Cytochemical, histochemical, and immunohistochemical analysis of the bone marrow. In: Knowles DM, ed. *Neoplastic hematopathology,* 2nd ed. Philadelphia: Lippincott Williams & Wilkins, 2001:1407–1445.
9. Lillie RD, Burtner HJ. Stable sudanophilia of human neutrophil leukocytes in relation to peroxidase and oxidase. *J Histochem Cytochem* 1953;1:8–26.
10. Bain BJ. *Leukemia diagnosis,* 2nd ed. Oxford: Blackwell Science, 1999.
11. Hayhoe FGJ. Acute leukemia: cellular morphology, cytochemistry, and fine structure. *Clin Hematol* 1972;1:49–94.
12. Hayhoe FGJ, Quaglino D. *Hematological cytochemistry,* 2nd ed. Edinburgh: Churchill Livingstone, 1988.
13. Fong TP, Okafor LA, Thomas W, Jr. Stainable iron in aspirated and needle-biopsy specimens of marrow: a source of error. *Am J Hematol* 1977;2:47–51.
14. Sundberg RD, Broman H. The application of the Prussian blue stain to previously stained films of blood and bone marrow. *Blood* 1955;10:160–166.
15. Bain BJ, Clark DM, Lampert IA, et al. *Bone marrow pathology,* 3rd ed. Oxford: Blackwell Science, 2001.
16. Gale E, Torrance J, Bothrell T. The quantitative estimation of total iron stores in human bone marrow. *J Clin Invest* 1963;42:1076–1082.
17. Lundin P, Persson E, Weinfeld A. Comparison of hemosiderin estimation in bone marrow sections and bone marrow smears. *Acta Med Scand* 1964;175:383–390.
18. Bainton DF, Finch CA. The diagnosis of iron deficiency anemia. *Am J Med* 1964;37:62–70.
19. Douglas AS, Dacie JV. The incidence and significance of iron-containing granules in human erythrocytes and their precursors. *J Clin Pathol* 1953;6:307–313.
20. Hansen HA, Weinfeld A. Hemosiderin estimations and sideroblast counts in the differential diagnosis of iron deficiency and other anemias. *Acta Med Scand* 1965;165:333–356.
21. Bauermeister DE. Quantification of bone marrow reticulin–a normal range. *Am J Clin Pathol* 1971;56:24–31.
22. Sheehan HL, Storey GW. An improved method of staining leukocyte granules with Sudan black B. *J Pathol* 1947:59:336–337.

Immunohistochemistry

1. Arber DA. Bone marrow. In: Weidner N, Cote RJ, Suster S, et al., eds. *Modern surgical pathology.* Philadelphia: WB Saunders, 2003:1597–1657.

2. Frizzera G, Wu CD, Inghrami G. The usefulness of immunophenotypic and genotypic studies in the diagnosis and classification of hematopoietic and lymphoid neoplasms: an update. *Am J Clin Pathol* 1999;111:S13–S39.
3. Ioachin HL, Ratech H, eds. *Ioachin's lymph node pathology*, 3rd ed. Philadelphia: Lipponcott Williams & Wilkins, 2002.
4. Bain BJ, Clark DM, Lampert IA, et al. *Bone marrow pathology*, 3rd ed. Oxford: Blackwell Science, 2001.
5. Arber DA, Jenkins KA. Paraffin section immunophenotyping of acute leukemias in bone marrow specimens. *Am J Clin Pathol* 1996;106:462–468.
6. Loyson SAJ, Rademakers LHPM, Joling P. Immunohistochemical analysis of decalcified paraffin-embedded human bone marrow biopsy with emphasis on MHC class 1 and CD34 expression. *Histopathology* 1997;31:412–419.
7. Pileri SA, Ascani S, Milani M. Acute leukemia immunophenotyping in bone marrow routine sections. *Br J Haematol* 1999; 105:394–401.

Flow Cytometry

1. Karen DF, CoCoy Jr JP, Carey JL. *Flow cytometry in clinical diagnosis*, 3rd ed. Chicago: ASCP Press, 2001.
2. U.S.-Canadian consensus recommendations on the immunophenotypic analysis of hematologic neoplasia by flow cytometry. *Cytometry* 1997;30:213–274.
3. Braylan RC, Atwater SK, Diamond L, et al. U.S.-Canadian consensus recommendations on the immunophenotypic analysis of hematologic neoplasia by flow cytometry: data reporting. *Cytometry* 1997;30:245–248.
4. Borowitz MT, Bray R, Gascoyne R, et al. U.S.-Canadian consensus recommendations on the immunophenotypic analysis of hematologic neoplasia by flow cytometry: data analysis and interpretation. *Cytometry* 1997;30:236–244.
5. Davis RH, Foucar K, Szczarkowski W, et al. US-Canadian consensus recommendations on the immunophenotypic analysis of hematologic neoplasia by flow cytometry: medical indications. *Cytometry* 1997;30:249–263.
6. Jennings CD, Foon KA. Recent advances in flow cytometry: application to the of hematologic malignancy. *Blood* 1997;90:2863–2892.
7. Matutes E, Polliack A. Morphological and immunophenotypic features of chronic lymphocytic leukemia. *Rev Clin Exp Hematol* 2000;4:22–47.
8. Rothe G, Schmitz G. Consensus protocol for the flow cytometric immunophenotyping of hematopoietic malignancy. *Leukemia* 1996;10:877–895.
9. Stelzer GT, Marti G, Hurley A, et al. U.S.-Canadian consensus recommendations on the immunophenotypic analysis of hematologic neoplasia by flow cytometry: standardization and validation of laboratory procedures. *Cytometry* 1997;30:214–230.
10. Stewart CC, Behm FG, Carey JL, et al. U.S.-Canadian consensus recommendations on the immunophenotypic analysis of hematologic neoplasia by flow cytometry: selection of antibody combinations. *Cytometry* 1997;30:231–235.
11. Borowitz MT, Guenther KL, Shults KE. Immunophenotyping of acute leukemia by flow cytometry analysis. Use of CD45 and right angle light scatter to gate on leukemic blasts in 3 color analysis. *Am J Clin Pathol* 1993;100:534–540.
12. Gratama JW, Bolhuis RLH, van's Veer MB. Quality assurance of flow cytometry immunophenotyping of hematologic malignancies. *Clin Lab Hematol* 1999;21:155–160.
13. Bain BJ, Clark DM, Lampert IA, et al. *Bone marrow pathology*, 3rd ed. Oxford: Blackwell Science, 2001.
14. Arber DA. Bone marrow. In: Weidner N, Cote RJ, Suster S, et al., eds. *Modern surgical pathology*. Philadelphia: WB Saunders, 2003:1597–1657.

Cytogenetics

1. Fonatsch C, Streubel B. Classical and molecular cytogenetics. In: Huhn D, ed. *New diagnostic methods in oncology and hematology*. Berlin: Springer, 1998.
2. Arber DA. Bone marrow. In: Weidner N, Cote RJ, Suster S, et al., eds. *Modern surgical pathology*. Philadelphia: WB Saunders, 2003:1597–1657.
3. Dimartino JF, Cleary ML. MLL rearrangements in hematologic malignancies: lessons from clinical and biological studies. *Br J Haematol* 1999;106:614–624.

Molecular Genetics

1. Pittaluga S, Tierous A, Dodoo YL. How reliable is histologic examination of bone marrow trephine biopsy specimens for the staging of non-Hodgkin's lymphoma? A study of hairy cell leukemia and mantle cell lymphoma involvement of the bone marrow trephine specimen by histology, immunohistochemistry, and PCR techniques. *Am J Clin Pathol* 1999;111:179–184.
2. Bagg A, Kallakury BVS. Molecular pathology of leukemia and lymphoma. *Am J Clin Pathol* 1999;112[Suppl 1]:S76–S92.
3. Neubauer A, Thiede C, Nagel S. Molecular biology. In: Huhn D, ed. *New diagnostic methods in oncology and hematology*. Berlin: Springer, 1998.
4. Wickham CI, Boyce M, Joyne MV. Amplification of PCR products in excess of 600 bp using DNA extracted from decalcified, paraffin wax embedded bone marrow trephine biopsy. *J Clin Pathol Mol Pathol* 2000;53:19–23.
5. Ioachin HL, Ratech H, eds. *Ioachin's lymph node pathology*, 3rd ed. Philadelphia: Lipponcott Williams & Wilkins, 2002.
6. Bain BJ, Clark DM, Lampert IA, et al. *Bone marrow pathology*, 3rd ed. Oxford: Blackwell Science, 2001.
7. Brauninger A, Yang W, Wacker HH, et al. B cell development in progressive transformation of germinal centers: similarities and differences compared with classical germinal center and lymphocyte predominant Hodgkin's lymphoma. *Blood* 2001;97:714–719.
8. Chang CC, Osipov V, Wheaton S, et al. Follicular hyperplasia, follicular lysis, and progressive transformation of germinal centers: a sequential spectrum of morphologic evolution in lymphoid hyperplasia. *Am J Clin Pathol* 2003;120:322–326.
9. Foroni L, Harrison CJ, Hoffbrand AV, et al. Investigation of minimal residual disease in childhood and adult acute lymphoblastic leukemia by molecular analysis. *Br J Haematol* 1999;105:7–24.
10. Yin JA, Tobal K. Detection of minimal residual disease in acute myelogenous leukemia: methodologies, clinical and biological significance. *Br J Haematol* 1999;106:578–590.
11. Yee K, Anglin P, Keating A. Molecular approaches to the detection and monitoring of chronic myelogenous leukemia: theory and practice. *Blood Rev* 1999:105–126.

Flourescence *In Situ* Hybridization

1. Fonatsch C, Streubel B. Classical and molecular cytogenetics. In: Huhn D, ed. *New diagnostic methods in oncology and hematology*. Berlin: Springer, 1998.

2. Fletcher JA. DNA in-situ hybridization as an adjunct to tumor diagnosis. *Am J Clin Pathol* 1999;112[Suppl 1]:S11–S18.

3. Kearney L. The impact of the new FISH technologies on the cytogenetics of hematological malignancies. *Br J Haematol* 1999;104:648–658.

4. Gozzetti A, Le Beau MM. FISH: uses and limitations. *Semin Hematol* 2000;37:320–333.

5. Schrock E, Padilla-Nash H. Spectral karyotyping and multicolor FISH reveal new tumor-specific chromosomal aberrations. *Semin Hematol* 2000:37:334–337.

6. Bain BJ, Barnett D, Linch D, et al. Revised guideline on immunophenotyping in acute leukemias and chronic lymphoproliferative disorders. *Clin Lab Hematol* 2002;24:1–13.

EXTRAMEDULLARY HEMATOPOIESIS

Extramedullary hematopoiesis (EMH) is found in conditions of excessive hematopoiesis and bone marrow replacement by other tissues and as a dystrophic element in tissue repair, tumors, and other rare conditions. It also occurs as a circumscribed or diffuse mass (myelolipoma). One or more hematopoietic cell lines may be present. EMH often occurs in myeloproliferative disorders, myelodysplastic syndromes, and acute leukemia; however, this chapter is concerned only with nonneoplastic causes of EMH.

EXCESSIVE HEMATOPOIESIS

In conditions of excessive hematopoiesis, blood-forming cells fill and expand the bone marrow cavity and eventually extend beyond the bone to involve adjacent areas, commonly the paravertebral and epidural spaces. The liver, spleen, and lymph nodes are also often involved. EMH may be diagnosed at any age in such patients.

Constitutional disorders causing excessive hematopoiesis and EMH include α and β thalassemia, hemoglobin C

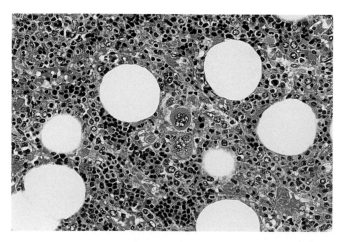

FIGURE 4-1. Posterior mediastinal mass, extramedullary hematopoiesis. A mass composed of hematopoietic tissue and adipose cells is seen in this specimen from a patient with long-standing thalassemia major. The findings are essentially indistinguishable from native bone marrow and myelolipoma.

disease, hemoglobin S disease, congenital dyserythropoietic anemia, hereditary spherocytosis, and pyruvate kinase deficiency (1–11) (Fig. 4-1).

Acquired disorders producing excessive hematopoiesis, some of which present in the neonatal period, include immune-mediated hemolytic anemia, cardiac disease, severe folate and vitamin B_{12} deficiency, and alcohol-related macrocytic anemia (12–18). Congenital syphilis may present with extramedullary hematopoiesis of the skin (see Dystrophic Hematopoiesis section). Therapy with hematopoietic growth factors can also produce EMH (19–21).

BONE MARROW REPLACEMENT

Replacement of bone marrow by nonhematopoietic tissue forces the redistribution of hematopoiesis to other sites, commonly the liver, spleen, and lymph nodes. Bone marrow may be occupied by histiocytes, granulomas, fibrous tissue, bone, and/or malignant cells. Peripheral blood often shows leukoerythroblastosis in this type of EMH.

Constitutional disorders causing bone marrow replacement and EMH include gray platelet syndrome, osteopetrosis, oxalosis, Gaucher disease, and pyknodysostosis (1–8).

Acquired disorders include Paget disease, renal osteodystrophy, hypertrophic osteoarthropathy, histoplasmosis, tuberculosis, sarcoidosis, multiple myeloma, metastatic carcinoma, and osteosarcoma (9–18).

DYSTROPHIC HEMATOPOIESIS

Foci of disordered growth, inflammation, repair, and age-related ossification may eventually develop EMH. This phenomenon has been reported in numerous sites (1–17) (Fig. 4-2).

Tumors may also show areas of EMH as a dystrophic element or as the result of tumor production of erythropoietin. EMH has been reported in tumors of the cardiovascular system, hepatic tissue, soft tissue, gonads, skin, uterus, central nervous system, kidney, and thyroid (18–34).

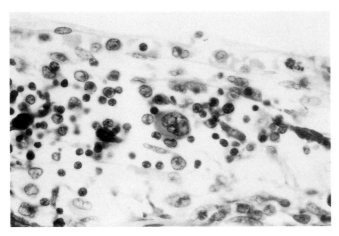

FIGURE 4-2. Choroid of the eye, dystrophic hematopoiesis. Extramedullary hematopoiesis is seen in this specimen from a patient with a traumatically damaged eye.

MYELOLIPOMA

Myelolipomas are extramedullary masses of hematopoietic tissue and fat (1–20) (Fig. 4-3). They are usually single but may be multiple and may occur as an isolated finding or within another pathologic lesion. They range from microscopic to massive in size and may or may not show distinct demarcation from surrounding tissue.

Myelolipomas have been associated with numerous constitutional and acquired conditions but are essentially of unknown origin. The most common site is the adrenal gland, followed by the presacral area, mediastinum, and retroperitoneum. Myelolipomas have less often been reported in the lung, pleura, liver, testis, kidney, lymph node, central nervous system, and ectopic adrenal tissue.

Histologic examination discloses trilineal hematopoiesis and adipose tissue, occasionally with benign lymphoid infiltrates, hemorrhage, trabecular bone, or fibromyxoid degeneration. Angiomyelolipoma has a significant vascular component. In the absence of an underlying hematologic disorder, bone marrow tissue is unremarkable. Genetic analysis has revealed a clonal abnormality in one case (21).

The differential diagnosis includes extramedullary myeloid disease, extramedullary hematopoiesis owing to chronic hemolysis, and adrenal cortical tumors containing adipose tissue (22,23). In myeloproliferative and myelodysplastic disorders, extramedullary sites show the same abnormal histology as the bone marrow. In chronic hemolytic disease, masses indistinguishable from idiopathic myelolipoma have been reported (24,25); therefore, a careful search for undiagnosed hematologic disease is warranted in cases of myelolipoma.

EMBOLIZATION FROM BONE MARROW

Bone marrow embolization is the relocation of bone marrow tissue from an intraosseous site to other sites, usually via the venous circulation (Fig. 4-4). Emboli are usually identified at postmortem examination as intravascular aggregates of hematopoietic cells, fat, and even cartilage and bone, most prominent in the lungs, kidneys, and brain. Fat or bone of marrow origin may be present without identifiable hematopoietic tissue.

Viable normal marrow embolizes under conditions of increased intraosseous pressure, such as marrow harvest and infusion, orthopedic surgery, resuscitation, asphyxia and other trauma, and hyperbarism (1–6).

Viable abnormal marrow embolizes primarily in the sickling disorders, usually in cases of sickle cell anemia but also in hemoglobin SC disease, hemoglobin S/β thalassemia, and storage disorders such as Gaucher disease (6–10).

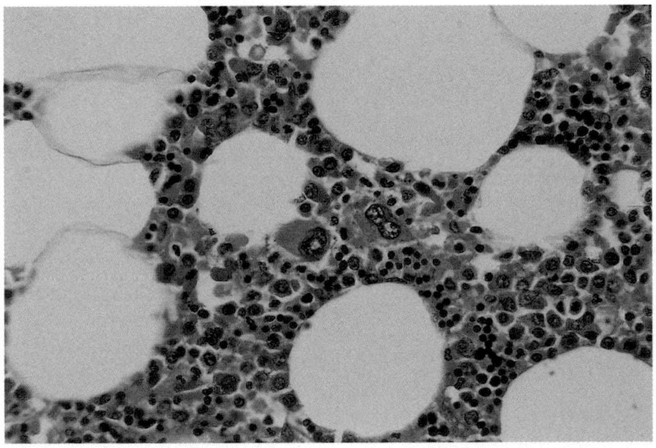

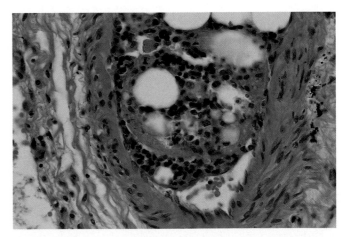

FIGURE 4-3. Retroperitoneum, myelolipoma. A mass composed of hematopoietic tissue and adipose cells is present in this specimen from a patient with an extraadrenal myelolipoma and no evidence of underlying hematopoietic disorder.

FIGURE 4-4. Lung, bone marrow embolus. A large pulmonary vessel is almost completely occluded by hematopoietic tissue in this specimen from a patient who underwent forceful resuscitation.

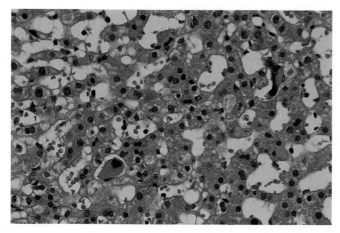

FIGURE 4-5. Liver, sinusoidal megakaryocytes. Two sinusoidal megakaryocytes are seen in this specimen from a patient with hepatomegaly owing to metastatic small cell undifferentiated carcinoma of the lung.

Necrotic marrow typically embolizes in sickling disorders and in hyperbarism. In hyperbarism, the emboli often consist only of fat and are accompanied by intravascular gas bubbles.

In autopsy cases, the differential diagnosis of *in vivo* marrow embolism includes the dislodging of marrow postmortem by the embalming process (11).

HEPATOSPLENOMEGALY

An enlarged liver or spleen often contains foci of EMH (Figs. 4-5 and 4-6). The most readily identifiable cells in such cases are megakaryocytes, followed by erythroid precursors, then myeloid precursors. The precise mechanism of this phenomenon is not known.

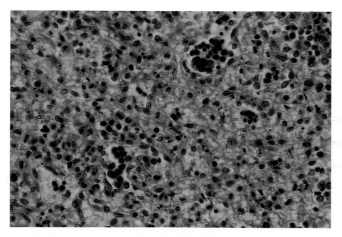

FIGURE 4-6. Spleen, sinusoidal hematopoiesis. Clusters of erythroid precursors are present in this specimen from a patient with splenomegaly secondary to ethanol-induced cirrhosis of the liver.

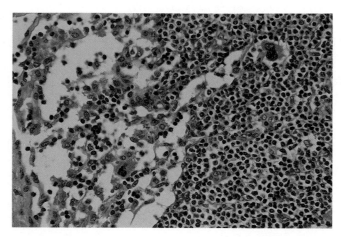

FIGURE 4-7. Lymph node, sinusoidal megakaryocytes. Two megakaryocytes are present in this specimen from a patient who underwent axillary lymph node dissection for breast carcinoma.

MEGAKARYOCYTES IN EXTRAMEDULLARY SITES

Isolated megakaryocytes may be found in extramedullary tissues in health and disease. They have been reported in the peripheral blood, lung, pleural and pericardial cavities, lymph nodes, spleen, liver, and renal glomerulus (1–6) (Fig. 4-7). Their regular occurrence in peripheral blood and pulmonary tissue suggests that these may be important sites of thrombopoiesis.

Care must be taken not to identify isolated megakaryocytes as metastatic tumor cells, especially in lymph nodes (7,8).

REFERENCES
Excessive Hematopoiesis

1. Aliberti B, Patrikiou A, Terentiou A, et al. Spinal cord compression due to extramedullary haematopoiesis in two patients with thalassaemia: complete regression with blood transfusion therapy. *J Neurol* 2001;248:18–22.
2. Calhoun SK, Murphy RC, Shariati N, et al. Extramedullary hematopoiesis in a child with hereditary spherocytosis: an uncommon cause of an adrenal mass. *Pediatr Radiol* 2001;31:879–881.
3. Chu KA, Lai RS, Lee CH, et al. Intrathoracic extramedullary haematopoiesis complicated by massive haemothorax in alpha-thalassaemia. *Thorax* 1999;54:466–468.
4. Hoyer JD, Fairbanks VF. Intrathoracic extramedullary hematopoietic tumor in hemoglobin C disease. *Arch Pathol Lab Med* 1997;121:355–356.
5. Granjo E, Bauerle R, Sampaio R, et al. Extramedullary hematopoiesis in hereditary spherocytosis deficient in ankyrin: a case report. *Int J Hematol* 2002;76:153–156.
6. Kapelushnik J, Shalev H, Schulman H, et al. Upper airway obstruction-related sleep apnea in a child with thalassemia intermedia. *J Pediatr Hematol Oncol* 2001;23:525–526.
7. Koudieh MS, Afzal M, Rasul K, et al. Intrathoracic extramedullary hematopoietic tumor in hemoglobin C disease. *Arch Pathol Lab Med* 1996;120:504–506.

8. Sandoval C, Stringel G, Weisberger J, et al. Failure of partial splenectomy to ameliorate the anemia of pyruvate kinase deficiency. *J Pediatr Surg* 1997;32:641–642.

9. Stokes GN, Thompson WC. Intrathoracic extramedullary hematopoietic tumor in hemoglobin C disease. *Arch Pathol Lab Med* 1997;121:355.

10. Taher A, Skouri H, Jaber W, et al. Extramedullary hematopoiesis in a patient with beta-thalassemia intermedia manifesting as symptomatic pleural effusion. *Hemoglobin* 2001;25:363–368.

11. Xiros N, Economopoulos T, Papageorgiou E, et al. Massive hemothorax due to intrathoracic extramedullary hematopoiesis in a patient with hereditary spherocytosis. *Ann Hematol* 2001;80:38–40.

12. Chang CS, Li CY, Liang YH, et al. Clinical features and splenic pathologic changes in patients with autoimmune hemolytic anemia and congenital hemolytic anemia. *Mayo Clin Proc* 1993;68:757–762.

13. De Geeter F, Van Renterghem D. Scintigraphic diagnosis of intrathoracic extramedullary hematopoiesis in alcohol-related macrocytosis. *J Nucl Med* 1996;37:473–475.

14. Fielding JR, Owens M, Naimark A. Intrathoracic extramedullary hematopoiesis secondary to B12 and folate deficiency: CT appearance. *J Comput Assist Tomogr* 1991;15:308–310.

15. Luban NL, Kapur S, DePalma L. Pericardial extramedullary hematopoiesis in a neonate with congenital heart disease. A case report. *Acta Cytol* 1993;37:729–731.

16. Pizarro A, Elorza D, Gamallo C, et al. Neonatal dermal erythropoiesis associated with severe rhesus immunization: amelioration by high-dose intravenous immunoglobulin. *Br J Dermatol* 1995;133:334–336.

17. Sherer DM, Abramowicz JS, Eggers PC, et al. Prenatal ultrasonographic diagnosis of intracranial teratoma and massive craniomegaly with associated high-output cardiac failure. *Am J Obstet Gynecol* 1993;168:97–99.

18. Taylor CL, Maynard F, Liebman J, et al. Extramedullary hematopoiesis causing paraparesis in congenital cyanotic heart disease. *Neurology* 1998;51:636–637.

19. Abdel-Dayem HM, Rosen G, El-Zeftawy H, et al. Fluorine-18 fluorodeoxyglucose splenic uptake from extramedullary hematopoiesis after granulocyte colony-stimulating factor stimulation. *Clin Nucl Med* 1999;24:319–322.

20. Friedman HD, Sanderson SO, Stein CK, et al. Extramedullary granulopoiesis mimicking recurrent lymphoma after prolonged administration of human recombinant granulocyte colony-stimulating factor. *Ann Hematol* 1998;77:79–83.

21. Vasef MA, Neiman RS, Meletiou SD, et al. Marked granulocytic proliferation induced by granulocyte colony-stimulating factor in the spleen simulating a myeloid leukemic infiltrate. *Mod Pathol* 1998;11:1138–1141.

Bone Marrow Replacement

1. Jantunen E, Hanninen A, Naukkarinen A, et al. Gray platelet syndrome with splenomegaly and signs of extramedullary hematopoiesis: a case report with review of the literature. *Am J Hematol* 1994;46:218–224.

2. Cure JK, Key LL, Goltra DD, et al. Cranial MR imaging of osteopetrosis. *AJNR Am J Neuroradiol* 2000;21:1110–1115.

3. Thelen MH, Eschmann SM, Moll-Kotowski M, et al. Bone marrow scintigraphy with technetium-99m anti-NCA-95 to monitor therapy in malignant osteopetrosis. *J Nucl Med* 1998;39:1033–1035.

4. Hricik DE, Hussain R. Pancytopenia and hepatosplenomegaly in oxalosis. *Arch Intern Med* 1984;144:167–168.

5. Ch'en IY, Lynch DA, Shroyer KR, et al. Gaucher's disease. An unusual cause of intrathoracic extramedullary hematopoiesis. *Chest* 1993;104:1923–1924.

6. Palestro CJ, Finn C. Indium-111-leukocyte imaging in Gaucher's disease. *J Nucl Med* 1993;34:818–820.

7. Tamm EP, Rabushka LS, Fishman EK, et al. Intrahepatic, extramedullary hematopoiesis mimicking hemangioma on technetium-99m red blood cell SPECT examination. *Clin Imaging* 1995;19:88–91.

8. Agarwal I, Kirubakaran C, Sridhar G. Pyknodysostosis: a report of two siblings with unusual manifestations. *Ann Trop Paediatr* 1999;19:301–305.

9. Relea A, Garcia-Urbon MV, Arboleya L, et al. Extramedullary hematopoiesis related to Paget's disease. *Eur Radiol* 1999;9:205–207.

10. Nomura S, Ogawa Y, Osawa G, et al. Myelofibrosis secondary to renal osteodystrophy. *Nephron* 1996;72:683–687.

11. Venencie PY, Blanchet P, Mallet V, et al. Pachydermoperiostosis with extramedullary hematopoiesis without myelofibrosis. *Ann Dermatol Venereol* 1998;125:193–195.

12. Harten P, Euler HH, Wolf E, et al. Disseminated histoplasmosis in a non-immunocompromised host. *Clin Invest* 1994;72:878–882.

13. Ben Rejeb A, Haouala H, Ben Hammadi F, et al. Pseudotumor extramedullary hematopoiesis. Report of 3 cases and review of the literature. *Ann Pathol* 1992;12:183–187.

14. Hill DA, Swanson PE. Myocardial extramedullary hematopoiesis: a clinicopathologic study. *Mod Pathol* 2000;13:779–787.

15. Brans B, Roland J, De Meyer P, et al. Generalized bone marrow metastases. High liver uptake on bone marrow immunoscintigraphy associated with extramedullary hematopoiesis. *Clin Nucl Med* 1996;21:40–42.

16. Yablonski-Peretz T, Sulkes A, Polliack A, et al. Secondary myelofibrosis with metastatic breast cancer simulating agnogenic myeloid metaplasia: report of a case and review of the literature. *Med Pediatr Oncol* 1985;13:92–96.

17. Creagh TM, Bain BJ, Evans DJ, et al. Endometrial extramedullary haemopoiesis. *J Pathol* 1995;176:99–104.

18. Ninomiya H, Hato T, Yamada T, et al. Multiple diffuse fibrosarcoma of bone associated with extramedullary hematopoiesis. *Intern Med* 1998;37:480–483.

Dystrophic Hematopoiesis

1. Arotcarena R, Hammel P, Terris B, et al. Regression of mesenteric lymph node cavitation syndrome complicating celiac disease after a gluten free diet. *Gastroenterol Clin Biol* 2000;24:579–581.

2. Bacchi CE, Rocha N, Carvalho M, et al. Immunohistochemical characterisation of probable intravascular haematopoiesis in the vasa rectae of the renal medulla in acute tubular necrosis. *Pathol Res Pract* 1994;190:1066–1070.

3. Crider S, Kroszer-Hamati A, Krishnan K. Isolated pancreatic extramedullary hematopoiesis. *Acta Haematol* 1998;99:38–40.

4. Fernandez Gonzalez AL, Montero JA, Martinez Monzonis A, et al. Osseous metaplasia and hematopoietic bone marrow in a calcified aortic valve. *Tex Heart Inst J* 1997;24:232.

5. Gilbert-Barness E, Barness LA. Isovaleric acidemia with promyelocytic myeloproliferative syndrome. *Pediatr Dev Pathol* 1999;2:286–291.

6. Goldman BI, Wurzel J. Hematopoiesis/erythropoiesis in myocardial infarcts. *Mod Pathol* 2001;14:589–594.

7. Hill DA, Swanson PE. Myocardial extramedullary hematopoiesis: a clinicopathologic study. *Mod Pathol* 2000;13:779–787.

8. Hinson DD, Rogers ZR, Hoffmann GF, et al. Hematological abnormalities and cholestatic liver disease in two patients with mevalonate kinase deficiency. *Am J Med Genet* 1998;78:408–412.

9. Kaim A, Ochsner P, Maurer T, et al. Ectopic hematopoietic bone marrow in the appendicular skeleton after trauma. *J Nucl Med* 1998;39:1980–1983.

10. Kazama T, Miyazawa M, Tsuchiya S, et al. Proliferation of macrophage-lineage cells in the bone marrow, severe thymic atrophy, and extramedullary hematopoiesis of possible donor origin in an autopsy case of post-transplantation graft-versus-host disease. *Bone Marrow Transplant* 1996;18:437–441.

11. Kuga T, Esato K, Kaneko J, et al. Congenital cystic adenomatoid malformation with extramedullary hematopoiesis of the lung: a case report. *J Pediatr Surg* 1997;32:1751–1753.

12. Lee KB, Kim BS, Cho JH. Focal hematopoietic hyperplasia of the rib. *Skeletal Radiol* 2002;31:175–178.

13. Levine Z, Sherer DM, Jacobs A, et al. Nonimmune hydrops fetalis due to congenital syphilis associated with negative intrapartum maternal serology screening. *Am J Perinatol* 1998;15:233–236.

14. Lew H, Shin DH, Lee SY, et al. Osseous metaplasia with functioning bone marrow in hydroxyapatite orbital implants. *Graefes Arch Clin Exp Ophthalmol* 2000;238:366–368.

15. Valeri RM, Ibrahim N, Sheaff MT. Extramedullary hematopoiesis in the endometrium. *Int J Gynecol Pathol* 2002;21:178–181.

16. Vega F, Diez S. Extramedullary hematopoiesis in juvenile polyposis coli. *Gastrointest Endosc* 2000;51:330.

17. Watson KE. Pathophysiology of coronary calcification. *J Cardiovasc Risk* 2000;7:93–97.

18. Alagappan A, Shattuck KE, Rowe T, et al. Massive intracranial immature teratoma with extracranial extension into oral cavity, nose, and neck. *Fetal Diagn Ther* 1998;13:321–324.

19. Ardito G, Fadda G, Revelli L, et al. Follicular adenoma of the thyroid gland with extensive bone metaplasia. *J Exp Clin Cancer Res* 2001;20:443–445.

20. Azua-Romeo J, Moreno E, Gomollon JP. Images in cardiology: Right atrial lithomyxoma with extramedullary hematopoiesis. *Heart* 2002;88:10.

21. Cha I, Cartwright D, Guis M, et al. Angiomyolipoma of the liver in fine-needle aspiration biopsies: its distinction from hepatocellular carcinoma. *Cancer* 1999;87:25–30.

22. Cribbs RK, Ishaq M, Arnold M, et al. Renal cell carcinoma with massive osseous metaplasia and bone marrow elements. *Ann Diagn Pathol* 1999;3:294–299.

23. de Montpreville VT, Serraf A, Aznag H, et al. Fibroma and inflammatory myofibroblastic tumor of the heart. *Ann Diagn Pathol* 2001;5:335–342.

24. Elgin VE, Connolly ES, Millar WS, et al. Extramedullary hematopoiesis within a frontoethmoidal encephalocele in a newborn with holoprosencephaly. *Pediatr Dev Pathol* 2001;4:289–297.

25. Falk S. EMH in pilomatricomas. *Am J Dermatopathol* 1996;18:218–219.

26. Herve S, Savoye G, Savoye-Collet C, et al. Intrahepatic extramedullary hematopoiesis as a manifestation of a malignant thymoma: an unusual cause of nodular hepatomegaly. *Gastroenterol Clin Biol* 2001;25:711–713.

27. Khalifa MA, Gersell DJ, Hansen CH, et al. Hepatic (hepatocellular) adenoma of the placenta: a study of four cases. *Int J Gynecol Pathol* 1998;17:241–244.

28. Kurosaki Y, Tanaka YO, Itai Y. Mature teratoma of the posterior mediastinum. *Eur Radiol* 1998;8:100–102.

29. Massa LR, Stone MS. An unusual hematopoietic proliferation seen in a nevus sebaceous. *J Am Acad Dermatol* 2000;42:881–882.

30. Neuhauser TS, Derringer GA, Thompson LD, et al. Splenic angiosarcoma: a clinicopathologic and immunophenotypic study of 28 cases. *Mod Pathol* 2000;13:978–987.

31. O'Connor JF, Levinthal GN, Sheets R, et al. Spinal extramedullary hematopoiesis secondary to hepatocellular carcinoma. Case report and literature review. *J Clin Gastroenterol* 1997;25:466–469.

32. Rowlands CG, Rapson D, Morell T. Extramedullary hematopoiesis in a pyogenic granuloma. *Am J Dermatopathol* 2000;22:434–438.

33. Saito A, Watanabe K, Kusakabe T, et al. Mediastinal mature teratoma with coexistence of angiosarcoma, granulocytic sarcoma and a hematopoietic region in the tumor: a rare case of association between hematological malignancy and mediastinal germ cell tumor. *Pathol Int* 1998;48:749–753.

34. Sciot R, Bekaert J. Spindle cell lipoma with extramedullary haematopoiesis. *Histopathology* 2001;39:215–216.

Myelolipoma

1. Adesokan A, Adegboyega PA, Cowan DF, et al. Testicular "tumor" of the adrenogenital syndrome: a case report of an unusual association with myelolipoma and seminoma in cryptorchidism. *Cancer* 1997;80:2120–2127.

2. Amin MB, Tickoo SK, Schultz D. Myelolipoma of the renal sinus. An unusual site for a rare extra-adrenal lesion. *Arch Pathol Lab Med* 1999;123:631–634.

3. Cappello F, Farina F, Di Felice V, et al. Defective apoptosis as potential mechanism in the tumorogenesis of myelolipoma. *Eur J Histochem* 1999;43:15–18.

4. Carazo ER, Herrera RO, de Fuentes TM, et al. Presacral extramedullary haematopoiesis with involvement of the sciatic nerve. *Eur Radiol* 1999;9:1404–1406.

5. d'Addessi A, Racioppi M, Fanasca A, et al. A rare case of perirenal myelolipoma. Diagnostic approach and therapeutic strategy. *Scand J Urol Nephrol* 1997;31:579–581.

6. Kawanami S, Watanabe H, Aoki T, et al. Mediastinal myelolipoma: CT and MRI appearances. *Eur Radiol* 2000;10:691–693.

7. Kenney PJ, Wagner BJ, Rao P, et al. Myelolipoma: CT and pathologic features. *Radiology* 1998;208:87–95.

8. Lamont JP, Lieberman ZH, Stephens JS. Giant adrenal myelolipoma. *Am Surg* 2002;68:392–394.

9. Merchant SH, Herman CM, Amin MB, et al. Myelolipoma associated with adrenal ganglioneuroma. *Arch Pathol Lab Med* 2002;126:736–737.

10. Nagai T, Imamura M, Honma M, et al. 17alpha-hydroxylase deficiency accompanied by adrenal myelolipoma. *Intern Med* 2001;40:920–923.

11. Reza-Albarran AA, Gomez-Perez FJ, Lopez JC, et al. Myelolipoma: a new adrenal finding in Carney's complex? *Endocr Pathol* 1999;10:251–257.

12. Rocher L, Youssef N, Tasu JP, et al. Adrenal pheochromocytoma and contralateral myelolipoma. *Clin Radiol* 2002;57:535–537.

13. Rossi A, Incensati R. Bone tissue in adrenal myelolipoma: a case report. *Tumori* 1998;84:90–93.

14. Sabate CJ, Shahian DM. Pulmonary myelolipoma. *Ann Thorac Surg* 2002;74:573–575.

15. Saboorian MH, Timmerman TG, Ashfaq R, et al. Fine-needle aspiration of a presacral myelolipoma: a case presentation with flow cytometry and immunohistochemical studies. *Diagn Cytopathol* 1999;20:47–51.

16. Spanta R, Saleh HA, Khatib G. Fine needle aspiration diagnosis of extraadrenal myelolipoma presenting as a pleural mass. A case report. *Acta Cytol* 1999;43:295–298.

17. Wat NM, Tse KK, Chan FL, et al. Adrenal extramedullary haemopoiesis: diagnosis by a non-invasive method. *Br J Haematol* 1998;100:725–727.

18. Wrightson WR, Hahm TX, Hutchinson JR, et al. Bilateral giant adrenal myelolipomas: a case report. *Am Surg* 2002;68:588–589.

19. Yeo W, Leong A, Ward SC, et al. Hepatic angiomyelolipoma and tuberous sclerosis. *J Gastroenterol Hepatol* 1996;11:196–198.

20. Yildiz L, Akpolat I, Erzurumlu K, et al. Giant adrenal myelolipoma: case report and review of the literature. *Pathol Int* 2000; 50:502–504.
21. Chang KC, Chen PI, Huang ZH, et al. Adrenal myelolipoma with translocation (3;21)(q25;p11). *Cancer Genet Cytogenet* 2002; 134:77–80.
22. Izumi M, Serizawa H, Iwaya K, et al. A case of myxoid adrenocortical carcinoma with extensive lipomatous metaplasia. *Arch Pathol Lab Med* 2003;127:227–230.
23. Lam KY, Lo CY. Adrenal lipomatous tumours: a 30 year clinicopathological experience at a single institution. *J Clin Pathol* 2001; 54:707–712.
24. Au WY, Tam PC, Ma SK, et al. Giant myelolipoma in a patient with thalassemia intermedia. *Am J Hematol* 2000;65:265–266.
25. Calhoun SK, Murphy RC, Shariati N, et al. Extramedullary hematopoiesis in a child with hereditary spherocytosis: an uncommon cause of an adrenal mass. *Pediatr Radiol* 2001;31:879–881.

Embolization from Bone Marrow

1. Fernandez LA, Romaguera R, Viciana AL, et al. Pulmonary embolism with bone fragments following vertebral body marrow infusion for tolerance induction. *Cell Transplant* 1996;5:513–516.
2. Jenny-Mobius U, Bruder E, Stallmach T. Recognition and significance of pulmonary bone embolism. *Int J Legal Med* 1999; 112:195–197.
3. Jones JP Jr, Ramirez S, Doty SB. The pathophysiologic role of fat in dysbaric osteonecrosis. *Clin Orthop* 1993;296:256–264.
4. Kim YH. Incidence of fat embolism syndrome after cemented or cementless bilateral simultaneous and unilateral total knee arthroplasty. *J Arthroplasty* 2001;16:730–739.
5. Mudd KL, Hunt A, Matherly RC, et al. Analysis of pulmonary fat embolism in blunt force fatalities. *J Trauma* 2000;48:711–715.
6. van Hoeven KH, Wanner JL, Ballas SK. Cytologic diagnosis of fat emboli in peripheral blood during sickle cell infarctive crisis. *Diagn Cytopathol* 1997;17:54–56.
7. Ballas SK, Pindzola A, Chang CD, et al. Postmortem diagnosis of hemoglobin SC disease complicated by fat embolism. *Ann Clin Lab Sci* 1998;28:144–149.
8. Eckardt P, Raez LE, Restrepo A, et al. Pulmonary bone marrow embolism in sickle cell disease. *South Med J* 1999;92:245–247.
9. Kolquist KA, Vnencak-Jones CL, Swift L, et al. Fatal fat embolism syndrome in a child with undiagnosed hemoglobin S/beta+ thalassemia: a complication of acute parvovirus B19 infection. *Pediatr Pathol Lab Med* 1996;16:71–82.
10. Smith RL, Hutchins GM, Sack GH Jr, et al. Unusual cardiac, renal and pulmonary involvement in Gaucher's disease. Interstitial glucocerebroside accumulation, pulmonary hypertension and fatal bone marrow embolization. *Am J Med* 1978;65:352–360.
11. Kramer M, Penners BM. Postmortem tissue embolisms. Report of 3 cases. *Arch Kriminol* 1989;183:29–36.

Megakaryocytes in Extramedullary Sites

1. Abati A, Landucci D, Danner RL, et al. Diagnosis of pulmonary microvascular metastases by cytologic evaluation of pulmonary artery catheter-derived blood specimens. *Hum Pathol* 1994;25: 257–262.
2. Behnke O, Forer A. From megakaryocytes to platelets: platelet morphogenesis takes place in the bloodstream. *Eur J Haematol Suppl* 1998;61:3–23.
3. Lunetta P, Penttila A. Pulmonary platelet production: physical fragmentation and platelet territories. *Eur J Haematol* 1997;59: 63–64.
4. Van Pampus FC, Huijgens PC, Zevenbergen A, et al. Circulating human megakaryocytes in cardiac diseases. *Eur J Clin Invest* 1994; 24:345–349.
5. Wilkins BS, Green A, Wild AE, et al. Extramedullary haemopoiesis in fetal and adult human spleen: a quantitative immunohistological study. *Histopathology* 1994;24:241–247.
6. Zucker-Franklin D, Philipp CS. Platelet production in the pulmonary capillary bed: new ultrastructural evidence for an old concept. *Am J Pathol* 2000;157:69–74.
7. Hoda SA, Resetkova E, Yusuf Y, et al. Megakaryocytes mimicking metastatic breast carcinoma. *Arch Pathol Lab Med* 2002;126:618–620.
8. Weeks DA, Beckwith JB, Mierau GW. Benign nodal lesions mimicking metastases from pediatric renal neoplasms: a report of the National Wilms' Tumor Study Pathology Center. *Hum Pathol* 1990;21:1239–1244.

5

CONSTITUTIONAL HEMATOPOIETIC DISORDERS

Many of the disorders described in this chapter show defects in more than one cell lineage. The following grouping is based on the predominant lineage in which defects are apparent (Tables 5-1 through 5-4).

CONSTITUTIONAL HEMATOPOIETIC STEM CELL DISORDERS

Congenital Hypoplastic Anemia (Diamond-Blackfan Anemia)

Congenital hypoplastic anemia (or Diamond-Blackfan anemia) is a genetically heterogeneous hematopoietic stem cell disorder transmitted in sporadic, autosomal dominant, and autosomal recessive forms (1–5) (Figs. 5-1 and 5-2). The most common genetic findings are mutations of *RPS19/DBA1*, located at chromosome 19q13, and *DBA2*, located at chromosome 8p23. *RPS19* mutations are associated with highly variable clinical findings, ranging from macrocytosis without anemia to overt congenital hypoplastic anemia. Patients typically present during infancy with anemia. Congenital malformations, predominantly of the head and upper limbs, occur in 33% of cases.

The peripheral blood shows moderate to marked macrocytic anemia, sometimes accompanied by neutropenia and thrombocytopenia. The bone marrow shows erythroid hypoplasia, progressing to aplastic anemia. Other findings include fibrosis, trilineal dysplasia, and erythrophagocytosis. Myelodysplastic syndrome and acute leukemia are late complications of congenital hypoplastic anemia. The differential diagnosis includes acquired erythroid hypoplasia, especially transient erythroblastopenia of childhood.

TABLE 5-1. CONSTITUTIONAL HEMATOPOIETIC STEM CELL DISORDERS

Congenital hypoplastic anemia (Diamond-Blackfan anemia)
Dyskeratosis congenita
Fanconi anemia

TABLE 5-2. CONSTITUTIONAL ERYTHROCYTE DISORDERS

Constitutional erythrocytosis
Congenital dyserythropoietic anemia
Congenital megaloblastic anemia
Congenital microcytic anemia
Congenital sideroblastic anemia
Erythrocyte membrane defects
Erythrocyte enzymopathies
Abnormal hemoglobins
Unbalanced globin chain production (thalassemia)

TABLE 5-3. CONSTITUTIONAL GRANULOCYTE DISORDERS

Alder-Reilly anomaly
Benign hereditary neutropenia
Chediak-Higashi syndrome
Cyclic neutropenia
Kostmann disease
Myelokathexis
Pelger-Hüet anomaly
Severe congenital neutropenia
Shwachman-Diamond syndrome

TABLE 5-4. CONSTITUTIONAL MEGAKARYOCYTE AND PLATELET DISORDERS

Bernard-Soulier syndrome
Congenital amegakaryocytic thrombocytopenia
Cyclic thrombocytopenia
Epstein and related syndromes
Gray platelet syndrome
Hermansky-Pudlak syndrome
Paris-Trousseau and related syndromes
Thrombocytopenia with absent radii syndrome
X-linked microthrombocytopenia and Wiskott-Aldrich syndrome
Other megakaryocyte and platelet disorders

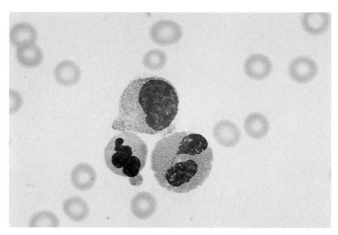

FIGURE 5-1. Peripheral blood smear, congenital hypoplastic (Diamond-Blackfan) anemia. Neutrophils show dysplastic changes.

Dyskeratosis Congenita

Dyskeratosis congenita (DC) is a genetically heterogeneous hematopoietic stem cell disorder transmitted in autosomal dominant and X-linked forms (6–9). Most cases are caused by mutations of *DKC1*, located at chromosome Xq28, which encodes dyskerin, an essential component of mRNA and telomere function. The *DKC1* mutation is associated with premature telomere shortening, and pathology evolves over time as the cell cycle number increases. The most affected tissues are therefore those with the highest proliferative rate: skin, mucous membranes, and bone marrow.

The age of onset, type, and severity of DC lesions are highly variable. Males with DC usually present at age 10 years or later with skin hyperpigmentation, nail dystrophy, and mucous membrane leukoplakia, followed by bone marrow failure. This sequence is sometimes reversed, with presentation of DC in early childhood as bone marrow failure without ectodermal abnormalities. Other findings in-

clude neurologic dysfunction, restrictive pulmonary disease, and severe immunodeficiency. Females heterozygous for the *DKC1* mutation show some clinical features of DC and marked skewing of X-chromosome inactivation, selecting for the normal *DKC1* allele.

The peripheral blood shows pancytopenia, with both neutropenia and lymphopenia. The bone marrow shows progressive trilineal hypoplasia, culminating in aplastic anemia in more than 90% of cases by the age of 20. Myelodysplastic syndrome and acute leukemia are late complications. Death results from hematopoietic failure, pulmonary disease, and malignancy.

Fanconi Anemia

Fanconi anemia is a genetically heterogeneous group of autosomal recessive disorders, linked by chromosomal instability (10–15) (Fig. 5-3). Many genetic mutations have been described, affecting different genes that encode functionally related proteins. Chromosome instability may be detected in the laboratory, by culturing patient lymphocytes with a DNA cross-linking agent (e.g., mitomycin). Most, but not all, cultured metaphase chromosomes show excessive and abnormal breaks.

Fanconi anemia is diagnosed from birth through adulthood, sometimes not until the development of acute leukemia. Patients present with cytopenias, hyperpigmentation, and a wide spectrum of congenital anomalies primarily involving the genitourinary and gastrointestinal tracts, limbs, and skeleton. The peripheral blood shows cytopenias in 70% of patients by age 7 and in nearly 100% by age 40. The bone marrow shows trilineal hypoplasia, progressing to aplastic anemia. Other findings include dyserythropoiesis and reactive mastocytosis. Major complications include aplastic anemia, leukemia, and other cancers. Hematopoietic clones

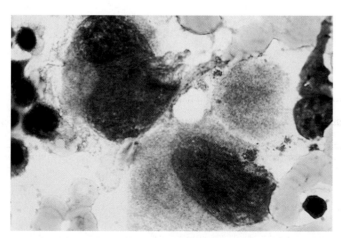

FIGURE 5-2. Bone marrow aspirate smear, congenital hypoplastic (Diamond-Blackfan) anemia. Dysplastic megakaryocytes are present.

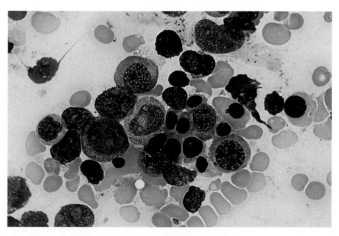

FIGURE 5-3. Bone marrow aspirate, Fanconi anemia. Erythroid hyperplasia with subtle dyserythropoiesis is seen in this patient with Fanconi anemia developing refractory anemia with ringed sideroblasts.

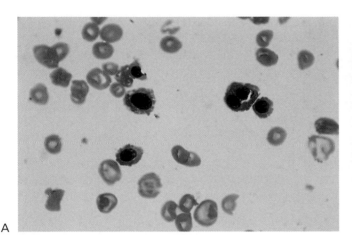 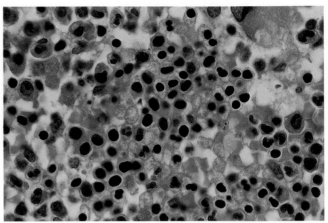

FIGURE 5-4. **A:** Peripheral blood smear, congenital dyserythropoietic anemia. A binucleated red blood cell is present. **B:** Bone marrow biopsy, congenital dyserythropoietic anemia. Erythroid hyperplasia is present.

arise frequently, showing expansion, evolution, regression, and even reversion to a normal genotype. By age 40, clonal hematopoiesis is found in nearly 100% of patients and recognizable myelodysplastic syndrome or acute leukemia in 50%.

CONSTITUTIONAL ERYTHROCYTE DISORDERS

Constitutional Erythrocytosis

Constitutional erythrocytosis is a genetically heterogeneous disorder occurring in autosomal dominant and sporadic forms (1–7). In approximately 10% of cases, a mutation at chromosome 19p13 involving *EpoR*, the gene encoding the erythropoietin (EPO) receptor, is found. This mutation results in EPO receptor truncation and EPO hypersensitivity of erythroid progenitors. Other cases show mutation of *FBP* (familial benign polycythemia gene) at 11q23. Patients are affected at birth, but the diagnosis may not be made until adulthood when unexpected erythrocytosis is discovered.

The red blood cell count, red blood cell mass, and hematocrit are increased. The serum EPO level is variable, and the arterial oxygen saturation is normal. The white blood cell and platelet counts are normal. The peripheral blood shows no morphologic abnormalities. The bone marrow shows erythroid hyperplasia.

The differential diagnosis includes high oxygen-affinity hemoglobinopathy and acquired erythrocytosis, either of which may present as congenital erythrocytosis. Hemoglobins with high oxygen-affinity usually result from mutations in the β-globin gene (8,9). In cases with unstable, high-affinity hemoglobins, hemolysis may reduce the hematocrit to near-normal levels, a state representing functional anemia.

Congenital Dyserythropoietic Anemia

Congenital dyserythropoietic anemia (CDA) comprises several rare disorders, usually presenting in infancy (10–15)

(Fig. 5-4). The most common types are CDA types I, II, and III.

CDA type I is an autosomal recessive disease linked to a genetic abnormality at chromosome 15q15 (16–20). The diagnosis is usually made at birth and occasionally in adulthood. Patients present with severe anemia and hyperbilirubinemia. Hemochromatosis eventually develops, exacerbated by transfusion and/or co-inheritance of Gilbert syndrome. The peripheral blood shows macrocytic anemia with marked anisopoikilocytosis, polychromasia, and basophilic stippling. The bone marrow demonstrates marked erythroid hyperplasia. Erythroid precursors exhibit megaloblastic change, binucleation, internuclear bridging, and uneven heterochromatin condensation, ultrastructurally appearing spongy or Swiss cheese–like. Ringed sideroblasts may be present but are not characteristic.

CDA type II [previously known as HEMPAS (hereditary erythroblastic multinuclearity associated with a positive acidified serum test)] is an autosomal recessive disease caused by a mutation of *CDAN2*, located at chromosome 20q11 (21–24). The mutation appears to result in defective glycosylation of red blood cell membrane proteins. The diagnosis is usually made at birth or during childhood. Patients present with anemia and eventually develop pigment cholelithiasis, splenomegaly, and hemochromatosis, exacerbated by transfusion and/or co-inheritance of other hematopoietic diseases. The peripheral blood shows normocytic to macrocytic, hemolytic anemia with microspherocytes. The bone marrow shows erythroid hyperplasia with bi- and multinucleated erythroid precursors. The differential diagnosis includes hereditary spherocytosis.

CDA type III is an autosomal dominant disease caused by a mutation of *CDAN3*, located at chromosome 15q21-25 (25–27). The diagnosis may be made at any age. Patients present with anemia-related cardiac failure and hepatosplenomegaly. The peripheral blood shows macrocytic anemia. The bone marrow shows erythroid hyperplasia with giant, multinucleated erythroid precursors.

Congenital Megaloblastic Anemia

This type of anemia encompasses a heterogeneous group of autosomal recessive conditions (28–33). The most common defects are lack of intrinsic factor and failure to absorb vitamin B_{12} (Gräsbeck-Imerslund disease). The peripheral blood shows profound pancytopenia with macroovalocytes and hypersegmented neutrophils. The bone marrow shows marked megaloblastic hematopoiesis. The differential diagnosis includes acquired megaloblastic anemia.

Congenital Microcytic Anemia

Severe microcytic hypochromic anemia is produced by autosomal recessive disorders affecting iron metabolism (34,35). The most common of these is congenital atransferrinemia. The bone marrow shows erythroid hyperplasia. Iron stores are increased, which distinguishes this disorder from iron deficiency anemia.

Congenital Sideroblastic Anemia

Congenital sideroblastic anemia is a broad term encompassing a heterogeneous group of anemias transmitted in autosomal, X-linked, and mitochondrial patterns of inheritance. Mitochondrial cytopathy and X-linked sideroblastic anemia (XLSA) are the most common entities in this group.

Mitochondrial cytopathy comprises a genetically heterogeneous group of disorders in which mitochondrial DNA shows large deletions and other mutations (36–44) (Fig. 5-5). The result of these mutations is intracellular adenosine triphosphate deficiency. The clinical course is highly variable but usually progressive and ultimately fatal. Mitochondrial cytopathy presents in the neonate as anemia and, in most cases, pancreatic insufficiency (Pearson marrow–pancreas syndrome). The peripheral blood shows severe macrocytic anemia, sometimes accompanied by neutropenia and/or thrombocytopenia. The bone marrow shows

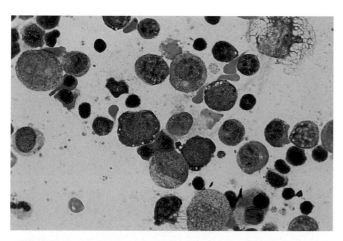

FIGURE 5-5. Bone marrow aspirate, Pearson syndrome. The erythroid precursors are vacuolated.

erythroid and myeloid precursors with distinctive vacuolation and ultrastructurally abnormal mitochondria. Ringed sideroblasts and increased iron stores are usually present. Survivors eventually develop progressive hematopoietic, neuroendocrine, and other systemic organ failure (Kearns-Sayre syndrome). The differential diagnosis includes acquired clonal sideroblastic anemia, which may show mtDNA deletions identical to those reported in hereditary mitochondrial cytopathy (45,46).

XLSA is caused by a mutation of *ALAS2*, located at chromosome Xq13 (47–51). The gene product, erythroid-specific 5-aminolevulinic synthase (ALAS2, ALAS-E), is located within mitochondria, where it catalyzes the rate-limiting step in heme synthesis. Thus, XLSA has features of both an X-linked disorder and a mitochondrial cytopathy. Anemia may be diagnosed at any age and in either gender. Disease in females is possible through mutations in both X chromosomes and, in older women, age-related skewing of X-chromosome inactivation in erythroid precursors. Hemochromatosis may be present because of transfusional iron overload and/or co-inheritance of hereditary hemochromatosis. The peripheral blood shows mild to severe microcytic hypochromic anemia. The bone marrow shows erythroid hyperplasia with numerous ringed sideroblasts. Anemia is ameliorated in most, but not all, cases by pyridoxine therapy. The differential diagnosis includes other sideroblastic anemias, especially the mitochondrial cytopathies in children and clonal myelodysplastic disease in adults.

XLSA with ataxia is caused by a mutation of *ABC7*, located at chromosome Xq13 (52–54). The gene product is a protein attached to the inner mitochondrial membrane, where it participates in iron metabolism. Thus, XLSA with ataxia has characteristics of both an X-linked disorder and a mitochondrial cytopathy. Male infants present with anemia and neuromuscular abnormalities. The peripheral blood shows mild microcytic hypochromic anemia with Pappenheimer bodies. The bone marrow shows erythroid hyperplasia with ringed sideroblasts. Carrier females are not anemic but may show red blood cell dimorphism and ringed sideroblasts.

Erythrocyte Membrane Defects

The main erythrocyte defects are hereditary elliptocytosis (HE) and the related disorder hereditary pyropoikilocytosis (HPP), hereditary spherocytosis (HS), and hereditary stomatocytosis.

HE is genetically and clinically heterogeneous, occurring as a *de novo*, autosomal dominant, and autosomal recessive disorder (55–58) (Fig. 5-6). HE is caused by mutations and polymorphisms of genes encoding linkage proteins between the erythrocyte cytoskeleton and the cell membrane: alpha spectrin, beta spectrin, protein 4.1, and glycophorin. Deficiencies in these proteins result in membrane destabilization, erythrocyte fragmentation and elongation (elliptocytosis), and increased osmotic fragility.

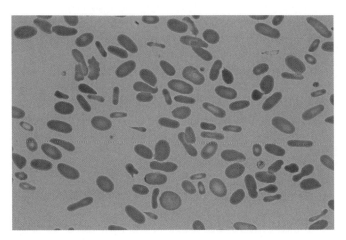

FIGURE 5-6. Peripheral blood smear, hereditary elliptocytosis. Numerous elliptocytes are present as well as microcytes and red blood cell fragments.

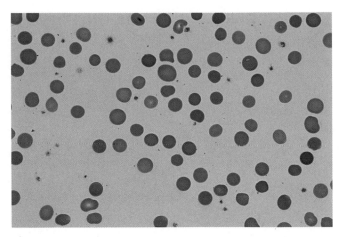

FIGURE 5-7. Peripheral blood smear, hereditary spherocytosis. Nearly all the red blood cells are microspherocytes or polychromatophilic cells.

HPP is a severe form of HE in which erythrocyte fragility and fragmentation are particularly marked on incubation at 37° to 48°C. Peripheral blood findings range from asymptomatic elliptocytosis to severe hemolytic anemia and may change over time. An individual may have HPP at birth, then hemolytic HE, followed by asymptomatic HE. In severely affected patients, the peripheral blood smear shows elliptocytes, microspherocytes, polychromasia, nucleated red blood cells, and fragmented erythrocytes. Bizarre erythrocyte morphology and nucleated red blood cells are especially prominent in infants with HPP. After splenectomy, erythrocytes may appear spiculated rather than elliptical. The bone marrow shows marked ineffective erythroid hyperplasia, which may be accompanied by dyserythropoiesis. The differential diagnosis includes erythrocyte abnormalities secondary to burns, microangiopathic hemolytic anemia, and clonal hematopoietic disease and artifactual erythrocyte fragmentation induced by storage at high temperatures (59,60).

HS, like HE, is genetically and clinically heterogeneous, occurring as a *de novo*, autosomal dominant and autosomal recessive disorder (61–69) (Fig. 5-7). HS is also caused by abnormalities in the genes encoding linkage proteins between the erythrocyte cytoskeleton and the cell membrane, specifically ankyrin, alpha spectrin, beta spectrin, anion exchanger 1 (band 3), and protein 4.2. Deficiencies in these proteins lead to microvesiculation or blistering of the membrane, microspherocytosis, hemolysis, and splenic sequestration and destruction. The peripheral blood demonstrates microcytic, hyperchromic anemia, with polychromasia and microspherocytes proportional to the degree of anemia. The bone marrow shows marked erythroid hyperplasia, and extramedullary hematopoiesis may occur. HS may be masked by concomitant folate or vitamin B_{12} deficiency and has been reported with hemoglobin S, β thalassemia, and hemochromatosis (70–72). HS predisposes patients to Parvovirus B19 infection. The differential diagnosis includes CDA and immune-mediated hemolytic anemia. CDA type II, like HS, is characterized by mild chronic hemolytic anemia, splenomegaly, increased osmotic fragility, microspherocytosis, and splenomegaly; but the red blood cell distribution width is higher and the mean corpuscular hemoglobin concentration is lower than in HS (73).

Hereditary stomatocytosis is an uncommon autosomal dominant disease characterized by defective erythrocyte membrane permeability to sodium and potassium ions, especially at room temperature or below (74–77). At these temperatures, potassium leaks out of the erythrocytes. Laboratory abnormalities occurring after storage at low temperature include pseudohyperkalemia, increased osmotic fragility, pseudomacrocytosis, macrospherocytosis, and marked autohemolysis. True (*in vivo*) hemolytic anemia is present in some cases. Parvovirus B19 infection with aplastic crisis has been reported, as in other chronic hemolytic anemias. The differential diagnosis includes hereditary spherocytosis.

Erythrocyte Enzymopathies

Numerous erythrocyte enzyme deficiencies have been described. The most commonly recognized are glucose-6-phosphate dehydrogenase (G6PD) deficiency and pyruvate kinase (PK) deficiency.

G6PD deficiency is a common disorder caused by various mutations of *G6PD*, located on the X chromosome (78–81) (Fig. 5-8). Females may be affected because of the variable clinical impact of different mutations and the possibility of inheriting two mutations. G6PD deficiency is thus genetically and clinically heterogeneous and may be exacerbated by co-inheritance of other hematopoietic disorders. Most patients are asymptomatic. Some experience episodic hemolysis triggered by fava bean ingestion (favism), oxidant drug exposure, fever, infection, and/or metabolic acidosis. Others manifest chronic moderate to severe hemolytic anemia. Favism by proxy occurs in newborns and nursing

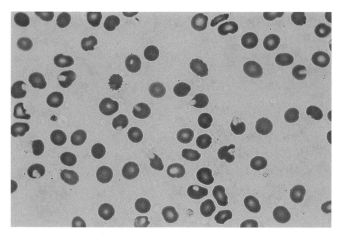

FIGURE 5-8. Peripheral blood smear, glucose-6-phosphate dehydrogenase deficiency. Numerous red blood cells with a peripheral crescentic defect (bite cells) are seen.

infants through maternal ingestion of fava beans. The peripheral blood shows anemia and abnormal red cell morphology during a hemolytic episode. Hemighosts are erythrocytes with a spherical concentration of hemoglobin at one end and colorless, closely apposed membranes at the other. Bite cells are erythrocytes with one or more peripheral concavities. The bone marrow demonstrates erythroid hyperplasia during and after a hemolytic episode. The differential diagnosis includes transient G6PD deficiency in typhoid fever (82).

PK deficiency is usually caused by a mutation of *PKLR* in combination with a *PKLR* polymorphism (83–85) (Fig. 5-9). Patients present with mild to severe hemolytic anemia and eventually develop hemochromatosis, exacerbated by transfusion and co-inheritance of other hematopoietic disorders and hemochromatosis. The peripheral blood shows nonspherocytic hemolytic anemia, and bone marrow shows marked but largely ineffective erythroid hyperplasia. Extramedullary hematopoiesis has been reported. PK defi-

ciency may be masked by infection and leukocytosis, which cause transient increases in PK activity.

Abnormal Hemoglobins

Many abnormal hemoglobins have been reported, the majority resulting from a single base-pair mutation in the β-globin gene. Inheritance of a single abnormal gene results in a trait, and inheritance of two abnormal genes results in disease. Abnormal hemoglobins are often inherited in combination with thalassemia or another hematopoietic disorder. The common abnormal hemoglobins C, E, and S are discussed below.

Hemoglobin C agglutinates and crystallizes under conditions of deoxygenation (86–88) (Fig. 5-10). The clinical findings are relatively mild, possibly because microcytosis offsets increased blood viscosity. The peripheral blood shows mild to moderate microcytic, hemolytic anemia with target cells and hemoglobin crystals. Hemoglobin C crystals are rectangular with tapered, slanted, or beveled ends and are found more often in hemoglobin C disease than in the trait. The bone marrow demonstrates erythroid hyperplasia.

Hemoglobin E is characterized by underproduction of an abnormal hemoglobin and thus shows features of both hemoglobinopathy and β thalassemia (Fig. 5-11). Anemia is present and characterized by shortened red blood cell survival.

Hemoglobin E/β thalassemia is relatively common (89, 90). The peripheral blood shows microcytic hypochromic anemia with numerous teardrop, target, and fragmented red blood cells. The bone marrow displays prominent erythroid hyperplasia with dyserythropoiesis in late erythrocyte precursors and prominent erythrophagocytosis. Erythroid precursors are prone to accelerated apoptosis owing to precipitation of α-globin chains.

Hemoglobin S agglutinates and polymerizes under conditions of deoxygenation and hypertonicity, causing the erythrocyte to assume a sickle shape (91–93) (Figs. 5-12

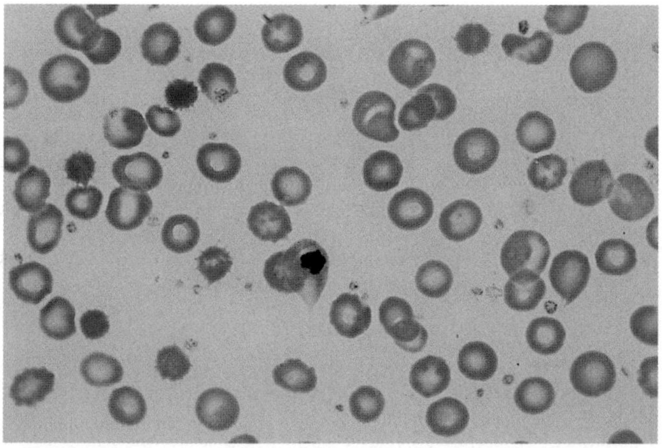

FIGURE 5-9. Peripheral blood smear, pyruvate kinase deficiency. Red blood cells with variable morphology and a dysplastic erythroid precursor are seen.

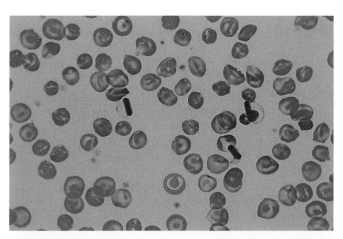

FIGURE 5-10. Peripheral blood smear, hemoglobin CC disease. Rectangular crystals with beveled edges are present in some of the red blood cells.

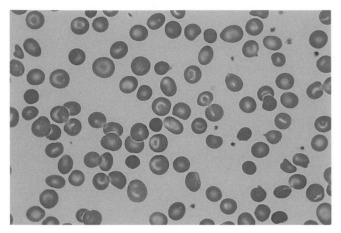

FIGURE 5-11. Peripheral blood smear, hemoglobin EE disease. Target cells and microcytes are present.

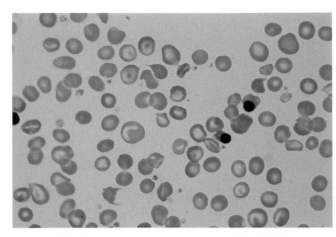

FIGURE 5-13. Peripheral blood smear, hemoglobin SS disease after a crisis. Sickle cells are absent, but numerous polychromatophilic cells and nucleated red blood cells are seen.

and 5-13). Sickling is reversible, but repeated sickling causes irreparable red blood cell damage and rapid clearance from peripheral blood. The clinical findings are highly variable. The hemoglobin S trait is characterized by mild anemia and occasional sickle cells. Hemoglobin S disease (sickle cell anemia) presents as severe hemolytic anemia with numerous sickle cells. Howell-Jolly bodies and other erythrocyte abnormalities appear with progressive splenic infarction and fibrosis. The bone marrow shows marked erythroid hyperplasia, with sickling of late erythrocyte precursors and erythrocytes. Megaloblastosis owing to folate deficiency, erythrophagocytosis, and bony changes secondary to chronic bone marrow expansion may also be present. Life-threatening events occurring in patients with hemoglobin S include aplastic crisis (a complication of Parvovirus B19 infection), hemolytic crisis triggered by infection or oxidant exposure in G6PD deficiency, pain crisis caused by deoxygenation and other unknown factors, and sequestration crisis marked by acute splenic engorgement and a rapid decrease in hematocrit. These events may be accompanied by bone marrow necrosis and embolism.

Combinations of hemoglobin S with other abnormal hemoglobins, thalassemia, and erythrocyte enzymopathies cause clinically significant disease. Hemoglobin SC disease is characterized by microcytic anemia with hyperchromia, hemoglobin C crystals, and sickled erythrocytes (94,95) (Fig. 5-14). Hemoglobin SE disease may be accompanied by bone marrow necrosis (96). Hemoglobin S/β thalassemia varies in severity, and results in death in some cases (97,98). Hemoglobin S/α thalassemia and hemoglobin S in association with an erythrocyte enzymopathy may cause severe anemia (99).

Unbalanced Globin Chain Production (Thalassemia)

Thalassemia, the most common inherited disease in the world, results from unbalanced globin chain production (100). Hemoglobin A1, the predominant adult hemoglobin, is composed of two α-globin and two β-globin chains. Thus, the thalassemias fall into two major groups: the α thalassemias and the β thalassemias. Thalassemia may be

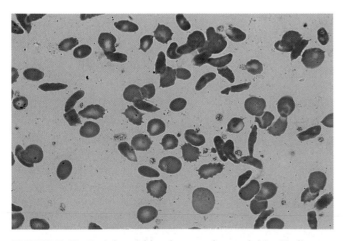

FIGURE 5-12. Peripheral blood smear, hemoglobin SS disease. Numerous sickle cells are present.

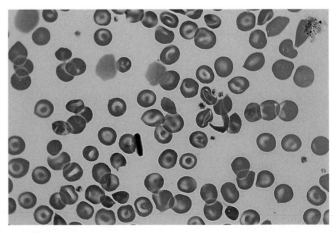

FIGURE 5-14. Peripheral blood smear, hemoglobin SC disease. A crystalline inclusion of hemoglobin C and a sickle cell are present.

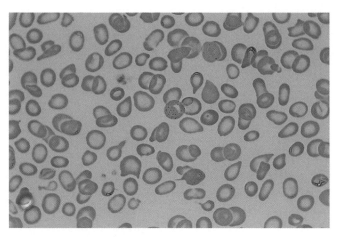

FIGURE 5-15. Peripheral blood smear, α thalassemia. Marked anisocytosis and poikilocytosis are present in this specimen from a patient with hemoglobin H disease.

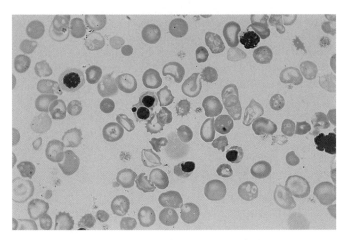

FIGURE 5-17. Peripheral blood smear, beta thalassemia major. Marked anisocytosis and poikilocytosis are present, with numerous target cells and nucleated red blood cells.

exacerbated by other hematopoietic disorders, including co-inheritance of α and β thalassemia (101).

α Thalassemia is caused by mutations in one or more of the four genes encoding α-globin chains (102,103) (Fig. 5-15). A single gene mutation produces a silent carrier state, with normal peripheral blood cell counts and red blood cell indices. Tetramers of γ-globin chains (hemoglobin Bart) may be present in neonatal blood, comprising 1% to 2% of hemoglobin. Two gene mutations result in the α thalassemia trait. The peripheral blood shows mild hypochromic microcytic anemia; neonatal blood may contain 2% to 6% hemoglobin Bart. Three gene mutations result in the formation of β-globin chain tetramers (hemoglobin H). The peripheral blood shows moderate to severe microcytic hemolytic anemia (hemoglobin H disease) with marked anisopoikilocytosis and polychromasia; neonatal blood may contain as much as 20% hemoglobin Bart. Four gene mutations result in lethal fetal hydrops, with 100% hemoglobin Bart. The bone marrow demonstrates erythroid hyperplasia, dyserythropoiesis, and reticulin fibrosis, proportional to

the degree of anemia. The differential diagnosis includes acquired thalassemia owing to a clonal myeloid disorder (104).

β Thalassemia is caused by mutations in one or both of the genes encoding β-globin chains (105–107) (Figs. 5-16 and 5-17). β Thalassemia is marked by precipitation of α-globin chain tetramers, which causes premature apoptosis of erythroid precursors and increased production of δ-globin chains, which join with α-globin chains to form hemoglobin A2. The peripheral blood shows microcytic hypochromic anemia. Anemia ranges from mild to moderate in cases with continued β-globin chain production ($\beta+$ thalassemia) to marked in cases with no β-globin chain production (β zero thalassemia). The bone marrow shows prominent, largely ineffective, erythroid hyperplasia with dyserythropoiesis. Other findings include megaloblastosis owing to folate deficiency, storage histiocytosis (pseudo-Gaucher cells), increased erythrophagocytosis, and bony abnormalities. Extramedullary hematopoiesis is common. The differential diagnosis includes increased hemoglobin A2 in the course of therapy with zidovudine (108).

CONSTITUTIONAL GRANULOCYTE DISORDERS

Alder-Reilly Anomaly

Alder-Reilly anomaly occurs as the result of mucopolysaccharidosis (1,2). Acid phosphatase–positive cytoplasmic inclusions (Alder-Reilly bodies) are found in neutrophils, monocytes, eosinophils, and basophils. The inclusions contain acid mucopolysaccharide. The differential diagnosis includes morphologically similar cells found in myeloperoxidase gene mutation and clonal hematopoietic disease (3,4).

Benign Hereditary Neutropenia

Benign hereditary (ethnic, familial) neutropenia is not a disorder but a normal finding in many African and some Middle

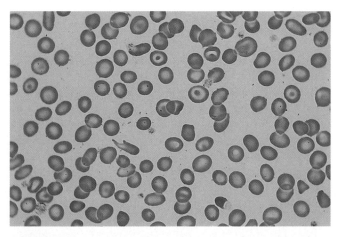

FIGURE 5-16. Peripheral blood smear, beta thalassemia minor. Mild anisocytosis and poikilocytosis are present, with occasional target cells.

Eastern populations (5–7). Compared with those of European and Asian origin, these populations show lower mean white blood cell and absolute neutrophil counts (ANC). In mixed populations of predominantly European origin, the lower limits of the normal white blood cell count and ANC may be set too high. Twenty-five percent to 50% of blacks, especially males, have white blood cell levels below the lower limit of "normal." The ANC is often less than 2.0×10^9/L and may be as low as 1.2×10^9/L without increased risk of infection.

The peripheral blood and bone marrow show no morphologic abnormalities.

The differential diagnosis includes true, or physiologically significant, neutropenia, which is associated with an increased risk of infection. Although common, benign hereditary neutropenia is often unrecognized and prompts fruitless efforts to discern the cause of neutropenia in these patients. The use of population-specific reference ranges has been suggested to eliminate this problem.

Chediak-Higashi Syndrome

Chediak-Higashi syndrome is a rare autosomal recessive disease caused by mutation of the *LYST* gene at chromosome 1q42 (8,9). The precise function of the encoded protein is unknown; however, it is apparently essential for the formation and/or trafficking of intracellular vesicles, including primary and secondary neutrophil granules, lysosomes, platelet dense bodies, and melanosomes. The effect of *LYST* mutation is fusion of multiple cytoplasmic vesicles into a single giant vesicle, with consequent impairment of cellular function. The abnormal vesicle appears as a huge cytoplasmic inclusion (as large as 1.5 microns in diameter) found in granulocytes, lymphocytes, platelets, megakaryocytes, Langerhans cells, and other cells.

Patients present from childhood through adulthood with oculocutaneous albinism, photophobia, neurologic dysfunction, coagulopathy, and recurrent infections. The peripheral blood shows neutropenia with characteristic inclusions in nucleated cells, and bone marrow is characterized by hematopoietic precursors with inclusions. An important fatal complication is an accelerated phase, which is characterized by systemic lymphohistiocytic infiltrates. The differential diagnosis includes Hermansky-Pudlak syndrome, the features of which include oculocutaneous albinism and a platelet storage pool defect.

Cyclic Neutropenia

Congenital cyclic neutropenia (CN) occurs as a sporadic disease and an autosomal dominant disorder (10–12). The most common genetic lesion is mutation of the *ELA2* gene at 19p13, which encodes neutrophil elastase. Congenital CN has also been reported in association with several other genetic disorders. The diagnosis may be made at any time

of life, from infancy to adulthood. Patients may be asymptomatic, but most present with recurrent bouts of fever, oral ulceration, lymphadenopathy, and skin and respiratory infections occurring at the nadir of the ANC.

The peripheral blood shows recurrent severe neutropenia, usually in a 21-day cycle (range, 14–22 days). Red and white blood cells and platelets are morphologically unremarkable. The ANC ranges from less than 0.3×10^9/L at the nadir to near-normal levels at the peak. The ANC nadir lasts 4 to 10 days. Oscillation of the neutrophil count may be accompanied by oscillation of the monocyte, lymphocyte, platelet, and/or eosinophil counts, usually in an inverse pattern (13). Granulocyte colony-stimulating factor therapy usually increases the ANC but does not eliminate the oscillation (14). Signs and symptoms may regress spontaneously during pregnancy and tend to lessen with age (15).

Bone marrow has a cyclic pattern of marked apoptosis affecting stem cells and early myeloid precursors (16). At the onset of peripheral neutropenia, promyelocytes, myelocytes, and the few segmented neutrophils present display autolytic changes. Near and at the neutrophil nadir, promyelocytes show marked apoptosis and nearly disappear. As the ANC recovers, promyelocytes regenerate normally, and macrophages show abundant neutrophilic debris. Monocytes, lymphocytes, eosinophils, and basophils do not demonstrate autolytic changes. Pre-B lymphocytes may oscillate synchronously but reciprocally to myeloid precursors, from normal to extraordinarily high levels.

Complications of congenital CN include life-threatening infection, reactive amyloidosis, and persistent neutropenia (17–19). Congenital CN does not carry an increased risk of acute leukemia (20).

The differential diagnosis includes acquired CN and other causes of congenital neutropenia, especially severe congenital neutropenia and Shwachman-Diamond syndrome. Acquired CN has been reported in autoimmune and inflammatory conditions and in clonal hematopoietic diseases (21–27).

Kostmann Disease

Kostmann disease is a rare autosomal recessive disorder (28–30). Shortly after birth, patients present with severe infections and abscesses, especially in the respiratory tract. Splenomegaly and severe osteopenia eventually occur. The peripheral blood shows severe neutropenia, sometimes accompanied by anemia. The bone marrow shows marked granulocytic hypoplasia, with a lack of differentiation beyond the promyelocyte/myelocyte stage. The disease is accompanied by an increased risk of myelodysplastic syndrome and acute leukemia. The emergence of clonal hematopoietic disease is closely linked to acquired mutation of *GCSFR*, which encodes the granulocyte colony-stimulating factor receptor. The differential diagnosis includes congenital CN and Shwachman-Diamond syndrome.

Myelokathexis

Myelokathexis is a rare inherited disorder, usually presenting in infancy or childhood with one or more components of the WHIM (warts, hypogammaglobulinemia, infection, and myelokathexis) syndrome (31–35). Recurrent bacterial infections of the respiratory tract are especially common. Other findings include growth retardation, skeletal anomalies, and phagocytic and immune dysfunction.

The peripheral blood is characterized by severe chronic neutropenia. The ANC increases sharply in response to infection, fever, or stress but quickly subsides. Neutrophil survival in peripheral blood is short, apparently because of prolonged retention in bone marrow. The bone marrow displays marked myeloid hyperplasia, largely owing to mature neutrophils. The neutrophils show signs of hypermaturity and degeneration, including vacuolated cytoplasm, nuclear hyperlobation, pyknotic changes, and interlobar chromatin filaments. Neutrophil precursors are decreased and show early and excessive apoptosis. Myelodysplastic syndrome has been reported as a possible late complication. The differential diagnosis includes acquired myelokathexis, a rare phenomenon seen in adults with malignancy (36,37).

Pelger-Hüet Anomaly

Pelger-Hüet anomaly (PHA) is an autosomal dominant disorder caused by mutation of *LBR* at chromosome 1q41-43, which encodes the laminin B receptor (38,39) (Fig. 5-18). The predominant findings are nuclear hypolobation in neutrophils and eosinophils, developmental delay, epilepsy, and skeletal abnormalities. Patients may also be at increased risk of tuberculosis (40–42).

The peripheral blood shows neutrophils with nonlobate, ovoid nuclei in homozygous PHA and bilobed nuclei in heterozygous PHA. The chromatin is condensed, as in a normal mature segmented neutrophil, but not pyknotic. Hypolobate neutrophils may be mistaken for band neutrophils. The

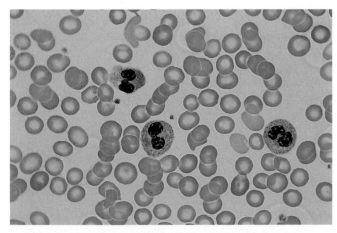

FIGURE 5-18. Peripheral blood smear, congenital Pelger-Hüet anomaly. Neutrophils show nuclear hyposegmentation.

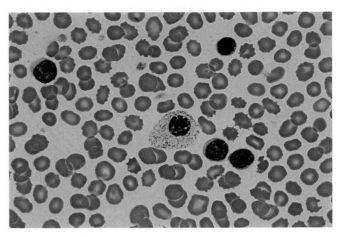

FIGURE 5-19. Peripheral blood smear, acquired Pelger-Hüet anomaly. A neutrophil shows complete lack of nuclear segmentation in this specimen from a patient with B-cell chronic lymphocytic leukemia.

bone marrow shows nuclear hypolobation in granulocytes and precursors. The differential diagnosis includes acquired PHA, a phenomenon seen in some types of infection and drug therapy, clonal B-cell disorders, and clonal myeloid disease, especially with the loss of chromosome 17p (43–54) (Fig. 5-19).

Severe Congenital Neutropenia

Severe congenital neutropenia occurs as a sporadic and autosomal dominant disorder, usually owing to mutations of the *ELA2* gene at chromosome 19p13, which encodes neutrophil elastase (55–58). Many different mutations have been identified, affecting both gene transcription and RNA splicing. Patients present with recurrent, severe infections. The peripheral blood shows marked and unremitting neutropenia, with an ANC of less than 0.5×10^9/L. The bone marrow demonstrates reduced and functionally abnormal myeloid precursors. Complications include life-threatening infection and clonal myeloid disease. The development of acute leukemia is linked to acquired mutation of the *G-CSFR* gene, which encodes the granulocyte colony-stimulating factor receptor.

The differential diagnosis includes congenital cyclic neutropenia, which involves a different *ELA2* site; Kostmann disease, an autosomal recessive disorder not involving *ELA2*; and Shwachman-Diamond syndrome, a disorder of unknown etiology characterized by pancreatic dysfunction and skeletal abnormalities in addition to neutropenia.

Shwachman-Diamond Syndrome

Shwachman-Diamond syndrome is a rare, probably autosomal recessive disorder associated with chromosome 7 anomalies (59–66). Patients present shortly after birth with recurrent infection, pancreatic exocrine insufficiency, growth retardation, and skeletal abnormalities. Laboratory studies show multiple functional abnormalities of neutrophils and lymphocytes and increased hemoglobin F, indicative of a stem cell disorder.

The peripheral blood shows neutropenia in all patients, anemia in 66%, and thrombocytopenia in 25%. Neutropenia may be constant or intermittent. The bone marrow shows decreased CD34-positive cells, increased CD5-positive precursor B cells, and prominent apoptosis. Complications include clonal hematopoietic disorders, seen in one-third of patients. The differential diagnosis includes congenital cyclic neutropenia, Kostmann disease, and severe congenital neutropenia.

CONSTITUTIONAL MEGAKARYOCYTE AND PLATELET DISORDERS

Bernard-Soulier Syndrome

Bernard-Soulier syndrome is a genetically heterogeneous, autosomal recessive disorder caused by mutations of the genes encoding glycoprotein (GP) Ib α, GP Ib β, and GP IX (1,2) (Fig. 5-20). Platelet aggregation studies are abnormal. The bleeding time is prolonged owing to defects in the platelet GP Ib-IX-V complex, a combination of GP Ib α, GP Ib β, GP IX, and GP V. Megakaryocytes fail to express the GP Ib-IX complex. The peripheral blood smear shows giant, round platelets. The bone marrow shows increased megakaryocytes with disordered maturation, increased cytoplasmic granularity, and increased ploidy.

Congenital Amegakaryocytic Thrombocytopenia

Congenital amegakaryocytic thrombocytopenia is an autosomal disorder caused by mutations of *c-mpl*, which encodes the thrombopoietin receptor (3–5). Both dominant and recessive mutations have been described. Some patients show double heterozygosity, inheriting an abnormal *c-mpl* allele from each parent. Hematopoietic cells fail to express surface c-Mpl, and serum thrombopoietin levels are increased. The disorder is apparent in the neonate and infant and presents as severe coagulopathy. Physical anomalies are absent, with rare exception. The peripheral blood shows thrombocytopenia, progressing to pancytopenia. The bone marrow may show adequate megakaryocytes initially but then progresses to megakaryocytic hypoplasia, followed by trilineal hypoplasia. Acute leukemia is a late complication.

Cyclic Thrombocytopenia

Cyclic thrombocytopenia has rarely been reported in the first year of life, when it may represent a congenital or hereditary disorder (6–9). Most patients with cyclic thrombocytopenia have an acquired disorder in association with menses, immune dysfunction, or clonal hematolymphoid disease (10–12). The peripheral blood shows episodic thrombocytopenia without morphologic abnormalities. The bone marrow may show cyclic changes in megakaryocyte number, with eventual amegakaryocytic thrombocytopenia developing in some patients.

Epstein and Related Syndromes

Epstein syndrome, Fechtner syndrome, May-Hegglin anomaly, and Sebastian syndrome are related autosomal dominant disorders (13–19) (Fig. 5-21). All but Epstein syndrome have been linked to mutations of *MYH9*, located at chromosome 22q12-13. Neutrophils often show blue, sometimes Döhle body–like, inclusions, apparently composed of MYH9 protein. Alport syndrome, a triad of chronic renal failure, sensorineural deafness, and ocular disease, is variably expressed. The reason for the disparity between genotype and clinical expression is not known.

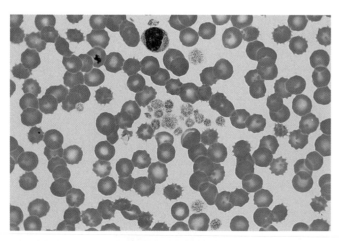

FIGURE 5-20. Peripheral blood smear, Bernard-Soulier syndrome. The platelets are larger than normal.

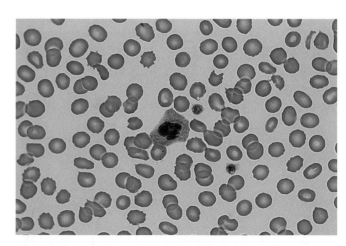

FIGURE 5-21. Peripheral blood smear, May-Hegglin anomaly. A neutrophil shows a slender, pale-blue cytoplasmic inclusion. Platelets are decreased and enlarged.

Epstein syndrome is characterized by chronic renal disease and deafness, but no neutrophil inclusions. Fechtner syndrome displays the complete Alport triad and neutrophil inclusions. May-Hegglin anomaly is characterized by chronic renal disease and neutrophil inclusions but not deafness or ocular disease. Sebastian syndrome has neutrophil inclusions but no features of Alport syndrome. The peripheral blood shows thrombocytopenia with large to giant platelets. The bone marrow has normal to increased megakaryocytes, which may contain giant intranuclear granules.

Gray Platelet Syndrome

Gray platelet syndrome is an autosomal disorder in which α granules fail to form within megakaryocytes but are released instead into the demarcation membrane system (20–23) (Fig. 5-22). Platelet aggregation study results are abnormal, and the bleeding time is prolonged. The peripheral blood shows mild to moderate thrombocytopenia with large, agranular, blue-gray platelets. Neutrophils may also show hypogranularity. The bone marrow shows adequate megakaryocytes with increased emperipolesis and mild reticulin fibrosis. The differential diagnosis includes acquired gray platelet syndrome, an ethylenediaminetetraacetic acid–dependent artifact.

Hermansky-Pudlak Syndrome

Hermansky-Pudlak syndrome is a genetically heterogeneous autosomal recessive disorder, usually owing to mutation of *HPS1* at chromosome 10q23, with a consequent lack of HPS1 protein production and defective lysosomes and melanosomes (24–26). The bleeding time is prolonged, consistent with platelet storage pool deficiency. Patients present with bruising and oculocutaneous albinism. The bone marrow contains increased storage-type histiocytes with pig-

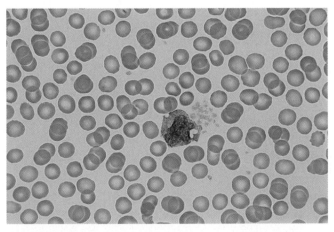

FIGURE 5-22. Peripheral blood smear, gray platelet syndrome. The platelets lack cytoplasmic granules.

mented lipid (ceroid lipofuscin). The differential diagnosis includes Chediak-Higashi syndrome, which also shows oculocutaneous albinism and a platelet storage pool defect.

Paris-Trousseau and Related Syndromes

Paris-Trousseau syndrome is a rare congenital disorder characterized by a deletion at chromosome 11q23 involving *ETS1*, a gene important in megakaryopoiesis (27,28). Patients present with mild coagulopathy and thrombocytopenia. Platelets contain giant chemically and functionally abnormal α granules. The bone marrow shows increased megakaryocytes, with numerous small forms, abnormal maturation, and excessive lysis. Similar syndromes have been described that affect the distal end of chromosome 11q, including Jacobsen syndrome, in which the features of Paris-Trousseau syndrome are accompanied by multiple congenital anomalies, cardiac defects, and psychomotor retardation.

Thrombocytopenia with Absent Radii Syndrome

Thrombocytopenia with absent radii syndrome occurs sporadically and as a hereditary disorder, usually transmitted in an autosomal dominant fashion (29–32). Neonates present with coagulopathy and a wide spectrum of genitourinary and limb anomalies, commonly bilateral absence of the radii. Other reported findings include periodic leukemoid reactions, eosinophilia, and impaired immunity. The peripheral blood shows severe thrombocytopenia. The bone marrow shows decreased megakaryocytes, with morphologic and functional abnormalities. The platelet count increases progressively after birth to reach normal levels. Acute leukemia has been reported as a late complication.

X-Linked Microthrombocytopenia and Wiskott-Aldrich Syndrome

X-linked microthrombocytopenia and Wiskott-Aldrich syndrome are related disorders caused by mutation of *WASP*, located at chromosome Xp11 (33–35). The gene product, WASP, is essential to the organization of actin filaments, major components of the cytoskeleton. Wiskott-Aldrich syndrome, but not X-linked microthrombocytopenia, also shows eczema and immunodeficiency. The peripheral blood shows thrombocytopenia and unusually small platelets.

Other Megakaryocyte and Platelet Disorders

A variety of other rare syndromes has been reported, some characterized by macrothrombocytopenia (36–43).

REFERENCES

Constitutional Hematopoietic Stem Cell Disorders

1. Giri N, Kang E, Tisdale JF, et al. Clinical and laboratory evidence for a trilineage haematopoietic defect in patients with refractory Diamond-Blackfan anaemia. *Br J Haematol* 2000;108:167–175.
2. Ramenghi U, Campagnoli MF, Garelli E, et al. Diamond-Blackfan anemia: report of seven further mutations in the RPS19 gene and evidence of mutation heterogeneity in the Italian population. *Blood Cells Mol Dis* 2000;26:417–422.
3. Santucci MA, Bagnara GP, Strippoli P, et al. Long-term bone marrow cultures in Diamond-Blackfan anemia reveal a defect of both granulomacrophage and erythroid progenitors. *Exp Hematol* 1999;27:9–18.
4. Vlachos A, Federman N, Reyes-Haley C, et al. Hematopoietic stem cell transplantation for Diamond Blackfan anemia: a report from the Diamond Blackfan Anemia Registry. *Bone Marrow Transplant* 2001;27:381–386.
5. Willig TN, Draptchinskaia N, Dianzani I, et al. Mutations in ribosomal protein S19 gene and Diamond Blackfan anemia: wide variations in phenotypic expression. *Blood* 1999;94:4294–4306.
6. Knight SW, Vulliamy TJ, Morgan B, et al. Identification of novel DKC1 mutations in patients with dyskeratosis congenita: implications for pathophysiology and diagnosis. *Hum Genet* 2001;108:299–303.
7. Vulliamy TJ, Knight SW, Heiss NS, et al. Dyskeratosis congenita caused by a 3′ deletion: germline and somatic mosaicism in a female carrier. *Blood* 1999;94:1254–1260.
8. Vulliamy TJ, Knight SW, Mason PJ, et al. Very short telomeres in the peripheral blood of patients with X-linked and autosomal dyskeratosis congenita. *Blood Cells Mol Dis* 2001;27:353–357.
9. Vulliamy T, Marrone A, Goldman F, et al. The RNA component of telomerase is mutated in autosomal dominant dyskeratosis congenita. *Nature* 2001;413:432–435.
10. Alter BP, Caruso JP, Drachtman RA, et al. Fanconi anemia: myelodysplasia as a predictor of outcome. *Cancer Genet Cytogenet* 2000;117:125–131.
11. De la Torre C, Pincheira J, Lopez-Saez JF. Human syndromes with genomic instability and multiprotein machines that repair DNA double-strand breaks. *Histol Histopathol* 2003;18:225–243.
12. Gregory JJ Jr, Wagner JE, Verlander PC, et al. Somatic mosaicism in Fanconi anemia: evidence of genotypic reversion in lymphohematopoietic stem cells. *Proc Natl Acad Sci U S A* 2001;98:2532–2537.
13. Medhurst AL, Huber PA, Waisfisz Q, et al. Direct interactions of the five known Fanconi anaemia proteins suggest a common functional pathway. *Hum Mol Genet* 2001;10:423–429.
14. Pang Q, Christianson TA, Keeble W, et al. The Fanconi anemia complementation group C gene product: structural evidence of multifunctionality. *Blood* 2001;98:1392–1401.
15. Pearson T, Jansen S, Havenga C, et al. Fanconi anemia. a statistical evaluation of cytogenetic results obtained from South African families. *Cancer Genet Cytogenet* 2001;126:52–55.

Constitutional Erythrocyte Disorders

1. Kralovics R, Prchal JT. Genetic heterogeneity of primary familial and congenital polycythemia. *Am J Hematol* 2001;68:115–121.
2. Percy MJ, McMullin MF, Roques AW, et al. Erythrocytosis due to a mutation in the erythropoietin receptor gene. *Br J Haematol* 1998;100:407–410.
3. Watowich SS, Xie X, Klingmuller U, et al. Erythropoietin receptor mutations associated with familial erythrocytosis cause hypersensitivity to erythropoietin in the heterozygous state. *Blood* 1999;94:2530–2532.
4. Kralovics R, Sokol L, Broxson EH Jr, et al. The erythropoietin receptor gene is not linked with the polycythemia phenotype in a family with autosomal dominant primary polycythemia. *Proc Assoc Am Physicians* 1997;109:580–585.
5. Vasserman NN, Karzakova LM, Tverskaya SM, et al. Localization of the gene responsible for familial benign polycythemia to chromosome 11q23. *Hum Hered* 1999;49:129–132.
6. Motohashi T, Nakamura Y, Osawa M, et al. Increased cell surface expression of C-terminal truncated erythropoietin receptors in polycythemia. *Eur J Haematol* 2001;67:88–93.
7. Athanasiou-Metaxa M, Economou M, Tsantali C, et al. Congenital erythrocytosis with increased erythropoietin level. *J Pediatr Hematol Oncol* 2002;24:234–236.
8. Bard H, Rosenberg A, Huisman TH. Hemoglobinopathies affecting maternal-fetal oxygen gradient during pregnancy: molecular, biochemical and clinical studies. *Am J Perinatol* 1998;15:389–393.
9. Imai K, Tientadakul P, Opartkiattikul N, et al. Detection of haemoglobin variants and inference of their functional properties using complete oxygen dissociation curve measurements. *Br J Haematol* 2001;112:483–487.
10. Delaunay J, Iolascon A. The congenital dyserythropoietic anaemias. *Baillieres Best Pract Res Clin Haematol* 1999;12:691–705.
11. Iolascon A, Martire B, Lee MJ, et al. Transfusion-dependent congenital dyserythropoietic anaemia with intraerythroblastic inclusions of a non-globin protein. *Eur J Haematol* 2000;65:140–143.
12. Majeed HA, Al-Tarawna M, El-Shanti H, et al. The syndrome of chronic recurrent multifocal osteomyelitis and congenital dyserythropoietic anaemia. Report of a new family and a review. *Eur J Pediatr* 2001;160:705–710.
13. Okajima K, Ito T, Wakita A, et al. Male siblings with dyserythropoiesis, microcephaly and intrauterine growth retardation. *Clin Dysmorphol* 2002;11:107–111.
14. Tekinalp G, Sarici SU, Erdinc AS, et al. Lethal hydrops fetalis due to congenital dyserythropoietic anemia in a newborn: association of a new skeletal abnormality. *Pediatr Hematol Oncol* 2001;18:537–542.
15. Wickramasinghe SN. Congenital dyserythropoietic anemias. *Curr Opin Hematol* 2000;7:71–78.
16. Kato K, Sugitani M, Kawataki M, et al. Congenital dyserythropoietic anemia type 1 with fetal onset of severe anemia. *J Pediatr Hematol Oncol* 2001;23:63–66.
17. Parez N, Dommergues M, Zupan V, et al. Severe congenital dyserythropoietic anaemia type I: prenatal management, transfusion support and alpha-interferon therapy. *Br J Haematol* 2000;110:420–423.
18. Shalev H, Moser A, Kapelushnik J, et al. Congenital dyserythropoietic anemia type I presenting as persistent pulmonary hypertension of the newborn. *J Pediatr* 2000;136:553–555.
19. Shamseddine A, Taher A, Jaafar H, et al. Interferon alpha is an effective therapy for congenital dyserythropoietic anaemia type I. *Eur J Haematol* 2000;65:207–209.
20. Tamary H, Shalmon L, Shalev H, et al. Localization of the gene for congenital dyserythropoietic anemia type I to a <1-cM interval on chromosome 15q15.1-15.3. *Am J Hum Genet* 1998;62:1062–1069.
21. Danise P, Amendola G, Nobili B, et al. Flow-cytometric analysis of erythrocytes and reticulocytes in congenital dyserythropoietic anaemia type II (CDA II): value in differential diagnosis with hereditary spherocytosis. *Clin Lab Haematol* 2001;23:7–13.

22. Fargion S, Valenti L, Fracanzani AL, et al. Hereditary hemochromatosis in a patient with congenital dyserythropoietic anemia. *Blood* 2000;96:3653–3655.

23. Iolascon A, Delaunay J, Wickramasinghe SN, et al. Natural history of congenital dyserythropoietic anemia type II. *Blood* 2001; 98:1258–1260.

24. Perrotta S, del Giudice EM, Carbone R, et al. Gilbert's syndrome accounts for the phenotypic variability of congenital dyserythropoietic anemia type II (CDA-II). *J Pediatr* 2000;136: 556–559.

25. Rohrig G, Kilter H, Beuckelmann D, et al. Congenital dyserythropoietic anemia type III associated with congenital atrioseptal defect has led to severe cardiac problems in a 32-year-old patient. *Am J Hematol* 2000;64:314–316.

26. Sandstrom H, Wahlin A. Congenital dyserythropoietic anemia type III. *Haematologica* 2000;85:753–757.

27. Sigler E, Shaft D, Shtalrid M, et al. New sporadic case of congenital dyserythropoietic anemia type III in an aged woman: detailed description of ultrastructural findings. *Am J Hematol* 2002;70:72–76.

28. Dugue B, Aminoff M, Aimone-Gastin I, et al. A urinary radioisotope-binding assay to diagnose Grasbeck-Imerslund disease. *J Pediatr Gastroenterol Nutr* 1998;26:21–25.

29. Grech V, Vella C, Mercieca V. Temporary myoclonus with treatment of congenital transcobalamin 2 deficiency. *Pediatr Neurol* 2001;24:75–76.

30. Gritli S, Omar S, Tartaglini E, et al. A novel mutation in the SLC19A2 gene in a Tunisian family with thiamine-responsive megaloblastic anaemia, diabetes and deafness syndrome. *Br J Haematol* 2001;113:508–513.

31. Kind T, Levy J, Lee M, et al. Cobalamin C disease presenting as hemolytic-uremic syndrome in the neonatal period. *J Pediatr Hematol Oncol* 2002;24:327–329.

32. Labrune P, Zittoun J, Duvaltier I, et al. Haemolytic uraemic syndrome and pulmonary hypertension in a patient with methionine synthase deficiency. *Eur J Pediatr* 1999;158:734–739.

33. Meire FM, Van Genderen MM, Lemmens K, et al. Thiamine-responsive megaloblastic anemia syndrome (TRMA) with conc-rod dystrophy. *Ophthalmic Genet* 2000;21:243–250.

34. Beutler E, Gelbart T, Lee P, et al. Molecular characterization of a case of atransferrinemia. *Blood* 2000;96:4071–4074.

35. Pearson HA, Lukens JN. Ferrokinetics in the syndrome of familial hypoferremic microcytic anemia with iron malabsorption. *J Pediatr Hematol Oncol* 1999;21:412–417.

36. Bader-Meunier B, Mielot F, Breton-Gorius J, et al. Hematologic involvement in mitochondrial cytopathies in childhood: a retrospective study of bone marrow smears. *Pediatr Res* 1999;46: 158–162.

37. Becher MW, Wills ML, Noll WW, et al. Kearns-Sayre syndrome with features of Pearson's marrow-pancreas syndrome and a novel 2905-base pair mitochondrial DNA deletion. *Hum Pathol* 1999;30:577–581.

38. Carelli V, Baracca A, Barogi S, et al. Biochemical-clinical correlation in patients with different loads of the mitochondrial DNA T8993G mutation. *Arch Neurol* 2002;59:264–270.

39. Fosslien E. Mitochondrial medicine—molecular pathology of defective oxidative phosphorylation. *Ann Clin Lab Sci* 2001;31: 25–67.

40. Lacbawan F, Tifft CJ, Luban NL, et al. Clinical heterogeneity in mitochondrial DNA deletion disorders: a diagnostic challenge of Pearson syndrome. *Am J Med Genet* 2000;95:266–268.

41. Leung TF, Hui J, Shoubridge E, et al. Aplastic anaemia in association with Kearns-Sayre syndrome. *J Inherit Metab Dis* 1999;22:86–87.

42. Muraki K, Sakura N, Ueda H, et al. Clinical implications of duplicated mtDNA in Pearson syndrome. *Am J Med Genet* 2001;98:205–209.

43. Naviaux RK. Mitochondrial DNA disorders. *Eur J Pediatr* 2000;159:S219–226.

44. Yanagihara I, Inui K, Yanagihara K, et al. Fluorescence in situ hybridization analysis of peripheral blood cells in Pearson marrow-pancreas syndrome. *J Pediatr* 2001;139:452–455.

45. Chan GC, Head DR, Wang WC. Refractory anemia with ringed sideroblasts in children: two diseases with a similar phenotype? *J Pediatr Hematol Oncol* 1999;21:418–423.

46. Wang YL, Choi HK, Aul C, et al. The MERRF mutation of mitochondrial DNA in the bone marrow of a patient with acquired idiopathic sideroblastic anemia. *Am J Hematol* 1999;60:83–84.

47. Cazzola M, May A, Bergamaschi G, et al. Familial-skewed X-chromosome inactivation as a predisposing factor for late-onset X-linked sideroblastic anemia in carrier females. *Blood* 2000;96:4363–4365.

48. Cotter PD, May A, Li L, et al. Four new mutations in the erythroid-specific 5-aminolevulinate synthase (ALAS2) gene causing X-linked sideroblastic anemia: increased pyridoxine responsiveness after removal of iron overload by phlebotomy and coinheritance of hereditary hemochromatosis. *Blood* 1999;93: 1757–1769.

49. Furuyama K, Sassa S. Interaction between succinyl CoA synthetase and the heme-biosynthetic enzyme ALAS-E is disrupted in sideroblastic anemia. *J Clin Invest* 2000;105:757–764.

50. May A, Bishop DF. The molecular biology and pyridoxine responsiveness of X-linked sideroblastic anaemia. *Haematologica* 1998;83:56–70.

51. Sadlon TJ, Dell'Oso T, Surinya KH, et al. Regulation of erythroid 5-aminolevulinate synthase expression during erythropoiesis. *Int J Biochem Cell Biol* 1999;31:1153–1167.

52. Bekri S, Kispal G, Lange H, et al. Human ABC7 transporter: gene structure and mutation causing X-linked sideroblastic anemia with ataxia with disruption of cytosolic iron-sulfur protein maturation. *Blood* 2000;96:3256–3264.

53. Hellier KD, Hatchwell E, Duncombe AS, et al. X-linked sideroblastic anaemia with ataxia: another mitochondrial disease? *J Neurol Neurosurg Psychiatry* 2001;70:65–69.

54. Lill R, Kispal G. Mitochondrial ABC transporters. *Res Microbiol* 2001;152:331–340.

55. Delaunay J. Molecular basis of red cell membrane disorders. *Acta Haematol* 2002;108:210–218.

56. DePalma L, Luban NL. Hereditary pyropoikilocytosis. Clinical and laboratory analysis in eight infants and young children. *Am J Dis Child* 1993;147:93–95.

57. Tse WT, Lux SE. Red blood cell membrane disorders. *Br J Haematol* 1999;104:2–13.

58. Wandersee NJ, Birkenmeier CS, Bodine DM, et al. Mutations in the murine erythroid alpha-spectrin gene alter spectrin mRNA and protein levels and spectrin incorporation into the red blood cell membrane skeleton. *Blood* 2003;101:325–330.

59. Perrotta S, del Giudice EM, Iolascon A, et al. Reversible erythrocyte skeleton destabilization is modulated by beta-spectrin phosphorylation in childhood leukemia. *Leukemia* 2001;15: 440–444.

60. Bain BJ, Liesner R. Pseudopyropoikilocytosis: a striking artefact. *J Clin Pathol* 1996;49:772–773.

61. Basseres DS, Duarte AS, Hassoun H, et al. beta-Spectrin S(ta) Barbara: a novel frameshift mutation in hereditary spherocytosis associated with detectable levels of mRNA and a germ cell line mosaicism. *Br J Haematol* 2001;115:347–353.

62. Bracher NA, Lyons CA, Wessels G, et al. Band 3 Cape Town (E90K) causes severe hereditary spherocytosis in combination with band 3 Prague III. *Br J Haematol* 2001;113:689–693.

63. Bruce LJ, Ghosh S, King MJ, et al. Absence of CD47 in protein 4.2-deficient hereditary spherocytosis in man: an interaction between the Rh complex and the band 3 complex. *Blood* 2002;100:1878–1885.

64. Delhommeau F, Cynober T, Schischmanoff PO, et al. Natural history of hereditary spherocytosis during the first year of life. *Blood* 2000;95:393–397.

65. Granjo E, Bauerle R, Sampaio R, et al. Extramedullary hematopoiesis in hereditary spherocytosis deficient in ankyrin: a case report. *Int J Hematol* 2002;76:153–156.

66. Miraglia del Giudice E, Nobili B, Francese M, et al. Clinical and molecular evaluation of non-dominant hereditary spherocytosis. *Br J Haematol* 2001;112:42–47.

67. Nakanishi H, Kanzaki A, Yawata A, et al. Ankyrin gene mutations in Japanese patients with hereditary spherocytosis. *Int J Hematol* 2001;73:54–63.

68. Reinhardt D, Witt O, Miosge N, et al. Increase in band 3 density and aggregation in hereditary spherocytosis. *Blood Cells Mol Dis* 2001;27:399–406.

69. Reliene R, Mariani M, Zanella A, et al. Splenectomy prolongs in vivo survival of erythrocytes differently in spectrin/ankyrin- and band 3-deficient hereditary spherocytosis. *Blood* 2002;100:2208–2215.

70. Ustun C, Kutlar F, Holley L, et al. Interaction of sickle cell trait with hereditary spherocytosis: splenic infarcts and sequestration. *Acta Haematol* 2003;109:46–49.

71. Akar N, Gokce H. Red blood cell indexes in patients with hereditary spherocytosis and beta-thalassemia combination. *Pediatr Hematol Oncol* 2002;19:569–573.

72. Brandenberg JB, Demarmels Biasiutti F, et al. Hereditary spherocytosis and hemochromatosis. *Ann Hematol* 2002;81:202–209.

73. Danise P, Amendola G, Nobili B, et al. Flow-cytometric analysis of erythrocytes and reticulocytes in congenital dyserythropoietic anaemia type II (CDA II): value in differential diagnosis with hereditary spherocytosis. *Clin Lab Haematol* 2001;23:7–13.

74. Chetty MC, Stewart GW. Pseudohyperkalaemia and pseudomacrocytosis caused by inherited red-cell disorders of the 'hereditary stomatocytosis' group. *Br J Biomed Sci* 2001;58:48–55.

75. Gore DM, Chetty MC, Fisher J, et al. Familial pseudohyperkalaemia Cardiff: a mild version of cryohydrocytosis. *Br J Haematol* 2002;117:212–214.

76. Grootenboer S, Barro C, Cynober T, et al. Dehydrated hereditary stomatocytosis: a cause of prenatal ascites. *Prenat Diagn* 2001;21:1114–1118.

77. Haines PG, Jarvis HG, King S, et al. Two further British families with the 'cryohydrocytosis' form of hereditary stomatocytosis. *Br J Haematol* 2001;113:932–937.

78. Jablonska-Skwiecinska E, Lewandowska I, Plochocka D, et al. Several mutations including two novel mutations of the glucose-6-phosphate dehydrogenase gene in Polish G6PD deficient subjects with chronic nonspherocytic hemolytic anemia, acute hemolytic anemia, and favism. *Hum Mutat* 1999;14:477–484.

79. Kaplan M, Vreman HJ, Hammerman C, et al. Favism by proxy in nursing glucose-6-phosphate dehydrogenase-deficient neonates. *J Perinatol* 1998;18:477–479.

80. Mehta A, Mason PJ, Vulliamy TJ. Glucose-6-phosphate dehydrogenase deficiency. *Bailliores Best Pract Res Clin Haematol* 2000;13:21–38.

81. Yoo D, Lessin LS. Drug-associated "bite cell" hemolytic anemia. *Am J Med* 1992;92:243–248.

82. Tanphaichitr VS, Suvatte V, Mahasandana C, et al. Transient, acquired glucose-6-phosphate dehydrogenase deficiency in Thai children with typhoid fever. *Southeast Asian J Trop Med Public Health* 1982;13:105–109.

83. Kugler W, Willaschek C, Holtz C, et al. Eight novel mutations and consequences on mRNA and protein level in pyruvate kinase-deficient patients with nonspherocytic hemolytic anemia. *Hum Mutat* 2000;15:261–272.

84. Nagai H, Takazakura E, Oda H, et al. An autopsy case of pyruvate kinase deficiency anemia associated with severe hemochromatosis. *Intern Med* 1994;33:56–59.

85. Zarza R, Alvarez R, Pujades A, et al. Molecular characterization of the PK-LR gene in pyruvate kinase deficient Spanish patients. Red Cell Pathology Group of the Spanish Society of Haematology (AEHH). *Br J Haematol* 1998;103:377–382.

86. Koudieh MS, Afzal M, Rasul K, et al. Intrathoracic extramedullary hematopoietic tumor in hemoglobin C disease. *Arch Pathol Lab Med* 1996;120:504–506.

87. Modiano D, Luoni G, Sirima BS, et al. Haemoglobin C protects against clinical *Plasmodium falciparum* malaria. *Nature* 2001;414:305–308.

88. Olson JF, Ware RE, Schultz WH, et al. Hemoglobin C disease in infancy and childhood. *J Pediatr* 1994;125:745–747.

89. Olivieri NF, De Silva S, Premawardena A, et al. Iron overload and iron-chelating therapy in hemoglobin E-beta thalassemia. *J Pediatr Hematol Oncol* 2000;22:593–597.

90. Pootrakul P, Sirankapracha P, Hemsorach S, et al. A correlation of erythrokinetics, ineffective erythropoiesis, and erythroid precursor apoptosis in Thai patients with thalassemia. *Blood* 2000;96:2606–2612.

91. Ataga KI, Orringer EP. Bone marrow necrosis in sickle cell disease: a description of three cases and a review of the literature. *Am J Med Sci* 2000;320:342–347.

92. Eckardt P, Raez LE, Restrepo A, et al. Pulmonary bone marrow embolism in sickle cell disease. *South Med J* 1999;92:245–247.

93. Hasegawa S, Rodgers GP, Dwyer N, et al. Sickling of nucleated erythroid precursors from patients with sickle cell anemia. *Exp Hematol* 1998;26:314–319.

94. Bain BJ. Blood film features of sickle cell-haemoglobin C disease. *Br J Haematol* 1993;83:516–518.

95. Ballas SK, Pindzola A, Chang CD, et al. Postmortem diagnosis of hemoglobin SC disease complicated by fat embolism. *Ann Clin Lab Sci* 1998;28:144–149.

96. Eichhorn RF, Buurke EJ, Blok P, et al. Sickle cell-like crisis and bone marrow necrosis associated with Parvovirus B19 infection and heterozygosity for haemoglobins S and E. *J Intern Med* 1999;245:103–106.

97. Hutchins KD, Ballas SK, Phatak D, et al. Sudden unexpected death in a patient with splenic sequestration and sickle cell-beta+-thalassemia syndrome. *J Forensic Sci* 2001;46:412–414.

98. Kolquist KA, Vnencak-Jones CL, Swift L, et al. Fatal fat embolism syndrome in a child with undiagnosed hemoglobin S/beta+ thalassemia: a complication of acute Parvovirus B19 infection. *Pediatr Pathol Lab Med* 1996;16:71–82.

99. Cohen-Solal M, Prehu C, Wajcman H, et al. A new sickle cell disease phenotype associating Hb S trait, severe pyruvate kinase deficiency (PK Conakry), and an alpha2 globin gene variant (Hb Conakry). *Br J Haematol* 1998;103:950–956.

100. Schrier SL. Pathophysiology of thalassemia. *Curr Opin Hematol* 2002;9:123–126.

101. Traeger-Synodinos J, Papassotiriou I, Vrettou C, et al. Erythroid marrow activity and functional anemia in patients with the rare interaction of a single functional a-globin and beta-globin gene. *Haematologica* 2001;86:363–367.

102. Bunyaratvej A, Fucharoen S, Butthep P, et al. Alterations and pathology of thalassemic red cells: comparison between alpha- and beta-thalassemia. *Southeast Asian J Trop Med Public Health* 1995;26:257–260.

103. Wickramasinghe SN, Hughes M, Fucharoen S, et al. The fate of excess beta-globin chains within erythropoietic cells in alpha-thalassaemia 2 trait, alpha-thalassaemia 1 trait, haemoglobin H

disease and haemoglobin Q-H disease: an electron microscope study. *Br J Haematol* 1984;56:473–482.

104. Higgs DR, Wood WG, Barton C, et al. Clinical features and molecular analysis of acquired hemoglobin H disease. *Am J Med* 1983;75:181–191.

105. Centis F, Tabellini L, Lucarelli G, et al. The importance of erythroid expansion in determining the extent of apoptosis in erythroid precursors in patients with beta-thalassemia major. *Blood* 2000;96:3624–3629.

106. Ho PJ, Wickramasinghe SN, Rees DC, et al. Erythroblastic inclusions in dominantly inherited beta thalassemias. *Blood* 1997;89:322–328.

107. Mathias LA, Fisher TC, Zeng L, et al. Ineffective erythropoiesis in beta-thalassemia major is due to apoptosis at the polychromatophilic normoblast stage. *Exp Hematol* 2000;28:1343–1353.

108. Routy JP, Monte M, Beaulieu R, et al. Increase of hemoglobin A2 in human immunodeficiency virus-1-infected patients treated with zidovudine. *Am J Hematol* 1993;43:86–90.

Constitutional Granulocyte Disorders

1. Clarke JT, Willard HF, Teshima I, et al. Hunter disease (mucopolysaccharidosis type II) in a karyotypically normal girl. *Clin Genet* 1990;37:355–362.

2. Peterson L, Parkin J, Nelson A. Mucopolysaccharidosis type VII. A morphologic, cytochemical, and ultrastructural study of the blood and bone marrow. *Am J Clin Pathol* 1982;78:544–548.

3. Presentey B. Alder anomaly accompanied by a mutation of the myeloperoxidase structural gene. *Acta Haematol* 1986;75:157–159.

4. Ghandi MK, Howard MR, Hamilton PJ. The Alder-Reilly anomaly in association with the myelodysplastic syndrome. *Clin Lab Haematol* 1996;18:39–40.

5. Bain BJ, Phillips D, Thomson K, et al. Investigation of the effect of marathon running on leucocyte counts of subjects of different ethnic origins: relevance to the aetiology of ethnic neutropenia. *Br J Haematol* 2000;108:483–487.

6. Haddy TB, Rana SR, Castro O. Benign ethnic neutropenia: what is a normal absolute neutrophil count. *J Lab Clin Med* 1999;133:15–22.

7. Rezvani K, Flanagan AM, Sarma U, et al. Investigation of ethnic neutropenia by assessment of bone marrow colony-forming cells. *Acta Haematol* 2001;105:32–37.

8. Huizing M, Anikster Y, Gahl WA. Hermansky-Pudlak syndrome and Chediak-Higashi syndrome: disorders of vesicle formation and trafficking. *Thromb Haemost* 2001;86:233–245.

9. Introne W, Boissy RE, Gahl WA. Clinical, molecular, and cell biological aspects of Chediak-Higashi syndrome. *Mol Genet Metab* 1999;68:283–303.

10. Dale DC, Person RE, Bolyard AA, et al. Mutations in the gene encoding neutrophil elastase in congenital and cyclic neutropenia. *Blood* 2000;96:2317–2322.

11. Palmer SE, Stephens K, Dale DC. Genetics, phenotype, and natural history of autosomal dominant cyclic hematopoiesis. *Am J Med Genet* 1996;66:413–422.

12. Peng HW, Chou CF, Liang DC. Hereditary cyclic neutropenia in the male members of a Chinese family with inverted Y chromosome. *Br J Haematol* 2000;110:438–440.

13. Engelhard D, Landreth KS, Kapoor N, et al. Cycling of peripheral blood and marrow lymphocytes in cyclic neutropenia. *Proc Natl Acad Sci U S A* 1983;80:5734–5738.

14. Heussner P, Haase D, Kanz L. G-CSF in the long-term treatment of cyclic neutropenia and chronic idiopathic neutropenia in adult patients. *Int J Hematol* 1998;62:225–234.

15. Kimura T, Takakura K, Nakagawa T, et al. Spontaneous remission of cyclic neutropenia during pregnancy. A case report. *J Reprod Med* 2001;46:141–143.

16. Aprikyan AA, Liles WC, Rodger E, et al. Impaired survival of bone marrow hematopoietic progenitor cells in cyclic neutropenia. *Blood* 2001;97:147–153.

17. Abe T, Azuma H, Watanabe A, et al. A patient with cyclic neutropenia complicated by severe persistent neutropenia successfully delivered a healthy baby. *Intern Med* 2000;39:663–666.

18. Bar-Joseph G, Halberthal M, Sweed Y, et al. Clostridium septicum infection in children with cyclic neutropenia. *J Pediatr* 1997;131:317–319.

19. Shiomura T, Ishida Y, Matsumoto N, et al. A case of generalized amyloidosis associated with cyclic neutropenia. *Blood* 1979;54:628–635.

20. Dale DC, Cottle TE, Fier CJ, et al. Severe chronic neutropenia: treatment and follow-up of patients in the Severe Chronic Neutropenia International Registry. *Am J Hematol* 2003;72:82–93.

21. Abe Y, Hirase N, Muta K, et al. Adult onset cyclic hematopoiesis in a patient with myelodysplastic syndrome. *Int J Hematol* 2000;71:40–45.

22. Bennett M, Grunwald AJ. Hydroxyurea and periodicity in myeloproliferative disease. *Eur J Haematol* 2001;66:317–323.

23. Goraya JS, Virdi VS, Marwaha N, et al. Acute lymphoblastic leukemia presenting as cyclic neutropenia. *Pediatr Hematol Oncol* 2002;19:279–282.

24. Fata F, Myers P, Addeo J, et al. Cyclic neutropenia in Crohn's ileocolitis: efficacy of granulocyte colony-stimulating factor. *J Clin Gastroenterol* 1997;24:253–256.

25. Heussner P, Haase D, Kanz L. G-CSF in the long-term treatment of cyclic neutropenia and chronic idiopathic neutropenia in adult patients. *Int J Hematol* 1998;62:225–234.

26. Hirase N, Abe Y, Muta K, et al. Autoimmune neutropenia with cyclic oscillation of neutrophil count after steroid administration. *Int J Hematol* 2001;73:346–350.

27. Moser C, Schlesier M, Drager R, et al. Transient CD80 expression defect in a patient with variable immunodeficiency and cyclic neutropenia. *Int Arch Allergy Immunol* 1997;112:96–99.

28. Carlsson G, Fasth A. Infantile genetic agranulocytosis, morbus Kostmann: presentation of six cases from the original "Kostmann family" and a review. *Acta Paediatr* 2001;90:757–764.

29. Freedman MH, Bonilla MA, Fier C, et al. Myelodysplasia syndrome and acute myeloid leukemia in patients with congenital neutropenia receiving G-CSF therapy. *Blood* 2000;96:429–436.

30. Zeidler C, Welte K, Barak Y, et al. Stem cell transplantation in patients with severe congenital neutropenia without evidence of leukemic transformation. *Blood* 2000;95:1195–1198.

31. Aprikyan AA, Liles WC, Park JR, et al. Myelokathexis, a congenital disorder of severe neutropenia characterized by accelerated apoptosis and defective expression of bcl-x in neutrophil precursors. *Blood* 2000;95:320–327.

32. Arai J, Wakiguchi H, Hisakawa H, et al. A variant of myelokathexis with hypogammaglobulinemia: lymphocytes as well as neutrophils may reverse in response to infections. *Pediatr Hematol Oncol* 2000;17:171–176.

33. Gorlin RJ, Gelb B, Diaz GA, et al. WHIM syndrome, an autosomal dominant disorder: clinical, hematological, and molecular studies. *Am J Med Genet* 2000;91:368–376.

34. Hord JD, Whitlock JA, Gay JC, et al. Clinical features of myelokathexis and treatment with hematopoietic cytokines: a case report of two patients and review of the literature. *J Pediatr Hematol Oncol* 1997;19:443–448.

35. Imashuku S, Miyagawa A, Chiyonobu T, et al. Epstein-Barr virus-associated T-lymphoproliferative disease with hemophagocytic syndrome, followed by fatal intestinal B lymphoma in a young adult female with WHIM syndrome. Warts, hypogammaglobulinemia, infections, and myelokathexis. *Ann Hematol* 2002;81:470–473.

36. Maran R, Mittelman M, Cohen AM, et al. Myelokathexis and monocytosis in a patient with gastric cancer. *Acta Haematol* 1992;87:210–212.

37. Rassam SM, Roderick P, al-Hakim I, et al. A myelokathexis-like variant of myelodysplasia. *Eur J Haematol* 1989;42:99–102.

38. Hoffmann K, Dreger CK, Olins AL, et al. Mutations in the gene encoding the laminin B receptor produce an altered nuclear morphology in granulocytes (Pelger-Hüet anomaly). *Nat Genet* 2002;31:410–414.

39. Waterham HR, Koster J, Mooyer P, et al. Autosomal recessive HEM/Greenberg skeletal dysplasia is caused by 3 beta-hydroxysterol delta 14-reductase deficiency due to mutations in the laminin B receptor gene. *Am J Hum Genet* 2003;72:1013–1017.

40. Cicchitto G, Parravicini M, De Lorenzo S, et al. Tuberculosis and Pelger-Hüet anomaly. Case report. *Panminerva Med* 1999;41:367–369.

41. Savage PJ, Dellinger RP, Barnes JV, et al. Pelger-Hüet anomaly of granulocytes in a patient with tuberculosis. *Chest* 1984;85:131–132.

42. Suzuki N, Yasutake T, Ushiyama O, et al. Familial Pelger-Hüet anomaly accompanied by tuberculosis and complicated by acute polyarthritis. *Scand J Rheumatol* 1995;24:319–320.

43. Deutsch PH, Mandell GL. Reversible Pelger-Hüet anomaly associated with ibuprofen therapy. *Arch Intern Med* 1985;145:166.

44. Gondo H, Okamura C, Osaki K, et al. Acquired Pelger-Hüet anomaly in association with concomitant tacrolimus and fluconazole therapy following allogeneic bone marrow transplantation. *Bone Marrow Transplant* 2000;26:1255–1257.

45. Juneja SK, Matthews JP, Luzinat R, et al. Association of acquired Pelger-Hüet anomaly with tactoid therapy. *Br J Haematol* 1996;93:139–141.

46. Kennedy GA, Kay TD, Johnson DW, et al. Neutrophil dysplasia characterised by a pseudo-Pelger-Hüet anomaly occurring with the use of mycophenolate mofetil and ganciclovir following renal transplantation: a report of five cases. *Pathology* 2002;34:263–266.

47. May RB, Sunder TR. Hematologic manifestations of long-term valproate therapy. *Epilepsia* 1993;34:1098–1101.

48. Kornberg A, Goldfarb A, Shalev O. Pseudo-Pelger-Hüet anomaly in chronic lymphocytic leukemia. *Acta Haematol* 1981;66:127–128.

49. Liesveld J, Smith BD. Acquired Pelger-Hüet anomaly in a case of non-Hodgkin's lymphoma. *Acta Haematol* 1988;79:46–49.

50. Fugazza G, Bruzzone R, Puppo L, et al. Granulocytes with segmented nucleus retain normal chromosomes 17 in Philadelphia chromosome-positive chronic myeloid leukemia with i(17q) and pseudo-Pelger anomaly. A case report studied with fluorescence in situ hybridization. *Cancer Genet Cytogenet* 1996;90:166–170.

51. O'Donnell JR, Farrell MA, Fitzgerald MX, et al. Agnogenic myeloid metaplasia preceded by repeated leukemoid reactions and persistent acquired Pelger-Hüet anomaly of granulocytes: case report with review of acquired Pelger-Hüet anomaly. *Cancer* 1982;50:1498–1505.

52. Shetty VT, Mundle SD, Raza A. Pseudo Pelger-Hüet anomaly in myelodysplastic syndrome: hyposegmented apoptotic neutrophil? *Blood* 2001;98:1273–1275.

53. van Hook L, Spivack C, Duncanson FP. Acquired Pelger-Hüet anomaly associated with *Mycoplasma pneumoniae* pneumonia. *Am J Clin Pathol* 1985;84:248–251.

54. Watson N, Dunlop L, Robson L, et al. 17p-syndrome arising from a novel dicentric translocation in a patient with acute myeloid leukemia. *Cancer Genet Cytogenet* 2000;118:159–162.

55. Dale DC, Cottle TE, Fier CJ, et al. Severe chronic neutropenia: treatment and follow-up of patients in the Severe Chronic Neutropenia International Registry. *Am J Hematol* 2003;72:82–93.

56. Germeshausen M, Ballmaier M, Welte K. Implications of mutations in hematopoietic growth factor receptor genes in congenital cytopenias. *Ann N Y Acad Sci* 2001;938:305–320.

57. Hunter MG, Avalos BR. Granulocyte colony-stimulating factor receptor mutations in severe congenital neutropenia transforming to acute myelogenous leukemia confer resistance to apoptosis and enhance cell survival. *Blood* 2000;95:2132–2137.

58. Nakamura K, Kobayashi M, Konishi N, et al. Abnormalities of primitive myeloid progenitor cells expressing granulocyte colony-stimulating factor receptor in patients with severe congenital neutropenia. *Blood* 2000;96:4366–4369.

59. Belkind-Gerson J, Ontiveros-Nevares P, Ocampo-Roosens V, et al. Shwachman-Diamond syndrome in a Mexican family. *Arch Med Res* 2001;32:318–323.

60. Cunningham J, Sales M, Pearce A, et al. Does isochromosome 7q mandate bone marrow transplant in children with Shwachman-Diamond syndrome? *Br J Haematol* 2002;119:1062–1069.

61. Dror Y, Freedman MH. Shwachman-Diamond syndrome marrow cells show abnormally increased apoptosis mediated through the Fas pathway. *Blood* 2001;97:3011–3016.

62. Ginzberg H, Shin J, Ellis L, et al. Segregation analysis in Shwachman-Diamond syndrome: evidence for recessive inheritance. *Am J Hum Genet* 2000;66:1413–1416.

63. Goobie S, Popovic M, Morrison J, et al. Shwachman-Diamond syndrome with exocrine pancreatic dysfunction and bone marrow failure maps to the centromeric region of chromosome 7. *Am J Hum Genet* 2001;68:1048–1054.

64. Jelic TM, Raj AB, Jin B, et al. Expression of CD5 on hematogones in a 7-year-old girl with Shwachman-Diamond syndrome. *Pediatr Dev Pathol* 2001;4:505–511.

65. Klupp N, Simonitsch I, Mannhalter C, et al. Emergence of an unusual bone marrow precursor B-cell population in fatal Shwachman-Diamond syndrome. *Arch Pathol Lab Med* 2000;124:1379–1381.

66. Spirito FR, Crescenzi B, Matteucci C, et al. Cytogenetic characterization of acute myeloid leukemia in Shwachman's syndrome. A case report. *Haematologica* 2000;85:1207–1210.

Constitutional Megakaryocyte and Platelet Disorders

1. Antonucci JV, Martin ES, Hulick PJ, et al. Bernard-Soulier syndrome: common ancestry in two African American families with the GP Ib alpha Leu129Pro mutation. *Am J Hematol* 2000;65:141–148.

2. Vanhoorelbeke K, Schlammadinger A, Delville JP, et al. Occurrence of the Asn45Ser mutation in the GPIX gene in a Belgian patient with Bernard Soulier syndrome. *Platelets* 2001;12:114–120.

3. Ballmaier M, Germeshausen M, Schulze H, et al. c-mpl mutations are the cause of congenital amegakaryocytic thrombocytopenia. *Blood* 2001;97:139–146.

4. Tonelli R, Scardovi AL, Pession A, et al. Compound heterozygosity for two different amino-acid substitution mutations in the thrombopoietin receptor (c-mpl gene) in congenital amegakaryocytic thrombocytopenia (CAMT). *Hum Genet* 2000;107:225–233.

5. van den Oudenrijn S, Bruin M, Folman CC, et al. Mutations in the thrombopoietin receptor, Mpl, in children with congenital amegakaryocytic thrombocytopenia. *Br J Haematol* 2000; 110:441–448.

6. Abe Y, Hirase N, Muta K, et al. Adult onset cyclic hematopoiesis in a patient with myelodysplastic syndrome. *Int J Hematol* 2000; 71:40–45.

7. Fureder W, Mitterbauer G, Thalhammer R, et al. Clonal T cell-mediated cyclic thrombocytopenia. *Br J Haematol* 2002;119: 1059–1061.

8. Junker AK, Poon MC, Hoar DI, et al. Severe combined immune deficiency presenting with cyclic hematopoiesis. *J Clin Immunol* 1991;11:369–377.

9. Wong LC, Rogers M, Lammi A. Severe cyclical thrombocytopenia in a patient with a large lymphatic-venous malformation: a potential association? *Australas J Dermatol* 2001;42: 38–42.

10. Fureder W, Mitterbauer G, Thalhammer R, et al. Clonal T cell-mediated cyclic thrombocytopenia. *Br J Haematol* 2002;119: 1059–1061.

11. Kojima K, Fujii N, Omoto E, et al. Cyclic thrombocytopenia and polycythemia vera. *Ann Hematol* 2003;82:61–63.

12. Rice L, Nichol JL, McMillan R, et al. Cyclic immune thrombocytopenia responsive to thrombopoietic growth factor therapy. *Am J Hematol* 2001;68:210–214.

13. Demeter J, Lelkes G, Nemes L, et al. Familial occurrence of the May-Hegglin anomaly: is the accompanying renal failure part of a new subentity? *Ann Hematol* 2001;80:368–371.

14. Kelley MJ, Jawien W, Ortel TL, et al. Mutation of MYH9, encoding non-muscle myosin heavy chain A, in May-Hegglin anomaly. *Nat Genet* 2000;26:106–108.

15. Kunishima S, Kojima T, Matsushita T, et al. Mutations in the NMMHC-A gene cause autosomal dominant macrothrombocytopenia with leukocyte inclusions (May-Hegglin anomaly/Sebastian syndrome). *Blood* 2001;97:1147–1149.

16. Kunishima S, Matsushita T, Kojima T, et al. Identification of six novel MYH9 mutations and genotype-phenotype relationships in autosomal dominant macrothrombocytopenia with leukocyte inclusions. *J Hum Genet* 2001;46:722–729.

17. McBane RD, Elliott MA, White JG, et al. Fechtner syndrome: physiologic analysis of macrothrombocytopenia. *Blood Coagul Fibrinolysis* 2000;11:243–247.

18. Seri M, Cusano R, Gangarossa S, et al. Mutations in MYH9 result in the May-Hegglin anomaly, and Fechtner and Sebastian syndromes. *Nat Genet* 2000;26:103–105.

19. Toren A, Rozenfeld-Granot G, Rocca B, et al. Autosomal-dominant giant platelet syndromes: a hint of the same genetic defect as in Fechtner syndrome owing to a similar genetic linkage to chromosome 22q11-13. *Blood* 2000;96:3447–3451.

20. Drouin A, Favier R, Masse JM, et al. Newly recognized cellular abnormalities in the gray platelet syndrome. *Blood* 2001;98: 1382–1391.

21. Falik-Zaccai TC, Anikster Y, Rivera CE, et al. A new genetic isolate of gray platelet syndrome (GPS): clinical, cellular, and hematologic characteristics. *Mol Genet Metab* 2001;74: 303–313.

22. Lages B, Sussman II, Levine SP, et al. Platelet alpha granule deficiency associated with decreased P-selectin and selective impairment of thrombin-induced activation in a new patient with gray platelet syndrome (alpha-storage pool deficiency). *J Lab Clin Med* 1997;129:364–375.

23. Toyota S, Nakamura N, Dan K. Pseudo gray platelet syndrome in a patient with acute myocardial infarction. *Int J Hematol* 2002;76:376–378.

24. Huizing M, Anikster Y, Gahl WA. Hermansky-Pudlak syndrome

25. Krisp A, Hoffman R, Happle R, et al. Hermansky-Pudlak syndrome. *Eur J Dermatol* 2001;11:372–373.

26. Sarangarajan R, Budev A, Zhao Y, et al. Abnormal translocation of tyrosinase and tyrosinase-related protein 1 in cutaneous melanocytes of Hermansky-Pudlak Syndrome and in melanoma cells transfected with anti-sense HPS1 cDNA. *J Invest Dermatol* 2001;117:641–646.

27. Krishnamurti L, Neglia JP, Nagarajan R, et al. Paris-Trousseau syndrome platelets in a child with Jacobsen's syndrome. *Am J Hematol* 2001;66:295–299.

28. Matheisel A, Babinska M, Wierzba J, et al. A case with 47,XXY,del(11)(q23) karyotype-coexistence of Jacobsen and Klinefelter syndromes. *Genet Couns* 2000;11:267–271.

29. al-Jefri AH, Dror Y, Bussel JB, et al. Thrombocytopenia with absent radii: frequency of marrow megakaryocyte progenitors, proliferative characteristics, and megakaryocyte growth and development factor responsiveness. *Pediatr Hematol Oncol* 2000; 17:299–306.

30. Bradshaw A, Donnelly LF, Foreman JW. Thrombocytopenia and absent radii (TAR) syndrome associated with horseshoe kidney. *Pediatr Nephrol* 2000;14:29–31.

31. Fadoo Z, Naqvi SM. Acute myeloid leukemia in a patient with thrombocytopenia with absent radii syndrome. *J Pediatr Hematol Oncol* 2002;24:134–135.

32. Letestu R, Vitrat N, Masse A, et al. Existence of a differentiation blockage at the stage of megakaryocyte precursor in the thrombocytopenia and absent radii (TAR) syndrome. *Blood* 2000;95:1633–1641.

33. Caron E. Regulation of Wiskott-Aldrich syndrome protein and related molecules. *Curr Opin Cell Biol* 2002;14:82–87.

34. El-Hakeh J, Rosenzweig S, Oleastro M, et al. Wiskott-Aldrich syndrome in Argentina: 17 unique, including nine novel, mutations. *Hum Mutat* 2002;19:186–187.

35. Snapper SB, Rosen FS. A family of WASPs. *N Engl J Med* 2003;348:4350–4351.

36. Drachman JG, Jarvik GP, Mehaffey MG. Autosomal dominant thrombocytopenia: incomplete megakaryocyte differentiation and linkage to human chromosome 10. *Blood* 2000;96: 118–125.

37. Fabris F, Cordiano I, Steffan A, et al. Indirect study of thrombopoiesis (TPO, reticulated platelets, glycocalicin) in patients with hereditary macrothrombocytopenia. *Eur J Haematol* 2000;64: 151–156.

38. Freson K, Devriendt K, Matthijs G, et al. Platelet characteristics in patients with X-linked macrothrombocytopenia because of a novel GATA1 mutation. *Blood* 2001;98:85–92.

39. Khabbaze Y, Karayalcin G, Paley C, et al. Thrombocytopenia absent corpus callosum syndrome: third case of a distinct clinical entity. *J Pediatr Hematol Oncol* 2001;23:469–471.

40. Kunishima S, Naoe T, Kamiya T, et al. Novel heterozygous missense mutation in the platelet glycoprotein Ib beta gene associated with isolated giant platelet disorder. *Am J Hematol* 2001;68:249–255.

41. Mhawech P, Saleem A. Inherited giant platelet disorders: classification and literature review. *Am J Clin Pathol* 2000;113:176–192.

42. Thompson AA, Woodruff K, Feig SA, et al. Congenital thrombocytopenia and radio-ulnar synostosis: a new familial syndrome. *Br J Haematol* 2001;113:866–870.

43. Willig TB, Breton-Gorius J, Elbim C, et al. Macrothrombocytopenia with abnormal demarcation membranes in megakaryocytes and neutropenia with a complete lack of sialyl-Lewis-X antigen in leukocytes—new syndrome? *Blood* 2001;97:826–828.

and Chediak-Higashi syndrome: disorders of vesicle formation and trafficking. *Thromb Haemost* 2001;86:233–245.

ERYTHROCYTES

CAROLYN CHILING CHAI

Red blood cells (RBCs) decrease in size as they mature and lose the nucleus. Cytoplasm changes from blue to pink-orange as it acquires hemoglobin (Hb). The average diameter of a mature RBC is 7–9 μm and the mean corpuscular volume (MCV) is 90 fL. The RBC membrane contains proteins, including cytoskeleton and cell antigens. The main function of the RBCs is to produce Hb.

RBCs with an enlarged central pallor are hypochromic. Defect in Hb synthesis usually leads to hypochromasia and decreased mean corpuscular Hb concentration (MCHC). A typical example is iron deficiency anemia. Hypochromasia may also be seen in lead poisoning and water artifact, although the central pallor in the latter is distinctly outlined. Hypochromic cells may not be microcytic (e.g., target cells). Conversely, normocytes or macrocytes may also be hypochromic. When RBCs are prematurely released to the circulation, they are large and polychromatic (blue-gray) owing to residual cytoplasmic RNA and are called reticulocytes. The normal value of the reticulocyte is 0.5% to 2.5%. During RBC regeneration (effective erythropoiesis) as in hemorrhage, hemolysis, or anemia treatment, the reticulocyte count and polychromasia are increased proportionately. Reticulocytes can be viewed with a supravital stain.

RED BLOOD CELL MORPHOLOGY AND IRON METABOLISM

The main hematopoietic sites in adults are the vertebrae, pelvis, ribs, sternum, skull, and proximal ends of the long bones. There, the RBCs originate from a pluripotent stem cell, the colony-forming unit stem. During differentiation, they become erythroid-committed burst-forming unit erythroids that mature into colony-forming unit erythroids. Erythropoietin stimulates burst-forming unit erythroids and colony-forming unit erythroids to differentiate to pronormoblasts, the first precursor recognizable by light microscope, which gives rise to 16 mature erythrocytes through four cell divisions in 72 hours. These four divisions, in sequential order, produce basophilic normoblasts, polychromatophilic normoblasts, orthochromatophilic normoblasts,

and reticulocytes. Reticulocytes eventually extrude RNA to become erythrocytes. Effective erythropoiesis is the rate of release of newly formed RBCs from bone marrow, and ineffective erythropoiesis is the rate of loss of potential erythrocytes as a result of phagocytosis (1–5).

Most RBCs are destroyed in the reticuloendothelial system. Extravascular hemolysis indicates RBC destruction by phagocytosis in the reticuloendothelial system. The spleen is the principal site of erythrocyte phagocytosis with normal aging. The liver plays a more active role in the removal of damaged RBCs. Extremely damaged cells may lyse within the circulation before reaching the liver or spleen, which is referred to as intravascular hemolysis.

OVERVIEW OF ERYTHROCYTE MORPHOLOGY

Red Blood Cell Size

A normal RBC is a biconcave disk with a diameter of 7–9 μm. A normocyte indicates a RBC with a mean corpuscular volume (MCV) of 75 to 100 fL (Fig. 6-1).

Microcytes are RBCs with an MCV of less than 80 fL. Any defect in Hb synthesis results in hypochromic microcytes

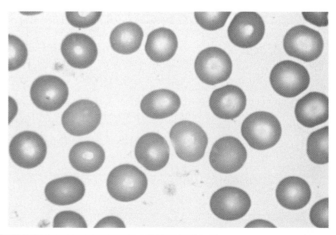

FIGURE 6-1. Normal red blood cell (normocytes) in peripheral blood.

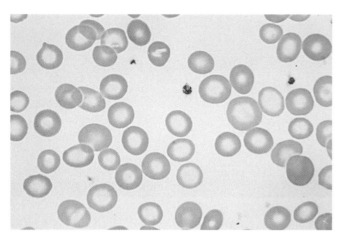

FIGURE 6-2. Hypochromic microcytic red blood cells in the peripheral blood smear from a patient with iron deficiency anemia.

(Fig. 6-2). The defect may be owing to the iron supply, absorption, release, or utilization, as in iron deficiency anemia, or globin synthesis, as in thalassemia and hemoglobinopathy. Although porphyrin synthesis is important for Hb synthesis, its deficiency typically does not cause decreased RBC size.

Macrocytes are RBCs with an MCV of more than 100 fL. Macrocyte formation may result from impaired DNA synthesis (megaloblastic erythropoiesis), accelerated erythropoiesis with early release of reticulocytes, or increased membrane cholesterol or lecithin, as found in liver disease. Macroovalocytes lack a central pallor and are characteristic of megaloblastic anemia (Fig. 6-3). Round macrocytes are seen in liver disease, chronic alcoholism, chemotherapy, hypothyroidism, and neonatal blood and after splenectomy. In patients with *Mycoplasma pneumoniae* infection or cold agglutinin disease, the MCV may be artificially elevated because of RBC doublets or triplets.

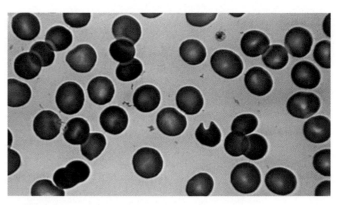

FIGURE 6-4. Normochromic normocytic red blood cells with a bite cell in the center of the field.

Red Blood Cell Shape

Acanthocytes (spur cells) are RBCs with pointed membrane spicules of uneven length. The most common inherited condition is abetalipoproteinemia. Acquired conditions include liver disease, splenectomy, and malabsorption. In contrast to burr cells, acanthocytes cannot regain a normal shape.

Bite cells are semicircle remnants of RBCs after being partially phagocytosed or after extrusion of the Heinz body from the RBC. They are seen in glucose-6-phosphate dehydrogenase deficiency, unstable Hb, and oxidant hemolysis in which the Heinz body is pitting by the spleen (Fig. 6-4).

Burr cells are an acquired RBC membrane abnormality with short, evenly spaced spicules. They are seen in uremia, liver disease, burns, pyruvate kinase deficiency, gastric ulcers, and cancer. They are difficult to distinguish from echinocytes. The spicules of burr cells may revert to normal (Fig. 6-5).

Codocytes (target cells) have a dense central Hb surrounded by a colorless ring owing to membrane redundancy. The osmotic fragility is reduced. Codocytes are characteristic of thalassemia, hemoglobinopathy, liver disease, and iron deficiency anemia and are seen after splenectomy (Fig. 6-5).

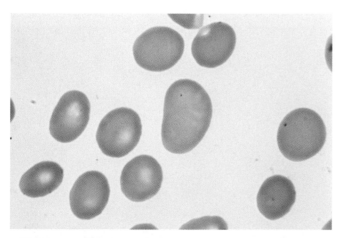

FIGURE 6-3. Macrocytes in the peripheral blood smear from a patient with vitamin B_{12} deficiency. A macroovalocyte is in the center of the field.

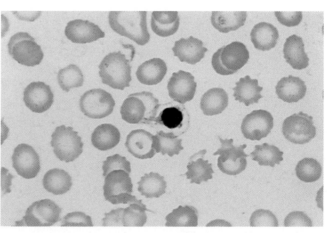

FIGURE 6-5. Peripheral blood smear contains burr cells and a target cell in the center of the field.

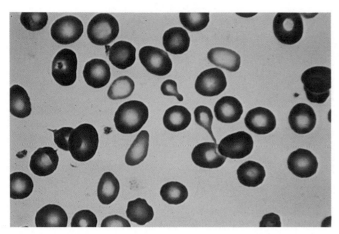

FIGURE 6-6. Peripheral blood smear contains occasional dacrocytes.

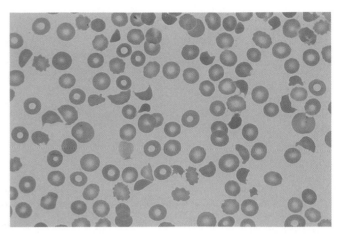

FIGURE 6-8. Peripheral blood smear contains schistocytes and increased reticulocytes in a patient with thrombotic thrombocytopenic purpura.

Dacrocytes (teardrop cells) are drop-shaped RBCs seen in myelofibrosis and myelopathies. They may also be seen in thalassemia, iron deficiency, and conditions in which Heinz bodies are formed (Fig. 6-6).

Drepanocytes (sickle cells) are crescent-shaped RBCs that are pointed at both ends as a result of Hb polymerization in low oxygen tension. They are typical of sickle cell disease. On oxygenation, most sickle cells revert to normal.

Echinocytes (crenated cells) have uniform blunt membrane spicules and represent artifact. They are difficult to distinguish from burr cells.

Elliptocytes are pencil-shaped RBCs similar to ovalocytes. They are most often seen in hereditary elliptocytosis (Fig. 6-7).

Ovalocytes are egg-shaped RBCs with varying Hb content. Although the exact mechanism is unclear, an ovalocyte is highly variable and may appear normochromic or hypochromic and normocytic or macrocytic. They are often seen in megaloblastic anemia (Fig. 6-3).

Schistocytes are RBC fragments caused by mechanical injury, commonly seen in malignant hypertension, vasculitis, thrombotic thrombocytopenic purpura, hemolytic uremic syndrome, disseminated intravascular coagulation, and heart valve replacement. Membrane defects such as spherocytes and antibody-binding RBCs may cause decreased cell survival and therefore increased schistocytes (Fig. 6-8).

Spherocytes are small, round RBCs with a decreased surface-to-volume ratio, a lower MCV, and no central pallor. The MCHC is elevated (>36%). They are characteristic of hereditary spherocytosis, immune hemolytic anemia, and transfusion reaction (Fig. 6-9).

Stomatocytes are RBCs with a slitlike central pallor. Some drugs (e.g., chlorpromazine and phenothiazine) may induce reversible stomatocytosis. They are seen in hereditary stomatocytosis, alcohol toxicity, liver disease, and the Rh null phenotype. More commonly, stomatocytes present as artifact (Fig. 6-10).

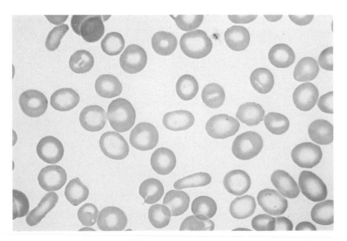

FIGURE 6-7. Peripheral blood smear contains occasional elliptocytes.

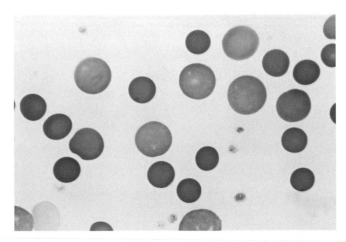

FIGURE 6-9. Peripheral blood smear contains spherocytes in a patient with autoimmune hemolytic anemia.

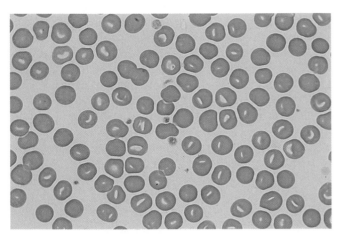

FIGURE 6-10. Peripheral blood smear contains stomatocytes in a patient with hereditary stomatocytosis.

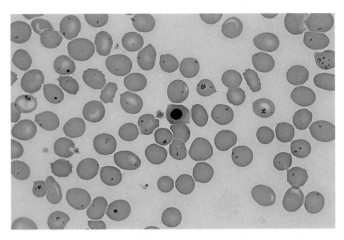

FIGURE 6-12. Peripheral blood smear contains many Howell-Jolly bodies in a patient after a splenectomy.

Red Blood Cell Inclusions

Basophilic stippling represents ribosomes and mitochondrial remnants distributed homogeneously over the cells. It is seen in arsenic and lead poisoning, thalassemia, megaloblastic anemia, alcoholism, and conditions causing accelerated heme synthesis (Fig. 6-11).

A Cabot ring is a ring or figure 8–like structure that appears reddish blue on Romanowsky stain. It contains arginine-rich histone and nonheme iron and represents mitotic spindles or microtubule remnants. It may be seen in megaloblastic anemia, hemolysis, overwhelming infection, lead poisoning, myelodysplasia, and thalassemia and after splenectomy.

Heinz bodies are 1–3 μm, denatured Hb attached to RBC membranes and are best visualized with crystal violet, brilliant cresyl blue, or methylene blue stains. They are seen in glucose-6-phosphate dehydrogenase deficiency, α thalassemia, unstable hemoglobinopathy syndromes, chemical insult, and oxidant stress. Multiple Heinz bodies give the RBC a golf ball appearance.

Howell-Jolly bodies are nuclear remnants. Normally, the spleen pits these fragments effectively. During stress, inclusion formation exceeds the splenic pitting mechanism and Howell-Jolly bodies appear. They are seen after splenectomy or in hemolytic anemia, thalassemia, megaloblastic anemia, and alcoholism (Fig. 6-12).

Pappenheimer bodies (siderotic granules) are nonheme iron at the cell periphery. Perls Prussian blue stain reveals siderotic granules as small magenta inclusions. On Wright stain, they are called Pappenheimer bodies. Siderotic granules are seen in sideroblastic anemia, hemoglobinopathy, hemochromatosis, and hemosiderosis and after splenectomy (Fig. 6-13).

Red Blood Cell Distribution

Agglutination appears as RBC clumping throughout the blood smear at room temperature. Sample warming may

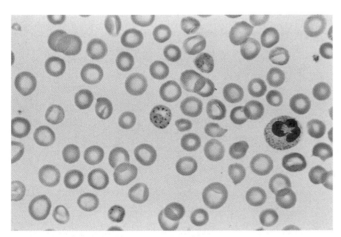

FIGURE 6-11. Peripheral blood smear from a patient with lead poisoning. The red blood cell in the center of the field shows basophilic stippling.

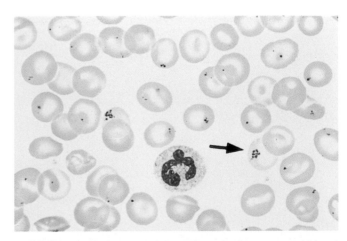

FIGURE 6-13. Peripheral blood smear contains many red blood cells with Pappenheimer bodies (siderotic granules) *(arrow).*

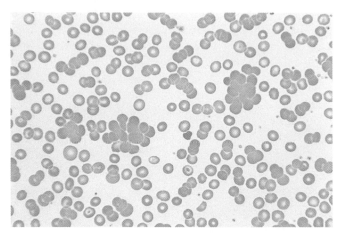

FIGURE 6-14. Peripheral blood smear shows red blood cell agglutination in a patient with cold agglutinin disease.

disperse agglutination, but saline dilution has no effect. It occurs when an antibody corresponding to a patient's RBC antigen is present in his or her plasma. This may be seen in cold agglutinin disease or paroxysmal cold hemoglutinuria (Fig. 6-14).

Rouleau formation results from elevated plasma globin. RBCs appear as stacks of coins. In contrast to agglutination, saline dilution disperses rouleaux. Rouleaux are common in multiple myeloma, Waldenström macroglobulinemia, chronic lymphocytic leukemia, and hyperproteinemia (Fig. 6-15).

HEMOLYTIC ANEMIA

Hemolytic anemia may be congenital or acquired. The congenital abnormalities include those of RBC membrane, enzymes, or Hb structure and synthesis and are discussed in Chapter 5. Acquired hemolytic anemia may be immune mediated drug-induced, infection-related, due to burns, or microangiopathic, which are characterized by macrocytosis,

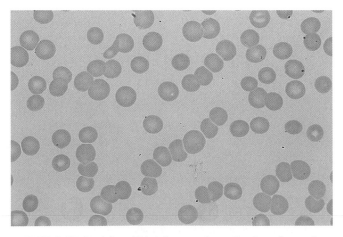

FIGURE 6-15. Peripheral blood smear shows Rouleau formation.

polychromasia, and reticulocytosis. Immune hemolytic anemia shows a positive Coombs or direct antiglobulin test and microspherocytosis. Microangiopathic hemolytic anemia is characterized by peripheral RBC fragments (schistocytes), a decreased serum haptoglobin level, and, in many cases, evidence of coagulopathy. The degree of erythropoiesis is commensurate with the degree of anemia and hemolysis. Concomitant megakaryocytic hyperplasia is often present. Macrophages and erythrophagocytic activity may be increased. Dyserythropoiesis may be present, likely owing to the stress of rapid erythrocyte production. Anemia develops when RBC destruction surpasses production.

Hemolysis can be intravascular (1) or extravascular. Most hemolysis is extravascular because of phagocytosis by mononuclear phagocytic cells, occurring in the liver, spleen, and bone marrow (2–4). Heme degradation produces bilirubin, which binds to albumin when entering the liver. In the liver, the water-insoluble bilirubin is converted to a soluble form and excreted in the bile, which is then converted to urobilinogen by the intestinal bacteria and eliminated in feces. Some urobilinogen is reabsorbed from the gut and excreted in urine. Patients with extravascular hemolysis have jaundice, elevated bilirubin, and elevated urine and fecal urobilinogen.

In intravascular hemolysis, Hb is released to bind haptoglobin; the resulting Hb-haptoglobin complex is then cleared by the liver. A reduction in plasma haptoglobin indicates intravascular hemolysis. When hemolysis exceeds the Hb-binding capacity of the haptoglobin, free Hb appears in the plasma and causes hemoglobinemia. Free Hb passes through renal glomeruli to cause hemoglobinuria. Heme from the circulating Hb binds hemopexin to form a heme-hemopexin complex, which is then removed by the liver. When hemopexin is exhausted, hematin is formed and binds albumin to produce methemalbumin. Methemalbumin gives plasma a brown color. Thus, in addition to reduced haptoglobin, other changes in intravascular hemolysis include reduced hemopexin, methemalbuminemia, hemoglobinemia, hemoglobinuria, and hemosiderinuria.

Immune Hemolytic Anemia

As the most common form of acquired hemolysis, immune hemolytic anemia can be classified as autoimmune, alloimmune, or drug induced (5). Whichever the etiology, the characteristic features are microspherocytes. Erythroid hyperplasia occurs in all hemolytic disorders, but bone marrow examination usually is not required.

Autoimmune Hemolytic Anemia

Autoimmune hemolytic anemia indicates premature RBC destruction by autoantibodies. It may be idiopathic or secondary to malignancy, infection, graft versus host disease, or drugs and can be induced by warm or cold antibodies.

Warm autoimmune hemolytic anemia accounts for as much as 70% of autoimmune hemolytic anemia; most cases are extravascular and do not cause autoagglutination. It is usually caused by immunoglobulin (Ig) G, although IgM and IgA may be detected. Fc receptor-mediated immune adherence to RBCs and complement-mediated hemolysis are proposed mechanisms. The presence of complement on RBCs facilitates IgG-mediated phagocytosis. The most useful test for diagnosing warm autoimmune hemolytic anemia is direct antiglobulin test (Coombs), using IgG, with or without complement C3d. Warm autoantibody usually has specificity for Rh antigen, although other antigens have been described. Spherocytosis in peripheral blood indicates hemolysis. Marked reticulocytosis reflects marrow compensation for RBC loss. The indirect Coombs test may detect circulating antibodies when hemolysis is active. Coombs-negative autoimmune hemolytic anemia may be caused by a low RBC antibody titer or hemolytic anemia with an antibody other than IgG.

Corticosteroids and splenectomy are used in the treatment of warm autoimmune hemolytic anemia. After undergoing a splenectomy, patients should be vaccinated against *Streptococcus pneumoniae*, meningococcus, and *Haemophilus influenzae*.

Cold autoimmune hemolytic anemia (cold agglutinin syndrome) is complement-mediated hemolysis at temperatures of 10° to 30°C and is most common in the elderly. Cold autoantibodies are usually IgM, with 15% being biphasic IgG (Donath-Landsteiner cold autoantibody), especially in pediatric patients. The most common antibody in cold autoimmune hemolytic anemia is anti-I in *M. pneumoniae* and infectious mononucleosis.

RBCs agglutinate at body extremities when the temperature is lower than 30°C. The complement is activated, and hemolysis is more likely when thermal reactivity is more than 30°C. Occasionally, blood films show neutrophil-RBC rosettes. A Coombs test is positive for C3d but negative for IgG. Pathologic anti-I antibody has a broad thermal range

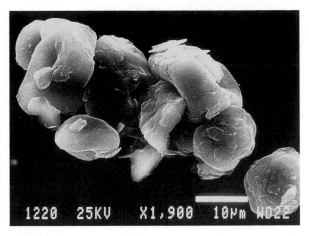

FIGURE 6-16. Scanning electron microscopy shows red blood cell agglutination.

(0°–32°C), whereas normal anti-I in healthy people has a thermal range of 0° to 22°C. This difference is significant because complement is most hemolytic at 22°C or higher and pathologic anti-I is able to cause hemolysis. Examined at room temperature, peripheral blood shows RBC agglutination (Fig. 6-16). At 37°C, the agglutination is reversed (Fig. 6-17).

Paroxysmal cold hemoglobinuria accounts for 35% to 40% of acute transient hemolytic anemia in children during viral infections (e.g., measles, mumps, influenza, chickenpox). Syphilis infection may also result in paroxysmal cold hemoglobinuria. It is caused by a cold biphasic IgG (Donath-Landsteiner cold autoantibody), mostly IgG3, against blood group P antigen. Antibody binds RBCs at cold temperatures in the peripheral circulation. The complement is activated, and intravascular hemolysis occurs when RBCs return to a warmer temperature (37°C).

Both direct and indirect antiglobulin tests are available. The indirect test has a higher sensitivity. The Coombs test is

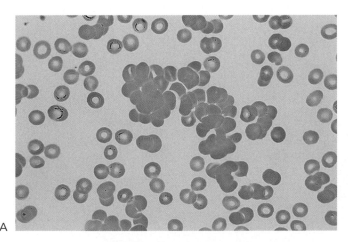

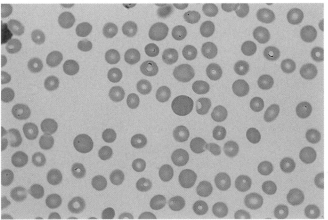

A   B

FIGURE 6-17. **A:** Peripheral blood smear shows red blood cell agglutination (room temperature) in a patient with cold agglutinin disease. **B:** Peripheral blood smear shows dissolution of red blood cell agglutination at 37°C in the same patient with cold agglutinin disease. Note the increased number of reticulocytes.

performed by incubating the sample at 0°C for 60 minutes and then at 37°C for 30 minutes. If Donath-Landsteiner cold autoantibody is present, it binds RBCs at cold temperatures and hemolysis occurs on warming. The indirect test is performed by mixing the patient's serum with P antigen–positive RBCs and then adding fresh serum as a complement source for hemolysis. Staying warm usually avoids hemolysis. Symptomatic patients may require transfusion.

Alloimmune Hemolytic Anemia

Alloimmune hemolytic anemia occurs when the immune system is sensitized to another individual's RBC antigen and an antibody is formed. The most common forms are hemolytic transfusion reaction and hemolytic disease of the newborn.

Hemolytic Transfusion Reaction

The acute transfusion reaction accounts for more than 80% of hemolytic transfusion reactions; most are owing to ABO incompatibility, usually caused by IgM (6,7). The blood film shows both agglutination and spherocytosis in massive hemolysis. If the antibody was not previously present, a less severe delayed hemolytic reaction occurs in 7 to 14 days. Although most patients were previously alloimmunized, this antibody becomes undetectable over time, and the only evidence may be a positive Coombs test result. The antibody in delayed reaction is usually IgG against Rh, Duffy, and Kidd blood groups, and hemolysis is extravascular.

Hemolytic disease of the newborn is also called erythroblastosis fetalis. During pregnancy, the maternal IgG is transferred to the fetus through the placenta. Hemolysis occurs when there is blood group incompatibility between the mother and the fetus. Antibodies against Rh, ABO, and Kell blood groups are the major causes, with anti-D antibody being more severe. This usually occurs in the second and subsequent pregnancies. Infants are anemic and jaundiced with hepatosplenomegaly. Severely affected infants have kernicterus. Stillbirths may occur. Rh-negative women should receive Rh Ig at 28 weeks' gestation and within 72 hours of exposure to RhD + RBCs. The Kleihauer-Betke test or flow cytometry analysis is useful in determining the amount of fetal cells in maternal blood so that the amount of Rh Ig can be adjusted.

Drug-Induced Hemolytic Anemia

Drug-induced hemolysis may be immune mediated or caused by oxidative injury. The former can be intravascular or extravascular hemolysis and is usually caused by one of three mechanisms: autoantibody production similar to warm autoimmune hemolytic anemia (e.g., α-methyldopa) in which the antibody directs against Rh antigen in many patients; hapten-dependent antibody formation (e.g., penicillin); and

formation of an antibody-protein complex (e.g., quinine, quinidine, rifampin). Hemolytic anemia is usually reversible on discontinuation of the drug. The Coombs test is positive in many patients and may continue to be positive for as long as 2 years after hemolysis resolves. The strength and blood level of the oxidant and the congenital deficiency of glucose-6-phosphate dehydrogenase or glutathione-dependent pathways determine the oxidative injury. Older RBCs are more prone to oxidative injury. The characteristic features of oxidative hemolysis include the formation of methemoglobin, sulfhemoglobin, and Heinz bodies.

Drugs likely causing oxidative hemolysis include nitrofurantoin, dapsone, aminosalicylic acid, and, rarely, high-dose oxygen treatment in vitamin E deficiency. Demonstration of drug-dependent hemagglutination with the Coombs test confirms the diagnosis.

Nonimmune Hemolytic Anemia

Infection

Infection-induced hemolysis may be caused by malaria, *Clostridium perfringens*, *Toxoplasma gondii*, or other microorganisms (Fig. 6-18). Microorganisms injure RBCs through different mechanisms including physical invasion, hemolysin secretion, antibody formation, and infection-associated disseminated intravascular coagulation. Antibiotics may also cause hemolysis. In some cases, multiple mechanisms coexist.

Mechanical Injury

Mechanical injury includes large-vessel hemolytic anemia (malignant hypertension, prosthetic heart valves) and microangiopathic hemolytic anemia seen in thrombotic thrombocytopenic purpura, hemolytic uremic syndrome, disseminated intravascular coagulation, autoimmune vasculitis, and

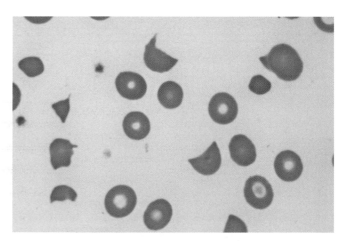

FIGURE 6-18. Peripheral blood smear contains schistocytes in a patient with meningococcal septicemia.

march hemoglobinuria. The peripheral blood smear usually contains burr cells and schistocytes.

Thermal and Osmotic Injury

RBCs are very fragile to high temperature exposure and changes in osmotic pressure. A burn results in fragmentation and membrane loss of RBCs with formation of microspherocytes, schistocytes, and burr cells. Hemoglobinemia and hemoglobinuria occur the first day after a burn. The morphologic damage is self-limiting. Freshwater or saltwater drowning causes hemolysis because of the abrupt osmotic change in pulmonary circulation.

Others

Nonimmune mechanisms occur in industrial toxins such as copper and arsine and do not involve antibody formation.

Other Causes of Hemolytic Anemia

Paroxysmal Nocturnal Hemoglobinuria

Paroxysmal nocturnal hemoglobinuria (PNH) is a rare acquired form of intravascular hemolysis caused by an abnormal clone of pluripotent stem cells with sensitivity to complement. All hematopoietic cell lines are affected (8).

Up to 20 proteins may be missing from the RBC surface in patients with PNH, with glycosyl-phosphatidylinositol being the essential glycolipid anchoring the proteins to the RBC membrane. The defect of glycosyl-phosphatidylinositol synthesis is caused by a mutation of the pig A gene at chromosome Xp22.1. Deficiency of the decay-accelerating factor (CD55), homologous restriction factor, or membrane inhibitor of reactive lysis (CD59) accelerates a complement complex and gives rise to episodic hemolysis, particularly at night when the pH is decreased (9). Three types of complement sensitivity are detected in PNH: RBCs in PNH-I react normally in the presence of complement, whereas PNH-II cells are three to five times more susceptible to lysis. PNH-III cells have 20 times or higher susceptibility to lysis. The level of deficiency provides information on the disease severity.

Peripheral blood shows pancytopenia and lower leukocyte alkaline phosphatase activity in the neutrophils. Bone marrow is hypoplastic despite significant hemolysis. Storage iron is deficient. The sucrose hemolysis test is the screening test, with more than 5% RBC lysis indicating PNH. The Ham test is confirmatory when the complement fixes the RBCs at a lower pH. RBCs from patients with PNH lyse, whereas normal RBCs are resistant to lysis. Flow cytometry provides a sensitive and specific measure. CD59 and CD55 detection may exclude other causes of hemolysis and quantitate the abnormal clones into partial or complete deficiency.

Cytogenetic analysis demonstrates the loss of chromosome Y and trisomy 9 in some patients.

Patients with PNH may progress to aplastic anemia or acute myelogenous leukemia, which can be complicated by thrombotic episodes at uncommon sites.

REVIEW OF IRON METABOLISM

The Hb molecule consists of iron, protoporphyrin IX, and globin. Deficiency of any of these results in Hb deficiency. Three major mechanisms are involved in abnormal iron metabolism: decreased iron supply (iron deficiency anemia), defective recycling of storage iron (anemia of chronic disease), and defective iron utilization (sideroblastic anemia, lead poisoning).

Animals and plants provide sufficient iron. Iron absorption depends on its supply, storage, and demand. A healthy adult absorbs 1 to 2 mg of iron daily. Dietary iron is in ferric form, converted to ferrous form in the stomach for absorption. Once in the blood, ferrous iron is reconverted to ferric form by ferroxidase and transported to transferrin. Once bound to transferrin, iron is delivered to tissue and organs freely. In the liver, iron is released from transferrin to form ferritin, the storage form. Hemosiderin is another storage iron in lysosomes of macrophages. Hemosiderin is typically visualized by Perls stain.

Each milliliter of RBC production requires 1 mg of iron. A healthy adult loses 20 to 25 mL of RBCs daily (1% of RBCs); therefore, 20 to 25 mg of iron is needed daily. Of these, 5% (1–2 mg) comes from the dietary supply and 95% comes from the recycling of senescent RBCs. This recycling recovers all iron except that lost from feces, urine, sweat, desquamation, and menstruation.

MICROCYTOSIS AND MICROCYTIC ANEMIA

Microcytic anemia is defined as the presence of small, often hypochromatic RBCs in the peripheral blood smear, characterized by a low MCV (<75 fL). Despite an abundant iron supply, iron deficiency anemia is the most common cause of microcytic anemia in the world. In adults, anemia of chronic disease is probably more common. The differential diagnosis includes thalassemia minor, hemoglobinopathy, and sideroblastic anemia.

Diagnosing iron deficiency in the elderly is difficult because of the common presence of chronic disease, which causes a high ferritin level. Recent studies suggested that the transferrin receptor–ferritin index is a more sensitive iron measurement and is able to diagnose iron deficiency anemia with a higher sensitivity (88%) (1–4). In microcytic or normocytic anemia, a bone marrow examination is still the gold standard to distinguish iron deficiency anemia from noniron deficiency anemia (5–13).

TABLE 6-1. DIFFERENTIAL DIAGNOSIS OF MICROCYTOSIS AND MICROCYTIC ANEMIA

Iron deficiency
Thalassemia and hemoglobinopathy
Sideroblastic anemia
Inflammation
Chronic renal failure

The main differential diagnosis of microcytosis includes, in decreasing frequency, iron deficiency anemia, thalassemia minor, inflammation, or chronic renal failure. In patients with normocytic anemia, disseminated malignancy and acute blood loss should always be considered (14,15) (Table 6-1).

Iron Deficiency Anemia

Iron deficiency anemia results from insufficient storage iron. It may be caused by inadequate intake, increased demand, or increased loss. Clinical manifestations range from asymptomatic to mild to severe. The process can be divided into three stages.

Stage 1 (iron depletion) starts when storage iron is used. Serum ferritin and marrow hemosiderin are decreased, and the latter may be absent. In response, iron absorption from the gastrointestinal mucosa is increased. Peripheral blood findings, including the RBC count, Hb level, reticulocyte count, and the serum iron level, are normal. A persistent negative balance leads to iron exhaustion and the development of iron-deficient erythropoiesis.

Stage 2 (iron-deficient erythropoiesis) starts when the serum iron level and transferrin saturation decrease. Serum transferrin (to increase iron absorption) and free erythrocyte protoporphyrin are elevated as a result of erythroid hyperplasia. The RBC count and morphology remain normal.

Stage 3 (iron deficiency anemia) is characterized by hypochromic microcytic anemia. Peripheral blood shows decreased Hb, MCV, MCHC, and an elevated RBC distribution width. RBCs are hypochromic microcytic with poikilocytosis (elliptocytes, ovalocytes, folded forms) (Fig. 6-19). The reticulocyte count is typically normal or slightly elevated, and the platelet count is often elevated. The bone marrow biopsy specimen shows ineffective erythropoiesis with small normoblasts containing scanty cytoplasm and ragged cytoplasmic borders. The dysplastic changes of the erythroid series are not prominent in patients with iron deficiency (Fig. 6-20). Perls stain reveals absent storage iron. When bleeding is the primary cause of iron deficiency anemia, leukocytosis and thrombocytosis may occur.

The classic signs include pallor, glossitis, koilonychias, and systolic heart murmur. Pica and angular stomatitis are common. Without treatment, patients may reveal decreased myeloperoxidase or T-cell activity, although these deficits are difficult to measure. Serum ferritin and free erythrocyte

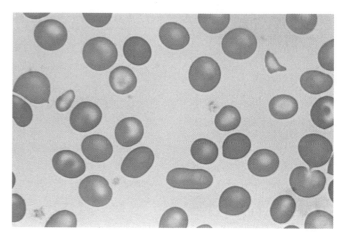

FIGURE 6-19. Peripheral blood smear shows hypochromic microcytic anemia with a patient with iron deficiency anemia.

protoporphyrin become abnormal early in the course, before morphologic and Hb changes. Measurement of serum iron, ferritin, total iron-binding capacity, and transferrin saturation provide an overall diagnosis of iron deficiency anemia. Serum iron and iron saturation are decreased. Free erythrocyte protoporphyrin and total iron-binding capacity are elevated.

The main differential diagnosis includes constitutional disorders of iron metabolism and defective iron reutilization syndrome, which shows hypochromic microcytic anemia, low serum iron, low to normal iron-binding capacity, high serum ferritin, and increased bone marrow iron without ringed sideroblasts.

Finding the underlying cause and providing an iron supplement are the mainstay of treatment. The reticulocyte count begins to increase in a few days and reaches a maximum in 7 to 10 days. The Hb normalizes in 2 months.

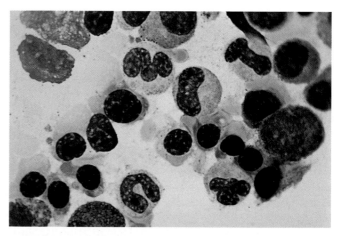

FIGURE 6-20. Bone marrow aspirate smear shows ineffective erythropoiesis with normoblasts containing ragged cytoplasmic borders in an iron-deficient patient.

Sideroblastic Anemia

Sideroblastic anemia is a diverse group of disorders with defective iron utilization in heme production and ineffective erythropoiesis. RBCs contain excessive iron in mitochondria owing to the inability to form heme. The iron-containing mitochondria often form a ring around the nucleus to give the pathognomonic ringed sideroblast (Fig. 6-21). Sideroblastic anemia may be hereditary or acquired. Most acquired forms are caused by copper deficiency (16–23), myelodysplastic syndrome, alcoholism, and drugs.

In addition to folate deficiency–related megaloblastic anemia, sideroblastic anemia is also common in alcoholics. RBCs are hypochromic microcytes with a normal to increased MCV. Peripheral blood shows dimorphism in 50% of patients and contains siderocytes in 33% of patients. The differential diagnosis includes myelodysplastic syndrome and acute leukemia. Patients with copper deficiency may have cytoplasmic vacuolization in the erythroid and myeloid precursors with ringed sideroblasts in bone marrow (24–27) (Fig. 6-22). Zinc supplementation (e.g., for acne-caused anemia, leukopenia, ulcer healing) causes copper deficiency by competing with copper for gastrointestinal absorption, with subsequent sideroblastic anemia. Zinc toxicity may present with anemia, leukopenia, and cytoplasmic vacuolization of myeloid and erythroid precursors (28,29). Occasional copper-deficient infants, because of a limited diet, may respond to a copper supplement with a quick increase in neutrophils and reticulocyte count. Some drugs (e.g., chloramphenicol, isoniazid) cause sideroblastic anemia by interfering with δ-aminolevulinic acid or heme synthase activity (16,25). Damage to bone marrow can occur in acute alcohol intoxication, drug reactions (30), nutritional deficiency, tuberculosis (31,32), myeloproliferative disorders, myelodysplastic syndrome, malignancy, some metabolic conditions, and chemotherapy.

Idiopathic sideroblastic anemia is a clonal disorder in adults and the elderly. According to French-American-

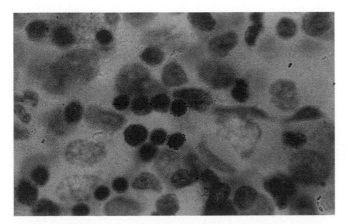

FIGURE 6-21. Bone marrow aspirate smear shows ringed sideroblasts in a patient with zinc-induced copper deficiency. (Copyright ASCP.)

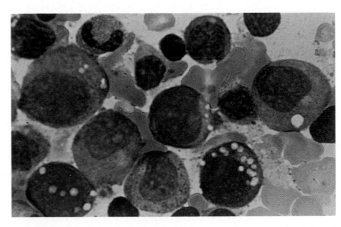

FIGURE 6-22. Bone marrow aspirate smear shows erythroid and myeloid precursors with cytoplasmic vacuoles. The patient has sideroblastic anemia. (Copyright ASCP.)

British and World Health Organization classifications, it corresponds to myelodysplastic syndrome, refractory anemia with ringed sideroblasts, with more than 15% of ringed sideroblasts. Chromosome abnormalities are detected in as many as 50% of the patients, with chromosomes 5, 7, 8, 20, and Y being the most frequently affected.

Laboratory results are consistent with iron overload with elevated transferrin saturation. Ringed sideroblasts usually disappear within 2 weeks after alcohol intake ceases. A pyridoxine supplement may be helpful (Table 6-2).

Anemia of Chronic Disease/Inflammation

Anemia of chronic disease is a common condition accompanying chronic infection, inflammation, and neoplastic disease (33–37). It is characterized by decreased serum iron with adequate storage iron. The pathogenesis is unclear but appears multifactorial and includes decreased RBC survival, impaired iron release from macrophages, and impaired bone marrow response. Active rheumatoid arthritis and systemic lupus erythematosus are associated with increased serum and marrow cytokine levels, antierythropoietin antibodies, decreased erythrocyte survival, and a reduced effect of erythropoietin on erythropoiesis (38–40). The burst-forming unit erythroids and colony-forming unit erythroids are inhibited by the inflammatory cytokine interleukin-1 and tumor necrosis factor-α through apoptosis. Hepcidin, an

TABLE 6-2. DIFFERENTIAL DIAGNOSIS OF SIDEROBLASTIC ANEMIA

Constitutional etiologies
   Constitutional sideroblastic anemia
   Mitochondrial cytopathy
Acquired etiologies
Copper deficiency
Ethanol abuse
Myelodysplastic syndrome

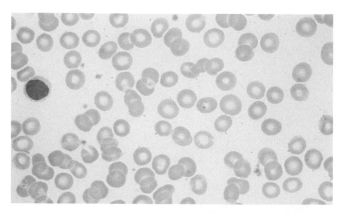

FIGURE 6-23. Peripheral blood smear shows normochromic normocytic anemia with no increase in reticulocytes in a patient with rheumatoid arthritis. (Copyright ASCP.)

antimicrobial protein produced by the liver in response to inflammation, has been reported to play a role in decreasing iron absorption and retention (41). Direct inhibition of erythropoietin production and increased requirement in inflammation decrease erythropoiesis in a combined fashion. Macrophage activation and increased erythrophagocytosis in inflammation also cause reduced RBC survival.

Laboratory studies show normochromic, normocytic anemia with reticulocytopenia (Fig. 6-23). Prolonged anemia may be hypochromic microcytic. Iron metabolism is altered, with decreased serum iron and total iron-binding capacity and increased serum ferritin. The bone marrow shows normal erythropoiesis or mild erythroid hyperplasia with increased iron stores (Fig. 6-24). Leukocyte and platelet counts vary with the underlying disease. The pattern of iron disturbance helps to confirm the diagnosis. Coexisting iron deficiency anemia may cause diagnostic difficulty (12,42). Serum ferritin and total iron-binding capacity distinguish the two conditions in some cases, but the sensitivity is relatively low. The absence of storage iron in bone marrow is the most definitive diagnosis of iron deficiency anemia.

Lead Intoxication

Lead intoxication occurs after exposure to or ingestion of excessive lead. Patients present with abdominal colic, peripheral neuropathy, and mild anemia. The central nervous system, kidney, and hematopoietic system are affected most often. Two important enzymes in heme synthesis, δ-aminolevulinic acid dehydratase and ferrochelatase, are inhibited. Basophilic stippling of RBCs is prominent. Bone marrow shows erythroid hyperplasia and ringed sideroblasts. An increased blood lead level confirms the diagnosis.

MACROCYTOSIS AND MACROCYTIC ANEMIA

Macrocytosis is defined as RBCs with an MCV of more than 100 fL and is seen in 2% to 4% of the patients. Macrocytosis and macrocytic anemia occurs in a broad spectrum of disorders and is not synonymous with vitamin B_{12} or folate deficiency (1–6). Megaloblastic anemia is a disorder of DNA synthesis. Nonmegaloblastic macrocytic anemia in North America is caused mainly by alcoholism, liver disease, hemolysis or bleeding, hypothyroidism, drugs (e.g., azathioprine) (7), and myelodysplastic syndrome (2). Alcoholic patients may also have megaloblastic anemia or sideroblastic anemia. In Japan, the most common cause of macrocytosis is B_{12} and folate deficiency, followed by alcoholism and liver disease. The initial evaluation of macrocytosis includes clinical history, complete blood count, reticulocyte count, and peripheral blood smear examination (5,8–10). Myelodysplastic syndromes are discussed in Chapter 21. The remaining syndromes are discussed below.

The blood smear differentiates megaloblastic from nonmegaloblastic anemia with neutrophil hypersegmentation (six or more lobes) being a sensitive and specific indicator of megaloblastic anemia (Fig. 6-25). Anisocytosis, macroovalocytosis, and the presence of teardrops are most common in

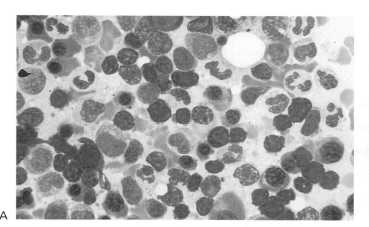

A

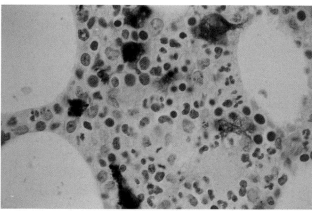

B

FIGURE 6-24. A: Bone marrow aspirate smear shows mild erythroid hyperplasia in a patient with rheumatoid arthritis (anemia of chronic disease). (Copyright ASCP.) **B:** Bone marrow particle section shows increased storage iron in the same patient.

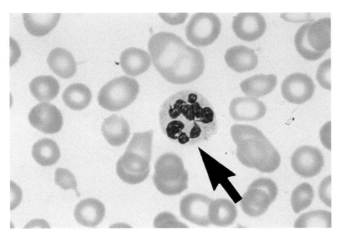

FIGURE 6-25. Peripheral blood smear shows a hypersegmented neutrophil *(arrow)* in a patient with folate deficiency.

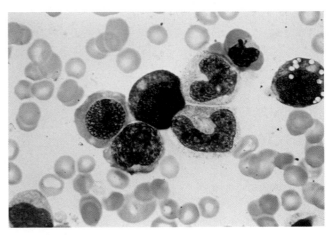

FIGURE 6-26. Bone marrow aspirate smear shows erythroid hyperplasia with megaloblastic change. A giant metamyelocyte is in the center of the field.

megaloblastic hematopoiesis (11). Hemorrhage and hemolysis are accompanied by an increased reticulocyte count, whereas alcoholism, liver disease (12), hypothyroidism, and myelodysplastic syndrome are accompanied by a normal to decreased reticulocyte count. A significant proportion of the elderly patients with idiopathic macrocytosis has findings suggestive of early myelodysplastic syndrome (13,14). Florid hypersegmentation of neutrophils may also be seen in acute pyogenic meningitis or epidural abscess with no megaloblastic anemia and likely represent a combination of infection and cytocentrifuge artifact.

Other causes of macrocytosis and macrocytic anemia include acute erythroleukemia (AML-M6) and drugs (e.g., antipurines, antipyrimidines, hydroxyurea, cyclophosphamide, and anticonvulsant) (11,15–20). Zidovudine may cause macrocytosis in patients with human immunodeficiency virus without anemia. Arsenic poisoning has also been reported. Dyserythropoietic changes are more marked. Patients with chronic alcoholism often contain ringed sideroblasts and proerythroblasts with cytoplasmic vacuolization in the bone marrow (Fig. 6-26). These abnormalities reverse quickly on discontinuation of alcohol. Some studies suggest that acetaldehyde produced by alcohol metabolism within macrophages plays an important role in bone marrow damage. In myelodysplastic syndrome and acute erythroleukemia, megaloblastic changes are usually confined to the erythroid series. Giant metamyelocytes or hypersegmented neutrophils are not present (Table 6-3).

The MCV is of little value in predicting megaloblastic change unless it is markedly elevated (>110 fL). A significant number of patients (37%) with megaloblastic bone marrow changes show a normal or decreased MCV. Meanwhile, many patients (60%) with an elevated MCV (100–110 fL) show no megaloblastic bone marrow changes. The presence of hypersegmented neutrophils and macroovalocytes provides a high sensitivity and specificity in diagnosing megaloblastic anemia. Neutrophil hypersegmentation was reported to be

95% specific and 78% sensitive in some studies. Meanwhile, macroovalocytosis was reported to be 90% sensitive with a lower specificity (68%). In comparison, the sensitivity and specificity of serum lactate dehydrogenase, plasma folate, and RBC folate are of little value. Among the three most common causes of macrocytosis, B_{12} and folate deficiency, liver disease, and reticulocytosis, the MCV rarely exceeds 110 fL in reticulocytosis, whereas in megaloblastic anemia, the MCV may be more than 150 fL. An MCV of more than 120 fL is relatively specific for megaloblastic anemia.

Vitamin B_{12} and Folate Deficiency

Megaloblastic hematopoiesis of B_{12} or folate deficiency results from defective DNA synthesis, with B_{12} deficiency from defective methionine formation and folate deficiency from the conversion of deoxyuridine diphosphate to deoxythymidine monophosphate (21–40). RNA synthesis is unaffected. Asynchrony between nuclear and cytoplasmic maturation occurs, with nuclear maturation lagging behind cytoplasmic maturation. There is ineffective erythroid hyperplasia with a relative increase in early erythroid precursors and a high rate of intramedullary cell death. The morphologic abnormality increases with the severity of anemia (Fig. 6-27).

TABLE 6-3. DIFFERENTIAL DIAGNOSIS OF MACROCYTOSIS AND MACROCYTIC ANEMIA

Anorexia nervosa
Chronic liver disease
Drugs (e.g., antivirals, azathioprine, chemotherapy)
Ethanol
Hypothyroidism
Megaloblastosis (vitamin B_{12} and folate deficiency)
Myelodysplastic syndrome
Reticulocytosis (hemorrhage, hemolysis)
Unknown

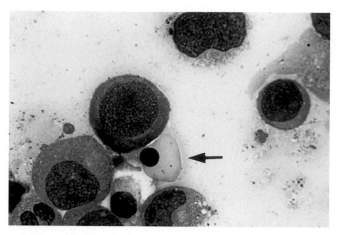

FIGURE 6-27. Bone marrow aspirate smear shows erythroid precursors with delayed nuclear maturation. A normoblast is in the center of the field *(arrow)*.

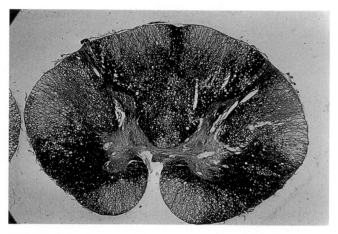

FIGURE 6-28. Section of the spinal cord shows demyelination of the posterior and lateral columns. The patient has pernicious anemia.

B_{12} is present in food of animal origin and is heat stable. It is stored in the amount of 2 to 3 μg; daily loss, and therefore requirement, is 1 to 2 μg. The body store is sufficient for 2 to 5 years. Folate, conversely, is heat labile, present mainly in green leafy vegetables and fruits. Because daily folate requirements are 100 to 200 μg, body stores (5–10 mg) are sufficient for only 2 to 5 months. Thus, folate deficiency is much more common. The liver is the main storage site of B_{12} and folate.

The main causes of B_{12} and folate deficiency include decreased dietary intake; malabsorption (e.g., pepsin deficiency, bacterial overgrowth); defective transportation (e.g., fish tapeworm); increased requirement as in pregnancy and lactation (41,42), malignancy (43), chronic hemolysis, or premature infants; and metabolic disorders. The most common cause of B_{12} deficiency is pernicious anemia owing to decreased intrinsic factor for absorption (44,45). The most common causes of folate deficiency are diet, chronic alcoholism, drug addiction, and malabsorption as in gluten enteropathy. Inadequate dietary folate is common in the poor and the elderly. The megaloblastic hematopoiesis in alcoholic patients may result from folate deficiency and the direct toxic effect of alcohol on erythroid precursors. Severe B_{12} deficiency may cause demyelination of the posterior and lateral columns of the spinal cord with associated peripheral neuropathy (46,47) (Fig. 6-28). Folate deficiency is reported to be associated with arteriosclerotic heart disease.

The peripheral blood shows normochromic macrocytic anemia and circulating macroovalocytes. Hypersegmented neutrophils are the initial and relatively specific morphologic findings followed by megaloblastic hematopoiesis (including macroovalocytes and giant metamyelocytes) (48–53). However, nuclear hypersegmentation has been reported to precede the increase in peripheral blood eosinophils in acute

eosinophilic pneumonia (51). Patients with concurrent iron deficiency anemia or anemia of chronic disease may have a normal MCV. The RBC distribution width is markedly increased. Howell-Jolly bodies and basophilic stippling may be present (Fig. 6-12). Severe cases are associated with neutropenia and thrombocytopenia (52). Megaloblastic erythropoiesis may be difficult to recognize in the blood. The blood smear shows macrocytic anemia, with pancytopenia in severe cases. Cabot rings and ring neutrophils are occasionally seen (53–59).

The bone marrow shows erythroid hyperplasia, with a relative increase in early erythroid precursors. Megaloblastic changes refer to the increased size of the hematopoietic precursors, the enlarged nucleus, and loose, poorly condensed chromatin persisting into the late stages of cell maturation (Fig. 6-29). Other findings include increased erythrophagocytosis and abundant mitoses typically arrested in metaphase

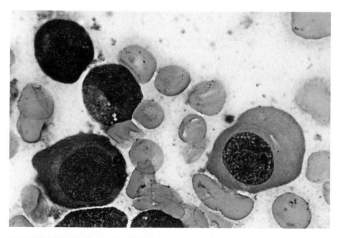

FIGURE 6-29. Bone marrow aspirate smear with erythroid precursors showing delayed nuclear maturation and nuclear cytoplasmic dyssynchrony. The patient has pernicious anemia.

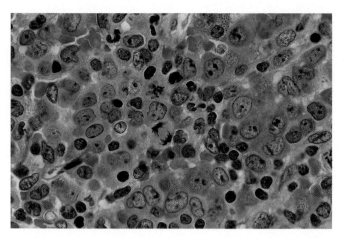

FIGURE 6-30. Trephine biopsy specimen shows erythroid hyperplasia with numerous early precursors in a patient with pernicious anemia. The section should be interpreted with caution and not mistaken for acute leukemia.

with large distinct chromosomes. This combination of marrow findings can produce a quite credible imitation of acute leukemia, a well-known pitfall for those examining sections without corresponding smears (60–62) (Fig. 6-30). In severe, untreated pernicious anemia, bone marrow megaloblasts exhibit periodic acid–Schiff positivity at all stages of maturation, resembling erythroleukemia. Patients have occasionally been misdiagnosed and treated.

To complicate matters, megaloblastic anemia may occur with other erythroid conditions and modify their interpretation, for example, with thalassemia, hemoglobinopathy, iron deficiency, or acute leukemia (63). Megaloblastic anemia in combination with the sickle cell trait produces the impression of sickle cell disease or sickle cell thalassemia because of the elevated HbA2 (64). The blood smear contains target cells, teardrop cells, and elliptocytes.

With B_{12} and folate supplementation, the hypersegmented neutrophils begin to reduce nuclear lobes at approximately day 11 and become normal by day 14. In patients with associated inflammatory disorders, the morphologic changes are usually more rapid. Pregnancy and lactation-related folate deficiency require folate supplementation. An interesting finding is the inverse relationship between hematologic and neurologic damage in B_{12} deficiency: Many patients with folate and B_{12} deficiency are hematologically normal, whereas those with subtle hematologic or neuropsychiatric symptoms may have early B_{12} deficiency. Quantitation of serum B_{12}, folate, and RBC folate levels provides a definitive diagnosis. Decreased serum levels usually occur before morphologic changes.

Serum vitamin B_{12} quantitation measures B_{12} storage. A decreased level indicates B_{12} deficiency. Patients with coexisting iron deficiency anemia, liver disease, myeloproliferative disorders, or hemoglobinopathy may have a normal or elevated B_{12} level, whereas those with transcobalamine deficiency or folate deficiency or women on estrogen therapy may have a falsely decreased B_{12} level. A concurrent low RBC folate level helps to confirm B_{12} deficiency.

Serum folate quantitation measures folate storage. A decreased level is seen in folate deficiency, whereas an elevated level may be seen in pernicious anemia. Patients with iron deficiency anemia may have normal serum folate levels. Diet may also influence folate level and mask true folate deficiency.

RBC folate quantitation is a more reliable measure of folate storage. A decreased level is seen in either B_{12} or folate deficiency. In patients with suspected folate deficiency, it is important to test the RBC folate level because the serum folate level may be normal or elevated in B_{12} deficiency.

Other Tests

The parietal cell antibody and the intrinsic factor antibody are common in patients with pernicious anemia, with the former being more sensitive and the latter more specific. The Schilling test provides an etiologic distinction when other test results are ambiguous. The urine excretion of radiolabeled B_{12} is low in patients with pernicious anemia but returns to normal when intrinsic factor is given. In patients with suspected intestinal bacterial overgrowth, antibiotics are given for bacterial destruction before B_{12} measurement. A deoxyuridine suppression test may be useful in selected patients when other tests fail to confirm B_{12} or folate deficiency. Serum lactate dehydrogenase, bilirubin, and storage iron are usually increased.

Distinguishing B_{12} from folate deficiency is important for treatment purposes because folate supplement may improve anemia of B_{12} deficiency, but neurologic symptoms persist (65). With the correct supplement, lactate dehydrogenase, bilirubin, and serum iron normalize promptly. The reticulocyte count starts to increase at days 3 to 5 and peaks at days 7 to 10, and megaloblastic changes return to normal a few days after. Then myeloid precursors revert to normal a few days later. The peripheral blood count returns to normal in 4 to 8 weeks. The neurologic symptoms improve significantly with B_{12} supplementation. Hematologic response to folate treatment is often poor because of associated acute and chronic diseases.

Other Causes of Megaloblastic Anemia

Megaloblastic anemias other than that from B_{12} or folate deficiency include anemias of abnormal nucleic acid synthesis and those of uncertain etiology (66–73). Most disorders with abnormal nucleic acid synthesis are inherited.

Orotic aciduria is a rare disorder of pyrimidine synthesis characterized by megaloblastic anemia with physical and mental retardation and excretion of a large amount of orotic acid in the urine. The inheritance pattern is autosomal recessive, and patients usually become symptomatic between the ages of 3 months and 7 years. The serum B_{12} and RBC folate levels are normal. Anemia and failure to thrive respond well to daily uridine supplementation.

Lesch-Nyhan syndrome is an X-linked disorder caused by deficiency of hypoxanthine phosphoribosyl transferase. It is characterized by mental retardation, choreoathetosis, self-mutilation, and gout. Children are more susceptible to infection because of impaired humoral immunity. Some patients have megaloblastic anemia that is responsive to adenine treatment.

ERYTHROID HYPOPLASIA

Transient Erythroblastopenia of Childhood

Transient erythroblastopenia of childhood (TEC) is a transient erythroid hypoplasia caused by Parvovirus B19, characterized by temporary cessation of erythropoiesis, normochromic normocytic anemia, reticulocytopenia, and bone marrow erythroblastopenia (1–5) (Fig. 6-31A). Some studies have also indicated an association of TEC with human herpesvirus type 6 (6,7). TEC occurs more commonly in patients younger than 6 months of age. Hereditary factors may be involved (8). The differential diagnosis includes Diamond-Blackfan anemia and pure red cell aplasia. Patients with TEC may have neurologic deficits (9) and often have concurrent neutropenia and thrombocytosis (10). Some patients may have reticulocytosis. Lymphoid aggregates and an increased number of lymphoid cells with B-precursor acute lymphoblastic leukemia phenotype (terminal deoxynucleotidyltransferase positive, CD10 positive, human leukocyte antigen D receptor positive, cytoplasmic μ positive) may be seen in TEC and should not be misdiagnosed as acute lymphoblastic leukemia (11–14). Spontaneous recovery is typical of TEC and helps to distinguish it from congenital dyserythropoietic anemia (Fig. 6-31B). Recognition of TEC in very young infants

helps to avoid an inappropriate diagnosis of Diamond-Blackfan anemia.

Pure Red Cell Aplasia

An uncommon disorder with selective decrease in erythroid precursors, pure red cell aplasia is characterized by severe normocytic or macrocytic anemia, a marked decrease in reticulocyte count, and a secondary increase in erythropoietin (15). The white blood cell and the platelet counts are usually normal. It has been associated with some medications (16–23), Parvovirus B19 (24–26), pregnancy (27–29), ABO-incompatible stem cell transplantation (30), chronic lymphocytic leukemia, diffuse large B-cell lymphoma, T-cell large granular cell lymphoma/leukemia, autoimmune hemolytic anemia (31), systemic lupus erythematosus (32–36), thymic hyperplasia, and thymoma (37–39) (Fig. 6-32). Immune mechanisms have been proposed in the development of pure red cell aplasia including thymoma and chronic lymphocytic leukemia (40), clonal proliferation of T cells (41–46), acquired circulating autoantibodies against erythropoietin, and Fas-associated dyserythropoiesis. Macrophages may become round and full of hemosiderin granules; erythroid and megakaryocytic hypoplasia may also occur (47,48). Vitamin K deficiency and chronic infection have been reported. Pure red cell aplasia may remit with therapy of an underlying condition or, in the case of pregnancy-associated disease, on delivery. Pure red cell aplasia may also evolve to myelodysplastic syndrome (49–54). Most patients require treatment (55–58).

Trilinear Hypoplasia or Aplastic Anemia

Aplastic anemia is characterized by peripheral blood pancytopenia and hypoplastic bone marrow (<25% or >50% cellularity with <30% hematopoietic cells) (59,60). The normal hematopoietic cells are replaced by fat (Fig. 6-33).

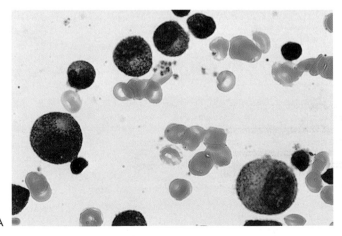
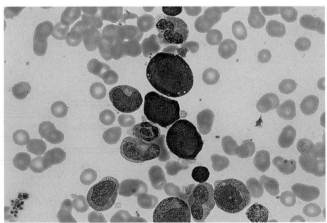

A   B

FIGURE 6-31. A: Bone marrow aspirate smear contains no erythroid precursors in a patient with transient erythroblastopenia of childhood. **B:** Bone marrow aspirate smear shows erythropoiesis in the same patient in recovery.

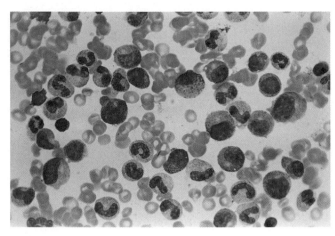

FIGURE 6-32. Bone marrow aspirate smear shows red blood cell aplasia in a patient with thymoma.

It is essential to confine the diagnosis of aplastic anemia to the absence of hematopoiesis at an age and biopsy site expected to show hematopoiesis (61). Biopsy specimens taken from elderly patients from sites other than central axial bone marrow or limited to subcortical bone marrow may not show hematopoiesis but do not fulfill the criteria of aplastic anemia.

Aplastic anemia may be congenital or acquired, with most cases being acquired. Hereditary aplastic anemia is rare and is referred as Fanconi anemia. Most acquired aplastic anemia is idiopathic, with a small proportion being secondary, and is associated with drugs (16,62–81), infection, malnutrition, hypothyroidism, pregnancy (82,83), herbal therapy, chemotherapy, radiation treatment, and transplantation (84,85).

Congenital Aplastic Anemias

These constitutional disorders are typically associated with other abnormalities (86) including bone and mucocutaneous

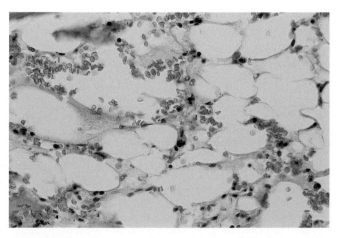

FIGURE 6-33. Bone marrow section shows markedly hypocellular marrow with few hematopoietic cells. The patient has aplastic anemia.

defects and mental retardation. Common types include Fanconi anemia, Diamond-Blackfan anemia, and dyskeratosis congenital, with Fanconi anemia being the best known. This chapter focuses on acquired disorders.

Acquired Aplastic Anemia

The main underlying abnormality in these patients is the destruction of CD34+ progenitor cells through cytotoxic T cell–induced apoptosis. Many drugs have been reported in the development of aplastic anemia, with chloramphenicol and phenylbutazone being the most common. Transient bone marrow suppression is often associated with vacuolization of marrow precursors and an increased serum iron level. Chemotherapy agents such as colchicine, insecticides, and aspirin have also been reported. Benzin and benzin derivatives inhibit DNA and RNA synthesis with resultant chromosomal abnormality and the eventual development of acute myelogenous leukemia. Penetrating radiation (gamma or x-ray) destroys stems cells, with high doses resulting in hematopoietic aplasia and lower doses causing reversible damage. Radiologists and patients with ankylosing spondylitis receiving radiation treatment have a much higher incidence of aplastic anemia than the general population. Many infectious agents are myelosuppressive (87). Epstein-Barr virus, cytomegalovirus, human immunodeficiency virus, Parvovirus B19 (88), and hepatitis viruses have been reported to cause aplastic anemia, with hepatitis C virus being the most common (89–92). The prognosis is poor, and the disease is often rapidly fatal. Tuberculosis, brucellosis, and alcohol toxicity (93,94) have also been reported. Malnutrition and pancreatic insufficiency are associated with stem cell necrosis and stromal cell degeneration, resulting in gelatinous transformation (95).

Secondary aplastic anemia has been reported as a prodrome of acute lymphoblastic leukemia and hairy cell leukemia (89,96–98). Trilinear hypoplasia may be the presenting sign of myelodysplastic syndrome (98–100). p53 Protein has recently been found in refractory anemia and Shwachman-Diamond syndrome with a similar prevalence but is rarely found in acquired aplastic anemia. It has been speculated that p53 overexpression may be an early indicator of significant DNA alteration, which is a crucial step in leukemogenesis (101,102). Anemia may develop after liver transplantation for hepatitis, recurrent cytomegalovirus infection, or Parvovirus B19 infection in children (88,103,104) or after drug treatment (e.g., indomethacin). Anemia may or may not resolve after discontinuation of the drug.

Clinical manifestations of aplastic anemia are related to pancytopenia (105). A normal spleen is important to distinguish aplastic anemia from other pancytopenic disorders. The peripheral blood demonstrates pancytopenia with reticulocytopenia (106). Platelet function is usually normal. Leukocyte alkaline phosphatase is elevated. HbF is increased in some patients with an uneven distribution on

TABLE 6-4. DIFFERENTIAL DIAGNOSIS OF ERYTHROID HYPOPLASIA

Transient erythroid hypoplasia of childhood

Pure red cell aplasia
  Parvovirus B19 infection
  Thymoma
  Myelodysplasic syndrome
  Diffuse large B-cell lymphoma
  Systemic lupus erythematosus
  Autoimmune hemolytic anemia
  Pregnancy
  Drugs
  T-cell large granular cell lymphoma/leukemia

Aplastic anemia

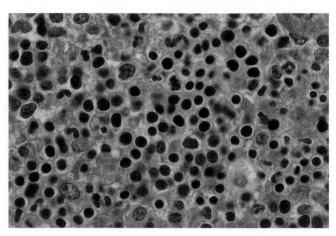

FIGURE 6-34. Bone marrow section shows erythroid hyperplasia in an erythroid colony.

the Kleihauer-Betke acid elution test. Serum iron is usually elevated because of adequate storage, decreased use, and delayed clearance. The erythropoietin level is normal or elevated. The bone marrow has decreased hematopoietic precursors with residual stromal cells, lymphocytes, and plasma cells. Small hematopoietic islands may be present (107–112). Multiple biopsies may be necessary before establishing the diagnosis (Table 6-4).

Most untreated patients with aplastic anemia undergo progressive pancytopenia (113). Bone marrow transplantation is the treatment of choice and has markedly improved survival. For this reason, transfusions should be minimized to decrease the chance of graft rejection (85,114).

ERYTHROID HYPERPLASIA AND ERYTHROCYTOSIS

Erythroid Hyperplasia

Erythroid hyperplasia is characterized by a shift in the ratio of early to late erythroid precursors with elevated early ones. This change is apparent in aspirate smears as a prominent increase in the number of proerythroblasts and basophilic erythroblasts. Trephine biopsy sections show numerous large, relatively well-demarcated erythroid colonies (Fig. 6-34). The peripheral blood may show erythrocytosis, anemia, or a normal RBC count, suggestive of compensated hemolytic anemia or polycythemia vera with iron deficiency.

Anemia is commonly found in erythroid hyperplasia. The differential diagnosis of erythroid hyperplasia and anemia includes the constitutional hematopoietic disorders, marrow replacement by clonal hematolymphoid disease, nonhematopoietic malignancy, and other space-occupying or infiltrative disorders. The anemia of chronic disease is not usually associated with erythroid hyperplasia (Table 6-5).

Erythrocytosis

Erythrocytosis indicates the possibility of familial (constitutional) erythrocytosis, high oxygen-affinity hemoglobinopa-

thy, hypoxia, erythropoietin, or rennin-producing tumors, tumors associated with von Hippel-Lindau disease (1,2), urogenital and hepatic tumors (3–9), and a variety of renal disorders (10–18). Cases not attributable to an underlying condition usually evolve into recognizable polycythemia vera (19,20). Features distinguishing reactive erythrocytosis from pernicious anemia include the platelet count and leukocyte alkaline phosphatase, lactate dehydrogenase, spleen size, and erythropoietin levels. Secondary polycythemia shows a minimal to slight increase in cellularity with a predominance of erythroid lineage and moderately enlarged erythroid islands. Granulocytopoiesis is prominent and left shifted. Small- to medium-size megakaryocytes without maturational defects are scattered throughout the marrow. Increased eosinophils, marked perivascular plasmacytosis, histiocytes with accumulated cell debris, and many iron-laden macrophages are also present. In contrast, early stage polycythemia vera shows splenomegaly, hypercellular bone marrow with trilineal proliferation, confluent sheets of erythropoiesis, and loose clusters of megakaryocytes without prominent inflammatory reactions. Megakaryocytes are typically pleomorphic. Lymphoid nodules are reported in some patients, with no conspicuous iron deposits. Most patients with secondary polycythemia have bronchopulmonary conditions, are frequently smokers, or rarely have renal disease (Table 6-6).

TABLE 6-5. DIFFERENTIAL DIAGNOSIS OF ERYTHROID HYPERPLASIA

Primary
  Polycythemia vera
  Other myeloproliferative disorder
Secondary
Erythroid hyperplasia with erythrocytosis
Erythroid hyperplasia with normal red blood cell count
Erythroid hyperplasia with anemia

TABLE 6-6. DIFFERENTIAL DIAGNOSIS OF ERYTHROCYTOSIS

Constitutional erythrocytosis
Familial (constitutional) erythrocytosis
High oxygen-affinity hemoglobinopathy
Acquired erythrocytosis
Primary
  Polycythemia vera
  Rare cases of other myeloproliferative disorders
Secondary
Hypoxia
Renal disease
Tumors associated with von Hippel-Lindau disease
  (hemangioblastomas, pheochromocytomas)
Urogenital and other tumors

REACTIVE ERYTHROCYTOSIS

Acquired erythrocytosis may be reactive or proliferative/neoplastic as in polycythemia vera. The latter disorder is discussed with myeloproliferative disorders.

Reactive erythrocytosis is characterized by an increased RBC count. The RBC indices (MCHC, MCV) and RBC distribution width are usually within normal limits. Exceptions include high oxygen-affinity hemoglobinopathies with hemolysis owing to unstable Hb. The white blood cells and platelets usually lack quantitative and qualitative abnormalities. The bone marrow shows erythroid hyperplasia without maturational abnormalities or increased blasts. Reactive erythrocytosis shows deposits of debris-containing histiocytes, iron-laden macrophages, plasmacytosis, and increased eosinophils (1,2).

CYCLIC HEMATOPOIESIS

Also called periodic oscillation of blood cell count, different etiologies have been proposed for cyclic hematopoiesis; in some cases, there are clearly acquired causes (1). Autoimmune (2), radiation (3), and drug (4–6) causes have been reported in the development of acquired cyclic hematopoiesis. Hydroxyurea treatment of polycythemia vera was indicated in the fluctuation of the platelet count in patients with polycythemia vera. The mean oscillation cycle ranges from 4 to 11 weeks, and cyclic changes include an increased or decreased number of neutrophils, platelets, and occasionally RBCs. Occasional cases of spontaneous remission has been reported in cyclic leukocytosis. The blood findings in cyclic hematopoiesis include periodic neutropenia (7), lymphocytopenia, monocytopenia, and thrombocytopenia. Bone marrow examination reveals intermittent hypoplasia. Most cases of periodic neutropenia indicate maturation arrest at the promyelocyte or myelocyte stage before neutropenia. Peripheral blood monocytes are usually normal or fluctuate out of the phase with neutrophils. Cases of infection-associated episodic panleukopenia have also been reported that involved neutrophils, monocytes, and lymphocytes, and Ig was an identified cytotoxin against myeloid stem cells.

Cyclic neutropenia is much better understood today than other types of cyclic hematopoiesis. It is characterized by a consistent cycle of 21 days of neutrophil oscillation, accompanied by fever, mouth ulcers, and infection at the nadir of neutrophil count. Most patients follow an autosomal dominant or sporadic pattern of inheritance. The genetic lesion responsible for cyclic neutropenia has recently been identified to occur at chromosome 19p13.3, which contains genes for three neutrophil serine proteases (azurocidin, proteinase 3, and neutrophil elastase). Mutations in or around the neutrophil elastase gene are the main cause of cyclic neutropenia. Interestingly, cyclic neutropenia shares many hematologic features with Kostmann syndrome, and 75% of patients with autosomal dominant Kostmann syndrome have a mutation in the same gene. Most patients respond to granulocyte-colony stimulating factor treatment.

IRON OVERLOAD

Iron overload may be primary or secondary. The primary form results from a genetically determined elevation in iron absorption (e.g., hereditary hemochromatosis) or impaired iron release (e.g., aceruloplasminemia). Secondary causes are a disturbance in erythropoiesis or environmental factors. Some disorders may have genetic and acquired components, and the distinction may not be clear-cut. RBC transfusion is a common secondary cause. Patients with the hemochromatosis gene with secondary iron overload experience more severe consequences. Iron overload has no direct effect on bone marrow function but causes liver damage with subsequent macrocytosis or cytopenia. Ineffective erythropoiesis may develop as a result of increased iron absorption and subsequent overload.

Primary Iron Overload

There are three main types of primary hemochromatosis: type 1, HFE gene–related hereditary hemochromatosis; type 2, non-HFE gene–related juvenile hemochromatosis; and type 3, non-HFE gene–related.

Type 1: HFE Gene–Related Hereditary Hemochromatosis

This type has an autosomal recessive pattern, one of the most common single gene defects in people of North European origin. The HFE gene is located at chromosome 6p with a C282Y point mutation responsible for a cysteine to tyrosine substitution at amino acid 282. Another mutation, H63D, which substitutes histidine with aspartic acid at amino acid 63, is the second most common abnormality and has a less defined role. A third mutation, S65C, is probably a mild form of the disease.

Sustained elevation in iron absorption leads to progressive iron overload with subsequent organ damage, usually starting in middle age. Arthralgia, impotence, and cardiac damage are common. Abnormal liver function tests and late-onset diabetes should trigger suspicion. The initial abnormality is the elevated transferrin saturation with a fasting transferrin saturation of more than 55% for men and postmenopausal women or more than 50% for premenopausal women. Measurement of serum ferritin allows the estimation of storage iron. If serum ferritin is elevated, phlebotomy and liver biopsy should be considered. Quantitative phlebotomy provides both diagnosis and treatment of iron overload.

Siblings are at 25% risk of having inherited hemochromatosis genes. Population screening remains controversial because the disease penetrance remains uncertain. Hepatocellular carcinoma is a major cause of death in patients with cirrhosis. Routine monitoring of serum α-fetoprotein and ultrasonography allow prompt identification and treatment. Patients treated before the development of cirrhosis have a normal life expectancy.

Type 2: Juvenile Hemochromatosis, Hereditary

Type 2 is a rare but severe form of iron overload. Patients have a wild-type HFE gene and usually present with gonadal failure and cardiomyopathy by the age of 30. The gene has not been identified but is mapped to the short arm of chromosome 1.

Type 3: Hereditary Hemochromatosis

This type results from inactivation of the transferrin receptor 2 gene located at chromosome 7q22, with a subsequent increase in iron absorption. Patients are homozygotes. One proposed mechanism is the impaired hepatic iron uptake and its subsequent decrease in hepcidin production, with uncontrollable iron absorption following.

Rare forms of primary iron overload have also been reported including ferroportin mutation, atransferrinemia with microcytic anemia, and aceruloplasminemia.

Secondary Iron Overload

Secondary iron overload occurs either through transfusion or increased absorption, with transfusion being much more common and pathologic effects occurring sooner. Patients may die of arrhythmia, cardiac failure, diabetes, or cirrhosis. Cirrhosis occurs early with mitochondrial and lysosomal damages.

Excess oral iron intake usually does not cause significant iron overload without additional factors. Some diseases (e.g.,

β-thalassemia intermedia, congenital dyserythroblastic anemia, congenital sideroblastic anemia) present with erythroid expansion in which iron load is proportional to the degree of erythroid expansion. The risk of iron loading in these patients may be concealed, and a liver biopsy should be considered to evaluate the iron loading and to avoid misguided oral iron supplement.

ACKNOWLEDGMENTS

The author gives sincere thanks to Dr. Diane Farhi for reviewing the chapter and for providing important suggestions, images, and references and to Bonnie Stephenson for providing references.

REFERENCES

Red Blood Cell Morphology and Iron Metabolism

1. Foucar K. *Bone marrow pathology*, 2nd ed. Chicago: ASCP Press, 2001.
2. Harmening DM. *Clinical hematology and fundamentals of hemostasis*, 4th ed. Philadelphia: FA Davis, 2002.
3. Steine-Martin EA, Lotspeich-Steininger CA, Keopke JA. *Clinical hematology, principles, procedures, correlations*, 2nd ed. Philadelphia: Lippincott–Raven Publishers, 1998.
4. Wickramasinghe SN, McCullough J. Blood and bone marrow pathology. New York: Churchill Livingstone, 2003.
5. Atlas of Clinical Hematology. Tkachuk DC, Hirschmann JV, McArthur JR. Philadelphia: WB Saunders, 2002.

Hemolytic Anemia

1. Chugh KS, Singhal PC, Sharma BK, et al. Acute renal failure due to intravascular hemolysis in the North Indian patients. *Am J Med Sci* 1977;274:139–146.
2. Beutler E, Coller BS, Kipps TJ, et al., eds. *Williams hematology*, 5th ed. New York: McGraw-Hill, 1995.
3. Kelton JG. Impaired reticuloendothelial function in patients treated with methyldopa. *N Engl J Med* 1985;313:596–600.
4. Lee GR, Foerster J, Lukens JN, et al., eds. *Wintrobe's clinical hematology*, 10th ed. Baltimore: Williams & Wilkins, 1999.
5. Petz LD. Drug-induced autoimmune hemolytic anemia. *Transfusion Med Rev* 1993;7:242–254.
6. Mollison PL. *Blood transfusion in clinical medicine*. Oxford: Blackwell, 1993.
7. Wickramasinghe SN, McCullough J. *Blood and bone marrow pathology*. New York: Churchill Livingstone, 2003.
8. Schrezenmeier H, Hildebrand A, Rojewski M, Hacker H, Heimpel H, Raghavachar A. Paroxysmal nocturnal haemoglobinuria: a replacement of haematopoietic tissue? *Acta Haematol* 2000;103:41–48.
9. Fores T, Bautista G, Steegmann JL, et al. De novo smoldering paroxysmal nocturnal hemoglobinuria: a flow cytometry diagnosis. *Hematologica* 1997;82:695–697.

Microcytosis and Microcytic Anemia

1. Mast A. The clinical utility of peripheral blood test in the diagnosis of iron deficiency anemia. *Bloodline Rev* 2001;1:7–9.

2. Rimon E, Levy S, Sapir A, et al. Diagnosis of iron deficiency anemia in the elderly by transferrin receptor-ferritin index. *Arch Intern Med* 2002;162:445–449.

3. Song JS, Park W, Bae SK, et al. The usefulness of serum transferrin receptor and ferritin for assessing anemia in rheumatoid arthritis: comparison with bone marrow iron study. *Rheumatol Int* 2001;21:24–29.

4. Suominen P, Punnonen K, Rajamaki A, et al. Serum transferrin receptor and transferrin receptor-ferritin index identify healthy subjects with subclinical iron deficits. *Blood* 1998;92:2934–2939.

5. Demiroglu H. Hypoferremia, absent bone marrow macrophage iron, and microcytic anemia with minimal response to iron therapy: an acquired disorder of iron metabolism. *Am J Hematol* 1998;57:260.

6. Farley PC, Foland J. Iron deficiency anemia. How to diagnose and correct. *Postgrad Med* 1990;87:89–93.

7. Green R, King R. A new red cell discriminant incorporating volume dispersion for differentiating iron deficiency anemia from thalassemia minor. *Blood Cells* 1989;15:481–491.

8. Navone R, Azzoni L, Valente G. Immunohistochemical assessment of ferritin in bone marrow trephine biopsies: correlation with marrow hemosiderin. *Acta Haematol* 1988;80:194–198.

9. Punnonen K, Irjala K, Rajamaki A. Serum transferrin receptor and its ratio to serum ferritin in the diagnosis of iron deficiency. *Blood* 1997;89:1052–1057.

10. Rozman M, Masat T, Feliu E, et al. Dyserythropoiesis in iron-deficiency anemia: ultrastructural reassessment. *Am J Hematol* 1992;41:147–150.

11. Thompson WG, Meola T, Lipkin M Jr, et al. Red cell distribution width, mean corpuscular volume, and transferrin saturation in the diagnosis of iron deficiency. *Arch Intern Med* 1988;148:2128–2130.

12. van Tellingen A, Kuenen JC, de Kieviet W, et al. Iron deficiency anaemia in hospitalised patients: value of various laboratory parameters. Differentiation between IDA and ACD. *Neth J Med* 2001;59:270–279.

13. Zago MA, Costa FF, Bottura C. Dyserythropoicsis in iron deficiency and in beta-thalassemia. *Braz J Med Biol Res* 1984;17:135–142.

14. Massey AC. Microcytic anemia. Differential diagnosis and management of iron deficiency anemia. *Med Clin North Am* 1992;76:549–566.

15. Mates M, Heyd J, Souroujon M, et al. The haematologist as watchdog of community health by full blood count. *Q J Med* 1995;88:333–339.

16. Kumar R, Kalra SP, Kumar H, et al. Pancytopenia—a six year study. *J Assoc Physicians India* 2001;49:1078–1081.

17. Llanos RM, Mercer JF. The molecular basis of copper homeostasis copper-related disorders. *DNA Cell Biol* 2002;21:259–270.

18. Naveh Y, Hazani A, Berant M. Copper deficiency with cow's milk diet. *Pediatrics* 198168:397–400.

19. Olivares M, Uauy R. Copper as an essential nutrient. *Am J Clin Nutr* 1996;63:791S–796S.

20. Prohaska JR. Effects of dietary copper deficiency on male offspring of heterozygous brindled mice. *Br J Nutr* 1989;62:177–184.

21. Spiegel JE, Willenbucher RF. Rapid development of severe copper deficiency in a patient with Crohn's disease receiving parenteral nutrition. *JPEN J Parenter Enteral Nutr* 1999;23:169–172.

22. Williams DM. Copper deficiency in humans. *Semin Hematol* 1983;20:118–128.

23. Yelin G, Taff ML, Sadowski GE. Copper toxicity following massive ingestion of coins. *Am J Forensic Med Pathol* 1987;8:78–85.

24. Ece A, Uyanik BS, Iscan A, et al. Increased serum copper and decreased serum zinc levels in children with iron deficiency anemia. *Biol Trace Elem Res* 1997;59:31–39.

25. Ramadurai J, Shapiro C, Kozloff M, et al. Zinc abuse and sideroblastic anemia. *Am J Hematol* 1993;42:227–228.

26. Summerfield AL, Steinberg FU, Gonzalez JG. Morphologic findings in bone marrow precursor cells in zinc-induced copper deficiency anemia. *Am J Clin Pathol* 1992;97:665–668.

27. Porea TJ, Belmont JW, Mahoney DH Jr. Zinc-induced anemia and neutropenia in an adolescent. *J Pediatr* 2000;136:688–690.

28. Bennett DR, Baird CJ, Chan KM, et al. Zinc toxicity following massive coin ingestion. *Am J Forensic Med Pathol* 1997;18:148–153.

29. Fiske DN, McCoy HE 3rd, Kitchens CS. Zinc-induced sideroblastic anemia: report of a case, review of the literature, and description of the hematologic syndrome. *Am J Hematol* 1994;46:147–150.

30. Rudek MA, Horne M, Figg WD, et al. Reversible sideroblastic anemia associated with the tetracycline analogue COL-3. *Am J Hematol* 2001;67:51–53.

31. Demiroglu H, Dundar S. Vitamin B6 responsive sideroblastic anaemia in a patient with tuberculosis. *Br J Clin Pract* 1997;51:51–52.

32. Tamura H, Hirose S, Watanabe O, et al. Anemia and neutropenia due to copper deficiency in enteral nutrition. *JPEN J Parenter Enteral Nutr* 1994;18:185–189.

33. Carmel R. Anemia and aging: an overview of clinical, diagnostic and biological issues. *Blood Rev* 2001;15:9–18.

34. Jongen-Lavrencic M, Peeters HR, Wognum A, et al. Elevated levels of inflammatory cytokines in bone marrow of patients with rheumatoid arthritis and anemia of chronic disease. *J Rheumatol* 1997;24:1504–1509.

35. Jurado RL. Iron, infections, and anemia of inflammation. *Clin Infect Dis* 1997;25:888–895.

36. Means RT Jr. Advances in the anemia of chronic disease. *Int J Hematol* 1999;70:7–12.

37. Pixley JS, MacKintosh FR, Smith EA, et al. Anemia of inflammation: role of T lymphocyte activating factor. *Pathobiology* 1992;60:309–315.

38. Voulgari PV, Kolios G, Papadopoulos GK, et al. Role of cytokines in the pathogenesis of anemia of chronic disease in rheumatoid arthritis. *Clin Immunol* 1999;92:153–160.

39. Voulgarelis M, Kokori SI, Ioannidis JP, et al. Anaemia in systemic lupus erythematosus: aetiological profile and the role of erythropoietin. *Ann Rheum Dis* 2000;59:217–222.

40. Weber J, Were JM, Julius HW, et al. Decreased iron absorption in patients with active rheumatoid arthritis, with and without iron deficiency. *Ann Rheum Dis* 1998;47:404–409.

41. Besa EC, Kim PW, Haurani FI. Treatment of primary defective iron-reutilization syndrome: revisited. *Ann Hematol* 2000;79:465–468.

42. Barron BA, Hoyer JD, Tefferi A. A bone marrow report of absent stainable iron is not diagnostic of iron deficiency. *Ann Hematol* 2001;80:166–169.

Macrocytosis and Macrocytic Anemia

1. Breedveld FC, Bieger R, van Wermeskerken RK. The clinical significance of macrocytosis. *Acta Med Scand* 1981;209:319–322.

2. Brigden ML. A systematic approach to macrocytosis. Sorting out the causes. *Postgrad Med* 1995;97:171–172.

3. Davenport J. Macrocytic anemia. *Am Fam Physician* 1996;53:155–162.

4. Geene D, Sudre P, Anwar D, et al. Causes of macrocytosis in

HIV-infected patients not treated with zidovudine. Swiss HIV Cohort Study. *J Infect* 2000;40:160–163.

5. Harkins LS, Sirel JM, McKay PJ, et al. Discriminant analysis of macrocytic red cells. *Clin Lab Haematol* 1994;16:225–234.

6. Keenan WF Jr. Macrocytosis as an indicator of human disease. *J Am Board Fam Pract* 1989;2:252–256.

7. Kissel JT, Levy RJ, Mendell JR, et al. Azathioprine toxicity in neuromuscular disease. *Neurology* 1986;36:35–39.

8. Seppa K, Sillanaukee P, Saarni M. Blood count and hematologic morphology in nonanemic macrocytosis: differences between alcohol abuse and pernicious anemia. *Alcohol* 1993;10: 343–347.

9. Snower DP, Weil SC. Changing etiology of macrocytosis. Zidovudine as a frequent causative factor. *Am J Clin Pathol* 1993;99:57–60.

10. Wymer A, Becker DM. Recognition and evaluation of red blood cell macrocytosis in the primary care setting. *J Gen Intern Med* 1990;5:192–197.

11. Savage DG, Ogundipe A, Allen RH, et al. Etiology and diagnostic evaluation of macrocytosis. *Am J Med Sci* 2000;319:343–352.

12. Maruyama S, Hirayama C, Yamamoto S, et al. Red blood cell status in alcoholic and non-alcoholic liver disease. *J Lab Clin Med* 2001;138:332–337.

13. Colon-Otero G, Menke D, Hook CC. A practical approach to the differential diagnosis and evaluation of the adult patient with macrocytic anemia. *Med Clin North Am* 1992;76:581–597.

14. Drabick JJ, Davis BJ, Byrd JC. Concurrent pernicious anemia and myelodysplastic syndrome. *Ann Hematol* 2001;80: 243–245.

15. Amos RJ, Amess JA. Megaloblastic haemopoiesis due to acyclovir. *Lancet* 1983;1:242–243.

16. Au WY, Ma ES, Kwong YL. Intravenous pentamidine induced megaloblastic anaemia. *Haematologica* 2002;87:ECR06.

17. Kim CJ, Park KI, Inoue H, et al. Azathioprine-induced megaloblastic anemia with pancytopenia 22 years after living-related renal transplantation. *Int J Urol* 1998;5:100–102.

18. Ozkara C, Dreifuss FE, Apperson Hansen C. Changes in red blood cells with valproate therapy. *Acta Neurol Scand* 1993;88: 210–212.

19. Sallah S, Hanrahan LR, Phillips DL. Intrathecal methotrexate-induced megaloblastic anemia in patients with acute leukemia. *Arch Pathol Lab Med* 1999;123:774–777.

20. Ward PC. Investigation of macrocytic anemia. *Postgrad Med* 1979;65:203–207.

21. Carmel R, Goodman SI. Abnormal deoxyuridine suppression test in congenital methylmalonic aciduria-homocystinuria without megaloblastic anemia: divergent biochemical and morphological bone marrow manifestations of disordered cobalamin metabolism in man. *Blood* 1982;59:306–311.

22. Carmel R. Subtle cobalamin malabsorption in a vegan patient: evolution into classic pernicious anemia with anti-intrinsic factor antibody. *Arch Intern Med* 1982;142:2206–2207.

23. Carmel R, Weiner JM, Johnson CS. Iron deficiency occurs frequently in patients with pernicious anemia. *JAMA* 1987;257: 1081–1083.

24. Carmel R, Sinow RM, Karnaze DS. Atypical cobalamin deficiency. Subtle biochemical evidence of deficiency is commonly demonstrable in patients without megaloblastic anemia and is often associated with protein-bound cobalamin malabsorption. *J Lab Clin Med* 1987;109:454–463.

25. Carmel R. Pernicious anemia. The expected findings of very low serum cobalamin levels, anemia, and macrocytosis are often lacking. *Arch Intern Med* 1988;148:1712–1714.

26. Carmel R. Subtle and atypical cobalamin deficiency states. *Am J Hematol* 1990;34:108–114.

27. Carmel R. Reversal by cobalamin therapy of minimal defects in the deoxyuridine suppression test in patients without anemia: further evidence for a subtle metabolic cobalamin deficiency. *J Lab Clin Med* 1992;119:240–244.

28. Carmel R, MacPhee RD Jr. Erythropoietin levels in cobalamin deficiency: comparison of anemic and non-anemic, subtly deficient patients. *Eur J Haematol* 1992;48:159–162.

29. Carmel R. Reassessment of the relative prevalences of antibodies to gastric parietal cell and to intrinsic factor in patients with pernicious anaemia: influence of patient age and race. *Clin Exp Immunol* 1992;89:74–77.

30. Carmel R, Perez-Perez GI, Blaser MJ. *Helicobacter pylori* infection and food-cobalamin malabsorption. *Dig Dis Sci* 1994;39: 309–314.

31. Carmel R. Megaloblastic anemias. *Curr Opin Hematol* 1994;1: 107–112.

32. Carmel R. Malabsorption of food cobalamin. *Baillieres Clin Haematol* 1995;8:639–655.

33. Carmel R. Prevalence of undiagnosed pernicious anemia in the elderly. *Arch Intern Med* 1996;156:1097–1100.

34. Carmel R, Green R, Jacobsen DW, et al. Neutrophil nuclear segmentation in mild cobalamin deficiency: relation to metabolic tests of cobalamin status and observations on ethnic differences in neutrophil segmentation. *Am J Clin Pathol* 1996;106: 57–63.

35. Carmel R. Current concepts in cobalamin deficiency. *Annu Rev Med* 2000;51:357–375.

36. Carmel R, Aurangzeb I, Qian D. Associations of food-cobalamin malabsorption with ethnic origin, age, *Helicobacter pylori* infection, and serum markers of gastritis. *Am J Gastroenterol* 2001; 96:63–70.

37. Chintagumpala MM, Dreyer ZA, Steuber CP, et al. Pancytopenia with chromosomal fragility: vitamin B12 deficiency. *J Pediatr Hematol Oncol* 1996;18:166–170.

38. Hines JD. Megaloblastic anemia in an adult vegan. *Am J Clin Nutr* 1966;19:260–268.

39. Green R, Miller JW. Folate deficiency beyond megaloblastic anemia: hyperhomocysteinemia and other manifestations of dysfunctional folate status. *Semin Hematol* 1999;36:47–64.

40. Kapadia CR. Vitamin B12 in health and disease: part I—inherited disorders of function, absorption, and transport. *Gastroenterologist* 1995;3:329–344.

41. Van de Velde A, Van Droogenbroeck J, Tjalma W, et al. Folate and vitamin B(12) deficiency presenting as pancytopenia in pregnancy: a case report and review of the literature. *Eur J Obstet Gynecol Reprod Biol* 2002;100:251–254.

42. Ingram CF, Fleming AF, Patel M, et al. Pregnancy- and lactation-related folate deficiency in South Africa—a case for folate food fortification. *S Afr Med J* 1999;89:1279–1284.

43. Vogelsang GB, Spivak JL. Unusual case of acute leukemia. Coexisting acute leukemia and pernicious anemia. *Am J Med* 1984;76:1144–1150.

44. Rabinowitz AP, Sacks Y, Carmel R. Autoimmune cytopenias in pernicious anemia: a report of four cases and review of the literature. *Eur J Haematol* 1990;44:18–23.

45. O'Brien HA, Sourial NA. Severe megaloblastic anaemia presenting as pancytopenia with red cell hypoplasia and elevated serum cobalamin and cobalamin binding proteins. *Clin Lab Haematol* 1991;13:307–310.

46. Licht DJ, Berry GT, Brooks DG, et al. Reversible subacute combined degeneration of the spinal cord in a 14-year-old due to a strict vegan diet. *Clin Pediatr (Phila)* 2001;40:413–415.

47. von Schenck U, Bender-Gotze C, Koletzko B. Persistence of neurological damage induced by dietary vitamin B-12 deficiency in infancy. *Arch Dis Child* 1997;77:137–139.

48. Bills T, Spatz L. Neutrophilic hypersegmentation as an indicator of incipient folic acid deficiency. *Am J Clin Pathol* 1977;68: 263–267.

49. Bunting RW, Selig MK, Dickersin GR. Ultrastructure of peripheral blood granulocytes from patients with low serum cobalamin. *J Submicrosc Cytol Pathol* 1996;28:187–195.

50. Lodge-Rigal RD, Novotny DB. Hypersegmentation of neutrophils in the cerebrospinal fluid: report of a case with hematologic correlation and review of the literature. *Diagn Cytopathol* 1994;11:56–59.

51. Maeno T, Maeno Y, Sando Y, et al. Nuclear hypersegmentation precedes the increase in blood eosinophils in acute eosinophilic pneumonia. *Intern Med* 2000;39:157–159.

52. Nath BJ, Lindenbaum J. Persistence of neutrophil hypersegmentation during recovery from megaloblastic granulopoiesis. *Ann Intern Med* 1979;90:757–760.

53. Thompson WG, Cassino C, Babitz L, et al. Hypersegmented neutrophils and vitamin B12 deficiency. Hypersegmentation in B12 deficiency. *Acta Haematol* 1989;81:186–191.

54. Kumar R, Kalra SP, Kumar H, et al. Pancytopenia—a six year study. *J Assoc Physicians India* 2001;49:1078–1081.

55. Craig A. Ring neutrophils in megaloblastic anaemia. *Br J Haematol* 1987;67:247–248.

56. Kass L. Origin and composition of Cabot rings in pernicious anemia. *Am J Clin Pathol* 1975;64:53–57.

57. Kass L, Gray RH. Ultrastructural visualization of Cabot rings in pernicious anemia. *Experientia* 1976;32:507–509.

58. Rothmann C, Malik Z, Cohen AM. Spectrally resolved imaging of Cabot rings and Howell-Jolly bodies. *Photochem Photobiol* 1998t;68:584–587.

59. Yalaburgi SB, Kapalanga NJ. Cabot's ring bodies in overwhelming infections. *S Afr Med J* 1983;64:1045–1046.

60. Levine PH, Hamstra RD. Megaloblastic anemia of pregnancy simulating acute leukemia. *Ann Intern Med* 1969;71:1141–1147.

61. Kass L. Unusual morphologic abnormalities of megaloblasts in pernicious anemia and folate deficiency. *Am J Clin Pathol* 1976;65:195–198.

62. Kass L. Periodic acid-Schiff-positive megaloblasts in pernicious anemia. *Am J Clin Pathol* 1977;67:371–373.

63. Spivak JL. Masked megaloblastic anemia. *Arch Intern Med* 1982;142:2111–2114.

64. Sinow RM, Johnson CS, Karnaze DS, et al. Unsuspected pernicious anemia in a patient with sickle cell disease receiving routine folate supplementation. *Arch Intern Med* 1987;147:1828–1829.

65. Karnaze DS, Carmel R. Neurologic and evoked potential abnormalities in subtle cobalamin deficiency states, including deficiency without anemia and with normal absorption of free cobalamin. *Arch Neurol* 1990;47:1008–1012.

66. Anttila P, Ihalainen J, Salo A, et al. Idiopathic macrocytic anaemia in the aged: molecular and cytogenetic findings. *Br J Haematol* 1995;90:797–803.

67. Grumbeck E, Aiginger P, Gisslinger B, et al. Macrocytic anemia and thrombocytosis associated with thymoma: a case report. *Am J Hematol* 2000;63:38–41.

68. Dan K, Ito T, Nomura T. Pure red cell aplasia following pernicious anemia. *Am J Hematol* 1990;33:148–150.

69. Hughes G Jr, Brown M, Martino R. Persistent megaloblastic anemia: a diagnostic dilemma. *South Med J* 1981;74:367–368.

70. Mahmoud MY, Lugon M, Anderson CC. Unexplained macrocytosis in elderly patients. *Age Ageing* 1996;25:310–312.

71. Mwanda OW, Dave P. Megaloblastic marrow in macrocytic anaemias at Kenyatta National and M P Shah Hospitals, Nairobi. *East Afr Med J* 1999;76:610–614.

72. Skacel PO, Hewlett AM, Lewis JD, et al. Studies on the haemopoietic toxicity of nitrous oxide in man. *Br J Haematol* 1983;53: 189–200.

73. Wickramasinghe SN. The wide spectrum and unresolved issues of megaloblastic anemia. *Semin Hematol* 1999;36:3–18.

Erythroid Hypoplasia

1. Cherrick I, Karayalcin G, Lanzkowsky P. Transient erythroblastopenia of childhood. Prospective study of fifty patients. *Am J Pediatr Hematol Oncol* 1994;16:320–324.

2. Gerrits GP, van Oostrom CG, de Vaan GA, et al. Transient erythroblastopenia of childhood. A review of 22 cases. *Eur J Pediatr* 1984;142:266–270.

3. Miller R, Berman B. Transient erythroblastopenia of childhood in infants <6 months of age. *Am J Pediatr Hematol Oncol* 1994; 16:246–248.

4. Skeppner G, Wranne L. Transient erythroblastopenia of childhood in Sweden: incidence and findings at the time of diagnosis. *Acta Paediatr* 1993;82:574–578.

5. Tamary H, Kaplinsky C, Shvartzmayer S, et al. Transient erythroblastopenia of childhood. Evidence for cell-mediated suppression of erythropoiesis. *Am J Pediatr Hematol Oncol* 1993; 15:386–391.

6. Penchansky L, Jordan JA. Transient erythroblastopenia of childhood associated with human herpesvirus type 6, variant B. *Am J Clin Pathol* 1997;108:127–132.

7. Skeppner G, Kreuger A, Elinder G. Transient erythroblastopenia of childhood: prospective study of 10 patients with special reference to viral infections. *J Pediatr Hematol Oncol* 2002;24: 294–298.

8. Skeppner G, Forestier E, Henter JI, et al. Transient red cell aplasia in siblings: a common environmental or a common hereditary factor? *Acta Paediatr* 1998;87:43–47.

9. Chan GC, Kanwar VS, Wilimas J. Transient erythroblastopenia of childhood associated with transient neurologic deficit: report of a case and review of the literature. *J Paediatr Child Health* 1998;34:299–301.

10. Hanada T, Ehara T, Nakahara S, et al. Simultaneous transient erythroblastopenia and agranulocytosis: IgG-mediated inhibition of erythrogranulopoiesis. *Eur J Haematol* 1987;38:200–203.

11. Farhi DC, Luebbers EL, Rosenthal NS. Bone marrow biopsy in childhood anemia. Prevalence of transient erythroblastopenia of childhood. *Arch Pathol Lab Med* 1998;122:638–641.

12. Foot AB, Potter MN, Ropner JE, et al. Transient erythroblastopenia of childhood with CD10, TdT, and cytoplasmic mu lymphocyte positivity in bone marrow. *J Clin Pathol* 1990;43: 857–859.

13. Leuschner S, Bodewaldt-Radzun S, Rister M. Increase of CALLA-positive stimulated lymphoid cells in transient erythroblastopenia of childhood. *Eur J Pediatr* 1990;149:551–554.

14. Mupanomunda OK, Alter BP. Transient erythroblastopenia of childhood (TEC) presenting as leukoerythroblastic anemia. *J Pediatr Hematol Oncol* 1997;19:165–167.

15. Charles RJ, Sabo KM, Kidd PG, et al. The pathophysiology of pure red cell aplasia: implications for therapy. *Blood* 1996;87:4831–4838.

16. Acharya S, Bussel JB. Hematologic toxicity of sodium valproate. *J Pediatr Hematol Oncol* 2000;22:62.

17. Auer J, Hinterreiter M, Allinger S, et al. Severe pancytopenia after leflunomide in rheumatoid arthritis. *Acta Med Austriaca* 2000;27:131–132.

18. Farkas V, Szabo M, Renyi I, et al. Temporary pure red-cell aplasia during valproate monotherapy: clinical observations and spectral

electroencephalographic aspects. *J Child Neurol* 2000;15: 485–487.

19. Lin YW, Okazaki S, Hamahata K, et al. PRCA associated with allopurinol therapy. *Am J Hematol* 1999;61:209–211.

20. Marseglia GL, Locatelli F. Isoniazid-induced pure red cell aplasia in two siblings. *J Pediatr* 1998;132:898–900.

21. Misra S, Moore TB, Ament ME, et al. Red cell aplasia in children on tacrolimus after liver transplantation. *Transplantation* 1998;65:575–577.

22. Tagawa T, Sumi K, Uno R, et al. Pure red cell aplasia during carbamazepine monotherapy. *Brain Dev* 1997;19:300–302.

23. Yamada O, Mizoguchi H, Oshimi K. Cyclophosphamide therapy for pure red cell aplasia associated with granular lymphocyte-proliferative disorders. *Br J Haematol* 1997;97:392–399.

24. Frickhofen N, Chen ZJ, Young NS, et al. Parvovirus B19 as a cause of acquired chronic pure red cell aplasia. *Br J Haematol* 1994;87:818–824.

25. Geetha D, Zachary JB, Baldado HM, et al. Pure red cell aplasia caused by Parvovirus B19 infection in solid organ transplant recipients: a case report and review of literature. *Clin Transpl* 2000;14:586–591.

26. Heegaard ED, Myhre J, Hornsleth A, et al. Parvovirus B19 infections in patients with chronic anemia. *Haematologica* 1997;82:402–405.

27. Baker RI, Manoharan A, de Luca E, et al. Pure red cell aplasia of pregnancy: a distinct clinical entity. *Br J Haematol* 1993;85: 619–622.

28. Sadahira Y, Sagihara T, Yawata Y. Expression of p53 and Ki67 in bone marrow giant proerythroblasts associated with human Parvovirus B19 infection. *Int J Hematol* 2001;74:147–152.

29. Tohda S, Nara N, Tanikawa S, et al. Pure red cell aplasia following autoimmune haemolytic anaemia. Cell-mediated suppression of erythropoiesis as a possible pathogenesis of pure red cell aplasia. *Acta Haematol* 1992;87:98–102.

30. Bolan CD, Leitman SF, Griffith LM, et al. Delayed donor red cell chimerism and pure red cell aplasia following major ABO-incompatible nonmyeloablative hematopoietic stem cell transplantation. *Blood* 2001;98:1687–1694.

31. Croisille L, Tchernia G, Casadevall N. Autoimmune disorders of erythropoiesis. *Curr Opin Hematol* 2001;8:68–73.

32. Choi BG, Yoo WH. Successful treatment of pure red cell aplasia with plasmapheresis in a patient with systemic lupus erythematosus. *Yonsei Med J* 2002;43:274–278.

33. Feng CS, Ng MH, Szeto RS, et al. Bone marrow findings in lupus patients with pancytopenia. *Pathology* 1991;23:5–7.

34. Kiely PD, McGuckin CP, Collins DA, et al. Erythrocyte aplasia and systemic lupus erythematosus. *Lupus* 1995;4:407–411.

35. Linardaki GD, Boki KA, Fertakis A, et al. Pure red cell aplasia as presentation of systemic lupus erythematosus: antibodies to erythropoietin. *Scand J Rheumatol* 1999;28:189–191.

36. Okada H, Suzuki H, Uchida H, et al. Acquired idiopathic pure red cell aplasia in a hemodialyzed patient with inactive systemic lupus erythematosus. *Intern Med* 1994;33:492–495.

37. Konstantopoulos K, Androulaki A, Aessopos A, et al. Pure red cell aplasia with true thymic hyperplasia. *Hum Pathol* 1995;26:1160–1162.

38. Kuo T, Shih LY. Histologic types of thymoma associated with pure red cell aplasia: a study of five cases including a composite tumor of organoid thymoma associated with an unusual lipofibroadenoma. *Int J Surg Pathol* 2001;9:29–35.

39. Wong KF, Chau KF, Chan JK, et al. Pure red cell aplasia associated with thymic hyperplasia and secondary erythropoietin resistance. *Am J Clin Pathol* 1995;103:346–347.

40. Katayama H, Takeuchi M, Yoshino T, et al. Epstein-Barr virus associated diffuse large B-cell lymphoma complicated by autoimmune hemolytic anemia and pure red cell aplasia. *Leuk Lymphoma* 2001;42:539–542.

41. Ergas D, Tsimanis A, Shtalrid M, et al. T-gamma large granular lymphocyte leukemia associated with amegakaryocytic thrombocytopenic purpura, Sjogren's syndrome, and polyglandular autoimmune syndrome type II, with subsequent development of pure red cell aplasia. *Am J Hematol* 2002;69:132–134.

42. Go RS, Li CY, Tefferi A, et al. Acquired pure red cell aplasia associated with lymphoproliferative disease of granular T lymphocytes. *Blood* 2001;98:483–485.

43. Kouides PA, Rowe JM. Large granular lymphocyte leukemia presenting with both amegakaryocytic thrombocytopenic purpura and pure red cell aplasia: clinical response to immunosuppressive therapy. *Am J Hematol* 1995;49:232–236.

44. Loughran TP Jr, Starkebaum G. Large granular lymphocyte leukemia. Report of 38 cases and review of the literature. *Medicine (Baltimore)* 1987;66:397–405.

45. Yamada O, Yun-Hua W, Motoji T, et al. Clonal T-cell proliferation causing pure red cell aplasia in chronic B-cell lymphocytic leukaemia: successful treatment with cyclosporine following in vitro abrogation of erythroid colony-suppressing activity. *Br J Haematol* 1998;101:335–337.

46. Yamada O. Clonal T cell proliferations in patients with pure red cell aplasia. *Leuk Lymphoma* 1999;35:69–82.

47. Canavan BF, Huhn RD, Kim HC, et al. Concurrent presentation of erythrocytic and megakaryocytic aplasia. *Am J Hematol* 1996;51:68–72.

48. Hanada T, Ehara T, Nakahara S, et al. Simultaneous transient erythroblastopenia and agranulocytosis: IgG-mediated inhibition of erythrogranulopoiesis. *Eur J Haematol* 1987;38:200–203.

49. Garcia-Suarez J, Pascual T, Munoz MA, et al. Myelodysplastic syndrome with erythroid hypoplasia/aplasia: a case report and review of the literature. *Am J Hematol* 1998;58:319–325.

50. Hirri HM, Green PJ. Pure red cell aplasia in a patient with chronic granulocytic leukaemia treated with interferon-alpha. *Clin Lab Haematol* 2000;22:53–54.

51. Keefer MJ, Solanki DL. Dyserythropoiesis and erythroblast-phagocytosis preceding pure red cell aplasia. *Am J Hematol* 1988;27:132–135.

52. Mijovic A, Rolovic Z, Novak A, et al. Chronic myeloid leukemia associated with pure red cell aplasia and terminating in promyelocytic transformation. *Am J Hematol* 1989;31:128–130.

53. Suvajdzic N, Marisavljevic D, Jovanovic V, et al. Pure red cell aplasia evolving through the hyperfibrotic myelodysplastic syndrome to the acute myeloid leukemia: some pathogenetic aspects. *Hematol Cell Ther* 1999;41:27–29.

54. Yokohama A, Murata N, Shimano S, et al. Myelodysplastic syndrome accompanied by i(17) (q10) anomaly following pure red cell aplasia and transient myeloproliferative stage [in Japanese]. *Rinsho Ketsueki* 1999;40:34–39.

55. de Vetten MP, van Gelder M, de Greef GE. Recovery of erythropoiesis following allogeneic bone marrow transplantation for chronic lymphocytic leukaemia-associated pure red cell aplasia. *Bone Marrow Transplant* 2001;27:771–773.

56. Kadikoylu G, Bolaman Z, Barutca S. High-dose methylprednisolone therapy in pure red cell aplasia. *Ann Pharmacother* 2002;36:55–58.

57. La Montagna G, Baruffo A, Abbadessa A, et al. Pure red cell aplasia in Felty's syndrome: a case report of successful reversal after cyclosporin A treatment. *Clin Rheumatol* 1999;18:244–247.

58. Zecca M, De Stefano P, Nobili B, et al. Anti-CD20 monoclonal antibody for the treatment of severe, immune-mediated, pure red cell aplasia and hemolytic anemia. *Blood* 2001;97:3995–3997.

59. Foucar K. *Bone marrow pathology,* 2nd ed. Chicago: ASCP Press, 2001.

60. Brunning RD, McKenna RW. Tumor of the bone marrow. Atlas of Tumor Pathology. 3rd series, fascicle 9. Washington, DC: AFIP, 1994.

61. Slater LM, Katz J, Walter B, et al. Aplastic anemia occurring

as amegakaryocytic thrombocytopenia with and without an inhibitor of granulopoiesis. *Am J Hematol* 1985;18:251–254.

62. Auer J, Hinterreiter M, Allinger S, et al. Severe pancytopenia after leflunomide in rheumatoid arthritis. *Acta Med Austriaca* 2000;27:131–132.

63. Bacon BR, Treuhaft WH, Goodman AM. Azathioprine-induced pancytopenia. Occurrence in two patients with connective-tissue diseases. *Arch Intern Med* 1981;141:223–226.

64. Baumelou E, Guiguet M, Mary JY. Epidemiology of aplastic anemia in France: a case-control study. I. Medical history and medication use. The French Cooperative Group for epidemiological Study of Aplastic Anemia. *Blood* 1993;81:1471–1478.

65. Blackburn SC, Oliart AD, Garcia Rodriguez LA, et al. Antiepileptics and blood dyscrasias: a cohort study. *Pharmacotherapy* 1998;18:1277–1283.

66. Critchley JA, Critchley LA, Yeung EA, et al. Granulocyte-colony stimulating factor in the treatment of colchicine poisoning. *Hum Exp Toxicol* 1997;16:229–232.

67. Escobar-Morreale HF, Bravo P, Garcia-Robles R, et al. Methimazole-induced severe aplastic anemia: unsuccessful treatment with recombinant human granulocyte-monocyte colony-stimulating factor. *Thyroid* 1997;7:67–70.

68. Finklestein M, Goldman L, Grace ND, et al. Granulocytopenia complicating colchicine therapy for primary biliary cirrhosis. *Gastroenterology* 1987;93:1231–1235.

69. Folpini A, Furfori P. Colchicine toxicity—clinical features and treatment. Massive overdose case report. *J Toxicol Clin Toxicol* 1995;33:71–77.

70. Hansen RM, Csuka ME, McCarty DJ, et al. Gold induced aplastic anemia. Complete response to corticosteroids, plasmapheresis, and N-acetylcysteine infusion. *J Rheumatol* 1985;12: 794–797.

71. Hoang C, Lavergne A, Bismuth C, et al. [Visceral histologic lesions of lethal acute colchicine poisoning. Apropos of 12 cases] [in French]. *Ann Pathol* 1982;2:229–237.

72. Hood RL. Colchicine poisoning. *J Emerg Med* 1994;12: 171–177.

73. Kornberg A, Rachmilewitz EA. Aplastic anemia after prolonged ingestion of indomethacin. *Acta Haematol* 1982;67:136–138.

74. Liu YK, Hymowitz R, Carroll MG. Marrow aplasia induced by colchicine. A case report. *Arthritis Rheum* 1978;21:731–735.

75. Malawista SE. Marrow aplasia induced by colchicine. A case report. Discussion. *Arthritis Rheum* 1978;21:735–736.

76. McIntyre IM, Ruszkiewicz AR, Crump K, et al. Death following colchicine poisoning. *J Forensic Sci* 1994;39:280–286.

77. Smith MT. Overview of benzene-induced aplastic anaemia. *Eur J Haematol Suppl* 1996;60:107–110.

78. Stanley MW, Taurog JD, Snover DC. Fatal colchicine toxicity: report of a case. *Clin Exp Rheumatol* 1984;2:167–171.

79. Stemmermann GN, Hayashi T. Colchicine intoxication. A reappraisal of its pathology based on a study of three fatal cases. *Hum Pathol* 1971;2:321–332.

80. Taher A, Ammash Z, Dabajah B, et al. Ticlopidine-induced aplastic anemia and quick recovery with G-CSF: case report and literature review. *Am J Hematol* 2000;63:90–93.

81. Wehr M, Schafer K, Bode JC. [Granulocytopenia with cimetidine therapy] [in German]. *Dtsch Med Wochenschr* 1980;105: 1571–1573.

82. Bourantas K, Makrydimas G, Georgiou I, et al. Aplastic anemia. Report of a case with recurrent episodes in consecutive pregnancies. *J Reprod Med* 1997;42:672–674.

83. Deka D, Banerjee N, Roy KK, et al. Aplastic anaemia during pregnancy: variable clinical course and outcome. *Eur J Obstet Gynecol Reprod Biol* 2001;94:152–154.

84. Goss JA, Schiller GJ, Martin P, et al. Aplastic anemia complicating orthotopic liver transplantation. *Hepatology* 1997;26: 865–869.

85. Hagglund H, Winiarski J, Ringden O, et al. Successful allogeneic bone marrow transplantation in a 2.5-year-old boy with ongoing cytomegalovirus viremia and severe aplastic anemia after orthotopic liver transplantation for non-A, non-B, non-C hepatitis. *Transplantation* 1997;64:1207–1208.

86. Schrezenmeier H, Hildebrand A, Rojewski M, et al. Paroxysmal nocturnal haemoglobinuria: a replacement of haematopoietic tissue? *Acta Haematol* 2000;103:41–48.

87. Pan KY, Lin JL, Chen JS. Severe reversible bone marrow suppression induced by *Selaginella doederleinii*. *J Toxicol Clin Toxicol* 2001;39:637–639.

88. Langnas AN, Markin RS, Cattral MS, et al. Parvovirus B19 as a possible causative agent of fulminant liver failure and associated aplastic anemia. *Hepatology* 1995;22:1661–1665.

89. Rafel M, Cobo F, Cervantes F, et al. Transient pancytopenia after non-A non-B non-C acute hepatitis preceding acute lymphoblastic leukemia. *Haematologica* 1998;83:564–566.

90. Pavone P, Greco F, Fisher A, et al. [Bone marrow hypoplasia associated with acute viral hepatitis in four children] [in English, Italian]. *Minerva Pediatr* 1999;51:319–324.

91. Nishioka SD. Aplastic anemia and viral hepatitis: a second look [Comment, Letter]. *Hepatology* 1997;26:1688–1689.

92. Paquette RL, Kuramoto K, Tran L, et al. Hepatitis C infection in acquired aplastic anemia. *Am J Hematol* 1998;58:122–126.

93. Ballard HS. Alcohol-associated pancytopenia with hypocellular bone marrow. *Am J Clin Pathol* 1980;73:830–834.

94. Nakao S, Harada M, Kondo K, et al. Reversible bone marrow hypoplasia induced by alcohol. *Am J Hematol* 1991;37:120–123.

95. Lampert F, Lau B. Bone marrow hypoplasia in anorexia nervosa. *Eur J Pediatr* 1976;124:65–71.

96. Krause JR. Aplastic anemia terminating in hairy cell leukemia. A report of two cases. *Cancer* 1984;53:1533–1537.

97. Sohn SK, Suh JS, Lee J, et al. Pancytopenic prodrome (pre-ALL) of acute lymphoblastic leukemia in adults: possible pathogenesis. *Korean J Intern Med* 1998;13:64–67.

98. Tooze JA, Marsh JC, Gordon-Smith EC. Clonal evolution of aplastic anaemia to myelodysplasia/acute myeloid leukaemia and paroxysmal nocturnal haemoglobinuria. *Leuk Lymphoma* 1999;33:231–241.

99. Ohara A, Kojima S, Hamajima N, et al. Myelodysplastic syndrome and acute myelogenous leukemia as a late clonal complication in children with acquired aplastic anemia. *Blood* 1997;90:1009–1013.

100. Orazi A, Albitar M, Heerema NA, et al. Hypoplastic myelodysplastic syndromes can be distinguished from acquired aplastic anemia by CD34 and PCNA immunostaining of bone marrow biopsy specimens. *Am J Clin Pathol* 1997;107:268–274.

101. Elghetany MT, Vyas S, Yuoh G. Significance of p53 overexpression in bone marrow biopsies from patients with bone marrow failure: aplastic anemia, hypocellular refractory anemia and hypercellular refractory anemia. *Ann Hematol* 1998;77: 261–264.

102. Elghetany MT. P53 overexpression in bone marrow biopsy in refractory anemia and aplastic anemia: impact of antibody selection. *Leuk Res* 2000;24:975–977.

103. Kaptan K, Beyan C, Ural AU, et al. Successful treatment of severe aplastic anemia associated with human Parvovirus B19 and Epstein-Barr virus in a healthy subject with allo-BMT. *Am J Hematol* 2001;67:252–255.

104. Sato S, Fuchinoue S, Abe M, et al. Successful cytokine treatment of aplastic anemia following living-related orthotopic liver transplantation for non-A, non-B, non-C hepatitis. *Clin Transpl* 1999;13:68–71.

105. Guinan EC. Clinical aspects of aplastic anemia. *Hematol Oncol Clin North Am* 1997;11:1025–1044.

106. Buttarello M, Bulian P, Farina G, et al. Five fully automated methods for performing immature reticulocyte fraction:

comparison in diagnosis of bone marrow aplasia. *Am J Clin Pathol* 2002;117:871–879.

107. Keung YK, Pettenati MJ, Cruz JM, et al. Bone marrow cytogenetic abnormalities of aplastic anemia. *Am J Hematol* 2001; 66:167–171.

108. Maciejewski JP, Selleri C, Sato T, et al. A severe and consistent deficit in marrow and circulating primitive hematopoietic cells (long-term culture-initiating cells) in acquired aplastic anemia. *Blood* 1996;88:1983–1991.

109. Maciejewski JP, Risitano A, Sloand EM, et al. Distinct clinical outcomes for cytogenetic abnormalities evolving from aplastic anemia. *Blood* 2002;99:3129–3135.

110. Maciejewski JP, Risitano A, Kook H, et al. Immune pathophysiology of aplastic anemia. *Int J Hematol* 2002;76[Suppl 1]: 207–214.

111. Mikhailova N, Sessarego M, Fugazza G, et al. Cytogenetic abnormalities in patients with severe aplastic anemia. *Haematologica* 1996;81:418–422.

112. Nakao S, Yamaguchi M, Takamatsu H, et al. Relative erythroid hyperplasia in the bone marrow at diagnosis of aplastic anaemia: a predictive marker for a favourable response to cyclosporine therapy. *Br J Haematol* 1996;92:318–323.

113. Brodsky RA. Biology and management of acquired severe aplastic anemia. *Curr Opin Oncol* 1998;10:95–99.

114. Kim SW, Rice L, Champlin R, et al. Aplastic anemia in eosinophilic fasciitis: responses to immunosuppression and marrow transplantation. *Haematologia (Budap)* 1997;28: 131–137.

Erythroid Hyperplasia and Erythrocytosis

1. Burns C, Levine PH, Reichman H, et al. Adrenal hemangioblastoma in von Hippel-Lindau disease as a cause of secondary erythrocytosis. *Am J Med Sci* 1987;293:119–121.

2. Trimble M, Caro J, Talalla A, et al. Secondary erythrocytosis due to a cerebellar hemangioblastoma: demonstration of erythropoietin mRNA in the tumor. *Blood* 1991;78:599–601.

3. Brewer CA, Adelson MD, Elder RC. Erythrocytosis associated with a placental-site trophoblastic tumor. *Obstet Gynecol* 1992;79:846–849.

4. Kohama T, Shinohara K, Takahura M, et al. Large uterine myoma with erythropoietin messenger RNA and erythrocytosis. *Obstet Gynecol* 2000;96:826–828.

5. Matsuyama M, Yamazaki O, Horii K, et al. Erythrocytosis caused by an erythropoietin-producing hepatocellular carcinoma. *J Surg Oncol* 2000;75:197–202.

6. Reman O, Reznik Y, Casadevall N, et al. Polycythemia and steroid overproduction in a gonadotropin-secreting seminoma of the testis. *Cancer* 1991;68:2224–2229.

7. Rothmann SA, Savage RA, Paul P. Erythropoietin-dependent erythrocytosis associated with hepatic angiosarcoma. *J Surg Oncol* 1982;20:105–108.

8. Sandler A, Rivlin L, Filler R, et al. Polycythemia secondary to focal nodular hyperplasia. *J Pediatr Surg* 1997;32:1386–1387.

9. Stephen MR, Lindop GB. A renin secreting ovarian steroid cell tumour associated with secondary polycythaemia. *J Clin Pathol* 1998;51:75–77.

10. Burton IE, Sambrook P, McWilliam LJ. Secondary polycythaemia associated with bilateral renal lymphocoeles. *Postgrad Med J* 1994;70:515–517.

11. Davis CJ Jr, Barton JH, Sesterhenn IA, et al. Metanephric adenoma. Clinicopathological study of fifty patients. *Am J Surg Pathol* 1995;19:1101–1114.

12. Gupta M, Miller BA, Ahsan N, et al. Expression of angiotensin II type I receptor on erythroid progenitors of patients with post transplant erythrocytosis. *Transplantation* 2000;70:1188–1194.

13. Konety BR, Hord JD, Weiner ES, et al. Embryonal adenoma of the kidney associated with polycythemia and von Willebrand disease. *J Urol* 1998;160:2171–2174.

14. Lim CS, Jung KH, Kim YS, et al. Secondary polycythemia associated with idiopathic membranous nephropathy. *Am J Nephrol* 2000;20:344–346.

15. Noguchi Y, Goto T, Yufu Y, et al. Gene expression of erythropoietin in renal cell carcinoma. *Intern Med* 1999;38:991–994.

16. Shih LY, Huang JY, Lee CT. Insulin-like growth factor I plays a role in regulating erythropoiesis in patients with end-stage renal disease and erythrocytosis. *J Am Soc Nephrol* 1999;10:315–322.

17. Wang AY, Yu AW, Lam CW, et al. Effects of losartan or enalapril on hemoglobin, circulating erythropoietin, and insulin-like growth factor-1 in patients with and without posttransplant erythrocytosis. *Am J Kidney Dis* 2002;39:600–608.

18. Yokoyama K, Ogura Y, Matsushita Y, et al. Hypererythropoietinemia and hyperreninemia in a continuous ambulatory peritoneal dialysis patient with chronic severe hypotension. *Clin Nephrol* 1998;50:60–63.

19. Pearson TC, Messinezy M. Idiopathic erythrocytosis, diagnosis and clinical management. *Pathol Biol (Paris)* 2001;49:170–177.

20. Shih LY, Lee CT, Ou YC. Prediction of clinical course in patients with idiopathic erythrocytosis by endogenous erythroid colony assay but not by serum erythropoietin levels. *Exp Hematol* 1997;25:288–292.

Reactive Erythrocytosis

1. Thiele J, Kvasnicka HM, Muehlhausen K, et al. Polycythemia rubra vera versus secondary polycythemias. A clinicopathological evaluation of distinctive features in 199 patients. *Pathol Res Pract* 2001;197:77–84.

2. Thiele J, Kvasnicka HM, Zankovich R, et al. The value of bone marrow histology in differentiation between early stage polycythemia vera and secondary polycythemias. *Haematologica* 2001;86:368–374.

Cyclic Hematopoiesis

1. Haurie C, Dale DC, Mackey MC. Cyclical neutropenia and other periodic hematological disorders: a review of mechanisms and mathematical models. *Blood* 1998;92:2629–2640.

2. Cline MJ, Opelz G, Saxon A, et al. Autoimmune panleukopenia. *N Engl J Med* 1976;295:1489–1493.

3. Crown JP, Jhanwar S, Haimi J, et al. Acquired cyclic haematopoiesis associated with a radiation-induced chromosomal abnormality with clonal, morphologically normal circulating leucocytes. *Acta Haematol* 1991;86:103–106.

4. Bennett M, Grunwald AJ. Hydroxyurea and periodicity in myeloproliferative disease. *Eur J Haematol* 2001;66:317–323.

5. Steensma DP, Harrison CN, Tefferi A. Hydroxyurea-associated platelet count oscillations in polycythemia vera: a report of four new cases and a review. *Leuk Lymphoma* 2001;42:1243–1253.

6. Tefferi A, Elliott MA, Kao PC, et al. Hydroxyurea-induced marked oscillations of platelet counts in patients with polycythemia vera. *Blood* 2000;96:1582–1584.

7. Adams WH, Liu YK. Periodic neutropenia and monocytopenia. *Am J Hematol* 1982;13:73–82.

7

NEUTROPHILS

NEUTROPENIA

Neutropenia is a frequent finding in the complete blood cell count (CBC). The time course may be transient, cyclic, or persistent. Transient neutropenia is a common complication of viral infection.

Cyclic neutropenia is an unusual disorder that may be constitutional or acquired; the two may be difficult to distinguish, especially in young patients. Constitutional cyclic neutropenia is discussed in Chapter 5. Acquired cyclic neutropenia may have a mild course, frequent cyclic fluctuation of other cell counts, a wide range of cycle length, variable cycle length in an individual patient, cyclic variation in the number of bone marrow granulocytic precursors, and cycling of body temperature (1–18) (Table 7-1). Associated conditions include autoimmune neutropenia, ankylosing spondylitis, Crohn's disease, phenylbutazone therapy, common variable immunodeficiency, myeloproliferative disorders, myelodysplastic syndrome, T-cell neoplasms, and acute lymphoblastic leukemia. The bone marrow may show cyclic variation in the number of neutrophilic precursors. Eventual development of persistent agranulocytosis has been reported.

Persistent or chronic neutropenia may be either constitutional or acquired. Constitutional neutropenia is discussed in Chapter 5. Acquired neutropenia has been reported in a variety of populations, from neonates to older adults (19–49) (Table 7-2). The clinical course ranges from benign (i.e.,

infection-free) to serious or fatal owing to life-threatening infection. Many cases respond to treatment with antibiotics, granulocyte colony-stimulating factor, and/or immune modulators; some show spontaneous remission.

Numerous mechanisms have been implicated in the pathogenesis of chronic neutropenia, including autoimmunity, alloimmunity, idiosyncratic and dose-dependent drug reactions, overwhelming infection, and premature birth. Transplacental passage of maternal antibodies may cause autoimmune or alloimmune neutropenia in the neonate. Conditions associated with chronic neutropenia include prior cyclic neutropenia, drug reactions, sepsis, bacterial and viral

TABLE 7-1. CONDITIONS ASSOCIATED WITH ACQUIRED CYCLIC NEUTROPENIA

Nonneoplastic conditions
  Autoimmune neutropenia
  Ankylosing spondylitis
  Crohn's disease
  Phenylbutazone therapy
  Common variable immunodeficiency

Neoplastic conditions
  Myeloproliferative disorders
  Myelodysplastic syndrome
  T-cell large granular lymphocytic leukemia
  Adult T-cell leukemia/lymphoma
  Acute lymphoblastic leukemia

TABLE 7-2. CONDITIONS ASSOCIATED WITH ACQUIRED PERSISTENT NEUTROPENIA

Nonneoplastic conditions
  Drug therapy
    Antibiotics
    Antithyroid medication
    Colchicine
    Gold
    Histamine 2 (H$_2$)-receptor antagonists
    Neuroleptic drugs

  Infection
    Bacterial infection
    Epstein-Barr virus infection
    Parvovirus B19 infection
    Sepsis

  Immune-mediated disorders
    Autoimmune neutropenia
    Alloimmune neutropenia
    Behçet disease
    Sjögren syndrome

  Neonatal conditions
    Premature birth
    Transplacental passage of maternal antibodies

  Prior cyclic neutropenia

Neoplastic conditions
  Prodrome to acute myeloid leukemia
  Hairy cell leukemia
  T-cell neoplasms
  Replacement of hematopoietic bone marrow by
    metastatic malignancy, fibrosis, or bone

infection, gold therapy, antibiotic therapy (which may both provoke and ameliorate neutropenia), antithyroid therapy, histamine 2 (H_2)-receptor antagonist therapy, colchicine intoxication, Epstein-Barr virus infection, parvovirus B19 infection, Behçet disease, Sjögren syndrome, T-cell neoplasms (especially T-cell large granular lymphocytic leukemia), hairy cell leukemia, acute myeloid leukemia, and replacement of bone marrow by fibrosis, bone, or metastatic malignancy. In many cases, no pathogenetic mechanism or underlying condition is apparent.

The peripheral blood shows an absolute neutrophil count (ANC) of less than the normal laboratory range, usually less than 1.5×10^9/L. Monocytosis is present in some cases. The platelet count may be decreased. Cases with neutropenia, thrombocytopenia, and anemia are discussed with aplastic anemia. Recovery from neutropenia may be attended by neutrophilia or a neutrophilic leukemoid reaction.

Bone marrow aspirate smears and histologic sections show variable cellularity. In most cases, neutrophils and precursors are increased, often with a pronounced increase in metamyelocytes, myelocytes, and promyelocytes (left shift) (see Neutrophilic Hyperplasia section). Phagocytosis of neutrophils by bone marrow macrophages has rarely been reported. Mature segmented neutrophils and band forms may be reduced or virtually absent, a condition termed granulocytic maturation arrest (see Neutrophilic Maturation Arrest section). This may be a misnomer because it is not clear in most cases whether the lack of mature neutrophils is actually owing to impaired maturation or to rapid clearance and destruction. Some cases of neutropenia show marked reduction in the entire neutrophil series (see Neutrophilic Hypoplasia section).

The differential diagnosis includes so-called benign ethnic neutropenia and pseudoneutropenia. Benign ethnic neutropenia is simply a lower normal range for the white blood cell (WBC) count and ANC found in some ethnic groups (50–54) (Table 7-3). Lower normal ranges for these values are found in some groups of Africans, African Americans, Arab Jordanians, and African and Yemenite Jews. The lower limit of a normal ANC in such groups is 1.2×10^9/L or possibly lower. This finding is of no clinical significance and should not be confused with true neutropenia, which is often complicated by serious infections. Individuals with benign ethnic neutropenia may be unnecessarily subjected to repeated laboratory testing, including bone marrow examination, in a futile effort to determine the cause of apparent neutropenia.

Pseudoneutropenia is an artifactual reduction in the ANC caused by neutrophil agglutination or, rarely, overfilled blood

TABLE 7-3. POPULATIONS WITH BENIGN ETHNIC NEUTROPENIA

Africans
African Americans
Arab Jordanians
African and Yemenite Jews

TABLE 7-4. CONDITIONS ASSOCIATED WITH PSEUDONEUTROPENIA

Neutrophil agglutination caused by immunoglobulin G or M antibodies against neutrophil surface antigens
High-dose γ-globulin therapy
Herpes simplex infection
Pneumonia caused by *Mycoplasma pneumoniae* and other organisms
Hepatic disorders
Vasculitis
Colon carcinoma
Overfilled blood vacuum tubes

vacuum tubes (55–62) (Table 7-4). Neutrophil agglutination is apparently mediated by immunoglobulin G or M antibodies against neutrophil surface antigens. Underlying conditions include high-dose γ-globulin therapy, herpes simplex infection, pneumonia caused by *Mycoplasma pneumoniae* and other organisms, hepatic disorders, vasculitis, and colon carcinoma; agglutination may disappear after treatment. Some subjects with neutrophil agglutination appear healthy. The physical conditions for neutrophil agglutination vary. In some cases, agglutination occurs with ethylenediaminetetraacetic acid, sodium citrate, lithium heparin, and/or acid citrate dextrose, at room temperature but not at 37°C. In other cases, agglutination occurs only with ethylenediaminetetraacetic acid, at both room temperature and 37°C. The CBC may also show pseudothrombocytopenia. The peripheral blood smear shows aggregates of neutrophils ranging from two to 80 or more cells and, in some cases, platelet satellitism around neutrophils.

REACTIVE NEUTROPHILIA AND LEUKEMOID REACTION

Reactive neutrophilia is a common peripheral blood finding (1–24) (Table 7-5). The WBC count and ANC exceed the upper limit of normal for the laboratory, approximately 11×10^9/L and 8×10^9/L, respectively. Leukemoid reaction is an imprecise term used for unusually brisk reactive leukocytosis that has been applied to increased numbers of neutrophils, monocytes, eosinophils, and lymphocytes. In most cases, the term refers to marked neutrophilia, in which the ANC exceeds 50×10^9/L.

Numerous underlying conditions may result in reactive neutrophilia. They include alcoholic hepatitis, diabetic ketoacidosis, drug reaction, ethylene glycol intoxication, infection, inflammatory disorders, inflammatory pseudotumor, labor and delivery, premature birth with chronic lung disease, rebound effect after neutropenia, retroperitoneal hemorrhage, surgery, trauma, Hodgkin lymphoma, plasma cell neoplasia, carcinoma, mesothelioma, and sarcoma. Reactive neutrophilia is mediated by increased cytokine production. Some cases of malignancy-related neutrophilia are caused by tumor cell production of granulocyte colony-stimulating factor.

TABLE 7-5. CONDITIONS ASSOCIATED WITH REACTIVE NEUTROPHILIA

Nonneoplastic conditions
  Alcoholic hepatitis
  Diabetic ketoacidosis
  Drug reaction
  Ethylene glycol intoxication
  Infection
  Inflammatory disorders
  Inflammatory pseudotumor
  Labor and delivery
  Premature birth with chronic lung disease
  Rebound effect after neutropenia
  Retroperitoneal hemorrhage
  Surgery
  Trauma
Neoplastic conditions
  Hodgkin lymphoma
  Plasma cell neoplasia
  Carcinoma
  Mesothelioma
  Sarcoma

TABLE 7-6. DIFFERENTIAL DIAGNOSIS OF REACTIVE NEUTROPHILIA

Corticosteroid-induced neutrophilia
Pseudoleukocytosis
  Cryoglobulin-induced pseudoleukocytosis with
    pseudothrombocytosis
  Anticoagulant-induced pseudoleukocytosis with
    pseudothrombocytopenia
Clonal myeloid disorders
  Chronic myeloid leukemia
  Chronic neutrophilic leukemia
  Myelodysplastic syndrome with neutrophilia

The peripheral blood smear shows increased neutrophils and neutrophil precursors, including bands, metamyelocytes, myelocytes, promyelocytes, and even occasional blasts (Fig. 7-1). Other cell counts are variable. The neutrophils may show signs of activation or early release from bone marrow: enhanced (toxic) granulation, vacuolation, and Döhle bodies. Dysplastic features are absent, and the neutrophil (leukocyte) alkaline phosphatase score is normal to increased. Bone marrow aspirate smears and histologic sections show increased cellularity and increased neutrophils and precursors. The myeloid-to-erythroid ratio is variable but usually increased. Other findings may include erythroid and megakaryocytic hyperplasia, benign lymphoid aggregates, and granulomas. In contrast to myeloproliferative and myelodysplastic disorders, bone marrow does not show evidence of hematopoietic dysplasia, fibrosis, or abnormal bony remodeling.

The differential diagnosis includes corticosteroid-induced neutrophilia, pseudoleukocytosis, and clonal myeloid disorders (Table 7-6).

Corticosteroid-induced neutrophilia is not reactive neutrophilia but an increase in the peripheral WBC count and ANC owing to demargination of neutrophils from the vascular endothelium to form part of the circulating neutrophil pool (25–27). At the same time, the absolute lymphocyte and eosinophil counts are reduced. The result is an increased WBC count, usually in the range of 15 to 20 × 10^9/L, an increased ANC, and an increased percentage of segmented neutrophils in the WBC differential count, usually in the range of 85% to 90%. Monocytes may be increased. Administration of both corticosteroid and granulocyte colony-stimulating factor for the purpose of peripheral blood neutrophil harvest may result in an ANC of more than 40 × 10^9/L. The neutrophils are unremarkable, without evidence of toxic granulation, vacuolation, or Döhle bodies. Neutrophilic precursors are absent, and bone marrow is unremarkable. Corticosteroid-related neutrophilia is a common occurrence. Failure to recognize this phenomenon may cause patients to be subjected to unnecessary tests, including bone marrow examination.

Pseudoleukocytosis is an artifactual increase in the WBC count and ANC (28–35). The mechanisms are cryoglobulinemia, in which cryoglobulin forms crystals or aggregates in peripheral blood, and anticoagulant-induced platelet aggregation. In both cases, automated hematology analyzers count the aggregates as WBCs. Pseudoleukocytosis may occur with pseudothrombocytosis, owing to small aggregates of cryoglobulin, or with pseudothrombocytopenia, owing to anticoagulant-induced platelet clumping. Correct diagnosis of pseudoleukocytosis caused by cryoglobulinemia permits further evaluation for an underlying inflammatory or neoplastic disorder.

Clonal myeloid disorders resembling reactive neutrophilia include myeloproliferative disorders (especially chronic neutrophilic leukemia) and myelodysplastic syndromes with neutrophilia. Reactive neutrophilia may antedate the discovery of an underlying carcinoma or plasma cell neoplasm by several years; in such cases, an erroneous diagnosis of chronic

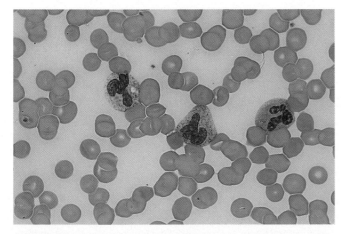

FIGURE 7-1. Peripheral blood smear, reactive neutrophilia. Neutrophils show prominent (toxic) granulation and vacuolation in this specimen from a patient with acute inflammation.

neutrophilic leukemia may be made. Clonality studies may be helpful in distinguishing reactive from neoplastic neutrophilia. It should be kept in mind that reactive neutrophilia and clonal myeloid disorders are not mutually exclusive, and some patients may have both.

LEUKOERYTHROBLASTOSIS

Leukoerythroblastosis or leukoerythroblastic reaction (formerly myelophthisic anemia) is a state in which immature neutrophils and red blood cells (RBCs) are found on peripheral blood smear examination (1–14) (Table 7-7). Numerous conditions produce leukoerythroblastosis, having in common hematopoietic stimulation or stress. These include alcoholic hepatitis, bone marrow fibrosis, bone marrow necrosis, granulocyte colony-stimulating factor therapy, hemolytic anemia, hemorrhage, infection, inflammatory disorders, iron and folate deficiencies, osteopetrosis, oxalosis, renal osteodystrophy, response to hematinics, steroid withdrawal, transient erythroblastopenia of childhood, myeloproliferative disorders, myelodysplastic syndromes, acute leukemia, malignant lymphoma in bone marrow, and nonhematolymphoid tumors in bone marrow.

The peripheral blood shows variable cell counts, depending on the underlying disorder. Automated hematology analyzers count nucleated RBCs as WBCs, and the WBC count should be corrected for this factor. In our laboratory, the correction is made when five or more nucleated RBCs are found during a 100-cell WBC differential count. The peripheral blood smear shows immature granulocytes and nucleated RBCs. Granulocytic fragments may be present and should be distinguished from schistocytes and large platelets. Bone marrow examination may show hematopoietic hypercellularity, necrosis, or replacement of hematopoietic tissue by bone, fibrous tissue, and/or malignancy.

NEUTROPHIL INCLUSIONS

Neutrophils may contain a variety of inclusions (1–14) (Fig. 7-2). Most are cytoplasmic and consist of ingested substances or organisms, accumulations of metabolites, or altered organelles.

Ingested substances may consist of cryoglobulins, found in connective tissue disorders and other conditions associated with cryoglobulinemia; denatured nucleic acid, producing the well-known LE cell of systemic lupus erythematosus; apoptotic nuclear fragments similar to Howell-Jolly bodies, seen in human immunodeficiency virus infection; immune complexes, seen in connective tissue disorders; malarial pigment; and melanin, seen in cells from patients with metastatic malignant melanoma.

Ingested microorganisms seen within neutrophils include bacteria (usually cocci), yeast, and protozoa (especially *Leishmania* species). Ehrlichiosis produces morules, or spherical aggregates, of organisms.

Accumulations of metabolites arise in the setting of inherited metabolic disease. These include acid mucopolysaccharide in mucopolysaccharidosis type VII (Alder-Reilly anomaly) and amylopectin in type IV glycogen storage disease.

Altered organelles include Döhle bodies, stacks of granule-free rough endoplasmic reticulum seen in cells from patients with active inflammation; Döhle body–like inclusions, found in May-Hegglin anomaly and related disorders; atypical and enlarged lysosomes, characteristic of Chediak-Higashi syndrome; abnormal granules resembling

TABLE 7-7. CONDITIONS ASSOCIATED WITH LEUKOERYTHROBLASTOSIS

Nonneoplastic conditions
  Alcoholic hepatitis
  Bone marrow fibrosis
  Bone marrow necrosis
  Granulocyte colony-stimulating factor therapy
  Hemolytic anemia
  Hemorrhage
  Infection
  Inflammatory disorders
  Iron and folate deficiency
  Osteopetrosis
  Oxalosis
  Renal osteodystrophy
  Response to hematinics
  Steroid withdrawal
  Transient erythroblastopenia of childhood
Neoplastic conditions
  Myeloproliferative disorders
  Myelodysplastic syndromes
  Acute leukemia
  Malignant lymphoma in bone marrow
  Nonhematolymphoid tumors in bone marrow

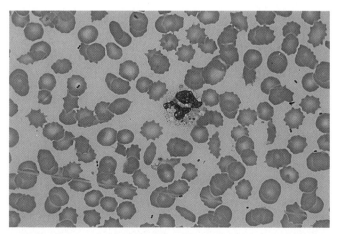

FIGURE 7-2. Peripheral blood smear, neutrophil containing diplococci. A reactive neutrophil shows vacuolation and contains two ingested bacteria (diplococci) in this specimen from a patient with sepsis.

Alder-Reilly anomaly, reported in the genetic mutation of the myeloperoxidase gene; multilamellar bodies, reported in amiodarone therapy; large, dark-staining inclusions, reported in colchicine intoxication; and small gray-blue inclusions composed of confronting cisternae, reported in chronic renal failure.

Intranuclear inclusions are uncommon in neutrophils. They have been reported in cells from patients receiving ganciclovir therapy.

NEUTROPHILIC HYPERPLASIA

Neutrophilic (or granulocytic) hyperplasia is a common bone marrow finding (1–4) (Table 7-8). Underlying conditions include autoimmune neutropenia, connective tissue disease, infection, inflammation, stress, trauma, and malignancy.

The peripheral blood may show neutrophilia or neutropenia. Other values in the CBC vary, depending on the underlying condition.

Bone marrow aspirate smears show increased neutrophilic precursors and mature segmented neutrophils (Figs. 7-3 through 7-6). The myeloid-to-erythroid ratio varies, depending on concomitant changes in the erythroid series. Among neutrophils, promyelocytes and myelocytes are relatively increased compared with later forms. Histologic sections show a diffuse increase in neutrophils and neutrophilic precursors throughout bone marrow and, in marked reactions, a homogeneous band of early myeloid precursors directly apposed to the surface of the trabecular bone. Other findings may include neutrophilic maturation arrest, phagocytosis of neutrophils by macrophages, and reactive plasmacytosis.

The differential diagnosis includes the myeloproliferative and myelodysplastic disorders, especially chronic myeloid leukemia and chronic myelomonocytic leukemia. These are distinguished from benign granulocytic hyperplasia by disordered myeloid architecture (atypical localization of immature precursors), dysplastic changes, increased blasts, and clonal cytogenetic anomalies. The bandlike paratrabecular population of early granulocytic precursors may be quite marked in some cases and resemble multiple myeloma or other tumors. Recognition of this pattern of myeloid hyperplasia is helpful in avoiding a mistaken diagnosis of malignancy.

TABLE 7-8. CONDITIONS ASSOCIATED WITH NEUTROPHILIC HYPERPLASIA

Autoimmune neutropenia
Connective tissue disease
Infection
Inflammation
Stress
Trauma
Malignancy

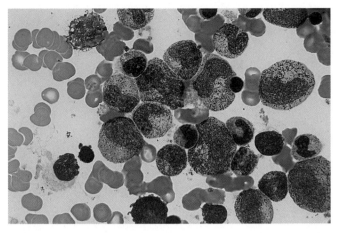

FIGURE 7-3. Bone marrow aspirate smear, neutrophilic hyperplasia. Neutrophils are increased and consist predominantly of immature forms in this specimen from a patient with chronic granulomatous disease.

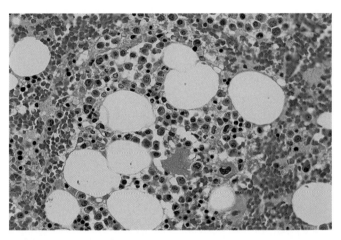

FIGURE 7-4. Bone marrow clot, neutrophilic hyperplasia. Neutrophils are increased in this specimen from a patient with autoimmune neutropenia and rheumatoid arthritis.

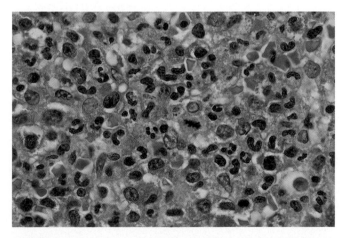

FIGURE 7-5. Bone marrow biopsy specimen, neutrophilic hyperplasia. Neutrophils of all maturational stages are markedly increased in this specimen from a patient with Hodgkin disease.

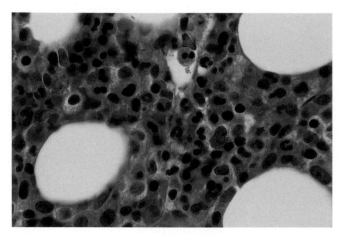

FIGURE 7-6. Bone marrow biopsy specimen, neutrophilic hyperplasia. Neutrophils, including bands and segmented neutrophils, are increased in this specimen from a patient with benign idiopathic neutropenia.

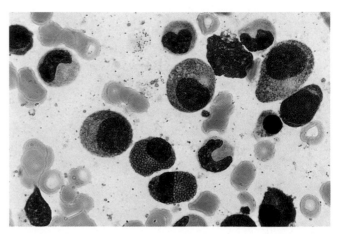

FIGURE 7-7. Bone marrow aspirate smear, neutrophilic maturation arrest. Numerous myelocytes are present in this specimen from a patient recovering after drug-induced neutropenia (agranulocytosis).

NEUTROPHILIC MATURATION ARREST

Neutrophilic maturation arrest is the presence of numerous early neutrophilic (granulocytic, myeloid) precursors in bone marrow with few, if any, band forms and mature segmented neutrophils (1–17) (Table 7-9). This term is probably a misnomer in most cases. Apparent maturation arrest is usually caused by synchronous regeneration of myeloid precursors after granulocytic aplasia or by immune-mediated clearance of mature segmented neutrophils from bone marrow. True failure of myeloid maturation is characteristic of some cases of severe congenital neutropenia and clonal myeloid disease.

Conditions under which maturation arrest have been reported include congenital neutropenia, infection, recovery after drug-induced agranulocytosis (with or without granulocyte colony-stimulating factor therapy), autoimmune neutropenia, connective tissue disorders, isovaleric acidemia, and T-cell large granular lymphocytic leukemia.

The peripheral blood usually shows neutropenia; myeloid precursors are sometimes present. Bone marrow aspirate smears and histologic sections show variable cellularity and a variable myeloid-to-erythroid ratio (Fig. 7-7). The myeloid series consists of promyelocytes, myelocytes, and possibly metamyelocytes. Mature neutrophils are reduced to absent.

TABLE 7-9. CONDITIONS ASSOCIATED WITH NEUTROPHILIC MATURATION ARREST

Nonneoplastic conditions
  Autoimmune neutropenia
  Congenital neutropenia
  Connective tissue disorders
  Infection
  Isovaleric acidemia
  Recovery after drug-induced agranulocytosis

Neoplastic conditions
  T-cell large granular lymphocytic leukemia

Other findings may be present, depending on the underlying etiology.

The differential diagnosis consists primarily of acute myeloid leukemia, especially acute promyelocytic leukemia. Recognition of the clinical setting helps to prevent a mistaken diagnosis of acute leukemia. Flow cytometry has shown expression of CD11b but not CD117 in recovering normal granulocytic precursors and the reverse phenotype in acute promyelocytic leukemia.

It should be kept in mind that the usual course of therapy for acute leukemia produces hematopoietic hypoplasia or aplasia, followed by synchronous regeneration of clonal and/or polyclonal myeloid precursors. In such cases, cytogenetic analysis is helpful in determining whether the myeloid precursors represent recurrent acute leukemia.

NEUTROPHILIC HYPOPLASIA

Neutrophilic (or granulocytic) hypoplasia occurs alone, in combination with pure red cell aplasia, or in aplastic anemia. As an isolated finding, it is often referred to as pure white cell aplasia (PWCA) (1–23) (Table 7-10). PWCA is

TABLE 7-10. CONDITIONS ASSOCIATED WITH PURE WHITE CELL APLASIA

Nonneoplastic conditions
  Excessive zinc intake
  Drug therapy
  Ethanol abuse
  Goodpasture syndrome
  Myasthenia gravis
  Nonimmune chronic neutropenia

Neoplastic conditions
  Malignant melanoma
  Thymoma
  Prodrome to hairy cell leukemia

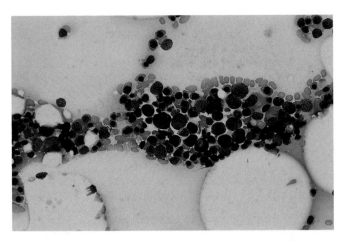

FIGURE 7-8. Bone marrow aspirate smear, pure white cell aplasia. No granulocytic precursors or segmented neutrophils are present in this specimen from a patient with Thorazine-induced agranulocytosis.

an uncommon disorder that may be transient, cyclic, or persistent. Conditions associated with PWCA include excessive zinc intake, drug therapy (especially antibiotics and antiepileptics), ethanol abuse, nonimmune chronic neutropenia, myasthenia gravis, thymoma, and Goodpasture disease. PWCA has also been reported as a prodrome to hairy cell leukemia. The mechanisms of PWCA include autoimmunity, increased apoptosis of neutrophilic precursors, reduction of lineage-specific CD34+ cells, increased production of cytokines inhibiting hematopoiesis, and increased splenic sequestration. The outcome is variable; some patients have been reported to develop clonal myeloid disease.

The peripheral blood usually shows neutropenia or frank agranulocytosis. Bone marrow aspirate smears and histologic sections show absence or near-absence of granulocytes and precursors (Figs. 7-8 and 7-9). Other possible

findings include reactive plasmacytosis and pure red cell aplasia.

The differential diagnosis includes neutropenia associated with neutrophilic hyperplasia rather than hypoplasia. This situation is found under conditions of increased peripheral clearance or destruction of neutrophils, as in the neutropenia of sepsis.

REFERENCES

Neutropenia

1. Abe Y, Hirase N, Muta K, et al. Adult onset cyclic hematopoiesis in a patient with myelodysplastic syndrome. *Int J Hematol* 2000; 71:40–45.
2. Adams WH, Liu YK. Periodic neutropenia and monocytopenia. *Am J Hematol* 1982;13:73–82.
3. Bennett M, Grunwald AJ. Hydroxyurea and periodicity in myeloproliferative disease. *Eur J Haematol* 2001;66:317–323.
4. Birgens HS, Karle H. Reversible adult-onset cyclic haematopoiesis with a cycle length of 100 days. *Br J Haematol* 1993;83:181–186.
5. Blanchong CA, Olshefski R, Kahwash S. Large granular lymphocyte leukemia: case report of chronic neutropenia and rheumatoid arthritis-like symptoms in a child. *Pediatr Dev Pathol* 2001;4: 94–99.
6. Boesen P. Cyclic neutropenia terminating in permanent agranulocytosis. *Acta Med Scand* 1988;223:89–91.
7. Fata F, Myers P, Addeo J, et al. Cyclic neutropenia in Crohn's ileocolitis: efficacy of granulocyte colony-stimulating factor. *J Clin Gastroenterol* 1997;24:253–256.
8. Goraya JS, Virdi VS, Marwaha N, et al. Acute lymphoblastic leukemia presenting as cyclic neutropenia. *Pediatr Hematol Oncol* 2002;19:279–282.
9. Haurie C, Dale DC, Mackey MC. Occurrence of periodic oscillations in the differential blood counts of congenital, idiopathic, and cyclical neutropenic patients before and during treatment with G-CSF. *Exp Hematol* 1999;27:401–409.
10. Heussner P, Haase D, Kanz L. G-CSF in the long-term treatment of cyclic neutropenia and chronic idiopathic neutropenia in adult patients. *Int J Hematol* 1995;62:225–234.
11. Hirase N, Abe Y, Muta K, et al. Autoimmune neutropenia with cyclic oscillation of neutrophil count after steroid administration. *Int J Hematol* 2001;73:346–350.
12. Kubota M, Nakamura K, Watanabe K, et al. A case of common variable immunodeficiency associated with cyclic thrombocytopenia. *Acta Paediatr Jpn* 1994;36:690–692.
13. Loughran TP Jr, Starkebaum G. Large granular lymphocyte leukemia. Report of 38 cases and review of the literature. *Medicine (Baltimore)* 1987;66:397–405.
14. Miyoshi I, Takemoto S, Taguchi H, et al. Adult T-cell leukemia with cyclic neutropenia in a seronegative patient carrying only the tax gene of HTLV-I. *Am J Hematol* 2002;71:137–138.
15. Moser C, Schlesier M, Drager R, et al. Transient CD80 expression defect in a patient with variable immunodeficiency and cyclic neutropenia. *Int Arch Allergy Immunol* 1997;112:96–99.
16. Rodgers GM, Shuman MA. Acquired cyclic neutropenia: successful treatment with prednisone. *Am J Hematol* 1982;13:83–89.
17. Rodriguez A, Yood RA, Condon TJ, et al. Recurrent uveitis in a patient with adult onset cyclic neutropenia associated with increased large granular lymphocytes. *Br J Ophthalmol* 1997; 81:415.
18. Storek J, Glaspy JA, Grody WW, et al. Adult-onset cyclic neutropenia responsive to cyclosporine therapy in a patient with ankylosing spondylitis. *Am J Hematol* 1993;43:139–143.

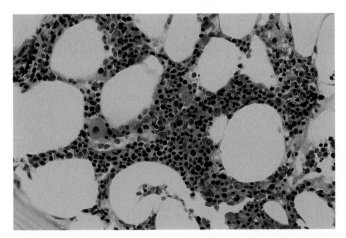

FIGURE 7-9. Bone marrow biopsy specimen, pure white cell aplasia. No granulocytic precursors or segmented neutrophils are present in this specimen from a patient with idiopathic agranulocytosis.

19. Aaron S, Davis P, Percy J. Neutropenia occurring during the course of chrysotherapy: a review of 25 cases. *J Rheumatol* 1985;12: 897–899.

20. Alliot C, Barrios M, Tabuteau S, et al. Autoimmune cytopenias associated with malignancies and successfully treated with intravenous immune globulins: about two cases. *Therapie* 2000;55:371–374.

21. Allo M, Silva J Jr. Antibiotic agranulocytosis: association with cephalothin and carbenicillin. *South Med J* 1977;70:1017–1019.

22. Auner HW, Klintschar M, Crevenna R, et al. Two case studies of chronic idiopathic neutropenia preceding acute myeloid leukaemia. *Br J Haematol* 1999;105:431–433.

23. Balkin MS, Buchholtz M, Ortiz J, et al. Propylthiouracil (PTU)-induced agranulocytosis treated with recombinant human granulocyte colony-stimulating factor (G-CSF). *Thyroid* 1993;3: 305–309.

24. Bjorkholm M, Pisa P, Arver S, et al. Haematologic effects of granulocyte-macrophage colony stimulating factor in a patient with thiamazole-induced agranulocytosis. *J Intern Med* 1992;232:443–445.

25. Bux J, Behrens G, Jaeger G, et al. Diagnosis and clinical course of autoimmune neutropenia in infancy: analysis of 240 cases. *Blood* 1998;91:181–186.

26. Calhoun DA, Rimsza LM, Burchfield DJ, et al. Congenital autoimmune neutropenia in two premature neonates. *Pediatrics* 2001;108:181–184.

27. Chirico G, Motta M, Villani P, et al. Late-onset neutropenia in very low birthweight infants. *Acta Paediatr Suppl* 2002;91: 104–108.

28. O'Connor CR, Schraeder PL, Kurland AH, et al. Evaluation of the mechanisms of antiepileptic drug-related chronic leukopenia. *Epilepsia* 1994;35:149–154.

29. Coppo P, Sibilia J, Maloisel F, et al. Primary Sjogren's syndrome associated agranulocytosis: a benign disorder? *Ann Rheum Dis* 2003;62:476–478.

30. Demiroglu H, Dundar S. Behcet's disease and chronic neutropenia. *Scand J Rheumatol* 1997;26:130–132.

31. Faurschou M, Hasselbalch HC, Nielsen OJ. Sustained remission of platelet counts following monoclonal anti-CD20 antibody therapy in two cases of idiopathic autoimmune thrombocytopenia and neutropenia. *Eur J Haematol* 2001;66:408–411.

32. Friedman J, Klepfish A, Miller EB, et al. Agranulocytosis in Sjogren's syndrome: two case reports and analysis of 11 additional reported cases. *Semin Arthritis Rheum* 2002;31:338–345.

33. Grohmann R, Schmidt LG, Spiess-Kiefer C, et al. Agranulocytosis and significant leucopenia with neuroleptic drugs: results from the AMUP program. *Psychopharmacology (Berl)* 1989;99 [Suppl]:S109–S112.

34. Harris R, Marx G, Gillett M, et al. Colchicine-induced bone marrow suppression: treatment with granulocyte colony-stimulating factor. *J Emerg Med* 2000;18:435–440.

35. Kameoka J, Funato T, Miura T, et al. Autoimmune neutropenia in pregnant women causing neonatal neutropenia. *Br J Haematol* 2001;114:198–200.

36. Karaaslan Y, Haznedaroglu S, Ozilkan E, et al. Granulocytopenia due to nifuroxazide followed by a G-CSF-induced leukemoid reaction. *Ann Pharmacother* 1999;33:1229–1230.

37. Kumar K, Kumar A. Reversible neutropenia associated with ampicillin therapy in pediatric patients. *Drug Intell Clin Pharm* 1981;15:802–806.

38. Lehmann HW, von Landenberg P, Modrow S. Parvovirus B19 infection and autoimmune disease. *Autoimmun Rev* 2003;2: 218–223.

39. Lyall EG, Lucas GF, Eden OB. Autoimmune neutropenia of infancy. *J Clin Pathol* 1992;45:431–434.

40. Marcus EL, Clarfield AM, Kleinman Y, et al. Agranulocytosis associated with initiation of famotidine therapy. *Ann Pharmacother* 2002;36:267–271.

41. Nahata MC. Lack of predictability of chloramphenicol toxicity in paediatric patients. *J Clin Pharm Ther* 1989;14:297–303.

42. Neel EU. Infectious mononucleosis. Death due to agranulocytosis and pneumonia. *JAMA* 1976;236:1493–1494.

43. Parmley RT, Crist WM, Ragab AH, et al. Phagocytosis of neutrophils by marrow macrophages in childhood chronic benign neutropenia. *J Pediatr* 1981;98:207–212.

44. Raizman MB, Fay AM, Weiss JS. Dapsone-induced neutropenia in patients treated for ocular cicatricial pemphigoid. *Ophthalmology* 1994;101:1805–1807.

45. Ross DW, Pryzwansky KB. Transient granulocyte maturation arrest: discovery by flow cytometry of a variant form of agranulocytosis. *Am J Pediatr Hematol Oncol* 1985;7:91–96.

46. Scheurlen W, Ramasubbu K, Wachowski O, et al. Chronic autoimmune thrombopenia/neutropenia in a boy with persistent Parvovirus B19 infection. *J Clin Virol* 2001;20:173–178.

47. Taniuchi S, Masuda M, Yamamoto A, et al. FcgammaRIII b and FcgammaRIIa polymorphism may affect the production of specific NA1 autoantibody and clinical course of autoimmune neutropenia of infancy. *Hum Immunol* 2001;62:408–413.

48. Taniuchi S, Masuda M, Yamamoto A, et al. Two cases of autoimmune neutropenia possibly induced by beta-lactam antibiotics in infants. *J Pediatr Hematol Oncol* 2000;22:533–538.

49. Valiaveedan R, Rao S, Miller S, et al. Transient neutropenia of childhood. *Clin Pediatr (Phila)* 1987;26:639–642.

50. Haddy TB, Rana SR, Castro O. Benign ethnic neutropenia: what is a normal absolute neutrophil count? *J Lab Clin Med* 1999;133:15–22.

51. Jumean HG, Sudah FI. Chronic benign idiopathic neutropenia in Jordanians. *Acta Haematol* 1983;69:59–60.

52. Rezvani K, Flanagan AM, Sarma U, et al. Investigation of ethnic neutropenia by assessment of bone marrow colony-forming cells. *Acta Haematol* 2001;105:32–37.

53. Shoenfeld Y, Alkan ML, Asaly A, et al. Benign familial leukopenia and neutropenia in different ethnic groups. *Eur J Haematol* 1988;41:273–277.

54. Weingarten MA, Pottick-Schwartz EA, Brauner A. The epidemiology of benign leukopenia in Yemenite Jews. *Isr J Med Sci* 1993;29:297–299.

55. Carr ME, Whitehead J, Carlson P, et al. Case report: immunoglobulin M-mediated, temperature-dependent neutrophil agglutination as a cause of pseudoneutropenia. *Am J Med Sci* 1996;311: 92–95.

56. Claviez A, Horst HA, Santer R, et al. Neutrophil aggregates in a 13-year-old girl: a rare hematological phenomenon. *Ann Hematol* 2003;82:251–253.

57. Galifi M, Schinella M, Nicoli M, et al. Instrumental reports and effect of anticoagulants in a case of neutrophil agglutination *in vitro*. *Haematologica* 1993;78:364–370.

58. Lazo-Langner A, Piedras J, Romero-Lagarza P, et al. Platelet satellitism, spurious neutropenia, and cutaneous vasculitis: casual or causal association? *Am J Hematol* 2002;70:246–249.

59. Moraglio D, Banfi G, Arnelli A. Association of pseudothrombocytopenia and pseudoleukopenia: evidence for different pathogenic mechanisms. *Scand J Clin Lab Invest* 1994;54:257–265.

60. Pewarchuk W, VanderBoom J, Blajchman MA. Pseudopolycythemia, pseudothrombocytopenia, and pseudoleukopenia due to overfilling of blood collection vacuum tubes. *Arch Pathol Lab Med* 1992;116:90–92.

61. Robbins SH, Conly MA, Oettinger J. Cold-induced granulocyte agglutination. A cause of pseudoleukopenia. *Arch Pathol Lab Med* 1991;115:155–157.

62. Zelster D, Fusman R, Chapman J, et al. Increased leukocyte aggregation induced by gamma-globulin: a clue to the presence of pseudoleukopenia. *Am J Med Sci* 2000;320:177–182.

Reactive Neutrophilia and Leukemoid Reaction

1. Arguelles-Grande C, Leon F, Matilla J, et al. Steroidal management and serum cytokine profile of a case of alcoholic hepatitis with leukemoid reaction. *Scand J Gastroenterol* 2002;37:1111–1113.
2. Au WY, Ma SK, Kwong YL. Disseminated hepatosplenic mycobacterial infection masking myeloproliferative diseases as leukemoid reaction: a diagnostic pitfall. *Leuk Lymphoma* 2001;42: 805–808.
3. Cohen Y, Rund D, Moualem E, et al. Carbamazepine-induced generalized "pseudoleukemia lymphoma"–like syndrome. *Isr Med Assoc J* 2003;5:457.
4. Ferrer A, Cervantes F, Hernandez-Boluda JC, et al. Leukemoid reaction preceding the diagnosis of colorectal carcinoma by four years. *Haematologica* 1999;84:671–672.
5. Hisaoka M, Tsuji S, Hashimoto H, et al. Dedifferentiated liposarcoma with an inflammatory malignant fibrous histiocytoma-like component presenting a leukemoid reaction. *Pathol Int* 1997;47:642–646.
6. Horii A, Shimamura K, Honjo Y, et al. Granulocyte colony stimulating factor-producing tongue carcinoma. *Head Neck* 1997;19:351–356.
7. Juturi JV, Hopkins T, Farhangi M. Severe leukocytosis with neutrophilia (leukemoid reaction) in alcoholic steatohepatitis. *Am J Gastroenterol* 1998;93:1013.
8. Karaaslan Y, Haznedaroglu S, Ozilkan E, et al. Granulocytopenia due to nifuroxazide followed by a G-CSF-induced leukemoid reaction. *Ann Pharmacother* 1999;33:1229–1230.
9. Kayashima T, Yamaguchi K, Akiyoshi T, et al. Leukemoid reaction associated with diabetic ketoacidosis—with measurement of plasma levels of granulocyte colony-stimulating factor. *Intern Med* 1993;32:869–871.
10. Kutluk T, Emir S, Karnak I, et al. Mesenteric inflammatory pseudotumor: unusual presentation with leukemoid reaction and massive calcified mass. *J Pediatr Hematol Oncol* 2002;24:158–159.
11. Lakhotia M, Shah PK, Gupta A, et al. Leukaemoid reaction in megaloblastic anemia during puerperium. *J Assoc Physicians India* 1996;44:744.
12. Marcus EL, Clarfield AM, Kleinman Y, et al. Agranulocytosis associated with initiation of famotidine therapy. *Ann Pharmacother* 2002;36:267–271.
13. Marinella MA. Extreme leukemoid reaction associated with retroperitoneal hemorrhage. *Arch Intern Med* 1998;158:300–301.
14. Mycyk MB, Drendel A, Sigg T, et al. Leukemoid response in ethylene glycol intoxication. *Vet Hum Toxicol* 2002;44:304–306.
15. Nakamura T, Ezaki S, Takasaki J, et al. Leukemoid reaction and chronic lung disease in infants with very low birth weight. *J Matern Fetal Neonatal Med* 2002;11:396–399.
16. Nimieri HS, Makoni SN, Madziwa FH, et al. Leukemoid reaction response to chemotherapy and radiotherapy in a patient with cervical carcinoma. *Ann Hematol* 2003;82:316–317.
17. Ohbayashi H, Nosaka H, Hirose K, et al. Granulocyte colony stimulating factor-producing diffuse malignant mesothelioma of pleura. *Intern Med* 1999;38:668–670.
18. Pradeepkumar VK, Rajadurai VS, Tan KW. Congenital candidiasis: varied presentations. *J Perinatol* 1998;18:311–316.
19. Saussez S, Heimann P, Vandevelde L, et al. Undifferentiated carcinoma of the nasopharynx and leukemoid reaction: report of case with literature review. *J Laryngol Otol* 1997;111:66–69.
20. Schmid C, Frisch B, Beham A, et al. Comparison of bone marrow histology in early chronic granulocytic leukemia and in leukemoid reaction. *Eur J Haematol* 1990;44:154–158.
21. Seebach JD, Morant R, Ruegg R, et al. The diagnostic value of the neutrophil left shift in predicting inflammatory and infectious disease. *Am J Clin Pathol* 1997;107:582–591.
22. Singh ZN, Kotwal J, Choudhry VP, et al. Leukemoid reaction simulating acute promyelocytic leukemia. *J Assoc Physicians India* 1999;47:1031–1032.
23. Watanabe M, Ono K, Ozeki Y, et al. Production of granulocyte-macrophage colony-stimulating factor in a patient with metastatic chest wall large cell carcinoma. *Jpn J Clin Oncol* 1998;28: 559–562.
24. Zanardo V, Savio V, Giacomin C, et al. Relationship between neonatal leukemoid reaction and bronchopulmonary dysplasia in low-birth-weight infants: a cross-sectional study. *Am J Perinatol* 2002;19:379–386.
25. Denison FC, Elliott CL, Wallace EM. Dexamethasone-induced leucocytosis in pregnancy. *Br J Obstet Gynaecol* 1997;104: 851–853.
26. Liles WC, Huang JE, Llewellyn C, et al. A comparative trial of granulocyte-colony-stimulating factor and dexamethasone, separately and in combination, for the mobilization of neutrophils in the peripheral blood of normal volunteers. *Transfusion* 1997;37:182–187.
27. Shoenfeld Y, Gurewich Y, Gallant LA, et al. Prednisone-induced leukocytosis. Influence of dosage, method and duration of administration on the degree of leukocytosis. *Am J Med* 1981;71: 773–778.
28. Di Giovanni S, De Matteis MA, Ciocca D, et al. Pseudothrombocytosis and pseudoleukocytosis in a case of essential mixed cryoglobulinemia (type II). *Clin Exp Rheumatol* 1986;4:143–145.
29. Fohlen-Walter A, Jacob C, Lecompte T, et al. Laboratory identification of cryoglobulinemia from automated blood cell counts, fresh blood samples, and blood films. *Am J Clin Pathol* 2002;117:606–614.
30. Lombarts AJ, de Kieviet W. Recognition and prevention of pseudothrombocytopenia and concomitant pseudoleukocytosis. *Am J Clin Pathol* 1988;89:634–639.
31. Patel KJ, Hughes CG, Parapia LA. Pseudoleucocytosis and pseudothrombocytosis due to cryoglobulinaemia. *J Clin Pathol* 1987;40:120–121.
32. Schrezenmeier H, Muller H, Gunsilius E, et al. Anticoagulant-induced pseudothrombocytopenia and pseudoleucocytosis. *Thromb Haemost* 1995;73:506–513.
33. Shah PC, Rao K, Noble V, et al. Transient pseudoleukocytosis caused by cryocrystalglobulinemia. *Arch Pathol Lab Med* 1978;102:172–173.
34. Shimasaki AK, Fujita K, Fujio S, et al. Pseudoleukocytosis without pseudothrombocytopenia induced by the interaction of EDTA and IgG(2)-kappa M-protein. *Clin Chim Acta* 2000;299: 119–128.
35. Taft EG, Grossman J, Abraham GN, et al. Pseudoleukocytosis due to cryoprotein crystals. *Am J Clin Pathol* 1973;60:669–671.

Leukoerythroblastosis

1. Arici M, Hazendaroglu IC, Erman M, et al. Leukoerythroblastosis following the use of G-CSF. *Am J Hematol* 1996;52:123–124.
2. Ataga KI, Orringer EP. Bone marrow necrosis in sickle cell disease: a description of three cases and a review of the literature. *Am J Med Sci* 2000;320:342–347.
3. Chang JC, Naqvi T. Thrombotic thrombocytopenic purpura associated with bone marrow metastasis and secondary myelofibrosis in cancer. *Oncologist* 2003;8:375–380.

4. Chen CJ, Lee MY, Hsu ML, et al. Malignant infantile osteopetrosis initially presenting with neonatal hypocalcemia: case report. *Ann Hematol* 2003;82:64–67.
5. Cooper BT, Evans DJ, Chadwick VS. Coeliac disease presenting with a leuco-erythroblastic anaemia. *Postgrad Med J* 1979;55:914–915.
6. Dalton RR, Krauss JS, Falls DG, et al. Clinical commentary: granulocytic fragments in sepsis. *Ann Clin Lab Sci* 2001;31:365–368.
7. Eichner ER. Spider bite hemolytic anemia: positive Coombs' test, erythrophagocytosis, and leukoerythroblastic smear. *Am J Clin Pathol* 1984;81:683–687.
8. Krauss JS, Dover RK, Khankhanian NK. Biochemical values, complement levels, and hemostatic data in septic leukoerythroblastosis. *Ann Clin Lab Sci* 1989;19:422–428.
9. Krauss JS, Dover RK, Khankhanian NK, et al. Granulocytic fragments in sepsis. *Mod Pathol* 1989;2:301–305.
10. Mathew P, Fleming D, Adegboyega PA. Myelophthisis as a solitary manifestation of failure from rectal carcinoma. A Batson phenomenon? *Arch Pathol Lab Med* 2000;124:1228–1230.
11. Mupanomunda OK, Alter BP. Transient erythroblastopenia of childhood (TEC) presenting as leukoerythroblastic anemia. *J Pediatr Hematol Oncol* 1997;19:165–167.
12. Nomura S, Ogawa Y, Osawa G, et al. Myelofibrosis secondary to renal osteodystrophy. *Nephron* 1996;72:683–687.
13. Simon D, Galambos JT. Leukoerythroblastosis with blasts in a patient with alcoholic hepatitis. *J Clin Gastroenterol* 1987;9:217–218.
14. Trenchard PM, Wells CE, Jarriwalla AG. Leuco-erythroblastosis following withdrawal from glucocorticoid therapy. *Postgrad Med J* 1977;53:391–393.

Neutrophil Inclusions

1. Adams PC, Sloan P, Morley AR, et al. Peripheral neutrophil inclusions in amiodarone treated patients. *Br J Clin Pharmacol* 1986;22:736–738.
2. Berkley CK, Parkin JD, Peterson LC. Confronting cisternae presenting as intracytoplasmic inclusions in monocytes. *Am J Clin Pathol* 1990;94:461–463.
3. Ghosh K, Muirhead D, Christie B, et al. Ultrastructural changes in peripheral blood neutrophils in a patient receiving ganciclovir for CMV pneumonitis following allogenic bone marrow transplantation. *Bone Marrow Transplant* 1999;24:429–431.
4. Gitzelmann R, Wiesmann UN, Spycher MA, et al. Unusually mild course of beta-glucuronidase deficiency in two brothers (mucopolysaccharidosis VII). *Helv Paediatr Acta* 1978;33:413–428.
5. Godwin JH, Stopeck A, Chang VT, et al. Mycobacteremia in acquired immune deficiency syndrome. Rapid diagnosis based on inclusions in the peripheral blood smear. *Am J Clin Pathol* 1991;95:369–375.
6. Hurd ER. Presence of leucocyte inclusions in spleen and bone marrow of patients with Felty's syndrome. *J Rheumatol* 1978;5:26–32.
7. Losito A, Lorusso L. Polymorphonuclear leucocyte fluorescence and cryoglobulin phagocytosis in systemic lupus erythematosus. *Clin Exp Immunol* 1979;35:376–379.
8. Maitra A, Ward PC, Kroft SH, et al. Cytoplasmic inclusions in leukocytes. An unusual manifestation of cryoglobulinemia. *Am J Clin Pathol* 2000;113:107–112.
9. Permin H, Wiik A, Djurup R. Phagocytosis by normal polymorphonuclear leukocytes of immune complexes from serum of patients with Felty's syndrome and rheumatoid arthritis with special reference to IgE immune complexes. *Acta Pathol Microbiol Immunol Scand [C]* 1984;92:37–42.
10. Powell HC, Wolf PL. Neutrophilic leukocyte inclusions in colchicine intoxication. *Arch Pathol Lab Med* 1976;100:136–138.
11. Presentey B. Alder anomaly accompanied by a mutation of the myeloperoxidase structural gene. *Acta Haematol* 1986;75:157–159.
12. Rosenthal P, Podesta L, Grier R, et al. Failure of liver transplantation to diminish cardiac deposits of amylopectin and leukocyte inclusions in type IV glycogen storage disease. *Liver Transpl Surg* 1995;1:373–376.
13. Slagel DD, Lager DJ, Dick FR. Howell-Jolly body-like inclusions in the neutrophils of patients with acquired immunodeficiency syndrome. *Am J Clin Pathol* 1994;101:429–431.
14. Weil SC, Holt S, Hrisinko MA, et al. Melanin inclusions in the peripheral blood leukocytes of a patient with malignant melanoma. *Am J Clin Pathol* 1985;84:679–681.

Neutrophilic Hyperplasia

1. Bux J, Behrens G, Jaeger G, et al. Diagnosis and clinical course of autoimmune neutropenia in infancy: analysis of 240 cases. *Blood* 1998;91:181–186.
2. Calhoun DA, Rimsza LM, Burchfield DJ, et al. Congenital autoimmune neutropenia in two premature neonates. *Pediatrics* 2001;108:181–184.
3. Min JK, Cho CS, Kim HY, et al. Bone marrow findings in patients with adult Still's disease. *Scand J Rheumatol* 2003;32:119–121.
4. Parmley RT, Crist WM, Ragab AH, et al. Phagocytosis of neutrophils by marrow macrophages in childhood chronic benign neutropenia. *J Pediatr* 1981;98:207–212.

Neutrophilic Maturation Arrest

1. Agnarsson BA, Loughran TP Jr, Starkebaum G, et al. The pathology of large granular lymphocyte leukemia. *Hum Pathol* 1989;20:643–651.
2. Ahmed MA. Promyelocytic leukaemoid reaction: an atypical presentation of mycobacterial infection. *Acta Haematol* 1991;85:143–145.
3. Allo M, Silva J Jr. Antibiotic agranulocytosis: association with cephalothin and carbenicillin. *South Med J* 1977;70:1017–1019.
4. Balkin MS, Buchholtz M, Ortiz J, et al. Propylthiouracil (PTU)-induced agranulocytosis treated with recombinant human granulocyte colony-stimulating factor (G-CSF). *Thyroid* 1993;3:305–309.
5. Bjorkholm M, Pisa P, Arver S, et al. Haematologic effects of granulocyte-macrophage colony stimulating factor in a patient with thiamazole-induced agranulocytosis. *J Intern Med* 1992;232:443–445.
6. Bux J, Behrens G, Jaeger G, et al. Diagnosis and clinical course of autoimmune neutropenia in infancy: analysis of 240 cases. *Blood* 1998;91:181–186.
7. Dreskin SC, Iberti TJ, Watson-Williams EJ. Pseudoleukemia due to infection. A case report. *J Med* 1983;14:147–155.
8. Friedman J, Klepfish A, Miller EB, et al. Agranulocytosis in Sjogren's syndrome: two case reports and analysis of 11 additional reported cases. *Semin Arthritis Rheum* 2002;31:338–345.
9. Gilbert-Barness E, Barness LA. Isovaleric acidemia with promyelocytic myeloproliferative syndrome. *Pediatr Dev Pathol* 1999;2:286–291.
10. Gursoy M, Haznedaroglu IC, Celik I, et al. Agranulocytosis, plasmacytosis and thrombocytosis followed by a leukemoid reaction due to acetaminophen toxicity. *Ann Pharmacother* 1996;30:762–765.
11. Kumar K, Kumar A. Reversible neutropenia associated with ampicillin therapy in pediatric patients. *Drug Intell Clin Pharm* 1981;15:802–806.

12. Lin SJ, Jaing TH. Thrombocytopenia in systemic-onset juvenile chronic arthritis: report of two cases with unusual bone marrow features. *Clin Rheumatol* 1999;18:241–243.
13. Miyachi H, Nakamura Y, Shimizu H, et al. Differential effects of IL-3, GM-CSF and G-CSF in an adult with congenital neutropenia. *Int J Hematol* 1992;56:113–118.
14. Rizzatti EG, Garcia AB, Portieres FL, et al. Expression of CD117 and CD11b in bone marrow can differentiate acute promyelocytic leukemia from recovering benign myeloid proliferation. *Am J Clin Pathol* 2002;118:31–37.
15. Ross DW, Pryzwansky KB. Transient granulocyte maturation arrest: discovery by flow cytometry of a variant form of agranulocytosis. *Am J Pediatr Hematol Oncol* 1985;7:91–96.
16. Sanal SM, Campbell EW Jr, Bowdler AJ, et al. Pseudoleukemia: when "leukemia" is not leukemia. *Postgrad Med* 1979;65:143–145.
17. Valiaveedan R, Rao S, Miller S, et al. Transient neutropenia of childhood. *Clin Pediatr (Phila)* 1987;26:639–642.

Neutrophilic Hypoplasia

1. Ackland SP, Bur ME, Adler SS, et al. White blood cell aplasia associated with thymoma. *Am J Clin Pathol* 1988;89:260–263.
2. Blackburn SC, Oliart AD, Garcia Rodriguez LA, et al. Antiepileptics and blood dyscrasias: a cohort study. *Pharmacotherapy* 1998;18:1277–1283.
3. Carmel R. An unusual case of autoimmune agranulocytosis with total absence of myeloid precursors: demonstration of diverse sources of R binder for cobalamin in plasma and secretions. *Am J Clin Pathol* 1983;79:611–615.
4. Firkin FC, Prewett EJ, Nicholls K, et al. Antithymocyte globulin therapy for pure white cell aplasia. *Am J Hematol* 1987;25:101–105.
5. Forsyth PD, Davies JM. Pure white cell aplasia and health food products. *Postgrad Med J* 1995;71:557–558.
6. Fumeaux Z, Beris P, Borisch B, et al. Complete remission of pure white cell aplasia associated with thymoma, autoimmune thyroiditis and type 1 diabetes. *Eur J Haematol* 2003;70:186–189.
7. Hanada T, Ehara T, Nakahara S, et al. Simultaneous transient erythroblastopenia and agranulocytosis: IgG-mediated inhibition of erythrogranulopoiesis. *Eur J Haematol* 1987;38:200–203.
8. Janka-Schaub GE, Raghavachar A, Rister M, et al. Treatment of chronic neutropenia of childhood responsive to cyclosporin A *in vitro* and *in vivo*. *Int J Hematol* 1992;55:157–163.

9. Julia A, Olona M, Bueno J, et al. Drug-induced agranulocytosis: prognostic factors in a series of 168 episodes. *Br J Haematol* 1991;79:366–371.
10. Levitt LJ. Chlorpropamide-induced pure white cell aplasia. *Blood* 1987;69:394–400.
11. Liu YK. Effects of alcohol on granulocytes and lymphocytes. *Semin Hematol* 1980;17:130–136.
12. Mamus SW, Burton JD, Groat JD, et al. Ibuprofen-associated pure white-cell aplasia. *N Engl J Med* 1986;314:624–625.
13. Marinone GM, Roncoli B. Selective myeloid aplasia: a long-lasting presentation of an unusual hairy cell leukemia variant? *Haematologica* 1993;78:239–241.
14. Mathieson PW, O'Neill JH, Durrant ST, et al. Antibody-mediated pure neutrophil aplasia, recurrent myasthenia gravis and previous thymoma: case report and literature review. *Q J Med* 1990;74:57–61.
15. Papadaki HA, Eliopoulos AG, Kosteas T, et al. Impaired granulocytopoiesis in patients with chronic idiopathic neutropenia is associated with increased apoptosis of bone marrow myeloid progenitor cells. *Blood* 2003;101:2591–2600.
16. Papadaki HA, Kosteas T, Gemetzi C, et al. Two patients with nonimmune chronic idiopathic neutropenia of adults developing acute myeloid leukemia with aberrant phenotype and complex karyotype but no mutations in granulocyte colony-stimulating factor receptor. *Ann Hematol* 2002;81:50–54.
17. Papadaki HA, Palmblad J, Eliopoulos GD. Non-immune chronic idiopathic neutropenia of adult: an overview. *Eur J Haematol* 2001;67:35–44.
18. Pisciotta AV. Agranulocytosis during antibiotic therapy: drug sensitivity or sepsis? *Am J Hematol* 1993;42:132–137.
19. Pisciotta AV. Drug-induced agranulocytosis. Peripheral destruction of polymorphonuclear leukocytes and their marrow precursors. *Blood Rev* 1990;4:226–237.
20. Pisciotta AV, Konings SA. 51Cr release assay of clozapine-induced cytotoxicity: evidence for immunogenic mechanism. *J Clin Psychiatry* 1994;55[Suppl B]:143–148.
21. Postiglione K, Ferris R, Jaffe JP, et al. Immune-mediated agranulocytosis and anemia associated with thymoma. *Am J Hematol* 1995;49:336–340.
22. Tohen M, Castillo J, Baldessarini RJ, et al. Blood dyscrasias with carbamazepine and valproate: a pharmacoepidemiological study of 2,228 patients at risk. *Am J Psychiatry* 1995;152:413–418.
23. White JD, MacPherson IR, Evans TR. Auto-immune neutropenia occurring in association with malignant melanoma. *Oncol Rep* 2003;10:249–251.

EOSINOPHILS AND BASOPHILS

EOSINOPENIA

Peripheral blood eosinopenia is an uncommon finding, diagnosed when the absolute eosinophil count is less than the normal range of the testing laboratory; in our laboratory, the lower limit of normal is 0.050×10^9/L.

Eosinopenia has been reported in vitiligo, corticosteroid therapy, Cushing syndrome, hemodialysis, infection, drugs, niacin deficiency (pellagra), pulmonary disease, acute inflammation, dysbarism, extreme exercise, heat exhaustion, stress, ovarian malignancy, and immunodeficiency syndromes, including Good syndrome (Table 8-1) (1–28).

REACTIVE EOSINOPHILIA

Peripheral Blood Eosinophilia

Peripheral blood eosinophilia is diagnosed when the absolute eosinophil count exceeds the normal range of the testing laboratory; in our laboratory, the upper limit of normal is 0.550×10^9/L. Persistent eosinophilia, whatever the cause,

TABLE 8-1. CONDITIONS ASSOCIATED WITH PERIPHERAL BLOOD EOSINOPENIA

Nonneoplastic conditions
  Acute inflammation
  Adult respiratory distress syndrome
  Asthma
  Corticosteroid excess
  Dysbarism
  Hemodialysis
  Immunodeficiency syndromes, including Good syndrome
  Infections, especially *Campylobacter* and human
    immunodeficiency virus infections, hyperinfective
    strongyloidiasis, malaria, and typhoid fever
  Drug reactions
  Niacin deficiency
  Stress, including extreme exercise and heat exhaustion
  Vitiligo
Neoplastic conditions
  Ovarian malignancy
  Thymoma

has serious clinical consequences, including thromboembolic disease, organ damage, and increased overall mortality.

Conditions in which reactive peripheral blood eosinophilia have been reported include adrenocorticoid and growth hormone deficiencies, angina pectoris, atopic disease, including asthma and allergies, autoimmune disease, cigarette smoking, cholesterol embolization, connective tissue disease, constitutional (familial) eosinophilia, drug reactions, eosinophilic gastroenteritis and pneumonitis, hemodialysis, hyperimmunoglobulin E syndrome, immunoglobulin A deficiency, infections (especially those caused by arthropods, flies, helminths, and viruses), ingestion of toxic substances (e.g., shiitake mushrooms, contaminated L-tryptophan), premature birth and neonatal infection, sarcoidosis, sinus histiocytosis with massive lymphadenopathy, solid organ transplant rejection, Wiskott-Aldrich syndrome, systemic mastocytosis, acute lymphoblastic leukemia, lymphoplasmacytic neoplasms, Hodgkin lymphoma, and carcinoma (Table 8-2) (1–41). When no underlying condition can be discovered, the disorder is called idiopathic hypereosinophilic syndrome.

The peripheral blood smear shows eosinophils that may be morphologically unremarkable or show dysplasia-like features such as nuclear hyperlobation (four or more lobes), hypogranularity, and clustering of eosinophil granules in one part of the cytoplasm (Figs. 8-1 through 8-4). Passage of time may be required for an accurate diagnosis because reactive eosinophilia may be morphologically indistinguishable from clonal eosinophilia.

Bone Marrow Eosinophilia

Eosinophilic hyperplasia of bone marrow is relatively common and may occur with or without peripheral blood eosinophilia. Definite numerical criteria have not been established, but it is probably safe to consider eosinophilic hyperplasia present when eosinophils and eosinophilic precursors exceed 5% of nucleated bone marrow cells.

Conditions under which reactive bone marrow eosinophilia has been reported are essentially similar to those causing peripheral blood eosinophilia.

TABLE 8-2. CONDITIONS ASSOCIATED WITH REACTIVE PERIPHERAL BLOOD EOSINOPHILIA

Nonneoplastic conditions
  Adrenocorticoid and growth hormone deficiencies
  Angina pectoris
  Atopic disease, including asthma and allergies
  Autoimmune and connective tissue disease
  Cigarette smoking
  Cholesterol embolization
  Constitutional (familial) eosinophilia
  Drug reactions
  Eosinophilic gastroenteritis and pneumonitis
  Hemodialysis
  Hyperimmunoglobulin E syndrome
  Immunoglobulin A deficiency
  Infections, especially caused by arthropods, flies,
    helminths, and viruses
  Ingestion of toxic substances (e.g., shiitake mushrooms)
  Premature birth and neonatal infection
  Sarcoidosis
  Sinus histiocytosis with massive lymphadenopathy
  Solid organ transplant rejection
  Wiskott-Aldrich syndrome
Neoplastic conditions
Systemic mastocytosis
Acute lymphoblastic leukemia
B-cell, plasma cell, and T cell neoplasms
Hodgkin disease
Carcinoma

Bone marrow aspirate smears and histologic sections show increased eosinophils and precursors. Mixed eosinophil-basophil precursors may be increased. Eosinophils may be distributed throughout bone marrow or located around benign lymphoid aggregates or other focal lesions, such as areas with systemic mastocytosis, malignant lymphoma, or Langerhans cell histiocytosis.

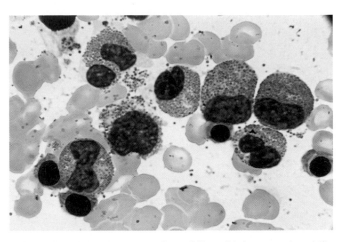

FIGURE 8-2. Bone marrow aspirate, idiopathic hypereosinophilic syndrome. Morphologically unremarkable eosinophils and eosinophilic precursors account for more than 50% of hematopoietic cells.

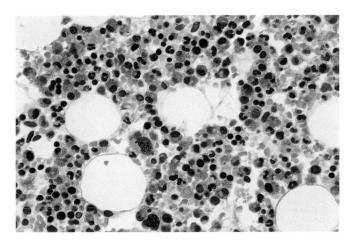

FIGURE 8-3. Bone marrow clot, idiopathic hypereosinophilic syndrome. Most granulocytes are eosinophils and eosinophilic precursors.

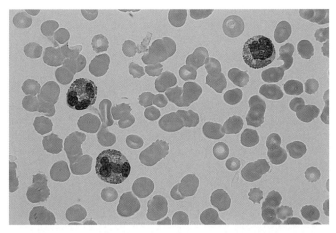

FIGURE 8-1. Peripheral blood, idiopathic hypereosinophilic syndrome. The eosinophils appear morphologically unremarkable.

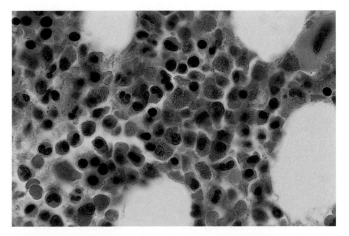

FIGURE 8-4. Bone marrow biopsy specimen, hypereosinophilia caused by adrenal insufficiency. The eosinophils are increased and morphologically unremarkable.

TABLE 8-3. CONDITIONS ASSOCIATED WITH PERIPHERAL BLOOD BASOPENIA

Nonneoplastic conditions
   Chronic urticaria
   Cigarette smoking
   Corticosteroid therapy
   Immunodeficiency syndromes, including Good syndrome
   Industrial chemical exposure
   Ovulation
   Renal transplantation
   Vitiligo
Neoplastic conditions
   Carcinoma

The differential diagnosis consists of clonal eosinophilia, as seen in myeloproliferative disorders; myelodysplastic syndromes; and acute myeloid leukemia.

BASOPENIA

Peripheral blood basopenia is an uncommon finding. It may be difficult to appreciate because basophils are so scarce in peripheral blood; in our laboratory, the lower limit of normal is 0.0×10^9/L (Table 8-3) (1–7).

Basopenia has been reported in Good syndrome and other immunodeficiency syndromes, chronic urticaria, cigarette smoking, corticosteroid therapy, industrial chemical exposure, ovulation, vitiligo, ovarian malignancy, and after renal transplantation (Table 8-4) (1–9).

REACTIVE BASOPHILIA

Peripheral Blood Basophilia

Peripheral blood basophilia is diagnosed when the absolute basophil count exceeds the normal range of the testing laboratory; in our laboratory, the upper limit of normal is 0.200×10^9/L.

Conditions under which reactive peripheral blood basophilia have been reported include atopic allergic rhinitis,

TABLE 8-4. CONDITIONS ASSOCIATED WITH REACTIVE PERIPHERAL BLOOD BASOPHILIA

Nonneoplastic conditions
   Acute rejection of solid organ transplant
   Anemia of undetermined cause
   Atopic disease, including asthma and allergies
   Autoimmune and connective tissue disease
   Chronic renal failure
   Drug reactions
   Helicobacter pylori infection
   Iron deficiency
Neoplastic conditions
Acute lymphoblastic leukemia
   Langerhans cell histiocytosis
   Carcinoma

TABLE 8-5. CONDITIONS ASSOCIATED WITH REACTIVE BONE MARROW BASOPHILIA

Anemia of chronic disease
Aplastic anemia
Iron deficiency anemia
Sideroblastic anemia

interleukin-3 therapy, stem cell factor therapy, asthma, rheumatoid arthritis, all-*trans*-retinoic acid ATRA therapy, eosinophilia-myalgia syndrome owing to contaminated L-tryptophan, *Helicobacter pylori* infection, iron deficiency, lung carcinoma, anemia of undetermined cause, chronic renal failure, acute lymphoblastic leukemia, granulocyte colony-stimulating factor therapy, acute rejection of solid organ transplants, and Langerhans cell histiocytosis (Table 8-4) (1–15).

The peripheral blood smear shows granulated and/or degranulated basophils; the latter may be difficult to identify. Degranulated basophils are characterized by red-purple chromatin (compared with the blue-purple of neutrophil chromatin), irregular lobation of the nucleus, and the presence of clear cytoplasmic vacuoles containing a small central violet dot.

The differential diagnosis includes clonal basophilia, as seen in myeloproliferative disorders; myelodysplastic syndromes; and acute myeloid leukemia.

Bone Marrow Basophilia

Basophilic hyperplasia of bone marrow is an uncommon reaction. Definite numerical criteria have not been established, but it is probably safe to consider basophilic hyperplasia present when basophils and basophilic precursors exceed 2% of nucleated bone marrow cells.

Conditions under which reactive bone marrow basophilia has been reported include anemia of chronic disease, aplastic anemia, iron deficiency anemia, and sideroblastic anemia (Table 8-5) (3,10).

Bone marrow aspirate smears and histologic sections show increased but morphologically unremarkable basophils and basophilic precursors. Eosinophils, eosinophilic precursors, and mast cells may also be increased.

The differential diagnosis consists of clonal basophilia and clonal mastocytosis, as seen in myeloproliferative disorders; myelodysplastic syndromes; and acute myeloid leukemia. Concurrent peripheral blood and bone marrow basophilia is highly associated with chronic myeloid leukemia.

REFERENCES

Eosinopenia

1. Abdalla SH. Peripheral blood and bone marrow leucocytes in Gambian children with malaria: numerical changes and evaluation of phagocytosis. *Ann Trop Paediatr* 1988;8:250–258.

2. Adedayo O, Grell G, Bellot P. Hyperinfective strongyloidiasis in the medical ward: review of 27 cases in 5 years. *South Med J* 2002;95:711–716.
3. Bergesio F, Monzani G, Manescalchi F, et al. Leukocytes, eosinophils and complement function during hemodialysis with polysulphone and polymethylmethacrylate membranes: comparison with cuprophan and polyacrylonitrile. *Blood Purif* 1988;6:16–26.
4. Bodner G, Peer G, Zakuth V, et al. Dialysis-induced eosinophilia. *Nephron* 1982;32:63–66.
5. Cooper PJ, Awadzi K, Ottesen EA, et al. Eosinophil sequestration and activation are associated with the onset and severity of systemic adverse reactions following the treatment of onchocerciasis with ivermectin. *J Infect Dis* 1999;179:738–742.
6. den Ouden M, Ubachs JM, Stoot JE, et al. Whole blood cell counts and leucocyte differentials in patients with benign or malignant ovarian tumours. *Eur J Obstet Gynecol Reprod Biol* 1997;72:73–77.
7. Derks MG, Koopmans RP, Oosterhoff E, et al. Prevention by theophylline of beta-2-receptor down regulation in healthy subjects. *Eur J Drug Metab Pharmacokinet* 2000;25:179–188.
8. Deshmukh CT, Nadkarni UB, Karande SC. An analysis of children with typhoid fever admitted in 1991. *J Postgrad Med* 1994;40:204–207.
9. Diagbouga S, Aldebert D, Fumoux F, et al. Relationship between interleukin-5 production and variations in eosinophil counts during HIV infection in West Africa: influence of *Mycobacterium tuberculosis* infection. *Scand J Immunol* 1999;49:203–209.
10. Donoghue AM, Sinclair MJ, Bates GP. Heat exhaustion in a deep underground metalliferous mine. *Occup Environ Med* 2000;57:165–174.
11. el-Shoura SM. *Falciparum* malaria in naturally infected human patients: IV–ultrastructural changes in peripheral white blood cells. *Ann Parasitol Hum Comp* 1993;68:169–175.
12. Francis H, Awadzi K, Ottesen EA. The Mazzotti reaction following treatment of onchocerciasis with diethylcarbamazine: clinical severity as a function of infection intensity. *Am J Trop Med Hyg* 1985;34:529–536.
13. Hallgren R, Borg T, Venge P, et al. Signs of neutrophil and eosinophil activation in adult respiratory distress syndrome. *Crit Care Med* 1984;12:14–18.
14. Jacey MJ, Gonzales A, Tappan DV. Hematologic changes after two exposures to 6.7 ATA air at three-day intervals. *J Appl Physiol* 1977;42:838–844.
15. Juhlin L, Michaelsson G. A new syndrome characterised by absence of eosinophils and basophils. *Lancet* 1977;1:1233–1235.
16. Juhlin L, Venge P. Total absence of eosinophils in a patient with chronic urticaria and vitiligo. *Eur J Haematol* 1988;40:368–370.
17. Khosla SN, Anand A, Singh U, et al. Haematological profile in typhoid fever. *Trop Doct* 1995;25:156–158.
18. Krause JR, Boggs DR. Search for eosinopenia in hospitalized patients with normal blood leukocyte concentration. *Am J Hematol* 1987;24:55–63.
19. Lee HK, Lim J, Kim M, et al. Immunological alterations associated with *Plasmodium vivax* malaria in South Korea. *Ann Trop Med Parasitol* 2001;95:31–39.
20. Leibovitz I, Zamir D, Polychuck I, et al. Recurrent pneumonia post-thymectomy as a manifestation of Good syndrome. *Eur J Intern Med* 2003;14:60–62.
21. Luksza AR, Jones DK. Comparison of whole-blood eosinophil counts in extrinsic asthmatics with acute and chronic asthma. *BMJ* 1982;285:1229–1231.
22. Mitchell EB, Platts-Mills TA, Pereira RS, et al. Acquired basophil and eosinophil deficiency in a patient with hypogammaglobulinaemia associated with thymoma. *Clin Lab Haematol* 1983;5:253–257.
23. Modig J, Hallgren R. Lethal adult respiratory distress syndrome after meningococcal septicemia biochemical markers in bronchoalveolar lavage. *Resuscitation* 1986;13:159–163.
24. Nieman DC, Berk LS, Simpson-Westerberg M, et al. Effects of long-endurance running on immune system parameters and lymphocyte function in experienced marathoners. *Int J Sports Med* 1989;10:317–323.
25. Pitkanen T, Pettersson T, Ponka A, et al. Clinical and serological studies in patients with *Campylobacter fetus* ssp. jejuni infection: I. Clinical findings. *Infection* 1981;9:274–278.
26. Ray D, Kanagasabapathy AS. Adrenal function and the pattern of glucocorticoid induced eosinopenia in tropical pulmonary eosinophilia. *Indian J Med Res* 1993;98:114–118.
27. Spivak JL, Jackson DL. Pellagra: an analysis of 18 patients and a review of the literature. *Johns Hopkins Med J* 1977;140:295–309.
28. Uchida K, Iwasaki R, Nakano S, et al. Non-obese Cushing's syndrome in an aged woman with non-insulin-dependent diabetes mellitus. *Intern Med* 1995;34:1089–1092.

Reactive Eosinophilia

1. Abali H, Altundag MK, Engin H, et al. Hypereosinophilia and metastatic anaplastic carcinoma of unknown primary. *Med Oncol* 2001;18:285–288.
2. Aglietta M, Sanavio F, Stacchini A, et al. Interleukin-3 *in vivo*: kinetic of response of target cells. *Blood* 1993;82:2054–2061.
3. Ballotta MR, Borghi L, Borin P. An unusual case of cytomegalovirus infection. *Pathologica* 1995;87:682–684.
4. Behnia M, Dowdeswell I, Vakili S. Pleural fluid and serum eosinophilia: association with fluoxetine hydrochloride. *South Med J* 2000;93:611–613.
5. Bhattacharyya N, Fried MP. Peripheral eosinophilia in the diagnosis of chronic rhinosinusitis. *Am J Otolaryngol* 2001;22:116–120.
6. Bodner G, Peer G, Zakuth V, et al. Dialysis-induced eosinophilia. *Nephron* 1982;32:63–66.
7. Brigden M, Graydon C. Eosinophilia detected by automated blood cell counting in ambulatory North American outpatients. Incidence and clinical significance. *Arch Pathol Lab Med* 1997;121:963–967.
8. Butterfield JH. Diverse clinical outcomes of eosinophilic patients with T-cell receptor gene rearrangements: the emerging diagnostic importance of molecular genetics testing. *Am J Hematol* 2001;68:81–86.
9. Calhoun DA, Sullivan SE, Lunoe M, et al. Granulocyte-macrophage colony-stimulating factor and interleukin-5 concentrations in premature neonates with eosinophilia. *J Perinatol* 2000;20:166–171.
10. Chamlin SL, McCalmont TH, Cunningham BB, et al. Cutaneous manifestations of hyper-IgE syndrome in infants and children. *J Pediatr* 2002;141:572–575.
11. Constantinescu M, Veillon DM, Nordberg ML, et al. Chronic allergic rhinitis in an adult male. *Lab Med* 2003;34:437–443.
12. Ehara A, Takeda Y, Kida T, et al. Time-course changes of eosinophil counts in premature infants: no effects of medical manipulation, except erythropoietin treatment, on eosinophilia. *Pediatr Int* 2000;42:58–60.
13. Gayraud M, Guillevin L, le Toumelin P, et al. Long-term followup of polyarteritis nodosa, microscopic polyangiitis, and Churg-Strauss syndrome: analysis of four prospective trials including 278 patients. *Arthritis Rheum* 2001;44:666–675.
14. Giacometti A, Cirioni O, Fortuna M, et al. Environmental and serological evidence for the presence of toxocariasis in the urban area of Ancona, Italy. *Eur J Epidemiol* 2000;16:1023–1026.

15. Hernandez D, Gutierrez L, Duque H, et al. Association of sinus histiocytosis with massive lymphadenopathy and idiopathic hypereosinophilic syndrome. *Histol Histopathol* 1987;2:239–242.
16. Hospers JJ, Schouten JP, Weiss ST, et al. Eosinophilia is associated with increased all-cause mortality after a follow-up of 30 years in a general population sample. *Epidemiology* 2000;11:261–268.
17. Huang ZS, Chien KL, Yang CY, et al. Peripheral differential leukocyte counts in humans vary with hyperlipidemia, smoking, and body mass index. *Lipids* 2001;36:237–245.
18. Jaffc JP, Gertner E, Miller W. Absent neutrophil alkaline phosphatase in the eosinophilia myalgia syndrome associated with L-tryptophan use. *Am J Hematol* 1991;36:280–281.
19. Jain P, Kumar R, Gujral S, et al. Granular acute lymphoblastic leukemia with hypereosinophilic syndrome. *Ann Hematol* 2000;79:272–274.
20. Kawada Y, Yamamoto Y, Noda M, et al. High prevalence of eosinophilia in growth hormone-deficient children. *Pediatr Int* 2001;43:141–145.
21. Koarada S, Tada Y, Aihara S, et al. Polyangiitis overlap syndrome with eosinophilia associated with an elevated serum level of major basic protein. *Intern Med* 1999;38:739–743.
22. Levy AM, Kita H, Phillips SF, et al. Eosinophilia and gastrointestinal symptoms after ingestion of shiitake mushrooms. *J Allergy Clin Immunol* 1998;101:613–620.
23. Lewis SA, Pavord ID, Stringer JR, et al. The relation between peripheral blood leukocyte counts and respiratory symptoms, atopy, lung function, and airway responsiveness in adults. *Chest* 2001;119:105–114.
24. Lin AY, Nutman TB, Kaslow D, et al. Familial eosinophilia: clinical and laboratory results on a U.S. kindred. *Am J Med Genet* 1998;19:229–237.
25. Maeda Y, Miyatake J, Naiki Y, et al. Transient eosinophilia by HIV infection. *Ann Hematol* 2000;79:99–101.
26. Maeno T, Maeno Y, Sando Y, et al. Nuclear hypersegmentation precedes the increase in blood eosinophils in acute eosinophilic pneumonia. *Intern Med* 2000;39:157–159.
27. Potter MB, Fincher RK, Finger DR. Eosinophilia in Wegener's granulomatosis. *Chest* 1999;116:1480–1483.
28. Renston JP, Goldman ES, Hsu RM, et al. Peripheral blood eosinophilia in association with sarcoidosis. *Mayo Clin Proc* 2000;75:586–590.
29. Rivers EP, Gaspari M, Saad GA, et al. Adrenal insufficiency in high-risk surgical ICU patients. *Chest* 2001;119:889–896.
30. Rosman HS, Davis TP, Reddy D, et al. Cholesterol embolization: clinical findings and implications. *J Am Coll Cardiol* 1990;15:1296–1299.
31. Sanchez PR, Guzman AP, Guillen SM, et al. Endemic strongyloidiasis on the Spanish Mediterranean coast. *Q J Med* 2001;94:357–363.
32. Sherer Y, Salomon O, Livneh A, et al. Thromboembolism in a patient with transient eosinophilia and thrombocytopenia. *Clin Lab Haematol* 2000;22:247–249.
33. Sezer O, Schmid P, Hallek M, et al. Eosinophilia during fludarabine treatment of chronic lymphocytic leukemia. *Ann Hematol* 1999;78:475–477.
34. Silvestri M, Oddera S, Spallarossa D, et al. In childhood asthma the degree of allergen-induced T-lymphocyte proliferation is related to serum IgE levels and to blood eosinophilia. *Ann Allergy Asthma Immunol* 2000;84:426–432.
35. Starr J, Pruett JH, Yunginger JW, et al. Myiasis due to Hypoderma lineatum infection mimicking the hypereosinophilic syndrome. *Mayo Clin Proc* 2000;75:755–759.
36. Teoh SC, Siow WY, Tan HT. Severe eosinophilia in disseminated gastric carcinoma. *Singapore Med J* 2000;41:232–234.
37. Thomeer M, Moerman P, Westhovens R, et al. Systemic lupus erythematosus, eosinophilia and Loffler's endocarditis. An unusual association. *Eur Respir J* 1999;13:930–933.
38. Trull A, Steel L, Cornelissen J, et al. Association between blood eosinophil counts and acute cardiac and pulmonary allograft rejection. *J Heart Lung Transplant* 1998;17:517–524.
39. Umemoto S, Suzuki N, Fujii K, et al. Eosinophil counts and plasma fibrinogen in patients with vasospastic angina pectoris. *Am J Cardiol* 2000;85:715–719.
40. Wong-Beringer A, Shriner K. Fluconazole-induced agranulocytosis with eosinophilia. *Pharmacotherapy* 2000;20:484–486.
41. Wynants H, Van Gompel A, Morales I, et al. The hypereosinophilic syndrome after residence in a tropical country: report of 4 cases. *Acta Clin Belg* 2000;55:334–340.

Basopenia

1. Biagini RE, Henningsen GM, Klincewicz SL. Immunologic analyses of peripheral leukocytes from workers at an ethical narcotics manufacturing facility. *Arch Environ Health* 1995;50:7–12.
2. den Ouden M, Ubachs JM, Stoot JE, et al. Whole blood cell counts and leucocyte differentials in patients with benign or malignant ovarian tumours. *Eur J Obstet Gynecol Reprod Biol* 1997;72:73–77.
3. Egido J, Sanchez Crespo M, Lahoz C, et al. Evidence of sensitized basophils in renal transplanted patients. *Transplantation* 1980;29:435–438.
4. Grattan CE, Dawn G, Gibbs S, et al. Blood basophil numbers in chronic ordinary urticaria and healthy controls: diurnal variation, influence of loratadine and prednisolone and relationship to disease activity. *Clin Exp Allergy* 2003;33:337–341.
5. Grattan CE, Walpole D, Francis DM, et al. Flow cytometric analysis of basophil numbers in chronic urticaria: basopenia is related to serum histamine releasing activity. *Clin Exp Allergy* 1997;27:1417–1424.
6. Juhlin L, Michaelsson G. A new syndrome characterised by absence of eosinophils and basophils. *Lancet* 1977;1:1233–1235.
7. Juhlin L, Venge P. Total absence of eosinophils in a patient with chronic urticaria and vitiligo. *Eur J Haematol* 1988;40:368–370.
8. Mitchell EB, Platts-Mills TA, Pereira RS, et al. Acquired basophil and eosinophil deficiency in a patient with hypogammaglobulinaemia associated with thymoma. *Clin Lab Haematol* 1983;5:253–257.
9. Soni R, Bose S, Gada D, et al. Basopenia as an indicator of ovulation (a short term clinical study). *Indian J Physiol Pharmacol* 1996;40:385–388.
10. Walter S, Nancy NR. Basopenia following cigarette smoking. *Indian J Med Res* 1980;72:422–425.

Reactive Basophilia

1. Aglietta M, Sanavio F, Stacchini A, et al. Interleukin-3 *in vivo*: kinetic of response of target cells. *Blood* 1993;82:2054–2061.
2. Andrews RG, Briddell RA, Appelbaum FR, et al. Stimulation of hematopoiesis in vivo by stem cell factor. *Curr Opin Hematol* 1994;1:187–196.
3. Arnalich F, Lahoz C, Larrocha C, et al. Incidence and clinical significance of peripheral and bone marrow basophilia. *J Med* 1987;18:293–303.
4. Azofra J, Sastre J, Gomez B, et al. Some cytological aspects of bronchial asthma. *Allergol Immunopathol (Madr)* 1986;14:295–301.
5. Isenberg DA, Martin P, Hajirousou V, et al. Haematological reassessment of rheumatoid arthritis using an automated method. *Br J Rheumatol* 1986;25:152–157.

6. Iwakiri R, Inokuchi K, Dan K, et al. Marked basophilia in acute promyelocytic leukaemia treated with all-trans retinoic acid: molecular analysis of the cell origin of the basophils. *Br J Haematol* 1994;86:870–872.

7. Jaffe JP, Gertner E, Miller W. Absent neutrophil alkaline phosphatase in the eosinophilia myalgia syndrome associated with L-tryptophan use. *Am J Hematol* 1991;36:280–281.

8. Karttunen TJ, Niemela S, Kerola T. Blood leukocyte differential in *Helicobacter pylori* infection. *Dig Dis Sci* 1996;41:1332–1336.

9. Lewis SA, Pavord ID, Stringer JR, et al. The relation between peripheral blood leukocyte counts and respiratory symptoms, atopy, lung function, and airway responsiveness in adults. *Chest* 2001;119:105–114.

10. May ME, Waddell CC. Basophils in peripheral blood and bone marrow. A retrospective review. *Am J Med* 1984;76:509–511.

11. Otsuka H, Dolovich J, Befus D, et al. Peripheral blood basophils, basophil progenitors, and nasal metachromatic cells in allergic rhinitis. *Am Rev Respir Dis* 1986;133:757–762.

12. Parker D, Graham-Pole J, Malpas JS, et al. Acute lymphoblastic leukemia with eosinophilia and basophilia. *Am J Pediatr Hematol Oncol* 1979;1:195–199.

13. Pedersen M, Kristensen KS, Clementsen P, et al. Increased numbers of circulating basophils with decreased releasability after administration of rhG-CSF to allergic patients. *Agents Actions* 1994;41:C24–C25.

14. Tikkanen J, Lemstrom K, Halme M, et al. Cytological monitoring of peripheral blood, bronchoalveolar lavage fluid, and transbronchial biopsy specimens during acute rejection and cytomegalovirus infection in lung and heart—lung allograft recipients. *Clin Transpl* 2001;15:77–88.

15. Zankowich R, Parwaresch MR, Lennert K. Blood findings in lymphogranulomatosis X. *Blut* 1984;48:99–107.

9

MONOCYTES AND HISTIOCYTES

MONOCYTOPENIA

Peripheral blood monocytopenia occurs in many of the same settings as neutropenia (Table 9-1) (1–19). Underlying conditions include acquired immunodeficiency syndrome, severe pulmonary tuberculosis, typhoid fever, aplastic anemia, connective tissue disease, cyclic leukopenia and cyclic neutropenia, hemodialysis, severe burns, B-cell chronic lymphocytic leukemia, hairy cell leukemia, myelodysplasia, and therapy with antineoplastic agents, corticosteroids, and infliximab (anti–tumor necrosis factor). The clinical consequence of monocytopenia is infection, primarily mycobacterial and fungal.

REACTIVE MONOCYTOSIS AND HISTIOCYTOSIS

The clinical settings for reactive monocytosis and histiocytosis include acute myocardial infarction, exercise, granulocyte-macrophage colony-stimulating factor and granulocyte colony-stimulating factor therapy, infectious disease, major

TABLE 9-1. CONDITIONS ASSOCIATED WITH PERIPHERAL BLOOD MONOCYTOPENIA

Nonneoplastic conditions
  Aplastic anemia
  Burn injury
  Connective tissue disease
  Cyclic leukopenia and cyclic neutropenia
  Hemodialysis
  Infection
  Acquired immunodeficiency syndrome
  Pulmonary tuberculosis
  Typhoid fever
  Therapeutic agents
  Antineoplastic agents
  Corticosteroids
  Infliximab (anti–tumor necrosis factor)

Neoplastic conditions
  B-cell chronic lymphocytic leukemia
  Hairy cell leukemia
  Myelodysplasia

TABLE 9-2. CONDITIONS ASSOCIATED WITH REACTIVE MONOCYTOSIS AND HISTIOCYTOSIS

Nonneoplastic conditions
  Acute myocardial infarction
  Exercise
  Granulocyte and granulocyte-macrophage colony-stimulating factor therapy
  Infectious disease
    Atypical mycobacteriosis
    Brucellosis
    Leishmaniasis
    Malaria
    Parvovirus B19 infection
    Syphilis
    Varicella virus infection
  Major depression
  Tissue damage
  Trauma

Neoplastic conditions
  Myelodysplastic syndrome
  Hodgkin lymphoma
  Adult T-cell leukemia/lymphoma
  Disseminated carcinoma

depression, tissue damage/trauma, myelodysplastic syndrome, Hodgkin disease, hairy cell leukemia, adult T-cell leukemia/lymphoma, and disseminated carcinoma (1–20) (Table 9-2). Monocytes, eosinophils, basophils, and mast cells are derived from a common precursor; thus, reactive monocytosis may accompany reactive eosinophilia, basophilia, and/or mastocytosis.

The peripheral blood smear shows absolute monocytosis exceeding the normal range, usually more than 1×10^9 cells/L. The monocytes may include mature and immature or activated forms (Fig. 9-1). Bone marrow aspirate smears show increased monocytes, monocytic precursors, and histiocytes (Figs. 9-2 and 9-3). Histologic sections of the bone marrow may appear less cellular than normal because of the increased number of monocytes and histiocytes with abundant pale-staining cytoplasm. Granulomas may be present.

The differential diagnosis consists of atypical lymphocytosis, myeloproliferative disorders, myelodysplastic syndromes, and acute leukemia.

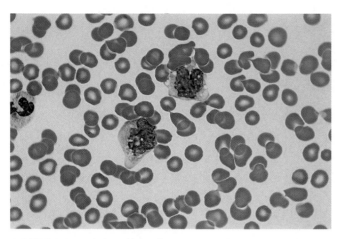

FIGURE 9-1. Peripheral blood smear, reactive monocytosis. Two monocytes with cytoplasmic vacuoles are present in this specimen from a patient with hairy cell leukemia.

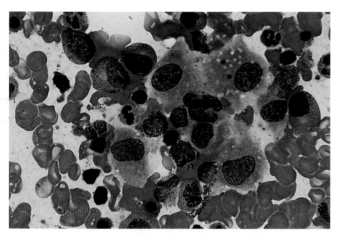

FIGURE 9-2. Bone marrow aspirate, reactive histiocytosis. Several histiocytes are present showing abundant pale basophilic, slightly granulated cytoplasm in this specimen from a patient with Hodgkin disease.

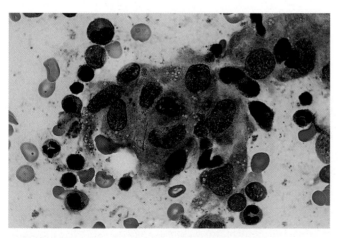

FIGURE 9-3. Bone marrow aspirate, reactive histiocytosis. A cluster of reactive histiocytes, apparently from a granuloma, is shown in this specimen from a patient with Hodgkin disease.

HEMOPHAGOCYTIC HISTIOCYTOSIS

Hemophagocytic disorders are characterized by increased bone marrow histiocytes with abundant cytoplasm containing ingested bone marrow cells and platelets.

Hemophagocytosis Caused by Increased and/or Ineffective Hematopoiesis

Histiocytes and hemophagocytic activity may be increased in the bone marrow under conditions of increased and/or ineffective hematopoiesis, such as megaloblastic anemia, hemoglobinopathy, immune-mediated cytopenias, myelodysplastic syndrome, sarcoidosis, vasculitis, and a variety of neoplasms (1–3) (Fig. 9-4). Aspirate smears show an increased number of morphologically benign histiocytes containing ingested hematopoietic cells, nuclear remnants, and/or blue-green granules. Histologic sections of the bone marrow show increased histiocytes scattered throughout the hematopoietic tissue. They are apparent on hematoxylin and eosin staining primarily because of their abundant pale, sometimes granular, cytoplasm.

No systemic signs or symptoms are associated with this type of hemophagocytic activity, in contrast to the findings in hemophagocytic syndrome (HPS).

Hemophagocytic Syndrome

HPS is a life-threatening disorder in which apparently normal histiocytes proliferate excessively in response to cytokine stimulation (Table 9-3) (Figs. 9-5 through 9-8). Patients present with fever, wasting, and hepatosplenomegaly. Most are immunosuppressed, but HPS has also been reported in apparently healthy individuals (4). Laboratory studies show a characteristic pattern of pancytopenia, abnormal liver

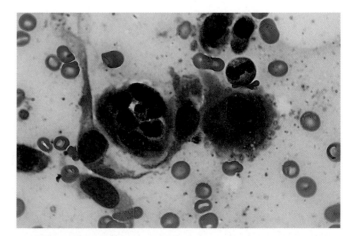

FIGURE 9-4. Bone marrow aspirate, increased hemophagocytosis. Two histiocytes are present, one showing hemophagocytosis. The patient had Hodgkin disease without the systemic manifestations of hemophagocytic syndrome.

TABLE 9-3. CONDITIONS ASSOCIATED WITH HEMOPHAGOCYTIC SYNDROME

Nonneoplastic conditions
    Constitutional immune defects (familial hemophagocytic
      lymphohistiocytosis)
    Lysinuric protein intolerance
    Connective tissue disorders
    Kikuchi disease (necrotizing lymphadenitis)
    Infectious diseases

Neoplastic conditions
    Langerhans cell histiocytosis
    Malignant lymphoma
    Carcinoma

function tests, hypertriglyceridemia, hyperferritinemia, and coagulopathy. Serum cytokine levels are increased.

Many underlying disorders can trigger HPS (Table 9-4). Constitutional defects in immunity produce HPS in infancy and early childhood (familial hemophagocytic lymphohistiocytosis) (5–8). Another hereditary cause of HPS is lysinuric protein intolerance (9). Acquired conditions associated with HPS include connective tissue disorders, Kikuchi disease (necrotizing lymphadenitis), many infectious diseases, Langerhans cell histiocytosis, malignant lymphoma, and carcinoma (10–42). Some cases do not have an identifiable antecedent triggering factor.

The peripheral blood shows pancytopenia. Bone marrow aspirate smears show variable numbers of histiocytes containing ingested hematopoietic cells (43). In infants, few histiocytes and little or no phagocytosis may be seen, and biopsy of the liver or other site may be required for diagnosis. Histologic sections of the bone marrow show increased histiocytes with abundant, eosinophilic, faintly granular cytoplasm and ingested nuclei. Iron stains may be helpful in identifying histiocytes. Hematopoietic precursors may show myelodysplastic changes, likely related to increased cell turnover

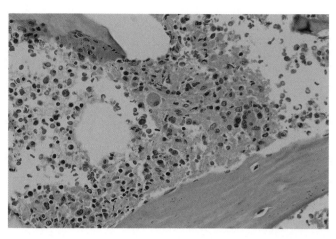

FIGURE 9-6. Bone marrow biopsy specimen, hemophagocytic syndrome. The bone marrow appears hypocellular owing to increased histocytes in this specimen from an infant with familial erythrophagocytic lymphohistiocytosis.

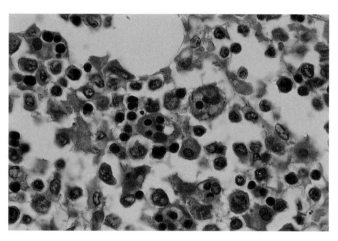

FIGURE 9-7. Bone marrow biopsy specimen, hemophagocytic syndrome. Histiocytes containing nucleated hematopoietic cells are seen in this autopsy specimen from a patient with hemophagocytic syndrome caused by Epstein-Barr virus infection.

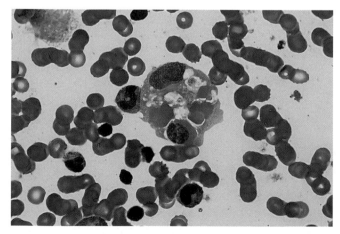

FIGURE 9-5. Bone marrow aspirate, hemophagocytic syndrome. A histiocyte has phagocytized red blood cells, a nucleated erythroid precursor, and platelets in this specimen from an infant with familial erythrophagocytic lymphohistiocytosis.

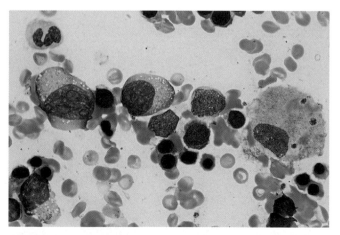

FIGURE 9-8. Bone marrow aspirate, hemophagocytic syndrome. A histiocyte containing red blood cells and platelets is seen adjacent to atypical lymphocytes in this specimen from a patient with hemophagocytic syndrome owing to peripheral T-cell lymphoma.

TABLE 9-4. CONDITIONS ASSOCIATED WITH ACQUIRED LIPID STORAGE HISTIOCYTOSIS IN THE BONE MARROW

Nonneoplastic conditions
  Chronic granulomatous disease
  Chronic lymphedema
  Hyperlipidemia
  Mineral oil lipidosis
  Prolonged total parenteral nutrition
  Takayasu arteritis

Neoplastic conditions
  Myeloproliferative disorders
  Myelodysplastic syndromes
  Acute lymphoblastic leukemia
  Monoclonal gammopathy of undetermined significance
  Malignant B-cell lymphoma

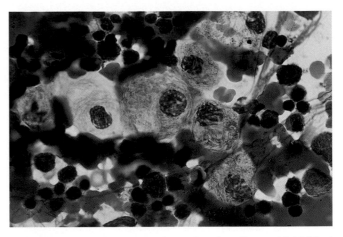

FIGURE 9-9. Bone marrow aspirate, Gaucher disease. Lipid-filled histiocytes show characteristic wrinkled or "crinkled tissue paper" cytoplasm.

(44,45). Infection-related HPS is characterized by interstitial T-cell infiltration. Malignancy-related HPS may show evidence of underlying leukemia, lymphoma, or carcinoma. HPS tends to mask underlying malignancy; thus, a specific and careful search for tumor cells is essential in evaluating bone marrow specimens with HPS.

Cytophagic Histiocytic Panniculitis

Cytophagic histiocytic panniculitis is a potentially lethal disorder of unknown etiology (46–49). Patients present with relapsing fever, subcutaneous nodules, and pancytopenia. The bone marrow shows prominent hemophagocytosis. No evidence of clonal proliferation is found in this disease, which distinguishes it from subcutaneous panniculitic T-cell lymphoma.

STORAGE HISTIOCYTOSIS

Storage histiocytosis may be owing to intracellular lipid, pigment, crystalline material, or foreign substances. Intracellular lipid and pigment are most frequently found. Histiocytes with intracellular lipid and/or pigment often stain blue to green; such cells have been termed "sea-blue histiocytes." Sea-blue histiocytosis is an imprecise term that has been applied both to constitutional and acquired storage disorders and does not represent a specific diagnosis.

Constitutional Lipid Storage Disorders

Constitutional storage disorders of the bone marrow are characterized by intrahistiocytic accumulation of lipid, often attributable to genetic defects in lysosomal transport and digestion (1–6). The morphologic findings are similar in many of these disorders and must be supplemented by enzymatic and genetic analysis for definitive diagnosis. Those most

likely to be encountered in the bone marrow are Gaucher disease, Niemann-Pick disease, and Hermansky-Pudlak syndrome.

Gaucher disease is a genetically heterogeneous group of autosomal recessive disorders characterized by defects in the gene encoding glucocerebrosidase (7–11) (Figs. 9-9 and 9-10). Prominent clinical findings include splenomegaly, bone pain, and, in some cases, neuropathy. The peripheral blood often shows thrombocytopenia and leukoerythroblastosis. Marrow aspirate smears show histiocytes with abundant, pale blue, faintly wrinkled or striated ("tissue-paper") cytoplasm. The cells are birefringent with polarized light and show positive reactions with Sudan black B, periodic acid–Schiff, Alcian blue, iron, and anti-CD68. Although striking, the histologic findings are not specific. Genetic and/or enzyme analysis is required for confirmation of the diagnosis. Complications include clonal B-cell and plasma cell disorders and light chain amyloidosis.

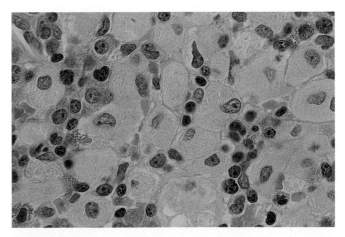

FIGURE 9-10. Bone marrow biopsy specimen, Gaucher disease. Lipid-filled histiocytes and lymphocytes virtually replace hematopoietic cells.

Niemann-Pick disease is a genetically heterogeneous group of autosomal recessive disorders caused by defects in the genes encoding sphingomyelinase and NPC-1 protein (12–14). Patients may present with neurologic symptoms, hepatosplenomegaly, cytopenias, and a leukoerythroblastic reaction. Aspirate smears show a combination of foamy and sea-blue histiocytes, with intermediate forms. The histiocytes are autofluorescent and show positive reactions with PAS, lipid, and acid-fast stains.

Hermansky-Pudlak syndrome is an autosomal recessive disorder characterized by oculocutaneous albinism, platelet storage pool deficiency, and histiocytosis (15–17). Pigmented lipid inclusions are found in circulating monocytes and marrow macrophages.

Acquired Lipid Storage Disorders

The acquired storage disorders resemble the constitutional disorders in showing increased histiocytes with blue-green, foamy, wrinkled, and/or granular cytoplasm (18–32) (Table 9-4). These cells are often referred to as sea-blue histiocytes or pseudo-Gaucher cells (Fig. 9-11). The histiocytes are usually not as numerous as those in the constitutional disorders.

Conditions in which sea-blue, foamy, or lipid-filled histiocytes have been reported include hyperlipidemia, mineral oil lipidosis, prolonged total parenteral nutrition, chronic lymphedema, chronic granulomatous disease, Takayasu arteritis, myeloproliferative disorders (especially chronic myeloid leukemia), myelodysplastic syndromes, acute lymphoblastic leukemia, monoclonal gammopathy of undetermined significance, and malignant B-cell lymphoma. In chronic myeloid leukemia, the storage histiocytes are part of the clonal population.

The differential diagnosis of lipid storage disease includes advanced mycobacterial infection in profoundly immuno-suppressed patients, as in acquired immunodeficiency syndrome (33). In this setting, histiocytes are proliferative and are distended by innumerable ingested mycobacteria. Histiocytosis resembling storage disease has also been described in the setting of stem cell transplantation with graft failure (34,35). This phenomenon is apparently caused by prolonged therapy with granulocyte or granulocyte-monocyte colony-stimulating factor.

Crystal Storage Histiocytosis

Crystal storage histiocytosis is a hallmark of cholesteryl ester storage disease, cystinosis, oxalosis, and clonal lymphoplasmacytic disorders. Histiocytes in the bone marrow and/or other organs contain phagocytized crystals. Clonal lymphoplasmacytic disorders produce crystal storage histiocytosis when the clonal immunoglobulin forms crystals; in such cases, crystals may be found both within the clonal cells and reactive histiocytes (Fig. 9-12).

Polyvinylpyrrolidone Storage Disease

Polyvinylpyrrolidone (PVP) storage disease is an uncommon disorder, resulting from the use of PVP as a plasma expander (36–39). PVP cannot be excreted from the body and is retained in the form of intrahistiocytic polymers. The peripheral blood may show severe anemia in advanced cases. Foamy histiocytes are prominent in the bone marrow and other organs. Histiocytes show positive reactions with mucicarmine, colloidal iron, and alkaline Congo red stains and negative reactions with periodic acid–Schiff and Alcian blue stains. Bone marrow fibrosis may be present.

In the absence of a clinical history of PVP exposure, these findings may be mistaken for a constitutional lipid storage disorder or metastatic signet-ring cell carcinoma.

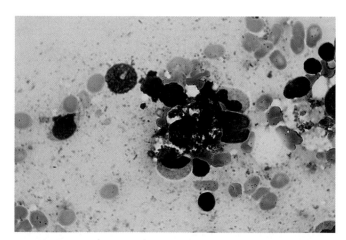

FIGURE 9-11. Bone marrow aspirate, sea-blue histiocyte. This histiocyte shows deeply staining blue-green to black granules in this specimen from a patient with human immunodeficiency virus infection.

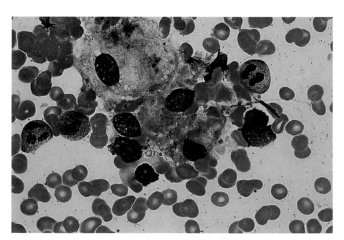

FIGURE 9-12. Bone marrow aspirate, crystal-storage histiocytosis. Reactive histiocytes contain ingested needle-like immunoglobulin crystals in this specimen from a patient with multiple myeloma.

SINUS HISTIOCYTOSIS WITH MASSIVE LYMPHADENOPATHY

Sinus histiocytosis with massive lymphadenopathy (Rosai-Dorfman disease) has rarely been reported in the bone and bone marrow (1–5). The peripheral blood may show eosinophilia. Bone marrow aspirate smears and histologic sections show foamy histiocytes containing intact lymphocytes, sometimes accompanied by eosinophilia or plasmacytosis.

REFERENCES
Monocytopenia

1. Adams WH, Liu YK. Periodic neutropenia and monocytopenia. *Am J Hematol* 1982;13:73–82.
2. Bethel KJ, Sharpe RW. Pathology of hairy-cell leukaemia. *Best Pract Res Clin Haematol* 2003;16:15–31.
3. Bloemena E, Koopmans RP, Weinreich S, et al. Pharmacodynamic modeling of lymphocytopenia and whole blood lymphocyte cultures in prednisolone-treated individuals. *Clin Immunol Immunopathol* 1990;57:374–386.
4. Chilcote RR, Rierden WJ, Baehner RL. Neutropenia, recurrent bacterial infections, and congenital deafness in patients with monocytopenia. Absence of peripheral blood colony-stimulating activity. *Am J Dis Child* 1983;137:964–967.
5. Cline MJ, Opelz G, Saxon A, et al. Autoimmune panleukopenia. *N Engl J Med* 1976;295:1489–1493.
6. Crown JP, Jhanwar S, Haimi J, et al. Acquired cyclic haematopoiesis associated with a radiation-induced chromosomal abnormality with clonal, morphologically normal circulating leucocytes. *Acta Haematol* 1991;86:103–106.
7. De Rossi G, Mauro FR, Ialongo P, et al. Monocytopenia and infections in chronic lymphocytic leukemia (CLL). *Eur J Haematol* 1991;46:119.
8. Isenberg DA, Martin P, Hajirousou V, et al. Haematological reassessment of rheumatoid arthritis using an automated method. *Br J Rheumatol* 1986;25:152–157.
9. Isenberg DA, Patterson KG, Todd-Pokropek A, et al. Haematological aspects of systemic lupus erythematosus: a reappraisal using automated methods. *Acta Haematol* 1982;67:242–248.
10. Kondo M, Oshita F, Kato Y, et al. Early monocytopenia after chemotherapy as a risk factor for neutropenia. *Am J Clin Oncol* 1999;22:103–105.
11. Kraut EH. Clinical manifestations and infectious complications of hairy-cell leukaemia. *Best Pract Res Clin Haematol* 2003;16:33–40.
12. Kurtin PJ, McKinsey DS, Gupta MR, et al. Histoplasmosis in patients with acquired immunodeficiency syndrome. Hematologic and bone marrow manifestations. *Am J Clin Pathol* 1990;93:367–372.
13. Lugering A, Schmidt M, Lugering N, et al. Infliximab induces apoptosis in monocytes from patients with chronic active Crohn's disease by using a caspase-dependent pathway. *Gastroenterology* 2001;121:1145–1157.
14. Morris CD, Bird AR, Nell H. The haematological and biochemical changes in severe pulmonary tuberculosis. *Q JM* 1989;73:1151–1159.
15. Nockher WA, Wiemer J, Scherberich JE. Haemodialysis monocytopenia: differential sequestration kinetics of CD14+ CD16+ and CD14++ blood monocyte subsets. *Clin Exp Immunol* 2001;123:49–55.
16. Peterson V, Hansbrough J, Buerk C, et al. Regulation of granulopoiesis following severe thermal injury. *J Trauma* 1983;23:19–24.
17. Spencer DC, Pienaar NL, Atkinson PM. Disturbances of blood coagulation associated with Salmonella typhi infections. *J Infect* 1988;16:153–161.
18. Weinberger M, Elattar I, Marshall D, et al. Patterns of infection in patients with aplastic anemia and the emergence of Aspergillus as a major cause of death. *Medicine (Baltimore)* 1992;71:24–43.
19. Wendland T, Herren S, Yawalkar N, et al. Strong alpha beta and gamma delta TCR response in a patient with disseminated Mycobacterium avium infection and lack of NK cells and monocytopenia. *Immunol Lett* 2000;72:75–82.

Reactive Monocytosis and Histiocytosis

1. Abdalla SH. Hematopoiesis in human malaria. *Blood Cells* 1990;16:401–416.
2. Ala-Houhala I, Makela S, Koivunen E, et al. Pronounced monocytosis in a case of nephropathia epidemica. *Scand J Infect Dis* 2000;32:419–420.
3. Blay JY, Rossi JF, Wijdenes J, et al. Role of interleukin-6 in the paraneoplastic inflammatory syndrome associated with renal-cell carcinoma. *Int J Cancer* 1997;72:424–430.
4. Ellaurie M, Rubinstein A. Elevated tumor necrosis factor-alpha in association with severe anemia in human immunodeficiency virus infection and *Mycobacterium avium intracellulare* infection. *Pediatr Hematol Oncol* 1995;12:221–230.
5. Galanakis E, Bourantas KL, Leveidiotou S, et al. Childhood brucellosis in north-western Greece: a retrospective analysis. *Eur J Pediatr* 1996;155:1–6.
6. Horiuchi Y. Mo2+ HLA-DR- monocytosis in varicella zoster virus infection. *J Dermatol* 1997;24:205–207.
7. Karayalcin G, Khanijou A, Kim KY, et al. Monocytosis in congenital syphilis. *Am J Dis Child* 1977;131:782–783.
8. Kawakami A, Fukunaga T, Usui M, et al. Visceral leishmaniasis misdiagnosed as malignant lymphoma. *Intern Med* 1996;35:502–506.
9. Maes M, Lambrechts J, Suy E, et al. Absolute number and percentage of circulating natural killer, non-MHC-restricted T cytotoxic, and phagocytic cells in unipolar depression. *Neuropsychobiology* 1994;29:157–163.
10. Meisel SR, Pauzner H, Schechter M, et al. Peripheral monocytosis following acute myocardial infarction: incidence and its possible role as a bedside marker of the extent of cardiac injury. *Cardiology* 1998;90:52–57.
11. Moraes M, Wilkes J, Lowder JN. Monocytic leukemoid reaction, glucocorticoid therapy, and myelodysplastic syndrome. *Cleve Clin J Med* 1990;57:571–574.
12. Rainer TH, Chan TY, Cocks RA. Do peripheral blood counts have any prognostic value following trauma? *Injury* 1999;30:179–185.
13. Ranaghan L, Drake M, Humphreys MW, et al. Leukaemoid monocytosis in M4 AML following chemotherapy and G-CSF. *Clin Lab Haematol* 1998;20:49–51.
14. Sen R, Tewari AD, Sehgal PK, et al. Clinico-haematological profile in acute and chronic *Plasmodium falciparum* malaria in children. *J Commun Dis* 1994;26:31–38.
15. Severs Y, Brenner I, Shek PN, et al. Effects of heat and intermittent exercise on leukocyte and sub-population cell counts. *Eur J Appl Physiol Occup Physiol* 1996;74:234–245.
16. Smith MB, Schnadig VJ, Boyars MC, et al. Clinical and pathologic features of *Mycobacterium fortuitum* infections. An emerging pathogen in patients with AIDS. *Am J Clin Pathol* 2001;116:225–232.

17. Togias AG. Systemic immunologic and inflammatory aspects of allergic rhinitis. *J Allergy Clin Immunol* 2000;106:S247–S250.
18. Warzocha K, Bienvenu J, Ribeiro P, et al. Plasma levels of tumour necrosis factor and its soluble receptors correlate with clinical features and outcome of Hodgkin's disease patients. *Br J Cancer* 1998;77:2357–2362.
19. Weitberg AB. A monocytic leukemoid reaction in a patient with myelodysplasia. *CA Cancer J Clin* 1985;35:308–310.
20. Yetgin S, Cetin M, Yenicesu I, et al. Acute Parvovirus B19 infection mimicking juvenile myelomonocytic leukemia. *Eur J Haematol* 2000;65:276–278.

Hemophagocytic Histiocytosis

1. Kumakura S, Ishikura H, Kondo M, et al. Hemophagocytosis associated with MPO-ANCA positive vasculitis in systemic sclerosis. *Clin Exp Rheumatol* 2002;20:411–414.
2. Shetty V, Hussaini S, Alvi S, et al. Excessive apoptosis, increased phagocytosis, nuclear inclusion bodies and cylindrical confronting cisternae in bone marrow biopsies of myelodysplastic syndrome patients. *Br J Haematol* 2002;116:817–825.
3. Taylor HG, Berenberg JL. Bone marrow phagocytosis in sarcoidosis. *Arch Intern Med* 1982;142:479–480.
4. Shirono K, Tsuda H. Virus-associated haemophagocytic syndrome in previously healthy adults. *Eur J Haematol* 1995;55:240–244.
5. Mullauer L, Gruber P, Sebinger D, et al. Mutations in apoptosis genes: a pathogenetic factor for human disease. *Mutat Res* 2001;488:211–231.
6. Allen M, De Fusco C, Legrand F, et al. Familial hemophagocytic lymphohistiocytosis: how late can the onset be? *Haematologica* 2001;86:499–503.
7. Goransdotter Ericson K, Fadeel B, Nilsson-Ardnor S, et al. Spectrum of perforin gene mutations in familial hemophagocytic lymphohistiocytosis. *Am J Hum Genet* 2001;68:590–597.
8. Graham GE, Graham LM, Bridge PJ, et al. Further evidence for genetic heterogeneity in familial hemophagocytic lymphohistiocytosis (FHLH). *Pediatr Res* 2000;48:227–232.
9. Duval M, Fenneteau O, Doireau V, et al. Intermittent hemophagocytic lymphohistiocytosis is a regular feature of lysinuric protein intolerance. *J Pediatr* 1999;134:236–239.
10. Stephan JL, Kone-Paut I, Galambrun C, et al. Reactive haemophagocytic syndrome in children with inflammatory disorders. A retrospective study of 24 patients. *Rheumatology (Oxford)* 2001; 40:1285–1292.
11. Sibilia J, Javier RM, Albert A, et al. Pancytopenia secondary to hemophagocytic syndrome in rheumatoid arthritis treated with methotrexate and sulfasalazine. *J Rheumatol* 1998;25:1218–1220.
12. Takahashi K, Kumakura S, Ishikura H, et al. Reactive hemophagocytosis in systemic lupus erythematosus. *Intern Med* 1998;37:550–553.
13. Kelly J, Kelleher K, Khan MK, et al. A case of haemophagocytic syndrome and Kikuchi-Fujimoto disease occurring concurrently in a 17-year-old female. *Int J Clin Pract* 2000;54:547–549.
14. Mahadeva U, Allport T, Bain B, et al. Haemophagocytic syndrome and histiocytic necrotising lymphadenitis (Kikuchi's disease). *J Clin Pathol* 2000;53:636–638.
15. Sakhalkar VS, Rao SP, Gottessman SR, et al. Hemophagocytosis and granulomas in the bone marrow of a child with Down syndrome. *J Pediatr Hematol Oncol* 2001;23:623–625.
16. Goto S, Aoike I, Shibasaki Y, et al. A successfully treated case of disseminated tuberculosis-associated hemophagocytic syndrome and multiple organ dysfunction syndrome. *Am J Kidney Dis* 2001;38:E19.
17. Mizukane R, Kadota Ji J, Yamaguchi T, et al. An elderly patient with hemophagocytic syndrome due to severe mycoplasma pneumonia with marked hypercytokinemia. *Respiration* 2002;69:87–91.
18. Chen YC, Chao TY, Chin JC. Scrub typhus-associated hemophagocytic syndrome. *Infection* 2000;28:178–179.
19. Marty AM, Dumler JS, Imes G, et al. Ehrlichiosis mimicking thrombotic thrombocytopenic purpura. Case report and pathological correlation. *Hum Pathol* 1995;26:920–925.
20. Pohl M, Niemeyer CM, Hentschel R, et al. Haemophagocytosis in early congenital syphilis. *Eur J Pediatr* 1999;158:553–555.
21. Rao RD, Morice WG, Phyliky RL. Hemophagocytosis in a patient with chronic lymphocytic leukemia and histoplasmosis. *Mayo Clin Proc* 2002;77:287–290.
22. Numata K, Tsutsumi H, Wakai S, et al. A child case of haemophagocytic syndrome associated with cryptococcal meningoencephalitis. *J Infect* 1998;36:118–119.
23. Finkielman JD, Grinberg AR, Paz LA, et al. Case report: reactive hemophagocytic syndrome associated with disseminated strongyloidiasis. *Am J Med Sci* 1996;312:37–39.
24. Tunc B, Ayata A. Hemophagocytic syndrome: a rare life-threatening complication of visceral leishmaniasis in a young boy. *Pediatr Hematol Oncol* 2001;18:531–536.
25. Marom D, Offer I, Tamary H, et al. Hemophagocytic lymphohistiocytosis associated with visceral leishmaniasis. *Pediatr Hematol Oncol* 2001;18:65–70.
26. Slovut DP, Benedetti E, Matas AJ. Babesiosis and hemophagocytic syndrome in an asplenic renal transplant recipient. *Transplantation* 1996;62:537–539.
27. Ohno T, Shirasaka A, Sugiyama T, et al. Hemophagocytic syndrome induced by *Plasmodium falciparum* malaria infection. *Int J Hematol* 1996;64:263–266.
28. Hashimoto H, Maruyama H, Fujimoto K, et al. Hematologic findings associated with thrombocytopenia during the acute phase of exanthem subitum confirmed by primary human herpesvirus-6 infection. *J Pediatr Hematol Oncol* 2002;24:211–214.
29. Luppi M, Barozzi P, Rasini V, et al. Severe pancytopenia and hemophagocytosis after HHV-8 primary infection in a renal transplant patient successfully treated with foscarnet. *Transplantation* 2002;74:131–132.
30. Sakamoto O, Ando M, Yoshimatsu S, et al. Systemic lupus erythematosus complicated by cytomegalovirus-induced hemophagocytic syndrome and colitis. *Intern Med* 2002;41:151–155.
31. To KF, Chan PK, Chan KF, et al. Pathology of fatal human infection associated with avian influenza A H5N1 virus. *J Med Virol* 2001;63:242–246.
32. Imashuku S, Tabata Y, Teramura T, et al. Treatment strategies for Epstein-Barr virus-associated hemophagocytic lymphohistiocytosis (EBV-HLH). *Leuk Lymphoma* 2000;39:37–49.
33. Takeoka Y, Hino M, Oiso N, et al. Virus-associated hemophagocytic syndrome due to rubella virus and varicella-zoster virus dual infection in patient with adult idiopathic thrombocytopenic purpura. *Ann Hematol* 2001;80:361–364.
34. Yagita M, Iwakura H, Kishimoto T, et al. Successful allogeneic stem cell transplantation from an unrelated donor for aggressive Epstein-Barr virus-associated clonal T-cell proliferation with hemophagocytosis. *Int J Hematol* 2001;74:451–454.
35. de Cremoux H, Monnet I, Fleury J, et al. Histiocytic medullary reticulosis occurring with small cell lung carcinoma. *Eur Respir J* 1991;4:122–124.
36. Sakai T, Shiraki K, Deguchi M, et al. Hepatocellular carcinoma associated with hemophagocytic syndrome. *Hepatogastroenterology* 2001;48:1464–1466.
37. Hesseling PB, Wessels G, Egeler RM, et al. Simultaneous occurrence of viral-associated hemophagocytic syndrome and

Langerhans cell histiocytosis: a case report. *Pediatr Hematol Oncol* 1995;12:135–141.

38. Klein A, Corazza F, Demulder A, et al. Recurrent viral associated hemophagocytic syndrome in a child with Langerhans cell histiocytosis. *J Pediatr Hematol Oncol* 1999;21:554–556.

39. Allory Y, Challine D, Haioun C, et al. Bone marrow involvement in lymphomas with hemophagocytic syndrome at presentation: a clinicopathologic study of 11 patients in a Western institution. *Am J Surg Pathol* 2001;25:865–874.

40. Chim CS, Hui PK. Reactive hemophagocytic syndrome and Hodgkin's disease. *Am J Hematol* 1997;55:49–50.

41. Dufau JP, Le Tourneau A, Molina T, et al. Intravascular large B-cell lymphoma with bone marrow involvement at presentation and haemophagocytic syndrome: two Western cases in favour of a specific variant. *Histopathology* 2000;37:509–512.

42. Imashuku S, Hibi S, Morinaga S, et al. Haemophagocytic lymphohistiocytosis in association with granular lymphocyte proliferative disorders in early childhood: characteristic bone marrow morphology. *Br J Haematol* 1997;96:708–714.

43. Florena AM, Iannitto E, Quintini G, et al. Bone marrow biopsy in hemophagocytic syndrome. *Virchows Arch* 2002;441:335–344.

44. Imashuku S, Kitazawa K, Ishii M, et al. Bone marrow changes mimicking myelodysplasia in patients with hemophagocytic lymphohistiocytosis. *Int J Hematol* 2000;72:353–357.

45. Macheta M, Will AM, Houghton JB, et al. Prominent dyserythropoiesis in four cases of haemophagocytic lymphohistiocytosis. *J Clin Pathol* 2001;54:961–963.

46. Craig AJ, Cualing H, Thomas G, et al. Cytophagic histiocytic panniculitis—a syndrome associated with benign and malignant panniculitis: case comparison and review of the literature. *J Am Acad Dermatol* 1998;39:721–736.

47. Huilgol SC, Fenton D, Pambakian H, et al. Fatal cytophagic panniculitis and haemophagocytic syndrome. *Clin Exp Dermatol* 1998;23:51–55.

48. Marzano AV, Berti E, Paulli M, et al. Cytophagic histiocytic panniculitis and subcutaneous panniculitis-like T-cell lymphoma: report of 7 cases. *Arch Dermatol* 2000;136:889–896.

49. Zollner TM, Podda M, Ochsendorf FR, et al. Monitoring of phagocytic activity in histiocytic cytophagic panniculitis. *J Am Acad Dermatol* 2001;44:120–123.

Storage Histiocytosis

1. Nam MH, Grande JP, Li CY, et al. Familial hypercholesterolemia with unusual foamy histiocytes. Report of a case with myelophthisic anemia and xanthoma of the maxillary sinus. *Am J Clin Pathol* 1988;89:556–561.

2. Nguyen TT, Kruckeberg KE, O'Brien JF, et al. Familial splenomegaly: macrophage hypercatabolism of lipoproteins associated with apolipoprotein E mutation [apolipoprotein E (delta149 Leu)]. *J Clin Endocrinol Metab* 2000;85:4354–4358.

3. Nowaczyk MJ, Feigenbaum A, Silver MM, et al. Bone marrow involvement and obstructive jaundice in Farber lipogranulomatosis: clinical and autopsy report of a new case. *J Inherit Metab Dis* 1996;19:655–660.

4. Horiuchi H, Saito N, Kobayashi S, et al. Avascular necrosis of the femoral head in a patient with Fabry's disease: identification of ceramide trihexoside in the bone by delayed-extraction matrix-assisted laser desorption ionization-time-of-flight mass spectrometry. *Arthritis Rheum* 2002;46:1922–1925.

5. Sergi C, Penzel R, Uhl J, et al. Prenatal diagnosis and fetal pathology in a Turkish family harboring a novel nonsense mutation in the lysosomal alpha-N-acetyl-neuraminidase (sialidase) gene. *Hum Genet* 2001;109:421–428.

6. Elleder M, Chlumska A, Ledvinova J, et al. Testis—a novel storage site in human cholesteryl ester storage disease. Autopsy report of an adult case with a long-standing subclinical course complicated by accelerated atherosclerosis and liver carcinoma. *Virchows Arch* 2000;436:82–87.

7. Cox TM. Gaucher disease: understanding the molecular pathogenesis of sphingolipidoses. *J Inherit Metab Dis* 2001;24:106–121.

8. Drugan C, Procopciuc L, Jebeleanu G, et al. Gaucher disease in Romanian patients: incidence of the most common mutations and phenotypic manifestations. *Eur J Hum Genet* 2002;10:511–515.

9. Pastores GM. Gaucher's disease. Pathological features. *Baillieres Clin Haematol* 1997;10:739–749.

10. Weinreb NJ, Charrow J, Andersson HC, et al. Effectiveness of enzyme replacement therapy in 1028 patients with type 1 Gaucher disease after 2 to 5 years of treatment: a report from the Gaucher Registry. *Am J Med* 2002;113:112–119.

11. Zhao H, Bailey LA, Elsas LJ 2nd, et al. Gaucher disease: *in vivo* evidence for allele dose leading to neuronopathic and nonneuronopathic phenotypes. *Am J Med Genet* 2003;116:52–56.

12. Candoni A, Grimaz S, Doretto P, et al. Sea-blue histiocytosis secondary to Niemann-Pick disease type B: a case report. *Ann Hematol* 2001;80:620–622.

13. Kennedy GA, Cobcroft R, Marlton P, et al. Type C Niemann-Pick disease. *Br J Haematol* 2000;111:718.

14. Kolodny EH. Niemann-Pick disease. *Curr Opin Hematol* 2000;7:48–52.

15. Gahl WA, Brantly M, Kaiser-Kupfer MI, et al. Genetic defects and clinical characteristics of patients with a form of oculocutaneous albinism (Hermansky-Pudlak syndrome). *N Engl J Med* 1998;25:380–385.

16. Krisp A, Hoffman R, Happle R, et al. Hermansky-Pudlak syndrome. *Eur J Dermatol* 2001;11:372–373.

17. Parker MS, Rosado Shipley W, de Christenson ML, et al. The Hermansky-Pudlak syndrome. *Ann Diagn Pathol* 1997;1:99–103.

18. Jacobs JW, Van der Weide FR, Kruijsen MW. Fatal cholestatic hepatitis caused by D-penicillamine. *Br J Rheumatol* 1994;33:770–773.

19. Yokoyama K, Shinohara N, Wada K. Osseous xanthomatosis and a pathologic fracture in a patient with hyperlipidemia. A case report. *Clin Orthop* 1988;236:307–310.

20. Bigorgne C, Le Tourneau A, Vahedi K, et al. Sea-blue histiocyte syndrome in bone marrow secondary to total parenteral nutrition. *Leuk Lymphoma* 1998;28:523–529.

21. Meiklejohn DJ, Baden H, Greaves M. Sea-blue histiocytosis and pancytopenia associated with chronic parenteral nutrition administration. *Clin Lab Haematol* 1997;19:219–221.

22. Heimpel H, Bierich JR, Herrmann JM, et al. Dysplasia of the lymphatics with lymphoedema, generalized lymphangiectasis, chylothorax and "pseudo-storage-disease." *Lymphology* 1979;12:228–240.

23. Tanaka T, Takahashi K, Morita H, et al. Chronic granulomatous disease of childhood and sea-blue histiocytosis. A pathologic study of an autopsy case. *Acta Pathol Jpn* 1984;34:1385–1401.

24. Tadmor R, Aghai E, Sarova-Pinhas I, et al. Sea-blue histiocytes in a case of Takayasu arteritis. *JAMA* 1976;235:2823–2853.

25. Regazzoli A, Pozzi A, Rossi G. Pseudo-Gaucher plasma cells in the bone marrow of a patient with monoclonal gammopathy of undetermined significance. *Haematologica* 1997;82:727.

26. Alterini R, Rigacci L, Stefanacci S. Pseudo-Gaucher cells in the bone marrow of a patient with centrocytic nodular non-Hodgkin's lymphoma. *Haematologica* 1996;81:282–283.

27. Lee KS, Tobin MS, Chen KT, et al. Acquired Gaucher's cells in Hodgkin's disease. *Am J Med* 1982;73:290–294.

28. Anastasi J, Musvee T, Roulston D, et al. Pseudo-Gaucher histiocytes identified up to 1 year after transplantation for CML are BCR/ABL-positive. *Leukemia* 1998;12:233–237.

29. Lang E, Uthman M. Pseudo-Gaucher cells in peritoneal fluid: an uncommon manifestation of extramedullary hematopoiesis. *Diagn Cytopathol* 1999;20:379–381.

30. Stewart AJ, Jones RD. Pseudo-Gaucher cells in myelodysplasia. *J Clin Pathol* 1999;52:917–918.

31. Knox-Macaulay H, Bhusnurmath S, Alwaily A. Pseudo-Gaucher's cells in association with common acute lymphoblastic leukemia. *South Med J* 1997;90:69–71.

32. Cruickshank B, Thomas MJ. Mineral oil (follicular) lipidosis: II. Histologic studies of spleen, liver, lymph nodes, and bone marrow. *Hum Pathol* 1984;15:731–737.

33. Argiris A, Maun N, Berliner N. *Mycobacterium avium* complex inclusions mimicking Gaucher's cells. *N Engl J Med* 1999;340:1372.

34. Al-Homaidhi A, Prince HM, Al-Zahrani H, et al. Granulocyte-macrophage colony-stimulating factor-associated histiocytosis and capillary-leak syndrome following autologous bone marrow transplantation: two case reports and a review of the literature. *Bone Marrow Transplant* 1998;21:209–214.

35. Rosenthal NS, Farhi DC. Failure to engraft after bone marrow transplantation: bone marrow morphologic findings. *Am J Clin Pathol* 1994;102:821–824.

36. Dunn P, Kuo T, Shih LY, et al. Bone marrow failure and myelofibrosis in a case of PVP storage disease. *Am J Hematol* 1998;57:68–71.

37. Bubis JJ, Cohen S, Dinbar J, et al. Storage of polyvinylpyrrolidone mimicking a congenital mucolipid storage disease in a patient with Munchausen's syndrome. *Isr J Med Sci* 1975;11:999–1004.

38. Dunn P, Kuo T, Shih LY, et al. Bone marrow failure and myelofibrosis in a case of PVP storage disease. *Am J Hematol* 1998;57:68–71.

39. Kuo TT, Hu S, Huang CL, et al. Cutaneous involvement in polyvinylpyrrolidone storage disease: a clinicopathologic study of five patients, including two patients with severe anemia. *Am J Surg Pathol* 1997;21:1361–1367.

Sinus Histiocytosis with Massive Lymphadenopathy

1. Grote HJ, Moesenthin M, Foss HD, et al. Osseous manifestation of Rosai-Dorfman disease (sinus histiocytosis with massive lymphadenopathy). A case report and review of the literature. *Gen Diagn Pathol* 1998;143:341–345.

2. Hernandez D, Gutierrez L, Duque H, et al. Association of sinus histiocytosis with massive lymphadenopathy and idiopathic hypereosinophilic syndrome. *Histol Histopathol* 1987;2:239–242.

3. Petschner F, Walker UA, Schmitt-Graff A, et al. Sinus histiocytosis with massive lymphadenopathy (Rosai-Dorfman disease) presenting with skeletal lesions. *Skeletal Radiol* 1998;27:115–117.

4. Pulsoni A, Anghel G, Falcucci P, et al. Treatment of sinus histiocytosis with massive lymphadenopathy (Rosai-Dorfman disease): report of a case and literature review. *Am J Hematol* 2002;69:67–71.

5. Rosai J, Dorfman RF. Sinus histiocytosis with massive lymphadenopathy: a pseudolymphomatous benign disorder. Analysis of 34 cases. *Cancer* 1972;30:1174–1188.

PLATELETS AND MEGAKARYOCYTES

THUY-LIEU THI VO
DIANE C. FARHI

THROMBOCYTOPENIA

Thrombocytopenia is a frequent finding in the complete blood cell count. The time course may be transient, cyclic, or persistent. Transient thrombocytopenia is a common complication of infection and hemorrhage. Cyclic thrombocytopenia is an uncommon disorder that may be constitutional or acquired. Constitutional cyclic thrombocytopenia is discussed in Chapter 5. Acquired cyclic thrombocytopenia is associated with antiplatelet antibody production, immunodeficiency, the menstrual cycle, myeloproliferative disorders, myelodysplastic syndromes, and malignant lymphoma (1–10) (Table 10-1). It may be accompanied by periodic fluctuations in other cell counts and in the number of bone marrow megakaryocytes.

Persistent thrombocytopenia may be constitutional or acquired. Constitutional persistent thrombocytopenia is discussed in Chapter 5. Acquired persistent thrombocytopenia may be attributable to bone marrow–related causes or peripheral blood–related causes (11–19) (Table 10-2). The bone marrow shows reduced platelet production in gold therapy, amegakaryocytic thrombocytopenic purpura, myelodysplastic syndromes, acute leukemia, and replacement of hematopoietic tissue by fibrous tissue, bone, malignant lymphoma, or metastatic malignancy. Peripheral blood–related causes may be categorized as increased platelet loss, consumption, destruction, or sequestration. Etiologies include cocaine use, drug- and immune-mediated thrombocytopenic purpura, hemorrhage, disseminated intravascular coagulation, hemolytic uremic syndrome, thrombotic thrombocytopenic purpura, phagocytosis by histiocytes (as

TABLE 10-1. CONDITIONS ASSOCIATED WITH ACQUIRED CYCLIC THROMBOCYTOPENIA

Antiplatelet antibody production
Immunodeficiency
Menstrual cycle
Myeloproliferative disorders
Myelodysplastic syndromes
Malignant lymphoma

TABLE 10-2. CONDITIONS ASSOCIATED WITH ACQUIRED PERSISTENT THROMBOCYTOPENIA

Bone marrow–related conditions with reduced platelet
     production and megakaryocytic hypoplasia
  Amegakaryocytic thrombocytopenic purpura
  Gold therapy
  Fibrosis
  Osteosclerosis
  Myelodysplastic syndrome
  Acute leukemia
  Malignant lymphoma
  Metastatic malignancy
Peripheral blood–related conditions with increased platelet
     loss, consumption, destruction, or sequestration and
     megakaryocytic hyperplasia
  Cocaine use
  Drug- and immune-mediated thrombocytopenic purpura
  Hemorrhage
  Disseminated intravascular coagulation
  Hemolytic uremic syndrome
  Thrombotic thrombocytopenic purpura
  Platelet phagocytosis by histiocytes (e.g., hemophagocytic
     syndrome)
  Platelet phagocytosis by neutrophils
  Splenomegaly with splenic sequestration

in hemophagocytic syndrome) or neutrophils, and excessive platelet sequestration in the spleen as a result of splenomegaly. Drug-related thrombocytopenia is usually attributable to heparin therapy but also occurs with c7E3Fab (abciximab), which is used to block platelet aggregation in patients with coronary artery disease.

The peripheral blood shows thrombocytopenia, sometimes with an increased mean platelet volume caused by the release of newly formed large platelets. The remaining complete blood cell count parameters are variable, depending on the etiology of the thrombocytopenia.

Bone marrow aspirate smears and histologic sections may show either increased, adequate, or decreased numbers of megakaryocytes. The megakaryocytes may be immature and/or mature. Compared with mature cells, immature megakaryocytes are relatively small, show fewer nuclear lobations, and possess less cytoplasm with more basophilia.

TABLE 10-3. DIFFERENTIAL DIAGNOSIS OF PSEUDOTHROMBOCYTOPENIA

Immunoglobulin M, G, and/or A anti-GPIIb/IIIa autoantibody reactive only in the presence of ethylenediaminetetraacetic acid and, in some cases, other anticoagulants
Immunoglobulin M anti-GPIIb/IIIa autoantibody reactive at room temperature independent of ethylenediaminetetraacetic acid
Giant platelet syndromes
Overfilling of vacuum blood container
Platelet satellitosis

TABLE 10-4. CONDITIONS ASSOCIATED WITH ETHYLENEDIAMINETETRAACETIC ACID–DEPENDENT PSEUDOTHROMBOCYTOPENIA

Antiphospholipid antibodies
Cryoglobulinemia
Drug exposure
Hepatic cirrhosis
Immunoglobulin A nephritis
Vasculitis
Viral infections (e.g., mumps, cytomegalovirus, Epstein-Barr virus)
Malignant lymphoma
Inadequate mixing of powdered ethylenediaminetetraacetic acid with the peripheral blood, especially in plastic collection tubes

The presence of increased megakaryocytes, including many immature forms, suggests peripheral platelet destruction or loss rather than failure of production. Conversely, a reduced number of megakaryocytes suggests failure of platelet production as the primary cause of thrombocytopenia. Abnormal megakaryocyte morphology suggests the possibility of a clonal hematopoietic disorder with ineffective and/or reduced platelet production.

The differential diagnosis includes pseudothrombocytopenia caused by various conditions (20–43) (Table 10-3). Of these, the most common by far is ethylenediaminetetraacetic acid (EDTA)–dependent pseudothrombocytopenia (EDTA-psTP), a condition of no clinical significance in which platelets clump on exposure to EDTA (Fig. 10-1). Most patients are healthy; some have associated laboratory test abnormalities, drug exposure, or diseases (Table 10-4). Laboratory studies show an artifactually decreased platelet count, and in some cases, artifactual increases in mean platelet volume and platelet distribution width. Artifactual decrease of the white blood cell count (pseudoleukopenia) may also be present. Platelet clumping occurs progressively over time in EDTA and is caused by the presence of immunoglobulin G, M, or A autoantibodies to the platelet glycoprotein IIb/IIIa complex that react in the presence of EDTA. Platelet clumping may occur at 37°C as well as at room temperature and with other anticoagulants (sodium citrate, sodium oxalate, lithium heparin, acid citrate dextrose) as well as with EDTA. In some cases, EDTA-psTP is associated with platelet phagocytosis by neutrophils and monocytes. EDTA-psTP may be detected by comparing platelet counts from an EDTA-anticoagulated specimen immediately after drawing and after a 4-hour delay; by comparing platelet counts from EDTA-anticoagulated specimens with and without the addition of aminoglycoside, a drug that abolishes EDTA-related platelet clumping; and, in some cases, by comparing platelet counts from specimens containing EDTA and other anticoagulant(s).

Other causes of pseudothrombocytopenia may be evaluated by various means. Giant platelet syndromes are apparent by peripheral blood smear examination. Clues to overfilling of vacuum blood containers are artifactual increases in hemoglobin and hematocrit and decreases in the platelet and white blood cell counts. Platelet aggregation caused by inadequate mixing of powdered EDTA with the peripheral blood may cause pseudothrombocytopenia, especially in plastic collection vials; this problem is solved by rapid and thorough mixing of the sample. EDTA-independent platelet agglutination is mediated by an immunoglobulin M autoantibody against the GPIIa/IIIb complex, which occurs with all anticoagulants at room temperature but not at 37°C.

Platelet satellitosis is an unusual and interesting cause of pseudothrombocytopenia (44–48) (Fig. 10-2). Underlying disorders include hereditary platelet disorders, hypogammaglobulinemia, vasculitis, myeloproliferative disorders, chronic lymphocytic leukemia, and mantle cell lymphoma. The phenomenon has been reported in specimens anticoagulated with EDTA, sodium citrate, and lithium heparin. Platelets may satellite around segmented neutrophils, eosinophils, basophils, monocytes, large granular lymphocytes, and/or clonal B cells, and in some cases have been ingested by neutrophils and/or monocytes.

It should be kept in mind that pseudothrombocytopenia may occur with, and thus mask, congenital platelet function

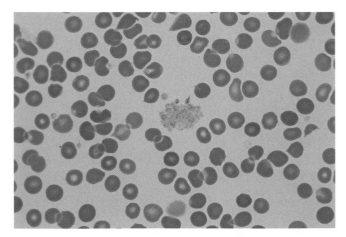

FIGURE 10-1. Peripheral blood smear, pseudothrombocytopenia caused by platelet clumping. The platelets are clumped together, causing artifactual reduction in the platelet count in this ethylenediaminetetraacetic acid–anticoagulated specimen.

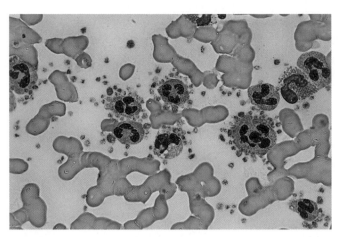

FIGURE 10-2. Peripheral blood smear, pseudothrombocytopenia caused by platelet satellitism. The platelets are bound to neutrophil membranes, causing artifactual reduction in the platelet count in this ethylenediaminetetraacetic acid–anticoagulated specimen.

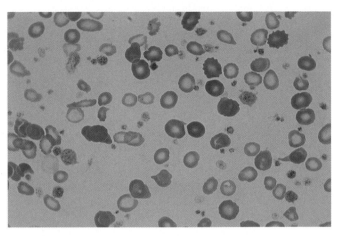

FIGURE 10-3. Peripheral blood smear, reactive thrombocytosis caused by iron deficiency anemia. Numerous immature and mature platelets are seen in this specimen from a woman with marked iron deficiency owing to excessive menstrual blood loss; the platelet count was $1,300 \times 10^9/L$.

disorders, constitutional giant platelet syndromes, and true thrombocytopenia owing to drugs or other causes.

REACTIVE THROMBOCYTOSIS

An increased peripheral blood platelet count is caused by reactive, or secondary, thrombocytosis in more than 80% of cases (1–7) (Table 10-5). Reactive thrombocytosis may be transient or persistent. Transient thrombocytosis is seen with hemorrhage, acute infection, and recovery after surgical procedures or other trauma. Persistent thrombocytosis is found in chronic infection, iron deficiency, chronic inflammatory diseases, and malignancy and after splenectomy (Fig. 10-3). In approximately 5% of cases of apparently reactive thrombocytosis, no etiology can be determined. In contrast to clonal thrombocytosis, the pathophysiology of reactive thrombocytosis is largely related to increased serum levels of thrombopoietin and other cytokines.

The clinical course is usually benign. Approximately 5% of patients sustain a bleeding episode and/or vasoocclusive event. Venous thromboembolism tends to occur in patients with underlying malignancy or recovering from surgery.

The peripheral blood shows increased platelets, exceeding the normal range for the laboratory performing the test, usually more than $450 \times 10^9/L$ and often more than $1,000 \times 10^9/L$. The platelet count is especially labile in children. Immature platelets are often present and display an increased size, generally round contour, and prominent reddish alpha granules. Bone marrow aspirate smears and histologic sections show increased megakaryocytes. Immature megakaryocytes are often increased, identifiable by their smaller size, fewer nuclear lobations, and relatively basophilic cytoplasm compared with mature megakaryocytes.

The differential diagnosis includes constitutional (hereditary) thrombocytosis, thrombocythemia accompanying clonal hematopoietic disorders, and pseudothrombocytosis. Constitutional thrombocytosis is a rare disorder, usually transmitted as an autosomal dominant disorder and rarely as an X-linked disorder (8,9). Patients typically show symptomatic, persistent thrombocytosis; the bone marrow shows increased numbers and size of both mature and immature megakaryocytes with no dysplastic changes. Clonal hematopoietic disorders with thrombocythemia are discussed elsewhere. Pseudothrombocytosis is usually caused by platelet-sized cryoglobulin aggregates or red blood cell fragments (10,11). Both are apparent on peripheral blood smear examination.

TABLE 10-5. CONDITIONS ASSOCIATED WITH REACTIVE THROMBOCYTOSIS

Chronic inflammatory diseases
Hemorrhage
Infection
Iron deficiency anemia
Surgery (especially splenectomy)
Trauma
Malignancy

MEGAKARYOCYTIC HYPERPLASIA

Reactive megakaryocytic hyperplasia is characterized by an increase in bone marrow megakaryocytes, usually both immature and mature forms (Figs. 10-4 and 10-5). It is often accompanied by reactive erythroid hyperplasia as megakaryocytes and erythroid cells arise from a common precursor. Many conditions are associated with megakaryocytic hyperplasia, including the peripheral blood–related causes of

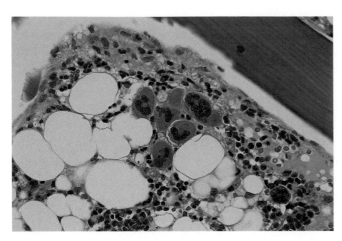

FIGURE 10-4. Bone marrow biopsy specimen, megakaryocytic hyperplasia. Morphologically normal megakaryocytes are increased and clustered in this specimen from a patient recovering from cytotoxic chemotherapy.

thrombocytopenia listed previously, the conditions associated with reactive thrombocytosis listed previously, and malignant lymphoma (1).

The peripheral blood may show an increased, normal, or decreased platelet count (Tables 10-2 and 10-5). Reactive megakaryocytic hyperplasia and thrombocytosis are found in chronic inflammatory diseases, tissue damage, infection, and malignancy. Megakaryocytic hyperplasia with thrombocytopenia is found in acute hemorrhage, immune-mediated thrombocytopenia, and splenic platelet sequestration.

Bone marrow aspirate smears and histologic sections show increased megakaryocytes. No standardized criteria for megakaryocytic hyperplasia have been in common use. In general, histologic sections of normal bone marrow show approximately one megakaryocyte per high-power (40×) field. In megakaryocytic hyperplasia, megakaryocytes are more frequently found, distributed singly and in small clus-

ters throughout the marrow. Both mature and immature megakaryocytes are found. They are morphologically normal, without evidence of dysplasia.

The differential diagnosis includes the clonal megakaryocytic hyperplasia seen in myeloproliferative disorders, myelodysplastic syndromes, and acute leukemia. It should be kept in mind that reactive megakaryocytic hyperplasia may coexist with primary and metastatic malignancies in bone marrow.

MEGAKARYOCYTIC HYPOPLASIA

Megakaryocytic hypoplasia, or amegakaryocytic thrombocytopenic purpura (AMTP), is an uncommon disorder that may be cyclic or persistent. Cyclic AMTP is a rare disorder of uncertain pathogenesis, immunologically mediated in at least some cases (1,2). Persistent AMTP is associated with several conditions, many involving autoimmunity or other immune disorders (3–28) (Table 10-6). These include anti-HLA antibodies, autoimmune hemolytic anemia, connective tissue disease, drug exposure, hepatic cirrhosis, hypogammaglobulinemia, mumps infection, vitamin B_{12} deficiency, CD8+ T-cell lymphocytosis, CD5+ B-cell lymphoma, and metastatic neuroblastoma. In some cases, no associated condition or etiology can be identified.

The clinical course is variable. Some cases respond to specific therapy or immunomodulators. Others progress to aplastic anemia or clonal hematopoietic disease.

The peripheral blood shows thrombocytopenia. Bone marrow aspirate smears and histologic sections show decreased or absent megakaryocytes. Other findings may include pure red cell aplasia, aplastic anemia, myelodysplastic syndrome, CD8+ T lymphocytosis, and malignant lymphoma.

The differential diagnosis includes, in neonates, the thrombocytopenia-absent radii (TAR) syndrome and other stem cell defects presenting as congenital amegakaryocytic thrombocytopenia (29). These syndromes should be distinguished from transient, autoantibody-mediated neonatal and childhood AMTP.

TABLE 10-6. CONDITIONS ASSOCIATED WITH AMEGAKARYOCYTIC THROMBOCYTOPENIC PURPURA

Anti-HLA antibodies
Autoimmune hemolytic anemia
Connective tissue disease
Drug exposure
Hepatic cirrhosis
Hypogammaglobulinemia
Mumps infection
Vitamin B_{12} deficiency
CD8+ T-cell lymphocytosis
CD5+ B-cell lymphoma
Metastatic tumor

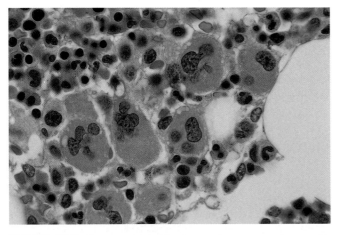

FIGURE 10-5. Bone marrow biopsy specimen, megakaryocytic hyperplasia. Morphologically normal megakaryocytes are increased and clustered in this specimen from a patient with malignant lymphoma.

REFERENCES

Thrombocytopenia

1. Abe Y, Hirase N, Muta K, et al. Adult onset cyclic hematopoiesis in a patient with myelodysplastic syndrome. *Int J Hematol* 2000;71: 40–45.
2. Fureder W, Mitterbauer G, Thalhammer R, et al. Clonal T cell-mediated cyclic thrombocytopenia. *Br J Haematol* 2002;119: 1059–1061.
3. Kashyap R, Choudhry VP, Pati HP. Danazol therapy in cyclic acquired amegakaryocytic thrombocytopenic purpura: a case report. *Am J Hematol* 1999;60:225–228.
4. Kojima K, Fujii N, Omoto E, et al. Cyclic thrombocytopenia and polycythemia vera. *Ann Hematol* 2003;82:61–63.
5. Kosugi S, Tomiyama Y, Shiraga M, et al. Cyclic thrombocytopenia associated with IgM anti-GPIIb-IIIa autoantibodies. *Br J Haematol* 1994;88:809–815.
6. Kubota M, Nakamura K, Watanabe K, et al. A case of common variable immunodeficiency associated with cyclic thrombocytopenia. *Acta Paediatr Jpn* 1994;36:690–692.
7. Nagasawa T, Hasegawa Y, Kamoshita M, et al. Megakaryopoiesis in patients with cyclic thrombocytopenia. *Br J Haematol* 1995; 91:185–190.
8. Rice L, Nichol JL, McMillan R, et al. Cyclic immune thrombocytopenia responsive to thrombopoietic growth factor therapy. *Am J Hematol* 2001;68:210–214.
9. Shirota T, Yamamoto H, Fujimoto H, et al. Cyclic thrombo cytopenia in a patient treated with cyclosporine for refractory idiopathic thrombocytopenic purpura. *Am J Hematol* 1997;56: 272–276.
10. Tomer A, Schreiber AD, McMillan R, et al. Menstrual cyclic thrombocytopenia. *Br J Haematol* 1989;71:519–524.
11. Burday MJ, Martin SE. Cocaine-associated thrombocytopenia. *Am J Med* 1991;91:656–660.
12. Greinacher A, Eichler P, Lubenow N, et al. Drug-induced and drug-dependent immune thrombocytopenias. *Rev Clin Exp Hematol* 2001;5:166–200.
13. Kobayashi I, Yamada M, Kawamura N, et al. Platelet-specific hemophagocytosis in a patient with juvenile dermatomyositis. *Acta Paediatr* 2000;89:617–619.
14. Lee JC, Tripathy K. Neutrophilic thrombophagocytosis. *Arch Pathol Lab Med* 2000;124:1545–1546.
15. Levin HA, McMillan R, Tavassoli M, et al. Thrombocytopenia associated with gold therapy. Observations on the mechanism of platelet destruction. *Am J Med* 1975;59:274–280.
16. Rutherford CJ, Frenkel EP. Thrombocytopenia. Issues in diagnosis and therapy. *Med Clin North Am* 1994;78:555–575.
17. Schell DA, Ganti AK, Levitt R, et al. Thrombocytopenia associated with c7E3 Fab (abciximab). *Ann Hematol* 2002;81:76–79.
18. White LA Jr, Brubaker LH, Aster RH, et al. Platelet satellitism and phagocytosis by neutrophils: association with antiplatelet antibodies and lymphoma. *Am J Hematol* 1978;4:313–323.
19. Yang R, Han ZC. Pathogenesis and management of chronic idiopathic thrombocytopenic purpura: an update. *Int J Hematol* 2000;71:18–24.
20. Ahn HL, Jo YI, Choi YS, et al. EDTA-dependent pseudothrombocytopenia confirmed by supplementation of kanamycin; a case report. *Korean J Intern Med* 2002;17:65–68.
21. Bartels PC, Schoorl M, Lombarts AJ. Screening for EDTA-dependent deviations in platelet counts and abnormalities in platelet distribution histograms in pseudothrombocytopenia. *Scand J Clin Lab Invest* 1997;57:629–636.
22. Bizzaro N. EDTA-dependent pseudothrombocytopenia: a clinical and epidemiological study of 112 cases, with 10-year follow-up. *Am J Hematol* 1995;50:103–109.
23. Bizzaro N, Brandalise M. EDTA-dependent pseudothrombocytopenia. Association with antiplatelet and antiphospholipid antibodies. *Am J Clin Pathol* 1995;103:103–107.
24. Cohen AM, Cycowitz Z, Mittelman M, et al. The incidence of pseudothrombocytopenia in automatic blood analyzers. *Haematologia (Budap)* 2000;30:117–121.
25. Criswell KA, Breider MA, Bleavins MR. EDTA-dependent platelet phagocytosis. A cytochemical, ultrastructural, and functional characterization. *Am J Clin Pathol* 2001;115:376–384.
26. Duschek EJ, Jonkhoff AR, Tol CA, et al. IgM auto-antibody thrombocytopenia simulating pseudothrombocytopenia. *Eur J Haematol* 1997;58:295–296.
27. Fiorin F, Steffan A, Pradella P, et al. IgG platelet antibodies in EDTA-dependent pseudothrombocytopenia bind to platelet membrane glycoprotein IIb. *Am J Clin Pathol* 1998;110: 178–183.
28. Hatzipantelis ES, Tsantali H, Athanassiou-Metaxa M, et al. Hereditary giant platelet disorder presented as pseudothrombocytopenia. *Eur J Haematol* 2001;67:330–331.
29. Hsieh AT, Chao TY, Chen YC. Pseudothrombocytopenia associated with infectious mononucleosis. *Arch Pathol Lab Med* 2003;127:e17–e18.
30. Jim RT. Case report. Pseudo pseudothrombocytopenia. *Hawaii Med J* 2001;60:108.
31. Matarazzo M, Conturso V, Di Martino M, et al. EDTA-dependent pseudothrombocytopenia in a case of liver cirrhosis. *Panminerva Med* 2000;42:155–157.
32. Nishioka T, Yokota M, Tsuda I, et al. Flow cytometric analysis of platelet activation under calcium ion-chelating conditions. *Clin Lab Haematol* 2002;24:115–119.
33. Pewarchuk W, VanderBoom J, Blajchman MA. Pseudopolycythemia, pseudothrombocytopenia, and pseudoleukopenia due to overfilling of blood collection vacuum tubes. *Arch Pathol Lab Med* 1992;116:90–92.
34. Sakurai S, Shiojima I, Tanigawa T, et al. Aminoglycosides prevent and dissociate the aggregation of platelets in patients with EDTA-dependent pseudothrombocytopenia. *Br J Haematol* 1997; 99:817–823.
35. Sawazaki A, Nakamura N, Jyokaji H, et al. Guillain-Barre syndrome and ethylene diamine tetraacetic acid-dependent pseudothrombocytopenia associated with mumps. *Intern Med* 1996; 35:996–999.
36. Schimmer A, Mody M, Sager M, et al. Platelet cold agglutinins: a flow cytometric analysis. *Transfus Sci* 1998;19:217–224.
37. Schrezenmeier H, Muller H, Gunsilius E, et al. Anticoagulant-induced pseudothrombocytopenia and pseudoleucocytosis. *Thromb Haemost* 1995;73:506–513.
38. Silvestri F, Masotti A, Pradella P, et al. More on false thrombocytopenias: EDTA-dependent pseudothrombocytopenia associated with a congenital platelet release defect. *Vox Sang* 1996;71: 27–29.
39. Silvestri F, Virgolini L, Savignano C, et al. Incidence and diagnosis of EDTA-dependent pseudothrombocytopenia in a consecutive outpatient population referred for isolated thrombocytopenia. *Vox Sang* 1995;68:35–39.
40. Takeuchi T, Yoshioka K, Hori A, et al. Cytomegalovirus mononucleosis with mixed cryoglobulinemia presenting transient pseudothrombocytopenia. *Intern Med* 1993;32:598–601.
41. Tu CH, Yang S. Olanzapine-induced EDTA-dependent pseudothrombocytopenia. *Psychosomatics* 2002;43:421–423.
42. van der Meer W, Allebes W, Simon A, et al. Pseudothrombocytopenia: a report of a new method to count platelets in a patient with EDTA- and temperature-independent antibodies of the IgM type. *Eur J Haematol* 2002;69:243–247.
43. Wool RL, Coleman TA, Hamill RL. Abciximab-associated pseudothrombocytopenia. *Am J Med* 2002;113:697–698.

44. Bizzaro N, Goldschmeding R, von dem Borne AE. Platelet satellitism is Fc gamma RIII (CD16) receptor-mediated. *Am J Clin Pathol* 1995;103:740–744.
45. Cesca C, Ben-Ezra J, Riley RS. Platelet satellitism as presenting finding in mantle cell lymphoma. A case report. *Am J Clin Pathol* 2001;115:567–570.
46. Espanol I, Muniz-Diaz E, Domingo-Claros A. The irreplaceable image: platelet satellitism to granulated lymphocytes. *Haematologica* 2000;85:1322.
47. Lazo-Langner A, Piedras J, Romero-Lagarza P, et al. Platelet satellitism, spurious neutropenia, and cutaneous vasculitis: casual or causal association? *Am J Hematol* 2002;70:246–249.
48. Morselli M, Longo G, Bonacorsi G, et al. Anticoagulant pseudothrombocytopenia with platelet satellitism. *Haematologica* 1999;84:655.

Reactive Thrombocytosis

1. Alexandrakis MG, Passam FH, Moschandrea IA, et al. Levels of serum cytokines and acute phase proteins in patients with essential and cancer-related thrombocytosis. *Am J Clin Oncol* 2003;26:135–140.
2. Buss DH, Cashell AW, O'Connor ML, et al. Occurrence, etiology and clinical significance of extreme thrombocytosis: a study of 280 cases. *Am J Med* 1994;96:247–253.
3. Chen HL, Chiou SS, Sheen JM, et al. Thrombocytosis in children at one medical center of southern Taiwan. *Acta Paediatr Taiwan* 1999;40:309–313.
4. Griesshammer M, Bangerter M, Sauer T, et al. Aetiology and clinical significance of thrombocytosis: analysis of 732 patients with an elevated platelet count. *J Intern Med* 1999;245:295–300.
5. Pearson TC. Diagnosis and classification of erythrocytosis and thrombocytosis. *Baillieres Clin Hematol* 1998;11:695–720.
6. Schafer AI. Thrombocytosis and thrombocythemia. *Blood Rev* 2001;15:159–166.
7. Wolach B, Morag H, Drucker M, et al. Thrombocytosis after pneumonia with empyema and other bacterial infections in children. *Pediatr Infect Dis J* 1990;9:718–721.
8. Stuhrmann M, Bashawri L, Ahmed MA, et al. Familial thrombocytosis as a recessive, possibly X-linked trait in an Arab family. *Br J Haematol* 2001;112:616–620.
9. Wiestner A, Padosch SA, Ghilardi N, et al. Hereditary thrombocythaemia is a genetically heterogeneous disorder: exclusion of TPO and MPL in two families with hereditary thrombocythaemia. *Br J Haematol* 2000;110:104–109.
10. Fohlen-Walter A, Jacob C, Lecompte T, et al. Laboratory identification of cryoglobulinemia from automated blood cell counts, fresh blood samples, and blood films. *Am J Clin Pathol* 2002;117:606–614.
11. Lawrence C, Atac B. Hematologic changes in massive burn injury. *Crit Care Med* 1992;20:1284–1288.

Megakaryocytic Hyperplasia

1. Lambertenghi-Deliliers G, Annaloro C, Soligo D, et al. Incidence and histological features of bone marrow involvement in malignant lymphomas. *Ann Hematol* 1992;65:61–65.

Megakaryocytic Hypoplasia

1. Kashyap R, Choudhry VP, Pati HP. Danazol therapy in cyclic acquired amegakaryocytic thrombocytopenic purpura: a case report. *Am J Hematol* 1999;60:225–228.
2. Zent CS, Ratajczak J, Ratajczak MZ, et al. Relationship between megakaryocyte mass and serum thrombopoietin levels as revealed by a case of cyclic amegakaryocytic thrombocytopenic purpura. *Br J Haematol* 1999;105:452–458.
3. Benedetti F, de Sabata D, Perona G. T suppressor activated lymphocytes (CD8+/DR+) inhibit megakaryocyte progenitor cell differentiation in a case of acquired amegakaryocytic thrombocytopenic purpura. *Stem Cells* 1994;12:205–213.
4. Ergas D, Tsimanis A, Shtalrid M, et al. T-gamma large granular lymphocyte leukemia associated with amegakaryocytic thrombocytopenic purpura, Sjogren's syndrome, and polyglandular autoimmune syndrome type II, with subsequent development of pure red cell aplasia. *Am J Hematol* 2002;69:132–134.
5. Evans DI. Immune amegakaryocytic thrombocytopenia of the newborn: association with anti-HLA-A2. *J Clin Pathol* 1987;40:258–261.
6. Geissler D, Thaler J, Konwalinka G, et al. Progressive preleukemia presenting amegakaryocytic thrombocytopenic purpura: association of the 5q-syndrome with a decreased megakaryocytic colony formation and a defective production of Meg-CSF. *Leuk Res* 1987;11:731–737.
7. Ghosh K, Sarode R, Varma N, et al. Amegakaryocytic thrombocytopenia of nutritional vitamin B12 deficiency. *Trop Geogr Med* 1988;40:158–160.
8. Katai M, Aizawa T, Ohara N, et al. Acquired amegakaryocytic thrombocytopenic purpura with humoral inhibitory factor for megakaryocyte colony formation. *Intern Med* 1994;33:147–149.
9. Katsumata Y, Suzuki T, Kuwana M, et al. Anti-c-Mpl (thrombopoietin receptor) autoantibody-induced amegakaryocytic thrombocytopenia in a patient with systemic sclerosis. *Arthritis Rheum* 2003;48:1647–1651.
10. King JA, Elkhalifa MY, Latour LF. Rapid progression of acquired megakaryocytic thrombocytopenia to aplastic anemia. *South Med J* 1997;90:91–94.
11. Kitano K, Shimodaira S, Ito T, et al. Liver cirrhosis with marked thrombocytopenia and highly elevated serum thrombopoietin levels. *Int J Hematol* 1999;70:52–55.
12. Koduri PR. Amegakaryocytic thrombocytopenia with a positive direct Coombs' test. *Am J Hematol* 1993;44:68–69.
13. Kouides PA, Rowe JM. Large granular lymphocyte leukemia presenting with both amegakaryocytic thrombocytopenic purpura and pure red cell aplasia: clinical course and response to immunosuppressive therapy. *Am J Hematol* 1995;49:232–236.
14. Leach JW, Hussein KK, George JN. Acquired pure megakaryocytic aplasia report of two cases with long-term responses to antithymocyte globulin and cyclosporine. *Am J Hematol* 1999;62:115–117.
15. Lonial S, Bilodeau PA, Langston AA, et al. Acquired amegakaryocytic thrombocytopenia treated with allogeneic BMT: a case report and review of the literature. *Bone Marrow Transplant* 1999;24:1337–1341.
16. Lugassy G. Non-Hodgkin's lymphoma presenting with amegakaryocytic thrombocytopenic purpura. *Ann Hematol* 1996; 73:41–42.
17. Manoharan A, Williams NT, Sparrow R. Acquired amegakaryocytic thrombocytopenia: report of a case and review of literature. *Q J Med* 1989;263:243–252.
18. Mills AE, Meyer JH, Karabus CD, et al. Transient dyserythropoiesis occurring during the involutional phase of stage IV-S neuroblastoma. *Am J Pediatr Hematol Oncol* 1989;11:23–27.
19. Nagasawa T, Sakurai T, Kashiwagi H, et al. Cell-mediated amegakaryocytic thrombocytopenia associated with systemic lupus erythematosus. *Blood* 1986;67:479–483.
20. Ninomiya N, Maeda T, Matsuda I. Thrombocytopenic purpura occurring during the early phase of a mumps infection. *Helv Paediatr Acta* 1977;32:87–89.

21. Peng CT, Kao LY, Tsai CH. Successful treatment with cyclosporin A in a child with acquired pure amegakaryocytic thrombocytopenic purpura. *Acta Paediatr* 1994;83:1222–1224.

22. Rovira M, Feliu E, Florensa L, et al. Acquired amegakaryocytic thrombocytopenic purpura associated with immunoglobulin deficiency. *Acta Haematol* 1991;85:34–36.

23. Sakurai T, Kono I, Kabashima T, et al. Amegakaryocytic thrombocytopenia associated with systemic lupus erythematosus successfully treated by a high-dose prednisolone therapy. *Jpn J Med* 1984;23:135–138.

24. Scarlett JD, Williams NT, McKellar WJ. Acquired amegakaryocytic thrombocytopaenia in a child. *J Paediatr Child Health* 1992;28:263–266.

25. Slater LM, Katz J, Walter B, et al. Aplastic anemia occurring as amegakaryocytic thrombocytopenia with and without an inhibitor of granulopoiesis. *Am J Hematol* 1985;18:251–254.

26. Trimble MS, Glynn MF, Brain MC. Amegakaryocytic thrombocytopenia of 4 years duration: successful treatment with antithymocyte globulin. *Am J Hematol* 1991;37:126–127.

27. Xue Y, Zhang R, Guo Y, et al. Acquired amegakaryocytic thrombocytopenic purpura with a Philadelphia chromosome. *Cancer Genet Cytogenet* 1993;69:51–56.

28. Yildiz BO, Haznedaroglu IC, Coplu L. Albendazole-induced amegakaryocytic thrombocytopenic purpura. *Ann Pharmacother* 1998;32:842.

29. Henter JI, Winiarski J, Ljungman P, et al. Bone marrow transplantation in two children with congenital amegakaryocytic thrombocytopenia. *Bone Marrow Transplant* 1995;15:799–801.

MAST CELLS

CONSTITUTIONAL MASTOCYTOSIS

Constitutional (familial) mastocytosis is a relatively common, probably autosomal dominant disorder characterized by occurrence in multiple generations, onset in neonatal life, and limitation of disease to the skin (1–7). The condition is typically indolent and may regress spontaneously. The peripheral blood and bone marrow show no pathologic findings. Genetic studies show no karyotypic abnormalities and no c-KIT mutations.

The differential diagnosis includes other rare constitutional syndromes with mast cell involvement (8), childhood mastocytosis with an inactivating c-KIT mutation, and neonatal presentation of systemic mastocytosis with an acquired activating c-KIT mutation (9–11). These disorders may show progressive mastocytosis and hematolymphoid, germ cell, and smooth muscle neoplasms.

CHILDHOOD-ONSET MASTOCYTOSIS

Childhood-onset mastocytosis is relatively common and characterized by sporadic occurrence, onset in childhood, and limitation of disease to the skin (1–5). The clinical course is indolent. The peripheral blood and bone marrow show no pathologic findings. Genetic studies may show inactivating c-KIT mutations.

The differential diagnosis includes constitutional mastocytosis, rare constitutional syndromes with mast cell involvement (6), and childhood presentation of systemic mastocytosis, which is characterized by an acquired activating c-KIT mutation (7–9). These disorders may show progressive mastocytosis and hematolymphoid, germ cell, and smooth muscle neoplasms.

REACTIVE MASTOCYTOSIS

Reactive mastocytosis, or mast cell hyperplasia, is a bone marrow response seen in a variety of conditions, especially low-grade B-cell neoplasms (Table 11-1) (1–13).

The peripheral blood may show eosinophilia and/or basophilia. Bone marrow aspirate smears show increased mast cells located within the particle and found scattered among hematopoietic cells in the area surrounding the particle (Figs. 11-1 through 11-4). Mast cells may be round, polygonal or angulated, or spindled. Flow cytometry shows an unremarkable mast cell phenotype, without CD2 or CD25 expression. Genetic studies show no c-KIT mutations.

The precise number of mast cells required for a diagnosis of mast cell hyperplasia is undefined. Examination of histologic sections of normal bone marrow have shown that mast cells comprise approximately 0.5% to 1% of nucleated cells per square millimeter or approximately one mast cell per high-power field. Flow cytometry corroborates these findings and demonstrates consistent expression of CD9, CD33, CD43, CD69, and CD117. Expression of CD11b, CD11c, CD13, CD22, and CD61 is variable, ranging from 40% to 70% of mast cells. Mast cell hyperplasia is probably present if the observer can easily find five or more morphologically unremarkable mast cells within and adjacent to a single bone marrow particle.

The differential diagnosis includes the clonal mast cell diseases: systemic mastocytosis, myelodysplastic syndromes with mast cell differentiation, aggressive mastocytosis, and

TABLE 11-1. CONDITIONS ASSOCIATED WITH REACTIVE BONE MARROW MASTOCYTOSIS

Nonneoplastic conditions
  Alcoholism
  Aplastic anemia
  Fanconi anemia
  Postmenopausal osteoporosis
  Renal osteodystrophy
  Stem cell factor therapy

Neoplastic conditions
  Chronic lymphocytic leukemia
  Follicular center cell lymphoma
  Hairy cell leukemia
  Lymphoplasmacytic lymphoma
  Multiple myeloma
  Myelodysplastic syndromes
  Acute leukemia

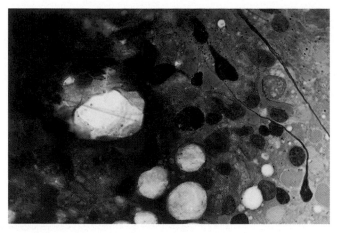

FIGURE 11-1. Bone marrow aspirate smear, reactive mastocytosis. Mast cells are typically found within and at the edges of the particle and are recognizable by their deep violet color and angular contours.

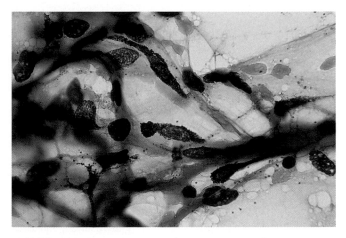

FIGURE 11-4. Bone marrow aspirate smear, reactive mastocytosis. Spindled mast cells with elongated nuclei are seen in this smear from a patient with aplastic anemia.

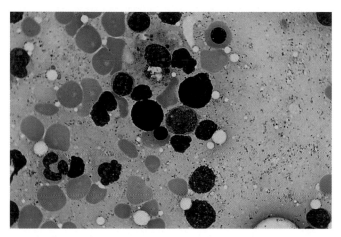

FIGURE 11-2. Bone marrow aspirate smear, reactive mastocytosis. Round mast cells with round nuclei are seen in this smear from a patient with aplastic anemia.

mast cell leukemia. Flow cytometry may be helpful in distinguishing reactive from clonal mastocytes because clonal (but not reactive) mast cells express CD2 and CD25. It should be kept in mind that both reactive mastocytosis and systemic mastocytosis are associated with malignant lymphoma, and mast cells accompanying clonal myeloid disease may be either reactive or clonal.

REFERENCES

Constitutional Mastocytosis

1. Buttner C, Henz BM, Welker P, et al. Identification of activating c-kit mutations in adult-, but not in childhood-onset indolent mastocytosis: a possible explanation for divergent clinical behavior. *J Invest Dermatol* 1998;111:1227–1231.
2. Chang A, Tung RC, Schlesinger T, et al. Familial cutaneous mastocytosis. *Pediatr Dermatol* 2001;18:271–276.
3. Hartmann K, Henz BM. Mastocytosis: recent advances in defining the disease. *Br J Dermatol* 2001;144:682–695.
4. Longley BJ Jr, Metcalfe DD, Tharp M, et al. Activating and dominant inactivating c-KIT catalytic domain mutations in distinct clinical forms of human mastocytosis. *Proc Natl Acad Sci U S A* 1999;96:1609–1614.
5. Middelkamp Hup MA, Heide R, Tank B, et al. Comparison of mastocytosis with onset in children and adults. *J Eur Acad Dermatol Venereol* 2002;16:115–120.
6. Rosbotham JL, Malik NM, Syrris P, et al. Lack of c-kit mutation in familial urticaria pigmentosa. *Br J Dermatol* 1999;140:849–852.
7. Valent P, Horny HP, Escribano L, et al. Diagnostic criteria and classification of mastocytosis: a consensus proposal. *Leuk Res* 2001;25:603–625.
8. Beghini A, Tibiletti MG, Roversi G, et al. Germline mutation in the juxtamembrane domain of the kit gene in a family with gastrointestinal stromal tumors and urticaria pigmentosa. *Cancer* 2001;92:657–662.
9. Kuint J, Bielorai B, Gilat D, et al. C-kit activating mutation in a neonate with in-utero presentation of systemic mastocytosis associated with myeloproliferative disorder. *Br J Haematol* 1999;106:838–839.

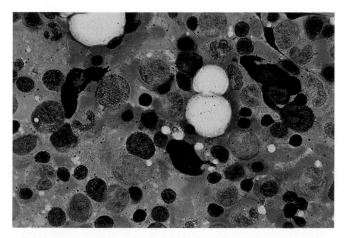

FIGURE 11-3. Bone marrow aspirate smear, reactive mastocytosis. Polygonal or angulated mast cells are seen in this smear from a patient with alcoholism.

10. Shah PY, Sharma V, Worobec AS, et al. Congenital bullous masto-cytosis with myeloproliferative disorder and c-kit mutation. *J Am Acad Dermatol* 1998;39:119–121.
11. Waxtein LM, Vega-Memije ME, Cortes-Franco R, et al. Diffuse cutaneous mastocytosis with bone marrow infiltration in a child: a case report. *Pediatr Dermatol* 2000;17:198–201.

Childhood-Onset Mastocytosis

1. Buttner C, Henz BM, Welker P, et al. Identification of activating c-kit mutations in adult-, but not in childhood-onset indolent mastocytosis: a possible explanation for divergent clinical behavior. *J Invest Dermatol* 1998;111:1227–1231.
2. Hartmann K, Henz BM. Mastocytosis: recent advances in defining the disease. *Br J Dermatol* 2001;144:682–695.
3. Longley BJ Jr, Metcalfe DD, Tharp M, et al. Activating and dom-inant inactivating c-KIT catalytic domain mutations in distinct clinical forms of human mastocytosis. *Proc Natl Acad Sci U S A* 1999;96:1609–1614.
4. Middelkamp Hup MA, Heide R, Tank B, et al. Comparison of mastocytosis with onset in children and adults. *J Eur Acad Der-matol Venereol* 2002;16:115–120.
5. Valent P, Horny HP, Escribano L, et al. Diagnostic criteria and classification of mastocytosis: a consensus proposal. *Leuk Res* 2001;25:603–625.
6. Beghini A, Tibiletti MG, Roversi G, et al. Germline mutation in the juxtamembrane domain of the kit gene in a family with gastrointestinal stromal tumors and urticaria pigmentosa. *Cancer* 2001;92:657–662.
7. Kuint J, Bielorai B, Gilat D, et al. C-kit activating mutation in a neonate with *in-utero* presentation of systemic mastocy-tosis associated with myeloproliferative disorder. *Br J Haematol* 1999;106:838–839.
8. Shah PY, Sharma V, Worobec AS, et al. Congenital bullous masto-cytosis with myeloproliferative disorder and c-kit mutation. *J Am Acad Dermatol* 1998;39:119–121.
9. Waxtein LM, Vega-Memije ME, Cortes-Franco R, et al. Diffuse cutaneous mastocytosis with bone marrow infiltration in a child: a case report. *Pediatr Dermatol* 2000;17:198–201.

Reactive Mastocytosis

1. Ellis HA, Peart KM, Pierides AM. Effect of renal transplantation on marrow mast cell hyperplasia of chronic renal failure. *J Clin Pathol* 1977;30:960–965.
2. Escribano L, Orfao A, Villarrubia J, et al. Immunophenotypic characterization of human bone marrow mast cells. A flow cyto-metric study of normal and pathological bone marrow samples. *Anal Cell Pathol* 1998;16:151–159.
3. Fallon MD, Whyte MP, Craig RB Jr, et al. Mast-cell proliferation in postmenopausal osteoporosis. *Calcif Tissue Int* 1983;35:29–31.
4. Fohlmeister I, Reber T, Fischer R. Bone marrow mast cell reaction in preleukaemic myelodysplasia and in aplastic anaemia. *Virchows Arch A Pathol Anat Histopathol* 1985;405:503–509.
5. Gozdasoglu S, Cavdar AO, Arcasoy A, et al. Fanconi's aplastic anemia, analysis of 18 cases. *Acta Haematol* 1980;64:131–135.
6. Jordan JH, Schernthaner GH, Fritsche-Polanz R, et al. Stem cell factor-induced bone marrow mast cell hyperplasia mimicking sys-temic mastocytosis (SM): histopathologic and morphologic eval-uation with special reference to recently established SM-criteria. *Leuk Lymphoma* 2002;43:575–582.
7. Macon WR, Kinney MC, Glick AD, et al. Marrow mast cell hyperplasia in hairy cell leukemia. *Mod Pathol* 1993;6:695–698.
8. Navone R, Pich A, Fiammotto M, et al. Bone marrow histopathology and prognosis in malignant lymphomas. *Tumori* 1992;78:176–180.
9. Prokocimer M, Polliack A. Increased bone marrow mast cells in preleukemic syndromes, acute leukemia, and lymphoproliferative disorders. *Am J Clin Pathol* 1981;75:34–38.
10. Ribatti D, Vacca A, Nico B, et al. Bone marrow angiogenesis and mast cell density increase simultaneously with progression of human multiple myeloma. *Br J Cancer* 1999;79:451–455.
11. Wilkins BS, Buchan SL, Webster J, et al. Tryptase-positive mast cells accompany lymphocytic as well as lymphoplasmacytic lym-phoma infiltrates in bone marrow trephine biopsies. *Histopathology* 2001;39:150–155.
12. Yoo D, Lessin LS. Bone marrow mast cell content in preleukemic syndrome. *Am J Med* 1982;73:539–542.
13. Yoo D, Lessin LS, Jensen WN. Bone-marrow mast cells in lym-phoproliferative disorders. *Ann Intern Med* 1978;88:753–757.

12

LYMPHOCYTES AND PLASMA CELLS

LYMPHOPENIA

Lymphopenia is a term usually applied to the peripheral blood rather than the bone marrow. A wide variety of medical conditions is associated with lymphopenia (Table 12-1). These include congenital immunodeficiency syndromes, acute pancreatitis, aging, aplastic anemia, autoimmune disorders, common variable immunodeficiency, chemotherapy and stem cell transplantation, chronic renal failure, corticosteroid therapy, ethanol, idiopathic T-cell lymphopenia syndrome, infection, nutritional deficiencies, sarcoidosis, stress, myeloproliferative disorders, myelodysplastic syndrome, malignant lymphoma, and multiple lymphangiomas (1–31). Mechanisms of lymphocytopenia include impaired lymphopoiesis, increased apoptosis, and alterations in lymphocyte trafficking and homing.

The peripheral blood and/or bone marrow show lymphopenia with analysis by automated instruments. Flow cytometry reveals decreases in B cells, T cells, and/or natural killer (NK) cells. No specific morphologic alterations accompany lymphopenia.

TABLE 12-1. CONDITIONS ASSOCIATED WITH LYMPHOPENIA

Nonneoplastic conditions
  Congenital immunodeficiency syndromes
  Acute pancreatitis
  Aging
  Aplastic anemia
  Autoimmune disorders
  Common variable immunodeficiency
  Chemotherapy and stem cell transplantation
  Chronic renal failure
  Corticosteroid therapy
  Ethanol
  Idiopathic T-cell lymphopenia syndrome
  Infection
  Nutritional deficiencies
  Posttransplantation lymphoproliferative disorder
  Sarcoidosis
  Stress

Neoplastic conditions
  Hematolymphoid malignancy
  Lymphangioma

REACTIVE LYMPHOCYTOSIS

Peripheral Blood Lymphocytosis

Peripheral blood lymphocytosis occurs under many conditions, including autoimmune disorders, connective tissue disease, strenuous exercise, hyperthermia, infection, malignancy, toxic industrial exposure, stress, trauma, and previous splenectomy (1–18) (Table 12-2). In some cases, no etiology is apparent. The peripheral blood smear may show unremarkable lymphocytes, lymphocytes with cleaved or convoluted nuclei, atypical lymphocytes, and/or immunoblasts. Flow cytometry may demonstrate T-cell, B-cell, and/or NK-cell immunophenotypes. Genetic studies usually reveal no clonal abnormalities. However, oligoclonal and monoclonal populations have been reported in some cases, without other

TABLE 12-2. CONDITIONS ASSOCIATED WITH REACTIVE PERIPHERAL BLOOD LYMPHOCYTOSIS

Nonneoplastic conditions
  Acquired autoimmune disorders
  Ataxia telangiectasia
  Autoimmune and connective tissue disorders
  Common variable immunodeficiency
  Connective tissue disease
  Drug hypersensitivity reaction
  Exercise
  Graft versus host disease
  Human immunodeficiency virus–related diffuse
    lymphocytosis syndrome
  Hyperreactive malarial splenomegaly
  Hyperthermia
  Infection
  Kikuchi disease
  Mosquito bite hypersensitivity
  Persistent polyclonal B lymphocytosis
  Splenectomy
  Stem cell transplantation
  Stress
  Toxic industrial exposure
  Trauma

Neoplastic conditions
  B-cell chronic lymphocytic leukemia
  Hairy cell leukemia
  Solid tumors
  Invasive thymoma

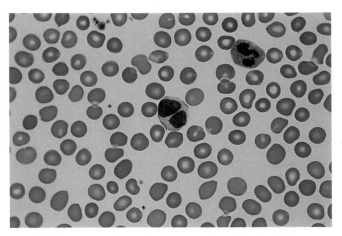

FIGURE 12-1. Peripheral blood smear, persistent polyclonal B lymphocytosis. A binucleated lymphocyte is seen in this specimen from a young woman who was a cigarette smoker.

signs of progression or malignant transformation. Specific clinicopathologic entities are described here.

Persistent polyclonal B-cell lymphocytosis is a rare disorder, usually found in young to middle-aged female cigarette smokers (19–25) (Fig. 12-1). It is associated with a polyclonal increase in serum immunoglobulin M level, serologic evidence of previous or chronic active Epstein-Barr virus infection, functional B-cell abnormalities, and HLA-DR7 phenotype. The peripheral blood characteristically shows binucleated lymphocytes. Flow cytometry shows a polyclonal, CD5-positive B-cell immunophenotype. Genetic studies have demonstrated clonal abnormalities in some cases, especially +i(3q) and *IgH* rearrangement. Evolution to malignant lymphoma has rarely been reported.

Chronic B-cell lymphocytosis also occurs in hyperreactive malarial splenomegaly (26–28). Genetic studies have revealed clonal *IgH* rearrangements in some cases, supporting an etiologic relationship between hyperreactive malarial splenomegaly and malignant B-cell lymphoma.

T-cell lymphocytosis has been reported after stem cell transplantation and in association with ataxia telangiectasia, autoimmune and connective tissue disease, graft versus host disease, infectious disease, common variable immunodeficiency, chronic B-cell lymphocytic leukemia, hairy cell leukemia, and invasive thymoma (29–59). Infectious agents associated with T-cell lymphocytosis include *Borrelia burgdorferi*, cytomegalovirus, Epstein-Barr virus, and human T lymphotropic virus type I. T-cell lymphocytosis may precede the diagnosis of invasive thymoma by years and may persist after resection of the tumor. The peripheral blood shows absolute lymphocytosis composed of small lymphocytes or large granular lymphocytes. Flow cytometry may show expression of CD4 and CD8, CD8 only, or neither CD4 nor CD8. Either T-cell receptor (TCR) α/β or TCR γ/δ may be expressed. Genetic studies may demonstrate polyclonal, oligoclonal, or monoclonal populations. Clonality appar-

ently arises owing to the expansion of clones with restricted TCR gene use but is not associated with other characteristics of progressive or malignant disease.

A specific type of T-cell lymphocytosis occurs as a complication of human immunodeficiency virus infection, termed diffuse lymphocytosis syndrome (60–65). This disorder is characterized by involvement of peripheral blood, nerves, salivary glands, and other organs. Flow cytometry reveals an activated suppressor T-cell phenotype, with expression of CD3, CD8, CD11c, CD57, and HLA-DR, but not CD4, CD16, or CD56. Genetic studies may show polyclonal, oligoclonal, or monoclonal TCR gene rearrangement. Clonality is apparently caused by expansion of one or more human immunodeficiency virus–specific clones with restricted TCR gene use.

NK-cell lymphocytosis has been reported in patients with infection, mosquito bite hypersensitivity, previous splenectomy, and clonal T-cell large granular lymphocytosis (43,66–73). The peripheral blood shows increased large granular lymphocytes indistinguishable from suppressor T cells. The differential diagnosis includes chronic NK-cell lymphocytic leukemia. Because no reliable method of determining NK-cell clonality yet exists, the distinction between reactive and clonal NK-cell disease must be made on clinical grounds.

Atypical lymphocytosis is seen in infectious mononucleosis, drug hypersensitivity reactions, and Kikuchi disease (74–79). Drug hypersensitivity reactions are usually accompanied by eosinophilia, fever, rash, hepatic disease, lymphadenopathy, and arthritis. Atypical lymphocytes are large cells with a relatively large, ovoid to folded nucleus showing moderately (not completely) condensed chromatin. A nucleolus may be present. The cytoplasm is usually abundant, agranular, and pale to moderately basophilic and may appear to flow around the surrounding red blood cells. Flow cytometry usually demonstrates a suppressor T-cell phenotype.

Immunoblasts may be found in drug hypersensitivity reactions, autoimmune disorders, and Epstein-Barr infection (17,80). They are usually accompanied by atypical lymphocytes, plasmacytoid lymphocytes, and plasma cells. Immunoblasts are large cells with round to ovoid nuclei and scant to moderately abundant, agranular, deeply basophilic cytoplasm.

The differential diagnosis includes clonal lymphoid disorders, acute leukemia, and malignant lymphoma in leukemic phase. Clinical judgment, immunophenotyping, and genotyping are essential in arriving at the correct diagnosis.

Bone Marrow Lymphoid Hyperplasia

Reactive lymphocytosis of the bone marrow occurs in association with peripheral lymphocytosis (see previously) and in aplastic anemia, autoimmune myelofibrosis, chronic renal failure, hypersplenism, infection, marrow regeneration after chemotherapy and/or stem cell transplantation, transient

TABLE 12-3. CONDITIONS ASSOCIATED WITH REACTIVE LYMPHOID HYPERPLASIA OF THE BONE MARROW

Nonneoplastic conditions
  Peripheral blood lymphocytosis
  Aplastic anemia
  Autoimmune and connective tissue disorders
  Chronic renal failure
  Hypersplenism
  Infection
  Marrow regeneration after chemotherapy and stem
    cell transplantation
  Transient erythroblastopenia of infancy

Neoplastic conditions
  Myeloproliferative disorders
  Myelodysplastic syndromes
  Acute leukemia
  Malignant lymphoma
  Invasive thymoma

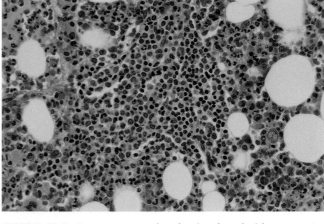

FIGURE 12-3. Bone marrow clot, benign lymphoid aggregate. Small, round to slightly irregular lymphocytes form an indistinct aggregate in the interstitial space.

erythroblastopenia of infancy, myeloproliferative disorders, myelodysplastic syndromes, acute leukemia, and malignant lymphoma (81–96) (Table 12-3). Flow cytometry may show a B-cell, T-cell, or NK-cell phenotype. Precursor B-cell lymphocytosis is discussed separately. Genetic studies usually indicate a polyclonal population.

Bone marrow aspirate smears show a higher percentage of lymphocytes than expected for age, in the range of 40% or more in young children and 20% or more in adults. Occasionally, only a single smear shows a high percentage of lymphocytes; this is usually attributable to aspiration and preparation of a benign lymphoid aggregate. Histologic sections of the bone marrow show interstitial lymphocytosis and/or benign lymphoid aggregates composed predominantly of small lymphocytes (Figs. 12-2 through 12-6). Interstitial lymphocytosis may be difficult to appreciate.

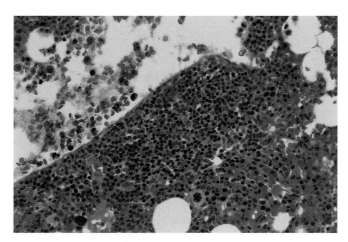

FIGURE 12-4. Bone marrow biopsy specimen, benign lymphoid aggregate. Another typical location for lymphoid aggregates is adjacent to the wall of a sinusoid.

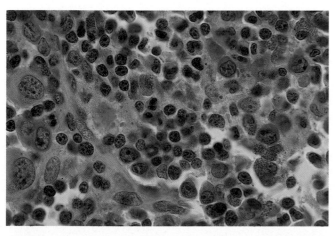

FIGURE 12-2. Bone marrow biopsy specimen, diffuse lymphocytosis. Small lymphocytes are distributed throughout the hematopoietic tissue.

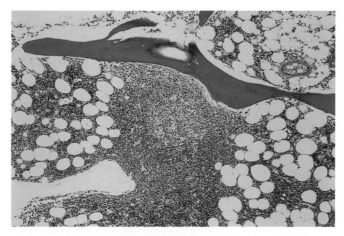

FIGURE 12-5. Bone marrow biopsy specimen, benign lymphoid aggregate with germinal center. Benign aggregates may occur next to trabecular bone but do not layer out along the bone as in follicular lymphoma.

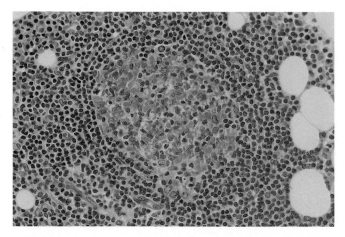

FIGURE 12-6. Bone marrow biopsy specimen, benign lymphoid aggregate with germinal center. The concentric rings of small lymphocytes and mixed population of central lymphocytes help to distinguish benign follicles from follicular lymphoma.

Benign lymphoid aggregates occur with increased frequency in women and elderly patients (97–103). They are often located adjacent to a sinusoid. When located near trabecular bone, they may resemble malignant lymphoma; however, they are not closely apposed to the bone and do not spread along the bone surface. Benign lymphoid aggregates are typically well-circumscribed in specimens from immunocompetent patients and are composed predominantly of small lymphocytes, sometimes with a small penetrating blood vessel and a ring of eosinophils. A germinal center may be present. In specimens from immunocompromised patients, benign lymphoid aggregates tend to be less well circumscribed and may consist of lymphocytes, histiocytes, plasma cells, and eosinophils. Staining for bcl-2 protein is usually, but not always, negative. Genetic studies show no evidence of clonality. Lack of evidence of clonality must be interpreted with caution because false-negative results sometimes occur in specimens with clear histologic evidence of malignant lymphoma.

Precursor B-cell (hematogone) hyperplasia occurs under conditions of hematopoietic stress and regeneration and may persist for months after resolution of the underlying condition (104–121) (Table 12-4). Associated conditions include marrow regeneration after chemotherapy and/or stem cell transplantation, immune-mediated cytopenias, infection, transient erythroblastopenia of infancy, Gaucher disease, acute leukemia, and malignant lymphoma. Bone marrow aspirate smears show precursor B cells comprising as much as 80% of nucleated cells. The cells are small to medium size and show round nuclei with small nuclear notches or cleaves, condensed homogeneous chromatin, and scant basophilic cytoplasm. Nucleoli are typically absent. Histologic sections of the bone marrow may show reactive lymphocytosis and/or lymphoid aggregates. Flow cytometry shows consistent, bright expression of CD10 and CD19. CD20, CD34, and terminal deoxynucleotidyl transferase are variably expressed. Surface immunoglobulin is typically not expressed.

TABLE 12-4. CONDITIONS ASSOCIATED WITH PRECURSOR B-CELL HYPERPLASIA OF THE BONE MARROW

Nonneoplastic conditions
    Connective tissue disease
    Gaucher disease
    Immune-mediated cytopenia
    Infection
    Marrow regeneration after chemotherapy and stem
        cell transplantation
    Transient erythroblastopenia of infancy

Neoplastic conditions
    Acute leukemia
    Malignant lymphoma

The differential diagnosis of reactive lymphocytosis includes drug reaction and malignant lymphoma (122–124). Morphologic features favoring a benign lymphoid aggregate include an interstitial location, well-defined borders, a central vessel, and a rim of plasma cells and/or eosinophils. After anti-CD20 therapy, deposits of malignant B-cell lymphoma may be reduced to aggregates of residual T cells, which may be mistaken for residual lymphoma (89). It should be kept in mind that reactive lymphocytosis and benign lymphoid aggregates may occur in conjunction with malignant lymphoma in the bone marrow.

The differential diagnosis of precursor B-cell hyperplasia includes acute leukemia and malignant lymphoma. Uniform CD10 and CD19 expression, lack of myeloid antigen expression, and lack of clonality help to distinguish reactive from neoplastic precursor B cells. It should be kept in mind that precursor B-cell hyperplasia may occur in conjunction with acute leukemia and malignant lymphoma.

REACTIVE PLASMACYTOSIS

Peripheral Blood Plasmacytosis

Reactive plasmacytosis of the peripheral blood is an uncommon phenomenon (Table 12-5). Underlying conditions include connective tissue disease, viral hepatitis, rubella virus infection, and reactions to sulfa drugs and streptokinase (1–4).

Bone Marrow Plasmacytosis

Reactive plasmacytosis of the bone marrow has been reported in a variety of settings (5–32) (Table 12-6). Underlying

TABLE 12-5. CONDITIONS ASSOCIATED WITH REACTIVE PERIPHERAL BLOOD PLASMACYTOSIS

Connective tissue disease
Drug reactions to sulfa and streptokinase
Rubella virus infection
Viral hepatitis

TABLE 12-6. CONDITIONS ASSOCIATED WITH REACTIVE BONE MARROW PLASMACYTOSIS

Nonneoplastic conditions
  Aplastic anemia
  Autoimmune disorders
  Chronic bronchopulmonary inflammation
  Connective tissue disease
  Drug reactions
  Granulocyte and granulocyte-monocyte colony-stimulating
    factor therapy
  Infection
  Multicentric giant lymph node hyperplasia (Castleman
    disease)
  Secondary erythrocytosis
  Sinus histiocytosis with massive lymphadenopathy
    (Rosai-Dorfman disease)
  Systemic plasmacytosis and immunoblastosis

Neoplastic conditions
  Hematolymphoid malignancy
  Clonal plasma cell disease
  Interleukin-6–producing solid tumors

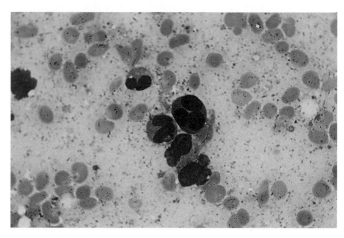

FIGURE 12-8. Bone marrow aspirate, reactive plasmacytosis. Reactive plasma cells may contain two, three, or four nuclei, each showing the condensed chromatin typical of a benign plasma cells.

conditions include autoimmune disorders, connective tissue disease, aplastic anemia, multicentric giant lymph node hyperplasia (Castleman disease), sinus histiocytosis with massive lymphadenopathy (Rosai-Dorfman disease), secondary erythrocytosis, drug reactions, and granulocyte and granulocyte-monocyte colony-stimulating factor therapy. Reactive plasmacytosis also occurs in chronic bronchopulmonary inflammation, viral hepatitis, leprosy, malaria, tuberculosis, and human herpesvirus 8, and human immunodeficiency virus infections. Neoplastic conditions characterized by reactive bone marrow plasmacytosis include myeloproliferative disorders, myelodysplastic syndromes, acute myeloid leukemia, Hodgkin disease, plasma cell dyscrasias, large granular lymphocytic leukemia, and interleukin-6–producing solid tumors.

Bone marrow aspirate smears may show plasma cells ranging from 2% to nearly 100% of nucleated cells (Figs. 12-7

through 12-10). Plasma cell morphology is usually unremarkable but has occasionally been described as abnormal, undifferentiated, or immunoblastic. Cytoplasmic inclusions may be present, occupying the cytoplasm as a large spherical mass (Russell body) or transforming the cytoplasm into a cluster of smaller spherical masses (Mott cells). Reactive plasma cells may contain as many as four nuclei, each resembling a normal plasma cell nucleus with condensed, clumped chromatin. Histologic sections of the bone marrow show plasma cells scattered among hematopoietic cells and lined up along small vessels, a phenomenon also observable in smears of marrow particles (33) (Figs. 12-7 through 12-10). Reactive lymphocytosis may also be present.

Flow cytometry and immunostaining show no abnormalities. With rare exceptions, genetic studies show no evidence of clonality (24,29).

The differential diagnosis includes posttransplantation lymphoproliferative disorder (which may be nonclonal or

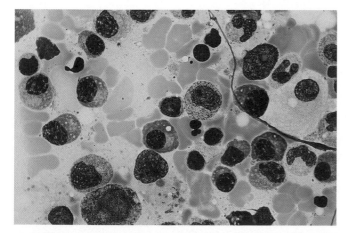

FIGURE 12-7. Bone marrow aspirate, reactive plasmacytosis. Numerous morphologically unremarkable plasma cells are seen in this specimen from a cigarette smoker.

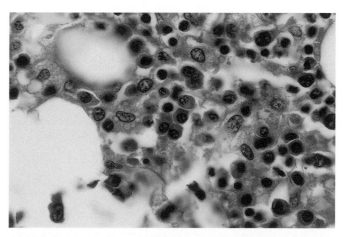

FIGURE 12-9. Bone marrow biopsy specimen, reactive plasmacytosis. Reactive plasma cells may be found in small clusters in the interstitial space.

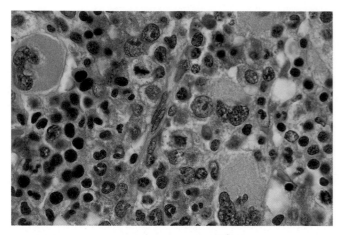

FIGURE 12-10. Bone marrow biopsy specimen, reactive plasmacytosis. Reactive plasma cells often line up along small blood vessels.

TABLE 12-7. CONDITIONS ASSOCIATED WITH BONE MARROW PLASMA CELL IRON

Nonneoplastic conditions
  Alcohol abuse
  Nonalcoholic hepatic cirrhosis
  Megaloblastic anemia
  Iron overload

Neoplastic conditions
  Multiple myeloma
  Malignant lymphoma
  Nasopharyngeal carcinoma

It should be kept in mind that reactive bone marrow plasmacytosis and clonal plasma cell disorders frequently coexist.

Bone Marrow Plasma Cell Iron

The plasma cells of the bone marrow occasionally contain cytoplasmic iron, visible with Prussian blue stain (35–44) (Table 12-7). This finding is of unknown pathogenesis but is usually a sign of systemic disease. The underlying condition is usually alcohol abuse, but iron-containing plasma cells have also been reported in marrow specimens from patients with nonalcoholic hepatic cirrhosis, megaloblastic anemia, iron overload, multiple myeloma, malignant lymphoma, and nasopharyngeal carcinoma.

Bone marrow aspirate smears show small plasma cells, without a significant increase in the number of plasma cells. Iron is visible within plasma cells with the Prussian blue stain (Fig. 12-12). Ultrastructural examination has shown that the iron is contained as ferritin within lysosomal vesicles. Intrahistiocytic iron stores may be absent, decreased, normal, or increased.

clonal), lymphoplasmacytic lymphoma, monoclonal gammopathy of undetermined significance, and multiple myeloma. Findings that support a diagnosis of reactive plasmacytosis are absence of monoclonal serum and urine protein, normal morphology, perivascular distribution, polyclonal phenotype, lack of CD117 expression (34), and lack of clonality. The percentage of bone marrow plasma cells per se is not a reliable criterion for distinguishing reactive from malignant plasmacytosis. In marked chronic inflammation, as in tuberculosis and leprosy, reactive plasma cells may constitute 50% or more of nucleated cells in the bone marrow. Likewise, plasma cell morphology is not always a reliable criterion; reactive plasma cells may be enlarged, contain a nucleolus, and show multinuclearity. It is particularly difficult to predict clonality in cases of posttransplantation lymphoproliferative disorder (Fig. 12-11).

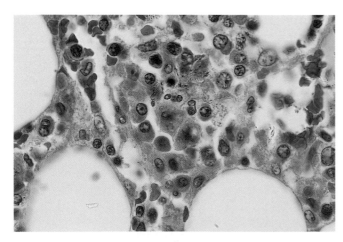

FIGURE 12-11. Bone marrow biopsy specimen, posttransplantation lymphoproliferative disorder. Plasma cells and lymphocytes are increased; additional studies are required to determine clonality.

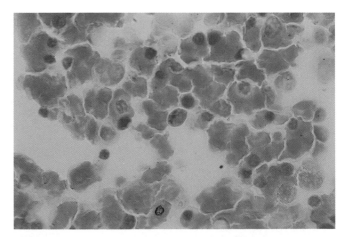

FIGURE 12-12. Bone marrow aspirate smear, iron-containing plasma cells (Prussian blue stain). The cytoplasm of a plasma cell is filled with coarse iron-containing granules in this specimen from an alcoholic.

REFERENCES

Lymphopenia

1. Abe Y, Hirase N, Muta K, et al. Adult onset cyclic hematopoiesis in a patient with myelodysplastic syndrome. *Int J Hematol* 2000; 71:40–45.
2. Amadori G, Micciolo R, Poletti A. A case of intra-abdominal multiple lymphangiomas in an adult in whom the immunological evaluation supported the diagnosis. *Eur J Gastroenterol Hepatol* 1999;11:347–351.
3. Brown KA. Nonmalignant disorders of lymphocytes. *Clin Lab Sci* 1997;10:329–235.
4. Cervantes F, Hernandez-Boluda JC, Villamor N, et al. Assessment of peripheral blood lymphocyte subsets in idiopathic myelofibrosis. *Eur J Haematol* 2000;65:104–108.
5. Fernandez-Fresnedo G, Ramos MA, Gonzalez-Pardo MC, et al. B lymphopenia in uremia is related to an accelerated in vitro apoptosis and dysregulation of Bcl-2. *Nephrol Dial Transplant* 2000;15:502–510.
6. Gubinelli E, Posteraro P, Girolomoni G. Idiopathic CD4+ T lymphocytopenia associated with disseminated flat warts and alopecia areata. *J Dermatol* 2002;29:653–656.
7. Gupta D, Rao VM, Aggarwal AN, et al. Haematological abnormalities in patients of sarcoidosis. *Indian J Chest Dis Allied Sci* 2002;44:233–236.
8. Gupta S. Molecular and biochemical pathways of apoptosis in lymphocytes from aged humans. *Vaccine* 2000;18:1596–1601.
9. Hequet O, Salles G, Espinousse D, et al. Multifocal progressive leukoencephalopathy occurring after refractory anemia and multiple infectious disorders consecutive to severe lymphopenia. *Ann Hematol* 2002;81:340–342.
10. Hotchkiss RS, Tinsley KW, Swanson PE, et al. Sepsis-induced apoptosis causes progressive profound depletion of B and CD4+ T lymphocytes in humans. *J Immunol* 2001;166:6952–6963.
11. Iglesias J, Matamoros N, Raga S, et al. CD95 expression and function on lymphocyte subpopulations in common variable immunodeficiency (CVID); related to increased apoptosis. *Clin Exp Immunol* 1999;117:138–146.
12. Jeon HJ, Lee MJ, Jeong YK, et al. Adult T cell leukemia/lymphoma with lymphopenia in a Korean. *J Korean Med Sci* 2000;15:233–239.
13. Jouen-Beades F, Joly P, Heron F, et al. Flow cytometry analysis of peripheral blood lymphocytes from patients with bullous pemphigoid. *Dermatology* 1998;197:137–140.
14. Kapasi AA, Patel G, Goenka A, et al. Ethanol promotes T cell apoptosis through the mitochondrial pathway. *Immunology* 2003;108:313–320.
15. Kemp K, Bruunsgaard H, Skinhoj P, et al. Pneumococcal infections in humans are associated with increased apoptosis and trafficking of type 1 cytokine-producing T cells. *Infect Immun* 2002;70:5019–5025.
16. Klinger J, Enriquez J, Arturo JA, et al. Comparison of immunophenotypes in the blood of patients on continuous ambulatory peritoneal dialysis, asymptomatic and with peritonitis. *Adv Perit Dial* 2002;18:165–169.
17. Lee N, Hui D, Wu A, et al. A major outbreak of severe acute respiratory syndrome in Hong Kong. *N Engl J Med* 2003;348:1986–1994.
18. Lim EJ, Peh SC. Bone marrow and peripheral blood changes in non-Hodgkin's lymphoma. *Singapore Med J* 2000;41:279–285.
19. Lin MT, Tseng LH, Frangoul H, et al. Increased apoptosis of peripheral blood T cells following allogeneic hematopoietic cell transplantation. *Blood* 2000;95:3832–3839.
20. McMurray DN. Cell-mediated immunity in nutritional deficiency. *Prog Food Nutr Sci* 1984;8:193–228.
21. Mert A, Bilir M, Tabak F, et al. Miliary tuberculosis: clinical manifestations, diagnosis and outcome in 38 adults. *Respirology* 2001;6:217–224.
22. Odendahl M, Jacobi A, Hansen A, et al. Disturbed peripheral B lymphocyte homeostasis in systemic lupus erythematosus. *J Immunol* 2000;165:5970–5979.
23. Okada H, Kobune F, Sato TA, et al. Extensive lymphopenia due to apoptosis of uninfected lymphocytes in acute measles patients. *Arch Virol* 2000;145:905–920.
24. Peake J, Waugh A, Le Deist F, et al. Combined immunodeficiency associated with increased apoptosis of lymphocytes and radiosensitivity fibroblasts. *Cancer Res* 1999;59:3454–3460.
25. Ray-Coquard I, Borg C, Bachelot T, et al. Baseline and early lymphopenia predict for the risk of febrile neutropenia after chemotherapy. *Br J Cancer* 2003;88:181–186.
26. Silva LM, Garcia AB, Donadi EA. Increased lymphocyte death by neglect-apoptosis is associated with lymphopenia and autoantibodies in lupus patients presenting with neuropsychiatric manifestations. *J Neurol* 2002;249:1048–1054.
27. Stricker RB, Winger EE. Decreased CD57 lymphocyte subset in patients with chronic Lyme disease. *Immunol Lett* 2001;76:43–48.
28. Takeyama Y, Takas K, Ueda T, et al. Peripheral lymphocyte reduction in severe acute pancreatitis is caused by apoptotic cell death. *J Gastrointest Surg* 2000;4:379–387.
29. Viguier M, Fouere S, de la Salmoniere P, et al. Peripheral blood lymphocyte subset counts in patients with dermatomyositis: clinical correlations and changes following therapy. *Medicine (Baltimore)* 2003;82:82–86.
30. Wang FZ, Linde A, Dahl H, et al. Human herpesvirus 6 infection inhibits specific lymphocyte proliferation responses and is related to lymphocytopenia after allogeneic stem cell transplantation. *Bone Marrow Transplant* 1999;24:1201–1206.
31. Zeng W, Maciejewski JP, Chen G, et al. Selective reduction of natural killer T cells in the bone marrow of aplastic anaemia. *Br J Haematol* 2002;119:803–809.

Reactive Lymphocytosis

1. Brown KA. Nonmalignant disorders of lymphocytes. *Clin Lab Sci* 1997;10:329–335.
2. Lim MS, Straus SE, Dale JK, et al. Pathological findings in human autoimmune lymphoproliferative syndrome. *Am J Pathol* 1998;153:1541–1550.
3. Ceddia MA, Price EA, Kohlmeier CK, et al. Differential leukocytosis and lymphocyte mitogenic response to acute maximal exercise in the young and old. *Med Sci Sports Exerc* 1999;31:829–836.
4. Gomez P, Matutes E, Sanchez J, et al. An unusual form of persistent polyclonal B lymphocytosis in an infant. *Br J Haematol* 2000;110:430–433.
5. Grossi A, Nozzoli C, Gheri R, et al. Pure red cell aplasia in autoimmune polyglandular syndrome with T lymphocytosis. *Haematologica* 1998;83:1043–1045.
6. Hristeva-Mirtcheva V. Changes in the peripheral blood of workers with occupational exposure to aromatic hydrocarbons. *Int Arch Occup Environ Health* 1998;71[Suppl]:S81–S83.
7. Hutchinson RE, Kurec AS, Davey FR. Lymphocytic surface markers in lymphoid leukemoid reactions. *Clin Lab Med* 1988;8:237–245.
8. Juneja S, Januszewicz E, Wolf M, et al. Post-splenectomy lymphocytosis. *Clin Lab Haematol* 1995;17:335–337.
9. Karandikar NJ, Hotchkiss EC, McKenna RW, et al. Transient stress lymphocytosis: an immunophenotypic characterization of the most common cause of newly identified adult lymphocytosis in a tertiary hospital. *Am J Clin Pathol* 2002;117:819–825.

10. Machii T, Yamaguchi M, Inoue R, et al. Polyclonal B-cell lymphocytosis with features resembling hairy cell leukemia-Japanese variant. *Blood* 1997;89:2008–2014.

11. Peterson L, Hrisinko MA. Benign lymphocytosis and reactive neutrophilia. Laboratory features provide diagnostic clues. *Clin Lab Med* 1993;13:863–877.

12. Radossi P, Dazzi F, De Franchis G, et al. Myasthenic syndrome and oligoclonal lymphocytosis: evolution into chronic lymphocytic leukemia. *Ann Hematol* 1998;76:45–47.

13. Rainer TH, Chan TY, Cocks RA. Do peripheral blood counts have any prognostic value following trauma? *Injury* 1999;30:179–185.

14. Rhind SG, Gannon GA, Shek PN, et al. Contribution of exertional hyperthermia to sympathoadrenal-mediated lymphocyte subset redistribution. *J Appl Physiol* 1999;87:1178–1185.

15. Sala P, Tonutti E, Feruglio C, et al. Persistent expansions of CD4+ CD8+ peripheral blood T cells. *Blood* 1993;82:1546–1552.

16. Siddiqui MA, Esmaili JH. Transient reactive lymphocytosis associated with acute middle cerebral artery aneurysmal rupture. *J Natl Med Assoc* 1997;89:283–284.

17. Ward PC. The lymphoid leukocytoses. *Postgrad Med* 1980;67:217–223.

18. Wulf GG, Schulz H, Hallermann C, et al. Reactive polyclonal T-cell lymphocytosis mimicking Sezary syndrome in a patient with hairy cell leukemia. *Haematologica* 2001;86:E27.

19. Delage R, Jacques L, Massinga-Loembe M, et al. Persistent polyclonal B-cell lymphocytosis: further evidence for a genetic disorder associated with B-cell abnormalities. *Br J Haematol* 2001;114:666–670.

20. Himmelmann A, Ruegg R, Fehr J. Familial persistent polyclonal B-cell lymphocytosis. *Leuk Lymphoma* 2001;41:157–160.

21. Lancry L, Roulland S, Roue G, et al. No BCL-2 protein over expression but BCL-2/IgH rearrangements in B cells of patients with persistent polyclonal B-cell lymphocytosis. *Hematol J* 2001;2:228–233.

22. Mossafa H, Malaure H, Maynadie M, et al. Persistent polyclonal B lymphocytosis with binucleated lymphocytes: a study of 25 cases. Groupe Francais d'Hematologie Cellulaire. *Br J Haematol* 1999;104:486–493.

23. Reimer P, Weissinger F, Tony HP, et al. Persistent polyclonal B-cell lymphocytosis—an important differential diagnosis of B-cell chronic lymphocytic leukemia. *Ann Hematol* 2000;79:327–331.

24. Roy J, Ryckman C, Bernier V, et al. Large cell lymphoma complicating persistent polyclonal B cell lymphocytosis. *Leukemia* 1998;12:1026–1030.

25. Salcedo I, Campos-Caro A, Sampalo A, et al. Persistent polyclonal B lymphocytosis: an expansion of cells showing IgVH gene mutations and phenotypic features of normal lymphocytes from the CD27+ marginal zone B-cell compartment. *Br J Haematol* 2002;116:662–666.

26. Bates I, Bedu-Addo G, Rutherford TR, et al. Circulating villous lymphocytes—a link between hyperreactive malarial splenomegaly and splenic lymphoma. *Trans R Soc Trop Med Hyg* 1997;91:171–174.

27. Bedu-Addo G, Bates I. Causes of massive tropical splenomegaly in Ghana. *Lancet* 2002;360:449–454.

28. Wallace S, Bedu-Addo G, Rutherford TR, et al. Serological similarities between hyperreactive malarial splenomegaly and splenic lymphoma in West Africa. *Trans R Soc Trop Med Hyg* 1998;92:463–467.

29. Barton AD. T-cell lymphocytosis associated with lymphocyte-rich thymoma. *Cancer* 1997;80:1409–1417.

30. Callan MF, Steven N, Krausa P, et al. Large clonal expansions of CD8+ T cells in acute infectious mononucleosis. *Nat Med* 1996;2:906–911.

31. de Jong D, Richel DJ, Schenkeveld C, et al. Oligoclonal peripheral T-cell lymphocytosis as a result of aberrant T-cell development in a cortical thymoma. *Diagn Mol Pathol* 1997;6:244–248.

32. Dow N. CD8/CD57 lymphocytosis in common variable immunodeficiency. *Blood* 1991;77:1400–1401.

33. Eiraku N, Hingorani R, Ijichi S, et al. Clonal expansion within CD4+ and CD8+ T cell subsets in human T lymphotropic virus type I-infected individuals. *J Immunol* 1998;161:6674–6680.

34. Goolsby CL, Kuchnio M, Finn WG, et al. Expansions of clonal and oligoclonal T cells in B-cell chronic lymphocytic leukemia are primarily restricted to the CD3(+)CD8(+) T-cell population. *Cytometry* 2000;42:188–195.

35. Grossi A, Nozzoli C, Gheri R, et al. Pure red cell aplasia in autoimmune polyglandular syndrome with T lymphocytosis. *Haematologica* 1998;83:1043–1045.

36. Hashino S, Mori A, Kobayashi S, et al. Proliferation of CD4+ lymphocytes in a patient with chronic graft-versus-host disease after allogeneic bone marrow transplantation. *Int J Hematol* 2000;71:389–393.

37. Horiuchi T, Hirokawa M, Satoh K, et al. Clonal expansion of gammadelta-T lymphocytes in an HTLV-I carrier, associated with chronic neutropenia and rheumatoid arthritis. *Ann Hematol* 1999;78:101–104.

38. Ichikawa M, Yanagisawa M, Kawai H, et al. Spontaneous improvement of juvenile rheumatoid arthritis after T lymphocytosis with suppressor phenotype and function. *J Clin Lab Immunol* 1988;27:197–201.

39. Ishii E, Kimura N, Kato K, et al. Clonal change of infiltrating T-cells in children with familial hemophagocytic lymphohistiocytosis: possible association with Epstein-Barr virus infection. *Cancer* 1999;85:1636–1643.

40. Katial RK, Lieberman MM, Muehlbauer SL, et al. Gamma delta T lymphocytosis associated with common variable immunodeficiency. *J Clin Immunol* 1997;17:34–42.

41. Katopodis O, Liossis SN, Viglis V, et al. Expansion of CD8+ T cells that express low levels of the B cell-specific molecule CD20 in patients with multiple myeloma. *Br J Haematol* 2003;120:478–481.

42. Khatri VP, Baiocchi RA, Peng R, et al. Endogenous CD8+ T cell expansion during regression of monoclonal EBV-associated posttransplant lymphoproliferative disorder. *J Immunol* 1999;163:500–506.

43. Kingreen D, Dalal BI, Heyman M, et al. Lymphocytosis of large granular lymphocytes in patients with Hodgkin's disease. *Am J Hematol* 1995;50:234–236.

44. Kluin-Nelemans JC, Kester MG, Melenhorst JJ, et al. Persistent clonal excess and skewed T-cell repertoire in T cells from patients with hairy cell leukemia. *Blood* 1996;87:3795–3802.

45. Kronenberg A, Seebach JD, Bossart W, et al. Polyclonal proliferation of large granular lymphocytes during cytomegalovirus primary infection in a human immunodeficiency virus-infected patient receiving antiretroviral therapy. *Clin Infect Dis* 2001;33:E34–E36.

46. Kvasnicka HM, Thiele J, Ahmadi T. Bone marrow manifestation of Lyme disease (Lyme borreliosis). *Br J Haematol* 2003;120:723.

47. Masci AM, Palmieri G, Perna F, et al. Immunological findings in thymoma and thymoma-related syndromes. *Ann Med* 1999;31[Suppl 2]:86–89.

48. Medeiros LJ, Bhagat SK, Naylor P, et al. Malignant thymoma associated with T-cell lymphocytosis. A case report with immunophenotypic and gene rearrangement analysis. *Arch Pathol Lab Med* 1993;117:279–283.

49. Mathew P, Hudnall SD, Elghetany MT, et al. T-gamma gene rearrangement and CMV mononucleosis. *Am J Hematol* 2001;66:64–66.

50. Mortreux F, Gabet AS, Wattel E. Molecular and cellular aspects of HTLV-1 associated leukemogenesis *in vivo*. *Leukemia* 2003;17:26–38.

51. Nakahara K, Utsunomiya A, Hanada S, et al. Transient appearance of CD3+CD8+ T lymphocytes with monoclonal gene rearrangement of T-cell receptor beta locus. *Br J Haematol* 1998;100:411–414.

52. Otton SH, Standen GR, Ormerod IE. T cell lymphocytosis associated with polymyositis, myasthenia gravis and thymoma. *Clin Lab Haematol* 2000;22:307–308.

53. Owen RG, Patmore RD, Smith GM, et al. Cytomegalovirus-induced T-cell proliferation and the development of progressive multifocal leucoencephalopathy following bone marrow transplantation. *Br J Haematol* 1995;89:196–198.

54. Sajeva MR, Greco MM, Cascavilla N, et al. Effective autologous peripheral blood stem cell transplantation in plasma cell leukemia followed by T-large granular lymphocyte expansion: a case report. *Bone Marrow Transplant* 1996;18:225–227.

55. Smith GP, Perkins SL, Segal GH, et al. T-cell lymphocytosis associated with invasive thymomas. *Am J Clin Pathol* 1994;102: 447–453.

56. Stern MH, Theodorou I, Aurias A, et al. T-cell nonmalignant clonal proliferation in ataxia telangiectasia: a cytological, immunological, and molecular characterization. *Blood* 1989;73:1285–1290.

57. Tamaoki J, Chiyotani A, Nagai A, et al. Invasive thymoma with CD4+CD8+ double-positive T cell lymphocytosis. *Respiration* 1997;64:176–178.

58. Witzens M, Mohler T, Willhauck M, et al. Detection of clonally rearranged T-cell-receptor gamma chain genes from T-cell malignancies and acute inflammatory rheumatic disease using PCR amplification, PAGE, and automated analysis. *Ann Hematol* 1997;74:123–130.

59. Wong KF, Yip SF, So CC, et al. Cytomegalovirus infection associated with clonal proliferation of T-cell large granular lymphocytes: causal or casual? *Cancer Genet Cytogenet* 2003;142: 77–79.

60. Franco-Paredes C, Rebolledo P, Folch E, et al. Diagnosis of diffuse CD8+ lymphocytosis syndrome in HIV-infected patients. *AIDS Read* 2002;12:408–413.

61. McArthur CP, Subtil-DeOliveira A, Palmer D, et al. Characteristics of salivary diffuse infiltrative lymphocytosis syndrome in West Africa. *Arch Pathol Lab Med* 2000;124:1773–1779.

62. Smith PR, Cavenagh JD, Milne T, et al. Benign monoclonal expansion of CD8+ lymphocytes in HIV infection. *J Clin Pathol* 2000;53:177–181.

63. Smith P, Helbert M, Raftery M, et al. Paraproteins and monoclonal expansion of CD3+CD8+ CD56−CD57+ T lymphocytes in a patient with HIV infection. *Br J Haematol* 1999;105:85–87.

64. Williams FM, Cohen PR, Jumshyd J, et al. Prevalence of the diffuse infiltrative lymphocytosis syndrome among human immunodeficiency virus type 1-positive outpatients. *Arthritis Rheum* 1998;41:863–868.

65. Zambello R, Trentin L, Agostini C, et al. Persistent polyclonal lymphocytosis in human immunodeficiency virus-1-infected patients. *Blood* 1993;81:3015–3021.

66. Ishiyama T, Koike M, Watanabe K, et al. Natural killer (NK) lymphocytosis induced by Epstein-Barr virus (EBV) reactivation in monoclonal gammopathy of undetermined significance (MGUS). *Clin Exp Immunol* 1996;105:46–51.

67. Kaito K, Otsubo H, Ogasawara Y, et al. Severe aplastic anemia associated with chronic natural killer cell lymphocytosis. *Int J Hematol* 2000;72:463–465.

68. Kondo H, Watanabe J, Iwasaki H. T-large granular lymphocyte leukemia accompanied by an increase of natural killer cells (CD3−) and associated with ulcerative colitis and autoimmune hepatitis. *Leuk Lymphoma* 2001;41:207–212.

69. Myers B, Speight EL, Huissoon AP, et al. Natural killer-cell lymphocytosis and strongyloides infection. *Clin Lab Haematol* 2000;22:237–238.

70. Orange JS, Chehimi J, Ghavimi D, et al. Decreased natural killer (NK) cell function in chronic NK cell lymphocytosis associated with decreased surface expression of CD11b. *Clin Immunol* 2001;99:53–64.

71. Otsuji A, Otsuji N, Ohno T, et al. Transient large granular lymphocytosis associated with pulmonary tuberculosis: a case report. *Rinsho Ketsueki* 1990;31:1955–1959.

72. Satoh M, Oyama N, Akiba H, et al. Hypersensitivity to mosquito bites with natural-killer cell lymphocytosis: the possible implication of Epstein-Barr virus reactivation. *Eur J Dermatol* 2002;12:381–384.

73. Vargas JA, Gea-Banacloche JC, Ramon y Cajal S, et al. Natural killer cell proliferation and renal disease: a functional and phenotypic study. *Cytometry* 1996;26:125–130.

74. Bessmertny O, Hatton RC, Gonzalez-Peralta RP. Antiepileptic hypersensitivity syndrome in children. *Ann Pharmacother* 2001;35:533–538.

75. Fujino Y, Nakajima M, Inoue H, et al. Human herpesvirus 6 encephalitis associated with hypersensitivity syndrome. *Ann Neurol* 2002;51:771–774.

76. Huh J, Kang GH, Gong G, et al. Kaposi's sarcoma-associated herpesvirus in Kikuchi's disease. *Hum Pathol* 1998;29:1091–1096.

77. MacNeil M, Haase DA, Tremaine R, et al. Fever, lymphadenopathy, eosinophilia, lymphocytosis, hepatitis, and dermatitis: a severe adverse reaction to minocycline. *J Am Acad Dermatol* 1997;36:347–350.

78. Sakai C, Takagi T, Oguro M, et al. Erythroderma and marked atypical lymphocytosis mimicking cutaneous T-cell lymphoma probably caused by phenobarbital. *Intern Med* 1993;32: 182–184.

79. Verrotti A, Feliciani C, Morresi S, et al. Carbamazepine-induced hypersensitivity syndrome in a child with epilepsy. *Int J Immunopathol Pharmacol* 2000;13:49–53.

80. Arce E, Jackson DG, Gill MA, et al. Increased frequency of pre-germinal center B cells and plasma cell precursors in the blood of children with systemic lupus erythematosus. *J Immunol* 2001;167:2361–2369.

81. Bass RD, Pullarkat V, Feinstein DI, et al. Pathology of autoimmune myelofibrosis. A report of three cases and a review of the literature. *Am J Clin Pathol* 2001;116:211–216.

82. Cervantes F, Pereira A, Marti JM, et al. Bone marrow lymphoid nodules in myeloproliferative disorders: association with the non-myelosclerotic phases of idiopathic myelofibrosis and immunological significance. *Br J Haematol* 1988;70:279–282.

83. Farhi DC, Luebbers EL, Rosenthal NS. Bone marrow biopsy findings in childhood anemia: prevalence of transient erythroblastopenia of childhood. *Arch Pathol Lab Med* 1998;122: 638–641.

84. Feng CS, Ng MH, Szeto RS, et al. Bone marrow findings in lupus patients with pancytopenia. *Pathology* 1991;23:5–7.

85. Franco V, Florena AM, Aragona F, et al. Immunohistochemical evaluation of bone marrow lymphoid nodules in chronic myeloproliferative disorders. *Virchows Arch* 1991;419:261–266.

86. Gottlieb CA, Maeda K, Hawley RC, et al. Myelodysplasia with bone marrow lymphocytosis and fibrosis mimicking recurrent Hodgkin's disease. *Am J Clin Pathol* 1989;91:6–11.

87. Horny HP, Wehrmann M, Griesser H, et al. Investigation of bone marrow lymphocyte subsets in normal, reactive, and neoplastic states using paraffin-embedded biopsy specimens. *Am J Clin Pathol* 1993;99:142–149.

88. Kiss TL, Spaner D, Daly AS, et al. Complete remission of tumour with interleukin 2 therapy in a patient with non-Hodgkin's lymphoma post allogeneic bone marrow transplant associated with polyclonal T-cell bone marrow lymphocytosis. *Br J Haematol* 2003;120:523–525.

89. Lim MS, Straus SE, Dale JK, et al. Pathological findings in human autoimmune lymphoproliferative syndrome. *Am J Pathol* 1998;153:1541–1550.

90. Mohty M, Faucher C, Gaugler B, et al. Large granular lymphocytes (LGL) following non-myeloablative allogeneic bone marrow transplantation: a case report. *Bone Marrow Transplant* 2001;28:1157–1160.

91. Navone R, Valpreda M, Pich A. Lymphoid nodules and nodular lymphoid hyperplasia in bone marrow biopsies. *Acta Haematol* 1985;74:19–22.

92. Papadaki HA, Chatzivassili A, Stefanaki K, et al. Morphologically defined myeloid cell compartments, lymphocyte subpopulations, and histological findings of bone marrow in patients with nonimmune chronic idiopathic neutropenia of adults. *Ann Hematol* 2000;79:563–570.

93. Rosenthal NS, Farhi DC. Reactive plasmacytosis and lymphocytosis in acute myeloid leukemia. *Hematol Pathol* 1994;8:43–51.

94. Rosenthal NS, Farhi DC. Bone marrow findings in connective tissue disease. *Am J Clin Pathol* 1989;92:650–654.

95. Sara E, Kotsakis A, Souklakos J, et al. Post-chemotherapy lymphopoiesis in patients with solid tumors is characterized by CD4+ cell proliferation. *Anticancer Res* 1999;19:471–476.

96. Upshaw JD Jr, Callihan TR. Spontaneous remission of B-cell chronic lymphocytic leukemia associated with T lymphocytic hyperplasia in bone marrow. *South Med J* 2002;95:647–649.

97. Ben-Ezra J, Hazelgrove K, Ferreira-Gonzalez A, et al. Can polymerase chain reaction help distinguish benign from malignant lymphoid aggregates in bone marrow aspirates? *Arch Pathol Lab Med* 2000;124:511–515.

98. Ben-Ezra JM, King BE, Harris AC, et al. Staining for Bcl-2 protein helps to distinguish benign from malignant lymphoid aggregates in bone marrow biopsies. *Mod Pathol* 1994;7:560–564.

99. Farhi DC. Germinal centers in the bone marrow. *Hematol Pathol* 1989;3:133–136.

100. Kremer M, Cabras AD, Fend F, et al. PCR analysis of IgH-gene rearrangements in small lymphoid infiltrates microdissected from sections of paraffin-embedded bone marrow biopsy specimens. *Hum Pathol* 2000;31:847–853.

101. Krober SM, Horny HP, Greschniok A, et al. Reactive and neoplastic lymphocytes in human bone marrow: morphological, immunohistological, and molecular biological investigations on biopsy specimens. *J Clin Pathol* 1999;52:521–526.

102. Rockman SP. Determination of clonality in patients who present with diagnostic dilemmas: a laboratory experience and review of the literature. *Leukemia* 1997;11:852–862.

103. Salisbury JR, Deverell MH, Cookson MJ. Three-dimensional reconstruction of benign lymphoid aggregates in bone marrow trephines. *J Pathol* 1996;178:447–450.

104. Callea V, Comis M, Iaria G, et al. Clinical significance of HLA-DR+, CD19+, CD10+ immature B-cell phenotype and CD34+ cell detection in bone marrow lymphocytes from children affected with immune thrombocytopenic purpura. *Haematologica* 1997;82:471–473.

105. D'Arena G, Bisceglia M, Ladogana S, et al. Expansion of hematogones in a patient with Gaucher disease. *Med Pediatr Oncol* 2001;36:657–668.

106. Davis RE, Longacre TA, Cornbleet PJ. Hematogones in the bone marrow of adults. *Am J Clin Pathol* 1994;102:202–211.

107. Farhi DC, Luebbers EL, Rosenthal NS. Bone marrow biopsy findings in childhood anemia: prevalence of transient erythroblastopenia of childhood. *Arch Pathol Lab Med* 1998;122:638–641.

108. Fisgin T, Yarali N, Duru F, et al. CMV-induced immune thrombocytopenia and excessive hematogones mimicking an acute B-precursor lymphoblastic leukemia. *Leuk Res* 2003;27:193–196.

109. Foot AB, Potter MN, Ropner JE, et al. Transient erythroblastopenia of childhood with CD10, TdT, and cytoplasmic mu lymphocyte positivity in bone marrow. *J Clin Pathol* 1990;43:857–859.

110. Gerrits GP, van Oostrom CG, de Vaan GA, et al. Transient erythroblastopenia of childhood. A review of 22 cases. *Eur J Pediatr* 1984;142:266–270.

111. Kallakury BV, Hartmann DP, Cossman J, et al. Posttherapy surveillance of B-cell precursor acute lymphoblastic leukemia. Value of polymerase chain reaction and limitations of flow cytometry. *Am J Clin Pathol* 1999;111:759–766.

112. Klupp N, Simonitsch I, Mannhalter C, et al. Emergence of an unusual bone marrow precursor B-cell population in fatal Shwachman-Diamond syndrome. *Arch Pathol Lab Med* 2000;124:1379–1381.

113. Leitenberg D, Rappeport JM, Smith BR. B-cell precursor bone marrow reconstitution after bone marrow transplantation. *Am J Clin Pathol* 1994;102:231–236.

114. Leuschner S, Bodewaldt-Radzun S, Rister M. Increase of CALLA-positive stimulated lymphoid cells in transient erythroblastopenia of childhood. *Eur J Pediatr* 1990;149:551–554.

115. McKenna RW, Washington LT, Aquino DB, et al. Immunophenotypic analysis of hematogones (B-lymphocyte precursors) in 662 consecutive bone marrow specimens by 4-color flow cytometry. *Blood* 2001;98:2498–2507.

116. Melillo LM, Cascavilla N, Musto P, et al. Increased CD10/TdT positive cells in the bone marrow of an infant with immune thrombocytopenia. *Haematologica* 1994;79:177–179.

117. Mizutani K, Azuma E, Komada Y, et al. An infantile case of cytomegalovirus induced idiopathic thrombocytopenic purpura with predominant proliferation of CD10 positive lymphoblast in bone marrow. *Acta Paediatr Jpn* 1995;37:71–74.

118. Richard G, Brody J, Sun T. A case of acute megakaryocytic leukemia with hematogones. *Leukemia* 1993;7:1900–1903.

119. Rimsza LM, Larson RS, Winter SS, et al. Benign hematogone-rich lymphoid proliferations can be distinguished from B-lineage acute lymphoblastic leukemia by integration of morphology, immunophenotype, adhesion molecule expression, and architectural features. *Am J Clin Pathol* 2000;114:66–75.

120. Vargas SO, Hasegawa SL, Dorfman DM. Hematogones as an internal control in flow cytometric analysis of suspected acute lymphoblastic leukemia. *Pediatr Dev Pathol* 1999;2:371–376.

121. Vandersteenhoven AM, Williams JE, Borowitz MJ. Marrow B-cell precursors are increased in lymphomas or systemic diseases associated with B-cell dysfunction. *Am J Clin Pathol* 1993;100:60–66.

122. Douglas VK, Gordon LI, Goolsby CL, et al. Lymphoid aggregates in bone marrow mimic residual lymphoma after rituximab therapy for non-Hodgkin lymphoma. *Am J Clin Pathol* 1999;112:844–853.

123. Kettaneh A, Fain O, Ziol M, et al. Minocycline-induced systemic adverse reaction with liver and bone marrow granulomas and Sezary-like cells. *Am J Med* 2000;108:353–354.

124. Thiele J, Zirbes TK, Kvasnicka HM, et al. Focal lymphoid

aggregates (nodules) in bone marrow biopsies: differentiation between benign hyperplasia and malignant lymphoma—a practical guideline. *J Clin Pathol* 1999;52:294–300.

Reactive Plasmacytosis

1. Arce E, Jackson DG, Gill MA, et al. Increased frequency of pre-germinal center B cells and plasma cell precursors in the blood of children with systemic lupus erythematosus. *J Immunol* 2001;167:2361–2369.
2. Gorden L, Smith C, Graber SE. Marked plasmacytosis and immunoglobulin abnormalities following infusion of streptokinase. *Am J Med Sci* 1991;301:186–189.
3. Shtalrid M, Shvidel L, Vorst E. Polyclonal reactive peripheral blood plasmacytosis mimicking plasma cell leukemia in a patient with staphylococcal sepsis. *Leuk Lymphoma* 2003;44:379–380.
4. Ward PC. The lymphoid leukocytoses. *Postgrad Med* 1980;67:217–223.
5. Agnarsson BA, Loughran TP Jr, Starkebaum G, et al. The pathology of large granular lymphocyte leukemia. *Hum Pathol* 1989;20:643–651.
6. Breier DV, Rendo P, Gonzalez J, et al. Massive plasmocytosis due to methimazole-induced bone marrow toxicity. *Am J Hematol* 2001;67:259–261.
7. Csaki C, Ferencz T, Sipos G, et al. Diffuse plasmacytosis in a child with brainstem glioma following multiagent chemotherapy and intensive growth factor support. *Med Pediatr Oncol* 1996;26:367–371.
8. Hyun BH, Kwa D, Gabaldon H, et al. Reactive plasmacytic lesions of the bone marrow. *Am J Clin Pathol* 1976;65:921–928.
9. Jego G, Avet-Loiseau H, Robillard N, et al. Reactive plasmacytoses in multiple myeloma during hematopoietic recovery with G- or GM-CSF. *Leuk Res* 2000;24:627–630.
10. Jourdan M, Bataille R, Seguin J, et al. Constitutive production of interleukin-6 and immunologic features in cardiac myxomas. *Arthritis Rheum* 1990;33:398–402.
11. Kass L, Votaw ML. Eosinophilia and plasmacytosis of the bone marrow in Hodgkin's disease. *Am J Clin Pathol* 1975;64:248–250.
12. Katsuki K, Shinohara K, Kameda N, et al. Two cases of myelodysplastic syndrome with extramedullary polyclonal plasma cell proliferation and autoantibody production: possible role of soluble Fas antigen for production of excessive self-reactive B cells. *Intern Med* 1998;37:973–977.
13. Kikuchi M, Ohsaka A, Chiba Y, et al. Bone marrow aplasia with prominent atypical plasmacytic proliferation preceding acute lymphoblastic leukemia. *Leuk Lymphoma* 1999;35:213–217.
14. Lim MS, Straus SE, Dale JK, et al. Pathological findings in human autoimmune lymphoproliferative syndrome. *Am J Pathol* 1998;153:1541–1550.
15. Luppi M, Barozzi P, Schulz TF, et al. Bone marrow failure associated with human herpesvirus 8 infection after transplantation. *N Engl J Med* 2000;343:1378–1385.
16. Miguel-Garcia A, Orero T, Matutes E, et al. bcl-2 expression in plasma cells from neoplastic gammopathies and reactive plasmacytosis: a comparative study. *Haematologica* 1998;83:298–304.
17. Molina T, Brouland JP, Bigorgne C, et al. Pseudo-myelomatous plasmacytosis of the bone marrow in a multicentric Castleman's disease. *Ann Pathol* 1996;16:133–136.
18. Nagase H, Agematsu K, Kitano K, et al. Mechanism of hypergammaglobulinemia by HIV infection: circulating memory B-cell reduction with plasmacytosis. *Clin Immunol* 2001;100:250–259.
19. Nishimoto Y, Iwahashi T, Nishihara T, et al. Hepatitis-associated aplastic anemia with systemic plasmacytosis. *Acta Pathol Jpn* 1987;37:155–166.
20. Ocqueteau M, Orfao A, Almeida J, et al. Immunophenotypic characterization of plasma cells from monoclonal gammopathy of undetermined significance patients. Implications for the differential diagnosis between MGUS and multiple myeloma. *Am J Pathol* 1998;152:1655–1665.
21. Papadaki HA, Chatzivassili A, Stefanaki K, et al. Morphologically defined myeloid cell compartments, lymphocyte subpopulations, and histological findings of bone marrow in patients with nonimmune chronic idiopathic neutropenia of adults. *Ann Hematol* 2000;79:563–570.
22. Poje EJ, Soori GS, Weisenburger DD. Systemic polyclonal B-immunoblastic proliferation with marked peripheral blood and bone marrow plasmacytosis. *Am J Clin Pathol* 1992;98:222–226.
23. Sen R, Chaudhary SD, Dixit VB, et al. Bone marrow cytomorphological changes in multibacillary leprosy. *Indian J Lepr* 1990;62:321–327.
24. Strobel ES, Fritschka E, Schmitt-Graff A, et al. An unusual case of systemic lupus erythematosus, lupus nephritis, and transient monoclonal gammopathy. *Rheumatol Int* 2000;19:235–241.
25. Tanvetyanon T, Leighton JC. Severe anemia and marrow plasmacytosis as presentation of Sjogren's syndrome. *Am J Hematol* 2002;69:233.
26. Tatsuno I, Nishikawa T, Sasano H, et al. Interleukin 6-producing gastric carcinoma with fever, hypergammaglobulinemia, and plasmacytosis in bone marrow. *Gastroenterology* 1994;107:543–547.
27. Terruzzi V, Minoli G, Levi C, et al. Medullary plasmocytosis in urologically silent Grawitz' tumor. *Minerva Med* 1978;69:2241–2248.
28. Thiele J, Kvasnicka HM, Muehlhausen K, et al. Polycythemia rubra vera versus secondary polycythemias. A clinicopathological evaluation of distinctive features in 199 patients. *Pathol Res Pract* 2001;197:77–84.
29. Turbat-Herrera EA, Hancock C, Cabello-Inchausti B, et al. Plasma cell hyperplasia and monoclonal paraproteinemia in human immunodeficiency virus-infected patients. *Arch Pathol Lab Med* 1993;117:497–501.
30. Wickramasinghe SN, Looareesuwan S, Nagachinta B, et al. Dyserythropoiesis and ineffective erythropoiesis in *Plasmodium vivax* malaria. *Br J Haematol* 1989;72:91–99.
31. Wulf GG, Jahns-Streubel G, Hemmerlein B, et al. Plasmacytosis in acute myeloid leukemia: two cases of plasmacytosis and increased IL-6 production in the AML blast cells. *Ann Hematol* 1998;76:273–277.
32. Yee TT, Murphy K, Johnson M, et al. Multiple myeloma and human immunodeficiency virus-1 (HIV-1) infection. *Am J Hematol* 2001;66:123–125.
33. Kass L, Kapadia IH. Perivascular plasmacytosis: a light-microscopic and immunohistochemical study of 93 bone marrow biopsies. *Acta Haematol* 2001;105:57–63.
34. Ocqueteau M, Orfao A, Garcia-Sanz R, et al. Expression of the CD117 antigen (c-Kit) on normal and myelomatous plasma cells. *Br J Haematol* 1996;95:489–493.
35. Blom J. The ultrastructural localization of iron in human bone marrow plasma cells. *Acta Pathol Microbiol Immunol Scand [A]* 1985;93:223–228.
36. Cook MK, Madden M. Iron granules in plasma cells. *J Clin Pathol* 1982;35:172–181.
37. D'Angelo G, Cueroni P, Cosini I. Iron granules in plasma cells: a particular morphologic aspect. *Am J Hematol* 1996;52:124–125.

38. Gruszecki AC, Audeh Y, Reddy VV. An unusual finding of plasma cell iron. *Arch Pathol Lab Med* 2002;126:873–874.
39. Karcioglu GL, Hardison JE. Iron-containing plasma cells. *Arch Intern Med* 1978;138:97–100.
40. Mattana RA, Du Plessis L, Stevens K. Iron uptake by plasma cells in haematological disorders. *Acta Haematol* 1994;92:126–129.
41. McCurley TL, Cousar JB, Graber SE, et al. Plasma cell iron—clinical and morphologic features. *Am J Clin Pathol* 1984;81:312–316.
42. Shanmugathasa M, Sobel HJ, Marquet E, et al. Plasma cells with inclusions containing iron. *Arch Pathol Lab Med* 1979;103:577–582.
43. Tsoi WC, Feng CS, Chew EC. Plasma cells with iron inclusions in two non-alcoholic Chinese women. *Pathology* 1996;28:125–127.
44. Wulfhekel U, Dullmann J. Storage of iron in bone marrow plasma cells. Ultrastructural characterization, mobilization, and diagnostic significance. *Acta Haematol* 1999;101:7–15.

STROMAL TISSUE AND EXTRACELLULAR SPACE

The stromal tissue of the bone marrow consists of adipose tissue, fibrous tissue, trabecular bone, and blood vessels. In addition, a potential space is present among the hematopoietic and connective tissue elements, known as the extracellular space. This space becomes apparent in some important conditions of the bone marrow.

ADIPOSE TISSUE

Fat Necrosis

Fat necrosis of the bone marrow is a sign of pancreatic disease or, less commonly, antiphospholipid antibody syndrome (1–3). In fat necrosis caused by pancreatitis, alcoholism is the most common underlying disorder. Histologic sections of the bone marrow show liquefactive necrosis of fat cells.

Lipomembranous Polycystic Osteodysplasia

Lipomembranous polycystic osteodysplasia (Nasu-Hakola disease) is an autosomal recessive disorder caused by mutations in genes encoding membrane receptor proteins of myeloid cells and natural killer cells (4–7). Pathologic findings are most prominent in the central nervous system and skeleton. The bone marrow shows a peculiar change of the adipose tissue, which is transformed into lipid-filled cystic spaces surrounded by a convoluted hyaline membrane. Bone cysts may be complicated by fractures.

Serous Fat Atrophy

Serous fat atrophy refers to the shrinkage of fat cells seen in gelatinous transformation of the marrow (see Extracellular Space section). In practice, these two terms are used interchangeably.

FIBROUS TISSUE

Fibrosis

Bone marrow fibrosis (myelofibrosis) is a relatively common phenomenon, produced by a wide variety of underlying conditions (Table 13-1) (Figs. 13-1 through 13-3). These include autoimmune disorders, drug therapy, graft versus host disease, hypertrophic osteoarthropathy, renal osteodystrophy, vitamin D–deficient rickets, systemic leishmaniasis, radiotoxicity, organic solvent toxicity, gray platelet syndrome, myeloproliferative disorders, myelodysplastic syndromes, acute leukemia, malignant lymphoma (especially Hodgkin lymphoma), multiple myeloma, and metastatic malignancy (1–18). Fibrosis is stimulated by increased production of cytokines in the marrow and appears to preceded by increased production of hyaluronan by marrow cells (19).

The peripheral blood smear may show leukoerythroblastosis in moderate to severe marrow fibrosis (20). Bone marrow aspirate smears may be hypocellular (dry tap) (21). Histologic sections show a patchy to diffuse increase in reticulin fibers, which may be thickened and/or elongated (22). The presence of increased reticulin may be suspected in hematoxylin and eosin–stained sections by a linear arrangement, or single filing, of hematopoietic cells. Close examination reveals the presence of delicate, eosinophilic strands between the aligned cells. A silver stain for reticulin is helpful and is often necessary to demonstrate increased reticulin in mild

TABLE 13-1. CONDITIONS ASSOCIATED WITH FIBROSIS OF THE BONE MARROW

Nonneoplastic conditions
  Autoimmune disorders
  Drug therapy
  Graft versus host disease
  Gray platelet syndrome
  Hypertrophic osteoarthropathy
  Leishmaniasis
  Organic solvent toxicity
  Radiotoxicity
  Renal osteodystrophy
  Vitamin D–deficient rickets

Neoplastic conditions
  Myeloproliferative disorders
  Myelodysplastic syndromes
  Acute leukemia
  Malignant lymphoma
  Multiple myeloma
  Metastatic malignancy

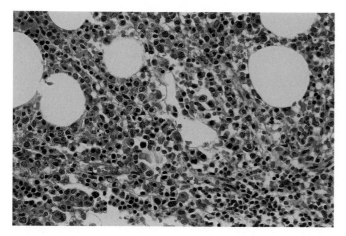

FIGURE 13-1. Bone marrow biopsy specimen, reticulin fibrosis. Delicate reticulin fibers constrain the hematopoietic cells into a single-file pattern in this specimen from a patient with myelodysplastic syndrome.

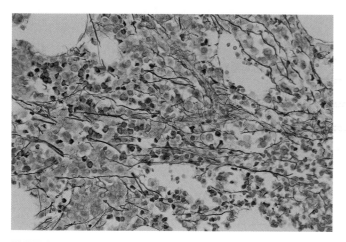

FIGURE 13-2. Bone marrow biopsy specimen, reticulin fibrosis (reticulin stain). The reticulin fibers are seen as fine black linear structures lying between hematopoietic cells in this specimen from a patient with myelodysplastic syndrome.

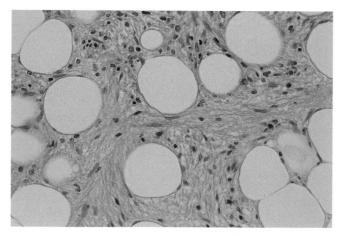

FIGURE 13-3. Bone marrow biopsy specimen, dense fibrosis. Large areas of hematopoietic tissue are replaced by dense fibrous tissue in this specimen from a patient with acute lymphoblastic leukemia.

fibrosis. Advanced fibrosis may be accompanied by collagen deposition, vascular proliferation, and osteosclerosis (23,24). Fibrosis and osteosclerosis may be so extensive as to nearly obliterate the marrow cavity. In such cases, a careful search for underlying malignancy should be made.

The differential diagnosis includes reparative changes caused by a previous biopsy in the same site (25).

Fibrous Tumors

Reactive bone marrow fibrosis may be difficult to distinguish from dysplastic and neoplastic fibrous tumors involving the bone marrow (26–29).

BLOOD VESSELS

Reactive Vascular Lesions

Bone marrow vessels, predominantly sinusoids, may show dilation and ectasia when the hematopoietic tissue has been depleted (Figs. 13-4 through 13-6). Thrombosis of small vessels may be seen in systemic disorders such as thrombotic thrombocytopenic purpura. Vasculitis has occasionally been reported in the small vessels of the bone marrow, in biopsy specimens from patients with giant cell arteritis, Churg-Strauss (allergic) angiitis, eosinophilia-myalgia syndrome, and Sjögren syndrome (1–5). Other reactive vascular lesions rarely reported in the bone marrow include peliosis, bacillary angiomatosis, and the destructive angiomatous proliferation associated with Gorham disease (6–8).

Vascular Tumors

Hemangiomas and lymphangiomas may be confined to the marrow space or involve the marrow together with adjacent tissues (9–14). These lesions usually affect the axial skeleton.

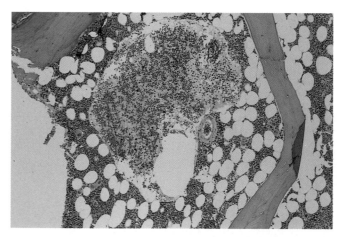

FIGURE 13-4. Bone marrow biopsy specimen, sinusoidal dilation. A sinusoid is dilated almost beyond recognition in this specimen from a patient with treated acute myeloid leukemia.

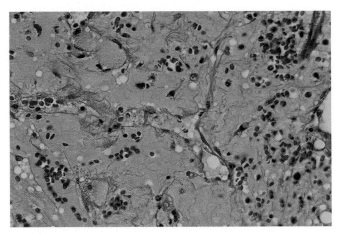

FIGURE 13-5. Bone marrow biopsy specimen, vascular proliferation and ectasia. Numerous thin-walled and ectatic vascular structures are seen in this specimen from a patient recovering from chemotherapy.

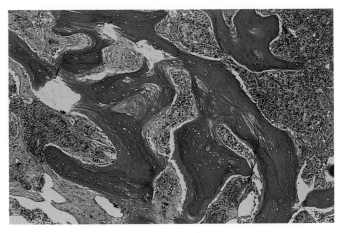

FIGURE 13-7. Bone marrow biopsy specimen, osteoblastosis. Trabecular bone is thickened and irregular in this specimen from a patient with metastatic adenocarcinoma of the prostate.

Rarely, the bone marrow is involved as part of systemic hemangiomatosis (15–17). Kaposi sarcoma has been reported in the bone marrow (18,19).

TRABECULAR BONE

Osteoblastosis

Osteoblastosis is the formation of new bone caused by an increase in osteoblasts, a phenomenon frequently seen in bone marrow involvement by clonal plasma cell disease and metastatic carcinoma (1) (Figs. 13-7 and 13-8). Bone marrow aspirate smears show the presence of osteoblasts, an abnormal finding in specimens from adults. Histologic sections of the bone marrow show plump osteoblasts lining the trabecular bone.

Osteolysis

Osteolysis is the destruction of trabecular bone, a common feature in metastatic carcinoma (2–4). Osteolysis is also a hallmark of Gorham disease, a constitutional disorder characterized by expansile, lytic bone lesions.

Bone marrow aspirate smears show the presence of osteoclasts, an abnormal finding in specimens from adults. Histologic sections of the bone marrow show increased osteoclasts on the surface of trabecular bone, overlying excavated and tunneled areas of bone resorption (Howship lacunae) (Fig. 13-9).

Osteomalacia and Renal Osteodystrophy

Osteomalacia is the defective mineralization of bone matrix or osteoid (Figs. 13-10 through 13-13). It occurs as the result

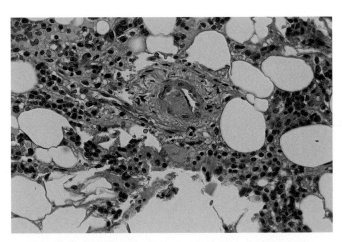

FIGURE 13-6. Bone marrow biopsy specimen, small vessel thrombosis. A small arteriole contains a partially endothelialized thrombus in this specimen from a patient with acute myeloid leukemia recovering from chemotherapy.

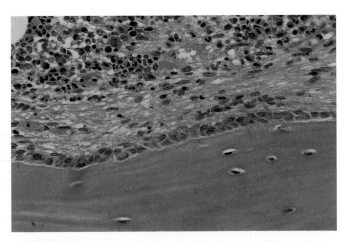

FIGURE 13-8. Bone marrow biopsy specimen, osteoblastosis. Trabecular bone is lined by a uniform row of plump osteoblasts in this specimen from a patient with metastatic adenocarcinoma of the prostate.

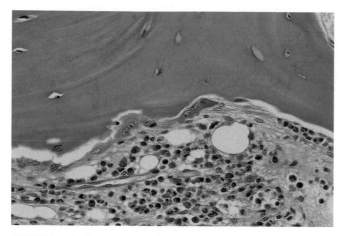

FIGURE 13-9. Bone marrow biopsy specimen, osteolysis. Trabecular bone shows focal excavation by osteoclasts in this specimen from a patient with renal osteodystrophy.

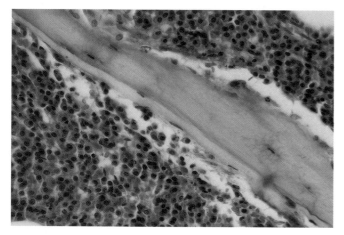

FIGURE 13-10. Bone marrow biopsy specimen, osteomalacia. The widened, uncalcified osteoid seam appears as a pink ribbon on the surface of trabecular bone in this specimen from a patient with multiple myeloma.

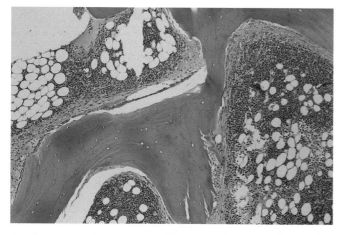

FIGURE 13-11. Bone marrow biopsy specimen, renal osteodystrophy. Trabecular bone is widened and irregular and surrounded by fibrous tissue in this specimen from a patient with uncontrolled chronic renal failure.

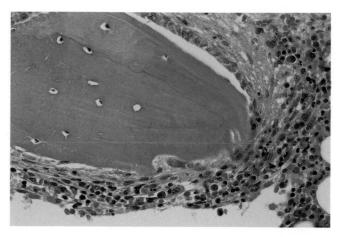

FIGURE 13-12. Bone marrow biopsy specimen, renal osteodystrophy. Trabecular bone shows the typical arrangement of osteoblasts on one surface and osteoclasts on the opposite surface in this specimen from a patient with uncontrolled chronic renal failure.

of disordered calcium and phosphate metabolism caused by renal phosphate wasting, high serum parathormone levels, or tumor production of parathormone-like protein. The most common underlying disorder is uncontrolled chronic renal failure (renal osteodystrophy), but osteomalacia is also seen as a complication of constitutional and vitamin D–dependent rickets, primary hyperparathyroidism, and primary and metastatic malignancies of the bone marrow (5–13).

Bone marrow aspirate smears often show osteoblasts. Histologic sections of the bone marrow show thickened trabeculae, with widened osteoid seams overlaid by plump osteoblasts. On the trabecular surface opposite the osteoid seam, osteoclasts may be found, creating superficial excavations (Howship lacunae) and penetrating tunnels in trabecular bone. Peritrabecular fibrosis may be present. In severe hyperparathyroidism, rapidly expanding osteolytic lesions

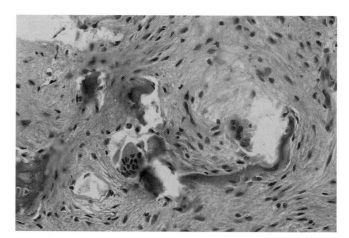

FIGURE 13-13. Bone marrow biopsy specimen, brown tumor. Trabecular bone has been nearly consumed by osteoclasts and replaced by fibrous tissue in this specimen from a patient with primary hyperparathyroidism.

(brown tumors) may be found, which may clinically mimic metastatic carcinoma. Specimens from adult patients without renal failure should be carefully examined for evidence of malignancy.

Osteoporosis

Osteoporosis is the loss of preexisting trabecular bone. Underlying conditions include aging, alcoholism, corticosteroid therapy, hypogonadism, hyperthyroidism, anticonvulsant therapy, Gaucher disease, myeloproliferative disorders, acute leukemia, and clonal B-cell and plasma cell disorders (14–20).

A bone marrow biopsy specimen may be difficult to obtain because of the loss of trabecular bone, rendering the marrow soft and collapsible. Histologic sections of the bone marrow show uniformly slender, widely spaced trabeculae. Excessive thinning of the trabeculae results in the presence of round to ovoid cross-sections of trabeculae appearing to "float" in the intertrabecular space (Fig. 13-14). Osteoblasts and osteoclasts are rare to absent. Other findings include hematopoietic hyperplasia or hypoplasia, increased adipose tissue, and benign lymphoid aggregates.

Osteosclerosis

Osteosclerosis is the presence of excessive trabecular bone. Osteosclerosis has been reported in SAPHO (synovitis, acne, pustulosis, hyperostosis, and osteitis) and other constitutional syndromes, primary hyperparathyroidism, chronic renal failure, fluoridosis and fluoride-treated osteoporosis, Paget disease of bone, hepatitis C infection, leishmaniasis, leprosy, Gaucher disease, oxalosis, sarcoidosis, Erdheim-Chester disease, myeloproliferative disorders, acute leukemia, hairy cell leukemia, clonal plasma cell disorders, and metastatic carcinoma (21–44).

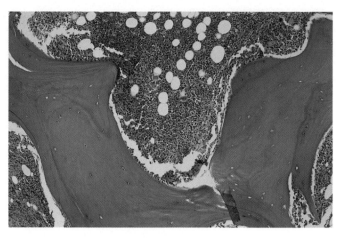

FIGURE 13-15. Bone marrow biopsy specimen, osteosclerosis. Trabecular bone is diffusely thickened in this specimen from a patient with chronic myeloid leukemia.

Histologic sections of the bone marrow show diffusely thickened trabeculae, sometimes with an increase in osteoid and flattened osteoblasts (Fig. 13-15). A careful search for an underlying malignancy should be made when osteosclerosis is noted. It is sometimes difficult to appreciate the presence of hematopoietic disease or carcinoma because of the compromise of the medullary space by bone and associated fibrosis.

Osteonecrosis

Osteonecrosis clinically and radiographically resembles bone marrow edema (see below), but trabecular bone appears nonviable (Fig. 13-16). Associated conditions include osteoarthritis, Gaucher disease, corticosteroid therapy, and radiotherapy (45–47).

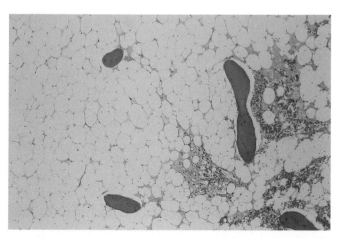

FIGURE 13-14. Bone marrow biopsy specimen, osteoporosis. Trabeculae are thinned and widely spaced in this specimen from a patient treated for malignant lymphoma.

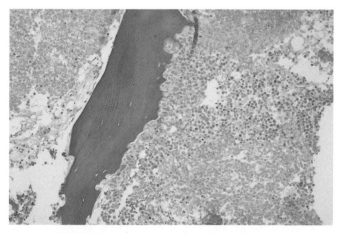

FIGURE 13-16. Bone marrow biopsy specimen, osteonecrosis. Trabecular bone shows focal disintegration and the spaces previously occupied by osteocytes are empty in this specimen from a patient with malignant lymphoma and bone marrow necrosis.

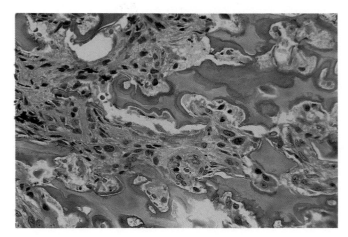

FIGURE 13-17. Bone marrow biopsy specimen, osteopetrosis. Trabecular bone is increased and irregular and hematopoietic tissue is absent in this specimen from a child with severe infantile osteopetrosis.

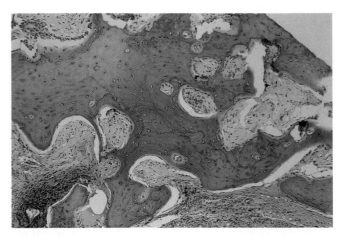

FIGURE 13-18. Bone marrow biopsy specimen, Paget disease of bone. Trabecular bone is irregular, thickened, and marked by prominent osteoid seams. The bone is surrounded by abundant fibrous tissue.

Osteopetrosis

Osteopetrosis occurs as a constitutional disorder of hematopoietic stem cells, in which normal bone growth and remodeling are impaired (48,49). It also occurs as a complication of carbonic anhydrase II deficiency. The correct diagnosis is usually known before the marrow specimen is obtained. Bone marrow aspirate smears may be hypocellular owing to reduced hematopoietic tissue. Histologic sections of the bone marrow show abnormally thickened trabeculae, with narrowing of the intertrabecular area and obliteration of hematopoietic tissue caused by encroaching bone (Fig. 13-17).

Paget Disease of Bone

Paget disease of bone is uncommonly found in bone marrow biopsy specimens (50–55). The diagnosis is usually known before bone marrow biopsy. This disease appears to arise from a combination of genetic factors and paramyxovirus infection of osteoclasts. The disorder begins as increased osteoclastic activity with osteolysis, progressing eventually to osteoblastosis and osteosclerosis.

Histologic sections of the bone marrow often show a mixed picture of osteoblastosis and osteolysis (Figs. 13-10 and 13-18). Trabecular bone exhibits prominent osteoid seams, increased and hypernucleated osteoclasts, abnormal new bone formation, and peritrabecular fibrosis. Complications of the disease include fracture and osteosarcoma.

Abnormal Bony Remodeling

Abnormal bony remodeling is an imprecise but useful term for mixed findings of osteoblastosis, osteolysis, osteomalacia, osteoporosis, and osteosclerosis. These findings are often seen after radiotherapy, in metabolic bone disease, and accompanying bone marrow involvement by hematolymphoid disorders and metastatic carcinoma (56–62). Bone marrow aspirate smears may show clusters of osteoblasts or an occasional osteoclast. Histologic sections of the bone marrow show trabeculae with irregular areas of thickening and thinning (Fig. 13-19). Osteoblasts and osteoclasts may be focally increased.

Healing Previous Biopsy Site

The bone marrow undergoes a reparative process after biopsy characterized by new bone formation and fibrosis, essentially resembling callus formation (25) (Fig. 13-20). These changes are likely to be seen in specimens from patients who have undergone multiple biopsies at the same site.

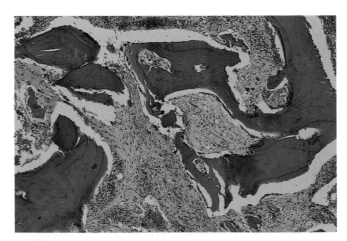

FIGURE 13-19. Bone marrow biopsy specimen, abnormal bony remodeling. Trabecular bone is markedly irregular and is surrounded by fibrous tissue in this specimen from a patient with treated acute myeloid leukemia.

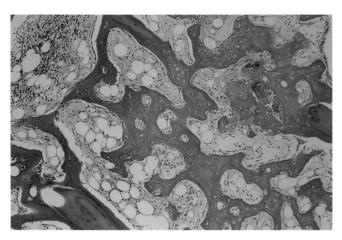

FIGURE 13-20. Bone marrow biopsy specimen, healing biopsy site. New bone formation and fibrosis are seen in this specimen from a patient with several previous bone marrow biopsies from the posterior iliac crest.

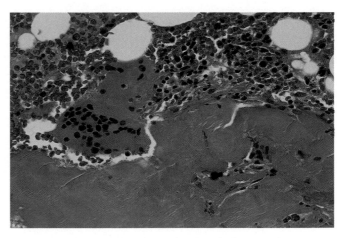

FIGURE 13-21. Bone marrow clot, amyloidosis. A large mass of amyloid is seen, with an accompanying foreign body giant cell reaction in this specimen from a patient with a plasma cell neoplasm.

EXTRACELLULAR SPACE

Amyloidosis

Amyloidosis is the deposition of a single type of protein, arranged in the form of a β-pleated sheet. The protein may be deposited because of a hereditary disorder, often traceable to a specific genetic mutation (1–5). Alternatively, the protein may be deposited because of an acquired disorder. In this category are amyloidosis owing to deposition of β_2-microglobulin in patients on renal dialysis (6), amyloidosis owing to deposition of serum amyloid A protein in patients with chronic inflammatory conditions (AA amyloidosis) (7–29), and amyloidosis owing to deposition of clonal immunoglobulin light chain or heavy chain (AL and AH amyloidosis) (see Chapter 26). Any of these may be found in the bone marrow.

The peripheral blood smear shows no findings specifically referable to amyloidosis. Bone marrow aspirate smears may show an amphophilic, acellular substance. Histologic sections of the bone marrow show perivascular and/or interstitial accumulation of amyloid (Fig. 13-21).

The differential diagnosis includes fibrin-platelet clots of intraoperative origin and immunoglobulin deposition disease.

Calcific Myelitis

Calcific myelitis, or calcification of the marrow space, occurs in constitutional tumoral calcinosis and in uremia (30–32). Focal dystrophic calcification also occurs in a setting of bone marrow repair. In tumoral calcinosis, laboratory studies reveal normocalcemia and hyperphosphatemia. Histologic sections of the bone marrow show patchy to diffuse calcium deposits (Figs. 13-21 through 13-23).

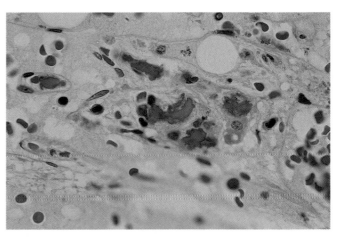

FIGURE 13-22. Bone marrow biopsy specimen, dystrophic calcification. Isolated foci of calcium deposition are seen in this specimen from a patient with treated acute myeloid leukemia.

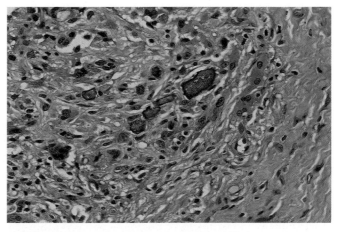

FIGURE 13-23. Bone marrow biopsy specimen, tumoral calcinosis. Focal calcification is seen in the fibrous wall of a tumoral calcinosis lesion.

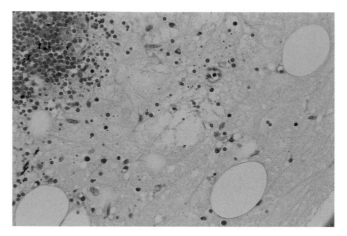

FIGURE 13-24. Bone marrow biopsy specimen, edema. Eosinophilic extracellular material replaces hematopoietic tissue in this specimen from a patient undergoing recent radiotherapy.

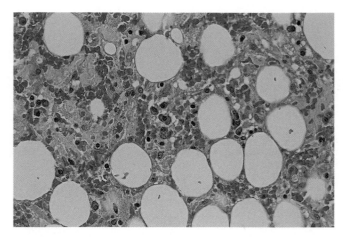

FIGURE 13-25. Bone marrow biopsy specimen, fibrinous myelitis. Granular extracellular material fills the spaces between remaining stromal cells and plasma cells in this specimen from a patient with recently treated acute myeloid leukemia.

Edema

Edema of the bone marrow is associated with osteoarthritis, osteomyelitis, corticosteroid therapy, gout, and acute and chronic bone injury (33–39). The main clinical findings are pain and an increased serum alkaline phosphatase level. The imaging findings in some cases may suggest a diagnosis of infiltrative malignancy of the bone marrow.

Histologic sections of the bone marrow show interstitial and intrasinusoidal fluid accumulation, sometimes accompanied by hemorrhage, focal marrow fibrosis, and loss of fat cells (Fig. 13-24). The trabecular bone is viable and often shows evidence of increased remodeling, including increased osteoid, decreased mineralization, and increased osteoblastic and osteoclastic activity. Bone marrow edema may resolve with rest and reduction of corticosteroid therapy, persist, or progress to osteonecrosis.

Fibrinous Myelitis

Fibrinous myelitis is an imprecise term applied to the marrow changes after cytotoxic chemotherapy or other acute stromal injury. Marrow aspirate smears show foamy histiocytes and relatively few hematopoietic cells. Histologic sections show loss of cellular architecture, sinusoidal dilation, and interstitial deposition of hyaluronidase-sensitive material (40) (Fig. 13-25).

Gelatinous Transformation

Gelatinous transformation is the accumulation of hyaluronic acid–rich mucopolysaccharides within the marrow. Gelatinous transformation is an uncommon finding of unknown pathogenesis, seen more often in specimens from men than women, and seems to be a complication of abnormal metabolism. Underlying conditions include alcoholism, anorexia nervosa and other forms of starvation, autoimmune disorders, chronic heart failure, malabsorption, acquired

TABLE 13-2. CONDITIONS ASSOCIATED WITH GELATINOUS TRANSFORMATION OF THE BONE MARROW

Nonneoplastic conditions
    Acquired immunodeficiency syndrome
    Alcoholism
    Anorexia nervosa and other forms of starvation
    Autoimmune disorders
    Chronic heart failure
    Malabsorption
    Systemic leishmaniasis
    Systemic lupus erythematosus
    Tuberculosis

Neoplastic conditions
    Myeloproliferative disorders
    Acute leukemia
    Malignant lymphoma
    Metastatic carcinoma

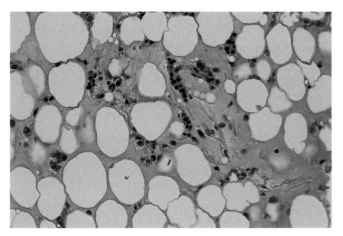

FIGURE 13-26. Bone marrow biopsy specimen, gelatinous transformation. Fat cells are separated by homogeneous, eosinophilic material in which residual hematopoietic cells appear to float in this specimen from a patient with profound cachexia.

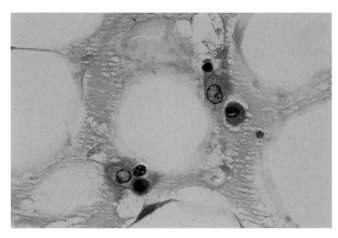

FIGURE 13-27. Bone marrow biopsy specimen, gelatinous transformation. The eosinophilic material has a smooth, solid appearance and characteristic chatter marks that create a likeness to gelatin in this specimen from a patient with profound cachexia.

immunodeficiency syndrome, systemic lupus erythematosus, tuberculosis, systemic leishmaniasis, myeloproliferative disorders, acute leukemia, malignant lymphoma, and metastatic carcinoma (41–50) (Table 13-2).

The peripheral blood may show anemia and acanthocytosis. Bone marrow smears show the presence of an indistinct, acellular amphophilic substance. Histologic sections show decreased fat cell number and volume (serous fat atrophy) and decreased hematopoiesis. The marrow space is replaced with a smooth, faintly granular to glassy, pale amphophilic acid mucopolysaccharide, in which the remaining hematopoietic cells appear to float (Figs. 13-26 and 13-27). This material is Alcian blue positive at pH 2.5 and is hyaluronidase sensitive.

Care should be taken not to overlook evidence of malignancy in the bone marrow when gelatinous transformation is found.

Scleromyxedema

Scleromyxedema is an uncommon complication of multiple myeloma, rarely involving the bone marrow (51). Histologic sections show accumulation of mucopolysaccharides in the bone marrow as well as evidence of the underlying clonal plasma cell disorder.

REFERENCES

Adipose Tissue

1. Ahn BC, Lee J, Suh KJ, et al. Intramedullary fat necrosis of multiple bones associated with pancreatitis. *J Nucl Med* 1998;39: 1401–1404.
2. Paycha F, Russ G, Bellivet C, et al. Solitary increased tibial uptake of 99mTc-diphosphonate unmasking pancreatic tumor-related medullary fat necrosis. *Eur J Nucl Med* 1989;15:678–679.
3. Dubost JJ, Kemeny JL, Soubrier M, et al. Primary antiphospholipid syndrome of fatal course and osteoarticular cytosteatonecrosis. *Rev Med Interne* 1994;15:535–540.
4. Kondo T, Takahashi K, Kohara N, et al. Heterogeneity of presenile dementia with bone cysts (Nasu-Hakola disease): three genetic forms. *Neurology* 2002;59:1105–1107.
5. Paloneva J, Manninen T, Christman G, et al. Mutations in two genes encoding different subunits of a receptor signaling complex result in an identical disease phenotype. *Am J Hum Genet* 2002; 71:656–662.
6. Sageshima M, Masuda H, Kawamura K, et al. Membranous lipodystrophy. Light and electron microscopic study of a biopsy case. *Acta Pathol Jpn* 1987;37:281–290.
7. Wood C. Membranous lipodystrophy of bone. *Arch Pathol Lab Med* 1978;102:22–27.

Fibrous Tissue

1. Bass RD, Pullarkat V, Feinstein DI, et al. Pathology of autoimmune myelofibrosis. A report of three cases and a review of the literature. *Am J Clin Pathol* 2001;116:211–216.
2. Kiss E, Gal I, Simkovics E, et al. Myelofibrosis in systemic lupus erythematosus. *Leuk Lymphoma* 2000;39:661–665.
3. Pullarkat V, Bass RD, Gong JZ, et al. Primary autoimmune myelofibrosis: definition of a distinct clinicopathologic syndrome. *Am J Hematol* 2003;72:8–12.
4. Douglas VK, Tallman MS, Cripe LD, et al. Thrombopoietin administered during induction chemotherapy to patients with acute myeloid leukemia induces transient morphologic changes that may resemble chronic myeloproliferative disorders. *Am J Clin Pathol* 2002;117:844–850.
5. Falk S, Seipelt G, Ganser A, et al. Bone marrow findings after treatment with recombinant human interleukin-3. *Am J Clin Pathol* 1991;95:355–362.
6. Hoffmann A, Kirn E, Krueger GR, et al. Bone marrow hypoplasia and fibrosis following interferon treatment. *In Vivo* 1994;8: 605–612.
7. Atkinson K, Dodds A, Concannon A, et al. Late onset transfusion-dependent anaemia with thrombocytopenia secondary to marrow fibrosis and hypoplasia associated with chronic graft-versus-host disease. *Bone Marrow Transplant* 1987;2:445–449.
8. Fontenay-Roupie M, Dupuy E, Berrou E, et al. Increased proliferation of bone marrow-derived fibroblasts in primitive hypertrophic osteoarthropathy with severe myelofibrosis. *Blood* 1995;85:3229–3238.
9. Nomura S, Ogawa Y, Osawa G, et al. Myelofibrosis secondary to renal osteodystrophy. *Nephron* 1996;72:683–687.
10. Stephan JL, Galambrun C, Dutour A, et al. Myelofibrosis: an unusual presentation of vitamin D-deficient rickets. *Eur J Pediatr* 1999;158:828–829.
11. Rocha Filho FD, Ferreira FV, Mendes F de O, et al. Bone marrow fibrosis (pseudo-myelofibrosis) in human kala-azar. *Rev Soc Bras Med Trop* 2000;33:363–366.
12. Kanberoglu K, Mihmanli I, Kurugoglu S, et al. Bone marrow changes adjacent to the sacroiliac joints after pelvic radiotherapy mimicking metastases on MRI. *Eur Radiol* 2001;11:1748–1752.
13. Bosch X, Campistol JM, Montoliu J, et al. Myelofibrosis and focal segmental glomerulosclerosis associated with toluene poisoning. *Hum Toxicol* 1988;7:357–361.
14. Tondel M, Persson B, Carstensen J. Myelofibrosis and benzene exposure. *Occup Med (Lond)* 1995;45:51–52.
15. Falik-Zaccai TC, Anikster Y, Rivera CE, et al. A new genetic isolate of gray platelet syndrome (GPS): clinical, cellular, and hematologic characteristics. *Mol Genet Metab* 2001;74:303–313.

16. Meadows LM, Rosse WR, Moore JO, et al. Hodgkin's disease presenting as myelofibrosis. *Cancer* 1989;64:1720–1726.
17. Ponzoni M, Fumagalli L, Rossi G, et al. Isolated bone marrow manifestation of HIV-associated Hodgkin lymphoma. *Mod Pathol* 2002;15:1273–1278.
18. Nowell PC, Kant JA, Finan JB, et al. Marrow fibrosis associated with a Philadelphia chromosome. *Cancer Genet Cytogenet* 1992;59:89–92.
19. Sundstrom G, Lofvenberg E, Hassan I, et al. Localisation and distribution of hyaluronan in normal bone marrow matrix: a novel method to evaluate impending fibrosis? *Eur J Haematol* 2002;68:194–202.
20. Rubins JM. The role of myelofibrosis in malignant leukoerythroblastosis. *Cancer* 1983;51:308–311.
21. Humphries JE. Dry tap bone marrow aspiration: clinical significance. *Am J Hematol* 1990;35:247–250.
22. Hernandez-Garcia MT, Hernandez-Nieto L, Brito-Barroso ML, et al. Bone marrow fibrosis: histomorphometric analysis and interobserver reproducibility of a simple optical method of assessing its intensity. *Clin Lab Haematol* 1993;15:129–135.
23. McGlave PB, Brunning RD, Hurd DD, et al. Reversal of severe bone marrow fibrosis and osteosclerosis following allogeneic bone marrow transplantation for chronic granulocytic leukaemia. *Br J Haematol* 1982;52:189–194.
24. Honma K, Nemoto K, Ohnishi Y. Chronic myelocytic leukemia with marked myelofibrosis and osteosclerosis. *Acta Pathol Jpn* 1983;33:599–607.
25. Salgado C, Feliu E, Blade J, et al. A second bone marrow biopsy as a cause of a false diagnosis of myelofibrosis. *Br J Haematol* 1992;80:407–409.
26. Craver RD, Heinrich S. Bone invasion by a recurrent digital fibroma of infancy in a child with Beckwith-Wiedemann syndrome. *Pediatr Pathol Lab Med* 1995;15:147–151.
27. Ippolito E, Corsi A, Grill F, et al. Pathology of bone lesions associated with congenital pseudarthrosis of the leg. *J Pediatr Orthop B* 2000;9:3–10.
28. Ninomiya H, Hato T, Yamada T, et al. Multiple diffuse fibrosarcoma of bone associated with extramedullary hematopoiesis. *Intern Med* 1998;37:480–483.
29. Williams W, Craver RD, Correa H, et al. Use of 2-chlorodeoxyadenosine to treat infantile myofibromatosis. *J Pediatr Hematol Oncol* 2002;24:59–63.

Blood Vessels

1. Cahalin PA, Pawade J. Giant cell arteritis detected by bone marrow trephine. *Br J Haematol* 2002;118:687.
2. Enos WF, Pierre RV, Rosenblatt JE. Giant cell arteritis detected by bone marrow biopsy. *Mayo Clin Proc* 1981;56:381–383.
3. Caluser I, Boieriu I, Olteanu L. A peculiar case of allergic angiitis. *Morphol Embryol (Bucur)* 1984;30:39–40.
4. de Oliveira JS, Auerbach SB, Sullivan KM, et al. Fatal eosinophilia myalgia syndrome in a marrow transplant patient attributed to total parenteral nutrition with a solution containing tryptophan. *Bone Marrow Transplant* 1993;11:163–167.
5. Poralla T, Trautmann F, Rumpelt HJ, et al. A case of Sjogren's syndrome with severe anemia due to myelitis. *Klin Wochenschr* 1986;64:92–95.
6. Asano S, Wakasa H, Kaise S, et al. Peliosis hepatis. Report of two autopsy cases with a review of literature. *Acta Pathol Jpn* 1982;32:861–877.
7. Fagan WA, Skinner SM, Ondo A, et al. Bacillary angiomatosis of the skin and bone marrow in a patient with HIV infection. *J Am Acad Dermatol* 1995;32:510–512.
8. Manisali M, Ozaksoy D. Gorham disease: correlation of MR

findings with histopathologic changes. *Eur Radiol* 1998;8:1647–1650.
9. Baudrez V, Galant C, Vande Berg BC. Benign vertebral hemangioma: MR-histological correlation. *Skeletal Radiol* 2001;30:442–446.
10. Ishida T, Dorfman HD, Steiner GC, et al. Cystic angiomatosis of bone with sclerotic changes mimicking osteoblastic metastases. *Skeletal Radiol* 1994;23:247–252.
11. Ling S, Rafii M, Klein M. Epithelioid hemangioma of bone. *Skeletal Radiol* 2001;30:226–229.
12. Park YW, Kim SM, Min BG, et al. Lymphangioma involving the mandible: immunohistochemical expressions for the lymphatic proliferation. *J Oral Pathol Med* 2002;31:280–283.
13. Baker LL, Dillon WP, Hieshima GB, et al. Hemangiomas and vascular malformations of the head and neck: MR characterization. *AJNR Am J Neuroradiol* 1993;14:307–314.
14. Niedt GW, Greco MA, Wieczorek R, et al. Hemangioma with Kaposi's sarcoma-like features: report of two cases. *Pediatr Pathol* 1989;9:567–575.
15. Maeda H, Matsuo T, Nagaishi T, et al. Diffuse hemangiomatosis, coagulopathy and microangiopathic hemolytic anemia. *Acta Pathol Jpn* 1981;31:135–142.
16. Sugimura H, Tange T, Yamaguchi K, et al. Systemic hemangiomatosis. *Acta Pathol Jpn* 1986;36:1089–1098.
17. Tsukagoshi H, Iwasaki Y, Toyoda M, et al. An autopsy case of systemic hemangiomatosis with honeycomb-like liver and focal splenic sarcomatoid changes. *Intern Med* 1998;37:847–852.
18. Isenbarger DW, Aronson NE. Lytic vertebral lesions: an unusual manifestation of AIDS-associated Kaposi's sarcoma. *Clin Infect Dis* 1994;19:751–755.
19. Teh BS, Lu HH, Lynch GR, et al. AIDS-related Kaposi's sarcoma involving bone and bone marrow. *South Med J* 1999;92:61–64.

Trabecular Bone

1. Cheville JC, Tindall D, Boelter C, et al. Metastatic prostate carcinoma to bone: clinical and pathologic features associated with cancer-specific survival. *Cancer* 2002;95:1028–1036.
2. Taube T, Elomaa I, Blomqvist C, et al. Histomorphometric evidence for osteoclast-mediated bone resorption in metastatic breast cancer. *Bone* 1994;15:161–166.
3. Yang TT, Sabokbar A, Gibbons CL, et al. Human mesenchymal tumour-associated macrophages differentiate into osteoclastic bone-resorbing cells. *J Bone Joint Surg Br* 2002;84:452–456.
4. Fujiu K, Kanno R, Suzuki H, et al. Chylothorax associated with massive osteolysis (Gorham's syndrome). *Ann Thorac Surg* 2002;73:1956–1957.
5. Gal-Moscovici A, Popovtzer MM. Parathyroid hormone-independent osteoclastic resorptive bone disease: a new variant of adynamic bone disease in haemodialysis patients. *Nephrol Dial Transplant* 2002;17:620–624.
6. Hruska KA, Teitelbaum SL. Renal osteodystrophy. *N Engl J Med* 1995;333:166–174.
7. Kato S, Yoshizawawa T, Kitanaka S, et al. Molecular genetics of vitamin D-dependent hereditary rickets. *Horm Res* 2002;57:73–78.
8. Abdullah MA, Salhi HS, Bakry LA, et al. Adolescent rickets in Saudi Arabia: a rich and sunny country. *J Pediatr Endocrinol Metab* 2002;15:1017–1025.
9. Kreiter SR, Schwartz RP, Kirkman HN Jr, et al. Nutritional rickets in African American breast-fed infants. *J Pediatr* 2000;137:153–157.
10. Gupta A, Horattas MC, Moattari AR, et al. Disseminated brown tumors from hyperparathyroidism masquerading as metastatic

cancer: a complication of parathyroid carcinoma. *Am Surg* 2001; 67:951–955.

11. Kao CL, Chang JP, Lin JW, et al. Brown tumor of the sternum. *Ann Thorac Surg* 2002;73:1651–1653.

12. Rowe PS, de Zoysa PA, Dong R, et al. MEPE, a new gene expressed in bone marrow and tumors causing osteomalacia. *Genomics* 2000;67:54–68.

13. Yamaguchi T, Hirano T, Kumagai K, et al. Osteitis fibrosa cystica generalizata with adult T-cell leukaemia: a case report. *Br J Haematol* 1999;107:892–894.

14. Chan GK, Duque G. Age-related bone loss: old bone, new facts. *Gerontology* 2002;48:62–71.

15. de Gennes C, Kuntz D, de Vernejoul MC. Bone mastocytosis. A report of nine cases with a bone histomorphometric study. *Clin Orthop* 1992;279:281–291.

16. Demeter J, Grotes HJ, Horvath C, et al. Bone densitometry and histomorphometry in patients with hairy cell leukemia. *Leuk Lymphoma* 1994;14:73–77.

17. Gallagher DJ, Phillips DJ, Heinrich SD. Orthopedic manifestations of acute pediatric leukemia. *Orthop Clin North Am* 1996;27:635–644.

18. Stowens DW, Teitelbaum SL, Kahn AJ, et al. Skeletal complications of Gaucher disease. *Medicine (Baltimore)* 1985;64: 310–322.

19. Verma S, Rajaratnam JH, Denton J, et al. Adipocytic proportion of bone marrow is inversely related to bone formation in osteoporosis. *J Clin Pathol* 2002;55:693–698.

20. Laroche M, Ludot I, Brousset P, et al. Osteoporosis with lymphoid nodules and hematopoietic marrow hyperplasia. *Clin Exp Rheumatol* 1999;17:457–460.

21. Beretta-Piccoli BC, Sauvain MJ, Gal I, et al. Synovitis, acne, pustulosis, hyperostosis, osteitis (SAPHO) syndrome in childhood: a report of ten cases and review of the literature. *Eur J Pediatr* 2000;159:594–601.

22. Whyte MP, Mills BG, Reinus WR, et al. Expansile skeletal hyperphosphatasia: a new familial metabolic bone disease. *J Bone Miner Res* 2000;15:2330–2344.

23. Boechat MI, Westra SJ, Van Dop C, et al. Decreased cortical and increased cancellous bone in two children with primary hyperparathyroidism. *Metabolism* 1996;45:76–81.

24. Weinstein RS, Sappington LJ. Qualitative bone defect in uremic osteosclerosis. *Metabolism* 1982;31:805–811.

25. Boivin G, Chavassieux P, Chapuy MC, et al. Skeletal fluorosis: histomorphometric findings. *J Bone Miner Res* 1990;5: S185–S189.

26. Aaron JE, de Vernejoul MC, Kanis JA. Bone hypertrophy and trabecular generation in Paget's disease and in fluoride-treated osteoporosis. *Bone Miner* 1992;17:399–413.

27. Shaker JL, Reinus WR, Whyte MP. Hepatitis C-associated osteosclerosis: late onset after blood transfusion in an elderly woman. *J Clin Endocrinol Metab* 1998;83:93–98.

28. Suvajdzic N, Pavlovic M, Misic S, et al. Secondary myelofibrosis in visceral leishmaniasis—case report. *Haematologia (Budap)* 2001;31:167–171.

29. Simone C, Racanelli A. Osteosclerosis in leprosy. *Ital J Orthop Traumatol* 1982;8:211–219.

30. Elmstahl B, Rausing A. A case of hyperoxaluria. Radiological aspects. *Acta Radiol* 1997;38:1031–1034.

31. Kirou KA, Bateman HE, Bansal M, et al. Sarcoidosis presenting with large vessel vasculitis and osteosclerosis-related bone and joint pain. *Clin Exp Rheumatol* 2000;18:401–403.

32. Murray D, Marshall M, England E, et al. Erdheim-Chester disease. *Clin Radiol* 2001;56:481–484.

33. Poulsen LW, Melsen F, Bendix K. A histomorphometric study of haematological disorders with respect to marrow fibrosis and osteosclerosis. *APMIS* 1998;106:495–499.

34. Janin A, Nelken B, Dufour S, et al. Acute monoblastic leukemia with osteosclerosis and extensive myelofibrosis. *Am J Pediatr Hematol Oncol* 1988;10:319–322.

35. Schenkein DP, O'Neill WC, Shapiro J, et al. Accelerated bone formation causing profound hypocalcemia in acute leukemia. *Ann Intern Med* 1986;105:375–378.

36. Demeter J, Grotes HJ, Horvath C, et al. Bone densitometry and histomorphometry in patients with hairy cell leukemia. *Leuk Lymphoma* 1994;14:73–77.

37. Kuo MC, Shih LY. Primary plasma cell leukemia with extensive dense osteosclerosis: complete remission following combination chemotherapy. *Ann Hematol* 1995;71:147–151.

38. Lacy MQ, Gertz MA, Hanson CA, et al. Multiple myeloma associated with diffuse osteosclerotic bone lesions: a clinical entity distinct from osteosclerotic myeloma (POEMS syndrome). *Am J Hematol* 1997;56:288–293.

39. Lipsker D, Veran Y, Grunenberger F, et al. The Schnitzler syndrome. Four new cases and review of the literature. *Medicine (Baltimore)* 2001;80:37–44.

40. Sternberg AJ, Davies P, Macmillan C, et al. Strontium-89: a novel treatment for a case of osteosclerotic myeloma associated with life-threatening neuropathy. *Br J Haematol* 2002;118:821–824.

41. Ghandur-Mnaymneh L, Broder LE, Mnaymneh WA. Lobular carcinoma of the breast metastatic to bone with unusual clinical, radiologic, and pathologic features mimicking osteopoikilosis. *Cancer* 1984;53:1801–1803.

42. Liel Y, Maor E, Ariad S, et al. Severe, diffuse osteosclerosis: A new manifestation of transitional cell carcinoma of the urinary bladder. *Calcif Tissue Int* 1998;63:471–474.

43. Yamashita K, Koyama H, Inaji H. Prognostic significance of bone metastasis from breast cancer. *Clin Orthop* 1995;312:89–94.

44. Chanchairujira K, Chung CB, Lai YM, et al. Intramedullary osteosclerosis: imaging features in nine patients. *Radiology* 2001; 220:225–230.

45. Mitchell MJ, Logan PM. Radiation-induced changes in bone. *Radiographics* 1998;18:1125–1136.

46. Ferrari P, Schroeder V, Anderson S, et al. Association of plasminogen activator inhibitor-1 genotype with avascular osteonecrosis in steroid-treated renal allograft recipients. *Transplantation* 2002; 74:1147–1152.

47. Wenstrup RJ, Roca-Espiau M, Weinreb NJ, et al. Skeletal aspects of Gaucher disease: a review. *Br J Radiol* 2002;75:A2–A12.

48. Frattini A, Orchard PJ, Sobacchi C, et al. Defects in TCIRG1 subunit of the vacuolar proton pump are responsible for a subset of human autosomal recessive osteopetrosis. *Nat Genet* 2000;25: 343–346.

49. McMahon C, Will A, Hu P, et al. Bone marrow transplantation corrects osteopetrosis in the carbonic anhydrase II deficiency syndrome. *Blood* 2001;97:1947–1950.

50. Hamadouche M, Mathieu M, Topouchian V, et al. Transfer of Paget's disease from one part of the skeleton to another as a result of autogenous bone-grafting: a case report. *J Bone Joint Surg Am* 2002;84:2056–2061.

51. Magitsky S, Lipton JF, Reidy J, et al. Ultrastructural features of giant cell tumors in Paget's disease. *Clin Orthop* 2002;402: 213–219.

52. McNairn JD, Damron TA, Landas SK, et al. Inheritance of osteosarcoma and Paget's disease of bone: a familial loss of heterozygosity study. *J Mol Diagn* 2001;3:171–177.

53. Mee AP, Dixon JA, Hoyland JA, et al. Detection of canine distemper virus in 100% of Paget's disease samples by in situ-reverse transcriptase-polymerase chain reaction. *Bone* 1998;23: 171–175.

54. Reddy SV, Kurihara N, Menaa C, et al. Paget's disease of bone: a disease of the osteoclast. *Rev Endocr Metab Disord* 2001;2: 195–201.

55. Smith SE, Murphey MD, Motamedi K, et al. From the archives of the AFIP. Radiologic spectrum of Paget disease of bone and its complications with pathologic correlation. *Radiographics* 2002;22: 1191–1216.

56. Abildgaard N, Glerup H, Rungby J, et al. Biochemical markers of bone metabolism reflect osteoclastic and osteoblastic activity in multiple myeloma. *Eur J Haematol* 2000;64:121–129.

57. Fukasawa H, Kato A, Fujigaki Y, et al. Hypercalcemia in a patient with B-cell acute lymphoblastic leukemia: a role of proinflammatory cytokine. *Am J Med Sci* 2001;322:109–112.

58. Hunt NC, Fujikawa Y, Sabokbar A, et al. Cellular mechanisms of bone resorption in breast carcinoma. *Br J Cancer* 2001;85: 78–84.

59. Kanis JA, McCloskey EV. Bone turnover and biochemical markers in malignancy. *Cancer* 1997;80:1538–1545.

60. Marcelli C, Chappard D, Rossi JF, et al. Histologic evidence of an abnormal bone remodeling in B-cell malignancies other than multiple myeloma. *Cancer* 1988;62:1163–1170.

61. Roebuck DJ. Skeletal complications in pediatric oncology patients. *Radiographics* 1999;19:873–885.

62. Vichinsky EP. The morbidity of bone disease in thalassemia. *Ann N Y Acad Sci* 1998;850:344–348.

Extracellular Space

1. Benson MD, Liepnieks JJ, Yazaki M, et al. A new human hereditary amyloidosis: the result of a stop-codon mutation in the apolipoprotein AII gene. *Genomics* 2001;72:272–277.

2. Ghiso JA, Holton J, Miravalle L, et al. Systemic amyloid deposits in familial British dementia. *J Biol Chem* 2001;276:43909–43914.

3. Gillmore JD, Stangou AJ, Tennent GA, et al. Clinical and biochemical outcome of hepatorenal transplantation for hereditary systemic amyloidosis associated with apolipoprotein AI Gly26Arg. *Transplantation* 2001;71:986–992.

4. Mansour I, Delague V, Cazeneuve C, et al. Familial Mediterranean fever in Lebanon: mutation spectrum, evidence for cases in Maronites, Greek orthodoxes, Greek Catholics, Syriacs and Chiites and for an association between amyloidosis and M694V and M694I mutations. *Eur J Hum Genet* 2001;9: 51–55.

5. Sousa MM, Cardoso I, Fernandes R, et al. Deposition of transthyretin in early stages of familial amyloidotic polyneuropathy: evidence for toxicity of nonfibrillar aggregates. *Am J Pathol* 2001;159:1993–2000.

6. Ohashi K. Pathogenesis of beta2-microglobulin amyloidosis. *Pathol Int* 2001;51:1–10.

7. Akcay S, Akman B, Ozdemir H, et al. Bronchiectasis-related amyloidosis as a cause of chronic renal failure. *Ren Fail* 2002;24: 815–823.

8. Akpolat T, Akpolat I, Kandemir B. Behcet's disease and AA-type amyloidosis. *Am J Nephrol* 2000;20:68–70.

9. Altiparmak MR, Tabak F, Pamuk ON, et al. Giant cell arteritis and secondary amyloidosis: the natural history. *Scand J Rheumatol* 2001;30:114–116.

10. Andronikou S, Kader E. Bronchial mucoepidermoid tumour in a child presenting with organomegaly due to secondary amyloidosis: case report and review of the literature. *Pediatr Radiol* 2001; 31:348–350.

11. Bakir AA, Dunea G. Drugs of abuse and renal disease. *Curr Opin Nephrol Hypertens* 1996;5:122–126.

12. Cosme A, Horcajada JP, Vidaur F, et al. Systemic AA amyloidosis induced by oral contraceptive-associated hepatocellular adenoma: a 13-year follow up. *Liver* 1995;15:164–167.

13. Delgado MA, Liu JY, Meleg Smith S. Systemic amyloidosis associated with hepatocellular carcinoma. Case report and literature review. *J La State Med Soc* 1999;151:474–478.

14. Gardyn J, Schwartz A, Gal R, et al. Waldenstrom's macroglobulinemia associated with AA amyloidosis. *Int J Hematol* 2001;74: 76–78.

15. Gillmore JD, Lovat LB, Persey MR, et al. Amyloid load and clinical outcome in AA amyloidosis in relation to circulating concentration of serum amyloid A protein. *Lancet* 2001;358: 24–29.

16. Joss N, McLaughlin K, Simpson K, et al. Presentation, survival and prognostic markers in AA amyloidosis. *QJM* 2000;93: 535–542.

17. Kagan A, Husza'r M, Frumkin A, et al. Reversal of nephrotic syndrome due to AA amyloidosis in psoriatic patients on long-term colchicine treatment. Case report and review of the literature. *Nephron* 1999;82:348–353.

18. Keven K, Nergizoglu G, Ates K, et al. Remission of nephrotic syndrome after removal of localized Castleman's disease. *Am J Kidney Dis* 2000;35:1207–1211.

19. Kovacsovics-Bankowski M, Zufferey P, So AK, et al. Secondary amyloidosis: a severe complication of ankylosing spondylitis. Two case-reports. *Joint Bone Spine* 2000;67:129–133.

20. Laiho K, Hannula S, Savolainen A, et al. Cervical spine in patients with juvenile chronic arthritis and amyloidosis. *Clin Exp Rheumatol* 2001;19:345–348.

21. Leidig P, Stolte M, Krakamp B, et al. Whipple's disease—a rare cause of secondary amyloidosis. *Z Gastroenterol* 1994;32: 109–112.

22. Lovat LB, Madhoo S, Pepys MB, et al. Long-term survival in systemic amyloid A amyloidosis complicating Crohn's disease. *Gastroenterology* 1997;112:1362–1365.

23. Moriguchi M, Terai C, Kaneko H, et al. A novel single-nucleotide polymorphism at the 5′-flanking region of SAA1 associated with risk of type AA amyloidosis secondary to rheumatoid arthritis. *Arthritis Rheum* 2001;44:1266–1272.

24. Nakayama EE, Ura S, Fleury RN, et al. Renal lesions in leprosy: a retrospective study of 199 autopsies. *Am J Kidney Dis* 2001;38: 26–30.

25. Rocken C, Radun D, Glasbrenner B, et al. Generalized AA-amyloidosis in a 58-year-old Caucasian woman with an 18-month history of gastrointestinal tuberculosis. *Virchows Arch* 1999;434:95–100.

26. Rocken C, Wieker K, Grote HJ, et al. Rosai-Dorfman disease and generalized AA amyloidosis: a case report. *Hum Pathol* 2000; 31:621–624.

27. Sungur C, Sungur A, Akpolat T, et al. Diagnostic value of bone marrow biopsy in patients with AA-type renal amyloidosis secondary to ankylosing spondylitis. *Nephrol Dial Transplant* 1996; 11:2520–2521.

28. Tanno S, Ohsaki Y, Osanai S, et al. Spontaneous rupture of the amyloid spleen in a case of usual interstitial pneumonia. *Intern Med* 2001;40:428–431.

29. Travis WD, Castile R, Vawter G, et al. Secondary (AA) amyloidosis in cystic fibrosis. A report of three cases. *Am J Clin Pathol* 1986; 85:419–424.

30. Blay P, Fernandez-Martinez JM, Diaz-Lopez B. Vertebral involvement in hyperphosphatemic tumoral calcinosis. *Bone* 2001;28: 316–318.

31. Apostolou T, Tziamalis M, Christodoulidou C, et al. Regression of massive tumoral calcinosis of the ischium in a dialysis patient after treatment with reduced calcium dialysate and i.v. administration. *Clin Nephrol* 1998;50:247–251.

32. Cofan F, Garcia S, Combalia A, et al. Uremic tumoral calcinosis in patients receiving longterm hemodialysis therapy. *J Rheumatol* 1999;26:379–385.

33. Felson DT, Chaisson CE, Hill CL, et al. The association of bone marrow lesions with pain in knee osteoarthritis. *Ann Intern Med* 2001;134:541–549.

34. Iida S, Harada Y, Shimizu K, et al. Correlation between bone marrow edema and collapse of the femoral head in steroid-induced osteonecrosis. *AJR Am J Roentgenol* 2000;174:735–743.

35. Koo KH, Ahn IO, Song HR, et al. Increased perfusion of the femoral head in transient bone marrow edema syndrome. *Clin Orthop* 2002;402:171–175.

36. Kubo T, Yamamoto T, Inoue S, et al. Histological findings of bone marrow edema pattern on MRI in osteonecrosis of the femoral head. *J Orthop Sci* 2000;5:520–523.

37. Papadopoulos EC, Papagelopoulos PJ, Boscainos PJ, et al. Bone marrow edema syndrome. *Orthopedics* 2001;24:69–73.

38. Robinson D, Kossashvili Y, Sandbank J, et al. Transient bone oedema of the tibia mimicking a tumorous process. *Acta Orthop Belg* 2002;68:157–162.

39. Yang I, Hayes CW, Biermann JS. Calcific tendinitis of the gluteus medius tendon with bone marrow edema mimicking metastatic disease. *Skeletal Radiol* 2002;31:359–361.

40. Feng CS. A variant of gelatinous transformation of marrow in leukemic patients post-chemotherapy. *Pathology* 1993;25:294–296.

41. Arranz R, Gil-Fernandez JJ, Acevedo A, et al. Gelatinous degeneration presenting as a preleukaemic syndrome. *J Clin Pathol* 1996;49:512–514.

42. Bohm J. Gelatinous transformation of the bone marrow: the spectrum of underlying diseases. *Am J Surg Pathol* 2000;24:56–65.

43. Bohm J, Schmitt-Graff A. Gelatinous bone marrow transformation in a case of idiopathic myelofibrosis: a morphological paradox. *Pathol Res Pract* 2000;196:775–779.

44. Feng CS, Ng MH, Szeto RS, et al. Bone marrow findings in lupus patients with pancytopenia. *Pathology* 1991;23:5–7.

45. Marie I, Levesque H, Heron F, et al. Gelatinous transformation of the bone marrow: an uncommon manifestation of intestinal lymphangiectasia (Waldmann's disease). *Am J Med* 1999;107:99–100.

46. Mehta K, Gascon P, Robboy S. The gelatinous bone marrow (serous atrophy) in patients with acquired immunodeficiency syndrome. Evidence of excess sulfated glycosaminoglycan. *Arch Pathol Lab Med* 1992;116:504–508.

47. Nonaka D, Tanaka M, Takaki K, et al. Gelatinous bone marrow transformation complicated by self-induced malnutrition. *Acta Haematol* 1998;100:88–90.

48. Riestra S, Dominguez F, Rodrigo L. Nodular regenerative hyperplasia of the liver in a patient with celiac disease. *J Clin Gastroenterol* 2001;33:323–326.

49. Varma N, Bhoria U, Bambery P, et al. Gelatinous transformation of the bone marrow and *Leishmania donovani* infection. *J Trop Med Hyg* 1991;94:310–312.

50. Wang C, Amato D, Fernandes B. Gelatinous transformation of bone marrow from a starch-free diet. *Am J Hematol* 2001;68:58–59.

51. Dowling JP, Griffiths JD, McLeish JA. Myeloma associated scleromyxedema with extensive involvement of small bowel. *Pathology* 1991;23:244–247.

14

INFECTIOUS DISEASE AND
RELATED TOPICS

The incidence of marrow disease, variety of organisms, and frequency of multiple infections has greatly increased in recent years because of the fast-growing population of immunosuppressed patients.

The range of reactive responses in the peripheral blood and bone marrow is limited, and morphologic findings are often nonspecific. Positive identification of the organism or specific serologic reaction is usually required for definitive diagnosis. Following are brief descriptions of the peripheral blood and bone marrow findings in response to various infectious agents (Table 14-1).

BACTERIA

Actinomyces spp may invade the bone marrow, especially that contained within the facial bones. Bone marrow necrosis and clusters of organisms may be found (Fig. 14-1).

Bartonella spp are the infectious agents of catscratch disease in the immunocompetent host and systemic bartonellosis in the immunosuppressed patient (1–3) (Figs. 14-2 and 14-3). Marrow sections may show bacillary angiomatosis or lymphohistiocytic aggregates without vascular proliferation. The diagnosis is made by detection of small, intracellular, gram-negative and silver-positive bacilli and identification of *Bartonella* spp by immunohistochemical and molecular studies.

Bordetella pertussis, parapertussis, and other species cause whooping cough and marked lymphocytosis (4–8). The white blood cell count may increase to more than $100 \times 10^9/$ L, consisting almost entirely of lymphocytes. Lymphocytosis is apparently caused by blockage of lymphocyte extravasation from blood vessels and stimulation of lymphocyte release from the thymus. The lymphocytes may show blastlike morphology and convoluted and cleaved nuclear membranes.

TABLE 14-1. INFECTIOUS AGENTS CAUSING PERIPHERAL BLOOD AND BONE MARROW CHANGES

Bacteria	Fungi	Viruses	Protozoa	Helminths
Actinomyces spp	*Candida* spp	Adenovirus	*Babesia microti*	*Mansonella perstans*
Bartonella spp	*Cryptococcus neoformans*	Coxsackievirus	*Leishmania* spp	*Wuchereria bancrofti*
Bordetella spp	*Histoplasma capsulatum*	Cytomegalovirus	Microsporidia spp	
Borrelia spp	*Paracoccidioides*	Dengue virus	*Plasmodium* spp	
Brucella spp	*brasiliensis*	Echovirus	*Toxocara canis*	
Coxiella burnetii	*Penicillium marneffei*	Enterovirus	*Toxoplasma gondii*	
Ehrlichia spp	*Pneumocystis jiroveci*	Epstein-Barr virus	*Trypanosoma* spp	
Klebsiella rhinoscleromatis		Hepatitis viruses		
Mycobacterium spp		Herpes simplex virus		
Rickettsia tsutsugamushi		Human herpesvirus 6		
Salmonella typhi		Human herpesvirus 7		
Shigella spp		Human herpesvirus 8		
Treponema pallidum		Human immunodeficiency		
Tropheryma whippelii		virus type 1		
		Human immunodeficiency		
		virus type 2		
		Human T lymphotropic virus I		
		Human T lymphotropic virus II		
		Influenza virus		
		Measles virus		
		Parvovirus B19		
		Rubella virus		
		Varicella-zoster virus		

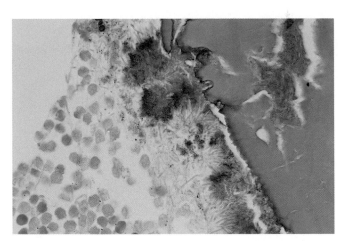

FIGURE 14-1. Bone marrow biopsy specimen, *Actinomyces* infection. The bone and hematopoietic tissue are necrotic; clouds (sulfur granules) of bacteria are seen along the bone surface.

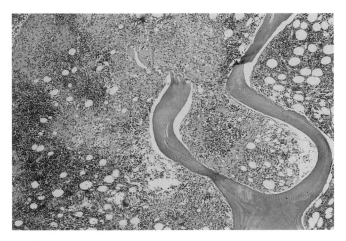

FIGURE 14-2. Bone marrow biopsy specimen, *Bartonella* infection (bacillary angiomatosis). The hematopoietic tissue is focally replaced by fibrovascular connective tissue.

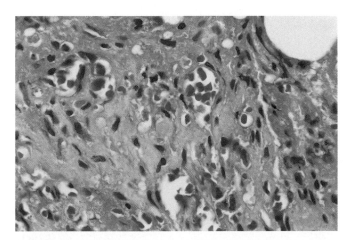

FIGURE 14-3. Bone marrow biopsy specimen, *Bartonella* infection (bacillary angiomatosis). The lesion is composed of multiple thin-walled blood vessels separated by connective tissue.

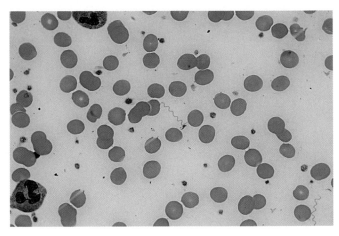

FIGURE 14-4. Peripheral blood smear, *Borrelia* infection (relapsing fever). A spirochete is present, floating in the plasma between red blood cells.

Flow cytometry shows a predominant population of CD3-positive T cells, with a normal CD4:CD8 ratio and no immunophenotypic abnormalities. The differential diagnosis includes acute lymphoblastic leukemia.

Borrelia spp cause Lyme disease, relapsing fever, and other clinical syndromes (9,10) (Fig. 14-4). In acute disease, the peripheral blood may show eosinophilia and free-floating spirochetes. The bone marrow may show T lymphocytosis and epithelioid granulomas, sometimes showing fibrin-ring morphology.

Brucella spp may cause disseminated infections with severe microangiopathic hemolytic anemia, especially in children and in immunocompromised patients (11–13) (Fig. 14-5). A peripheral blood smear may show pancytopenia. The bone marrow shows erythroid and megakaryocytic hyperplasia, eosinophilia, reactive plasmacytosis, granulomas, and reactive histiocytosis. Hemophagocytic syndrome has been reported.

Coxiella burnetii, the agent of Q fever, may be accompanied by cytopenias, hematopoietic hypoplasia, and bone

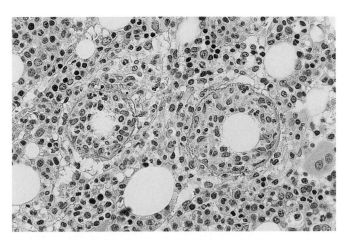

FIGURE 14-5. Bone marrow biopsy specimen, *Coxiella* infection (Q fever). Fibrin-ring granulomas are present.

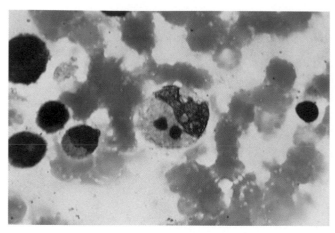

FIGURE 14-6. Bone marrow aspirate smear, *Ehrlichia* infection (human monocytic ehrlichiosis). A monocyte containing cytoplasmic inclusions or morules is present.

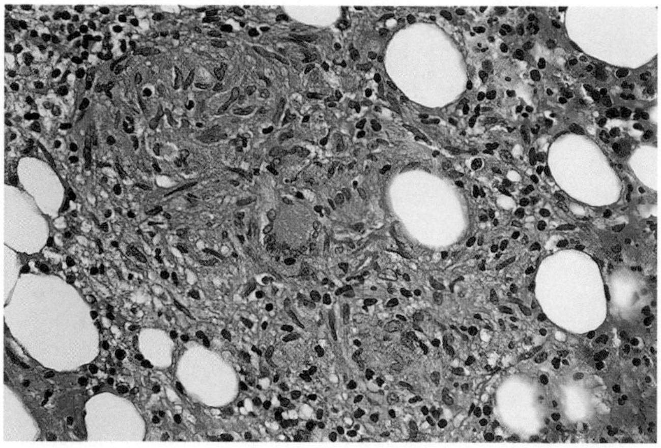

FIGURE 14-7. Bone marrow biopsy specimen, *Mycobacterium tuberculosis* infection. A large, well-formed granuloma is present and composed of histiocytes and giant cells.

marrow granulomas (14–18). The granulomas are composed of a clear central space or vacuole rimmed by fibrin and neutrophils and surrounded by a collar of histiocytes (ring granuloma); however, this histologic appearance is not specific for Q fever. Hemophagocytic syndrome has been reported.

Ehrlichia spp, the agents of human granulocytic and monocytic ehrlichiosis, may infect both immunocompetent and immunocompromised patients (19–22) (Fig. 14-6). Cytopenias and coagulopathies are often present. Peripheral blood and bone marrow aspirate smears show cytoplasmic inclusions, predominantly in either granulocytes or monocytes, rarely in lymphocytes. The inclusions are aggregates (morulae) of intracellular organisms. Histologic sections of the bone marrow show myeloid and megakaryocytic hyperplasia or, less often, trilineal hypoplasia; other findings include reactive histiocytosis, perivascular lymphohistiocytic aggregates, and granulomas, with or without fibrin-ring morphology. Hemophagocytic syndrome has been reported.

Klebsiella rhinoscleromatis is the agent of rhinoscleroma. In disseminated disease, the bone marrow shows proliferation of large histiocytes with bacillus-filled cytoplasm (Mikulicz cells) (23).

Mycobacterium bovis (*bacille Calmette-Guérin*) causes disseminated infection in vaccinated immunodeficient patients and those undergoing intravesical bacille Calmette-Guérin therapy (24–27). Depending on the level of immunosuppression, histologic sections of the bone marrow may show granulomas, loose lymphohistiocytic aggregates, or sheets of bacillus-laden histiocytes.

Mycobacterium leprae, the agent of leprosy, may become disseminated and involve the bone marrow (28–31). The peripheral blood often shows anemia of chronic disease. The bone marrow shows megaloblastic erythropoiesis, reactive plasmacytosis, granulomas, and histiocytosis. Acid-fast bacilli may be both intracellular and lying free in the interstitial space. Depending on the stage of disease and level of immunocompetence, bacilli may be scant or numerous.

In overwhelming disease, bacillus-filled histiocytes (Virchow cells) are seen, with little or no granulomatous reaction.

Mycobacterium tuberculosis is an important cause of bone marrow granulomas, especially in immunosuppressed patients (32–35) (Fig. 14-7). The peripheral blood may show a wide variety of findings, with increases or decreases in total white blood cell count, neutrophils, lymphocytes, and monocytes. Disseminated disease is accompanied by cytopenias. Depending on the level of immunity, marrow sections show granulomas with rare acid-fast bacilli, lymphohistiocytic aggregates with more numerous bacilli, or sheets of bacillus-laden histiocytes. Caseation is uncommon in marrow granulomas. Hemophagocytic syndrome has been reported.

Mycobacteria of other species (atypical mycobacteria) cause disseminated infection in immunosuppressed patients (36–39) (Figs. 14-8 through 14-11). The peripheral blood

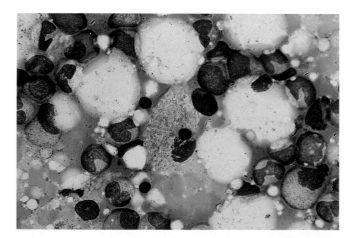

FIGURE 14-8. Bone marrow aspirate smear, *Mycobacterium avium-intracellulare complex* infection (atypical tuberculosis). A histiocyte is present, and its cytoplasm is filled and distended by organisms, which are seen as negative (nonstaining) rods.

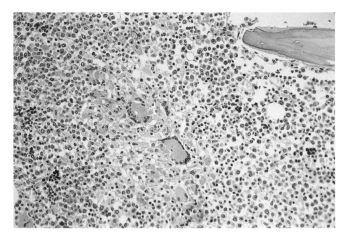

FIGURE 14-9. Bone marrow biopsy, *Mycobacterium avium-intracellulare complex* infection (atypical tuberculosis). A very large, poorly circumscribed granuloma is present that is composed of histiocytes, lymphocytes, and giant cells.

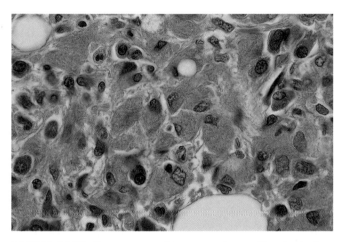

FIGURE 14-10. Bone marrow biopsy specimen, *Mycobacterium avium-intracellulare complex* infection (atypical tuberculosis). A sheet of bacillus-filled histiocytes is present, without evidence of granuloma formation, in this specimen from a patient infected with human immunodeficiency virus.

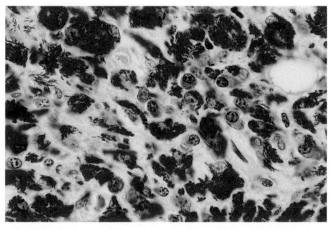

FIGURE 14-11. Bone marrow biopsy specimen, *Mycobacterium avium-intracellulare complex* infection (atypical tuberculosis). A sheet histiocytes shows massive infection with acid-fast bacilli in this specimen from a patient infected with human immunodeficiency virus.

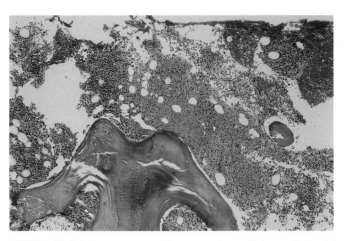

FIGURE 14-12. Bone marrow biopsy specimen, *Salmonella typhi* infection (typhoid fever). A well-formed granuloma is present in this specimen from a patient who had traveled and lived in Mexico.

often shows cytopenias. The degree of tissue reaction in the bone marrow depends on the level of immunosuppression. With relatively intact immunity, well-formed granulomas with few acid-fast bacilli are found. In profound immunosuppression, indistinct lymphohistiocytic aggregates or sheets of bacillus-laden histiocytes are found.

Rickettsia tsutsugamushi, the agent of scrub typhus, may cause atypical lymphocytosis and hemophagocytic syndrome (40,41).

Salmonella typhi, the agent of typhoid fever, causes neutropenia, eosinopenia, lymphopenia, and thrombocytopenia (42–47) (Fig. 14-12). In acute disease, the bone marrow may show granulocytic hyperplasia, myeloid maturation arrest, decreased erythroid precursors and megakaryocytes, and increased hemophagocytic activity. Frank hemophagocytic syndrome has been reported. Chronic disease is characterized by bone marrow granulomas.

Shigella spp cause dysentery, pancytopenia, and hematopoietic hypoplasia (48,49).

Treponema pallidum, the etiologic agent of syphilis, can cause hematopoietic complications in the fetus and infant (50–53). These include fetal hydrops, anemia, peripheral monocytosis, extramedullary hematopoiesis, and hemophagocytic syndrome.

Tropheryma whippelii, the agent of Whipple disease, may cause disseminated infection and anemia (54–57). The bone marrow shows increased monocytes and macrophages, filled with periodic acid–Schiff-positive bacilli.

FUNGI

Candida spp may appear in the peripheral blood but rarely cause bone marrow granulomas (1) (Fig. 14-13).

Cryptococcus neoformans may infect the bone marrow in immunosuppressed patients, especially those with reduced T-cell immunity (2–5) (Figs. 14-14 and 14-15). Peripheral

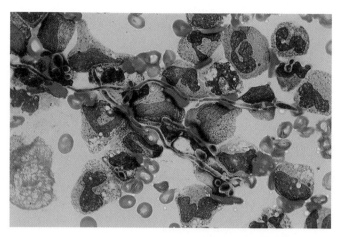

FIGURE 14-13. Peripheral blood smear, *Candida albicans* infection. Yeast forms and branching pseudohyphae are seen in this specimen from a patient with an indwelling catheter.

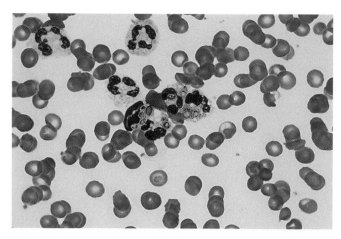

FIGURE 14-16. Peripheral blood smear, *Histoplasma capsulatum* infection. Neutrophils containing ingested yeast forms are present in this specimen from a patient infected with human immunodeficiency virus.

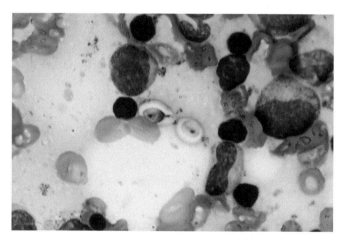

FIGURE 14-14. Bone marrow aspirate smear, *Cryptococcus neoformans* infection. Encapsulated, free-floating yeast forms are present in this specimen from a patient infected with human immunodeficiency virus.

blood and bone marrow aspirate smears may show ingested organisms in phagocytic cells. Depending on the level of immunosuppression, histologic sections of the bone marrow show granulomas, lymphohistiocytic aggregates, or diffuse histiocytic infiltrates. Hemophagocytic syndrome has been reported.

Histoplasma capsulatum may disseminate to involve the marrow in infants and immunosuppressed patients (6–10) (Figs. 14-16 and 14-17). Peripheral blood and bone marrow aspirate smears show organisms within phagocytic cells. Depending on the level of immunosuppression, histologic sections of the bone marrow show granulomas, lymphohistiocytic aggregates, or sheets of histiocytes with abundant intracellular and free-lying organisms. Hemophagocytic syndrome has been reported.

Paracoccidioides brasiliensis, the agent of South American blastomycosis, affects normal individuals and immunocompromised patients in endemic areas (11,12). The peripheral

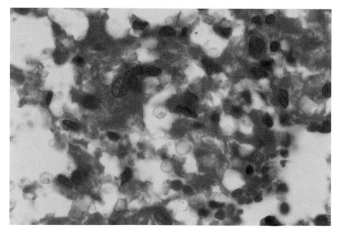

FIGURE 14-15. Bone marrow biopsy specimen, *Cryptococcus neoformans* infection. Encapsulated free-floating yeast forms appear among histiocytes in this specimen from a patient infected with human immunodeficiency virus.

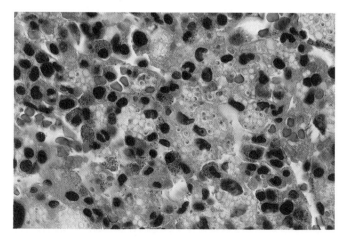

FIGURE 14-17. Bone marrow biopsy specimen, *Histoplasma capsulatum* infection. Histiocytes filled with yeast forms are present in this specimen from a patient infected with human immunodeficiency virus.

blood may show anemia, leukocytosis, and eosinophilia. The bone marrow may show eosinophilic hyperplasia, increased histiocytes with phagocytic activity, and granulomas containing yeast forms.

Penicillium marneffei is an important opportunistic pathogen of immunosuppressed patients traveling or residing in Southeast Asia (13–16). The peripheral blood may show cytopenias. The bone marrow shows granulomas, lymphohistiocytic aggregates, or sheets of yeast-laden histiocytes, depending on the degree of immunosuppression. Hemophagocytic syndrome has been reported. The morphologic appearance of the organism may be mistaken for *Histoplasma capsulatum;* a differential point is that *Histoplasma* organisms divide by budding and *Penicillium* organisms by fission.

Pneumocystis jiroveci (formerly *Pneumocystis carinii*) may disseminate to involve the bone marrow in immunosuppressed patients (17–20). Bone marrow aspirate smears and histologic sections show a foamy exudate containing rare unicellular organisms. Hemophagocytic syndrome has been reported.

VIRUSES

Adenovirus has been reported to cause hemophagocytic syndrome (1).

Coxsackievirus has been associated with acute infectious lymphocytosis, atypical lymphocytosis, and hemophagocytic syndrome (2–4).

Cytomegalovirus causes primary infection followed by latency and possible reactivation (5–13) (Fig. 14-18). The peripheral blood may show atypical lymphocytosis, large granular T-cell lymphocytosis, neutropenia, and thrombocytopenia. The bone marrow may show myelodysplastic changes, eosinophilic hyperplasia, lymphoid hyperplasia,

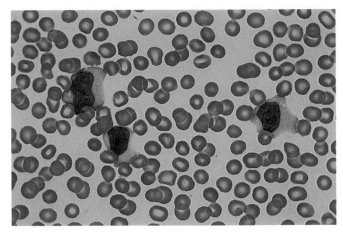

FIGURE 14-19. Peripheral blood smear, Epstein-Barr virus infection. Atypical lymphocytes are present, showing large nuclei and abundant, pale blue, spreading cytoplasm.

granulomas, and increased hemophagocytosis. Cells containing intranuclear "owl's-eye" viral inclusions have been described in the peripheral blood and bone marrow. Precursor B-cell hyperplasia may be marked in the bone marrow of infected infants. Hematologic complications of infection include pancytopenia, hematopoietic hypoplasia, large granular cell lymphocytosis, bone marrow necrosis, and hemophagocytic syndrome.

Dengue virus causes neutropenia, thrombocytopenia, and lymphocytosis (14–16). The bone marrow is hypocellular and hematopoiesis is suppressed, with erythroid hypoplasia and megakaryocytic degeneration. Regeneration of hematopoietic cells parallels remission of symptoms.

Echovirus has been reported as a cause of acute infectious lymphocytosis and hemophagocytic syndrome (17,18).

Enterovirus has been associated with acute infectious lymphocytosis (19).

Epstein-Barr virus causes primary infection followed by latency and possible reactivation (20–32) (Figs. 14-19

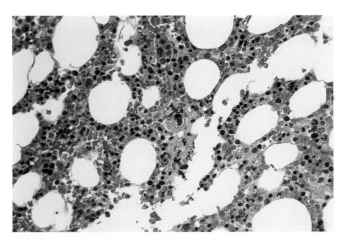

FIGURE 14-18. Bone marrow biopsy specimen, cytomegalovirus infection. A large cell in the center contains an intranuclear viral inclusion in this specimen from a patient infected with human immunodeficiency virus.

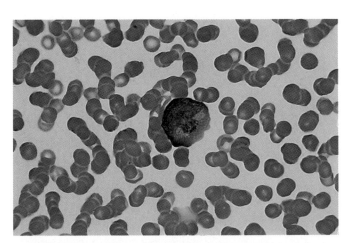

FIGURE 14-20. Peripheral blood smear, Epstein-Barr virus infection. An immunoblast is present, showing a large nucleus, condensed chromatin, and deeply basophilic cytoplasm.

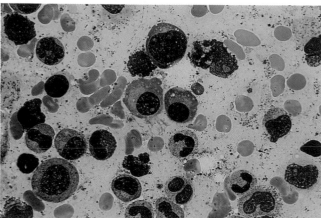

FIGURE 14-21. Bone marrow aspirate, Epstein-Barr virus infection. Reactive plasmacytosis is present.

through 14-22). The peripheral blood shows absolute and atypical lymphocytosis. Both T cells and B cells are increased. The atypical lymphocytes are primarily CD8-positive T cells but also CD4-positive T cells and natural killer cells. Apoptotic lymphocytes and neutrophils may be present. Smudge cells and lymphocytes with cloverleaf nuclei are characteristic. The bone marrow may show megaloblastic maturation, atypical lymphocytosis, and/or granulomas. Complications of infection include pancytopenia and death during acute infection, aplastic anemia, hemophagocytic syndrome, persistent polyclonal B-cell lymphocytosis, clonal lymphoproliferative disorders, and acute leukemia.

Hepatitis virus infections have been linked to numerous hematologic abnormalities. Hepatitis A virus is associated with thrombocytopenia and increased megakaryocytic emperipolesis (33). Hepatitis B virus is associated with pancytopenia and hemophagocytic syndrome (34,35). Hepatitis C virus is associated with pure red cell aplasia, aplastic anemia, hemophagocytic syndrome, and clonal B-cell and plasma cell

disorders (35–37). Non-A, non-B, non-C viral hepatitis is associated with aplastic anemia (38).

Herpes simplex virus infection has been reported to cause bone marrow necrosis and hemophagocytic syndrome (1,39).

Human herpesvirus 6 causes primary infection followed by latency and possible reactivation (40–53). In primary infection, the peripheral blood may show atypical lymphocytosis, neutropenia, reticulocytopenia, and thrombocytopenia. Apoptotic lymphocytes may be present. The bone marrow may show transient erythroid hypoplasia, myelodysplastic changes, atypical lymphocytosis, and increased hemophagocytosis. Complications of infection include death during the acute phase, persistent atypical lymphocytosis, transient erythroblastopenia, generalized lymphoproliferation, marrow suppression, triggering of drug hypersensitivity syndrome, hemophagocytic syndrome, and possibly clonal lymphoproliferative disorders and acute leukemia.

Human herpesvirus 7 causes primary infection followed by latency and possible reactivation (54–56). Little is known about the pathology of primary infection, although it may be accompanied by atypical lymphocytosis. The long-term consequences of infection are unclear.

Human herpesvirus 8 causes primary infection followed by latency and possible reactivation (57–64). Little is known regarding the pathology of primary infection, although it may be attended by severe pancytopenia and increased bone marrow hemophagocytosis in an immunocompromised host. Complications of chronic infection include multicentric plasma cell Castleman disease and clonal B-cell and plasma cell disorders.

Human immunodeficiency virus type 1 causes primary infection and chronic disease (65–75) (Figs. 14-23 through 14-26). In primary infection, the peripheral blood shows atypical lymphocytosis with CD4-positive T-cell depletion and CD8-positive T-cell lymphocytosis. Chronic infection

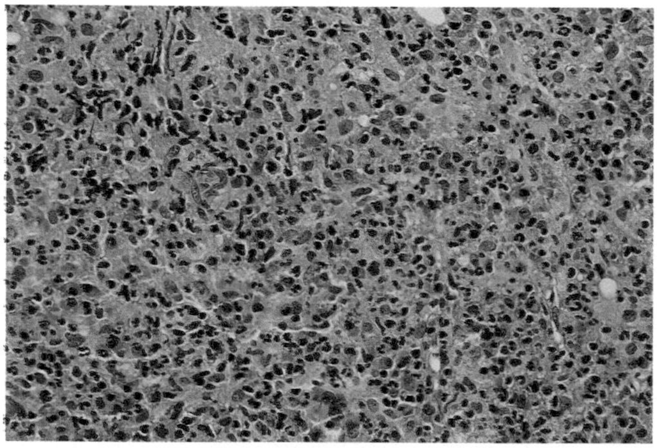

FIGURE 14-22. Bone marrow biopsy specimen, Epstein-Barr virus infection. Cellularity is increased owing to a diffuse infiltrate of lymphocytes and plasma cells.

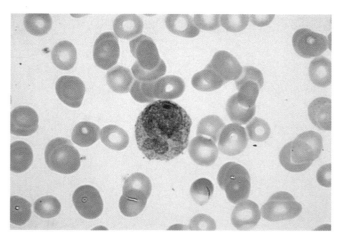

FIGURE 14-23. Peripheral blood smear, human immunodeficiency virus infection. A dysplastic neutrophil is unusually large and shows abnormal nuclear lobation.

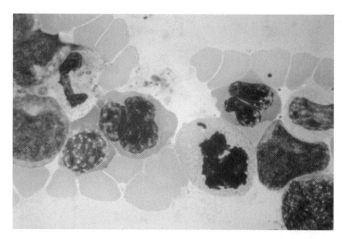

FIGURE 14-24. Bone marrow aspirate smear, human immunodeficiency virus infection. Marked dyserythropoiesis is evident.

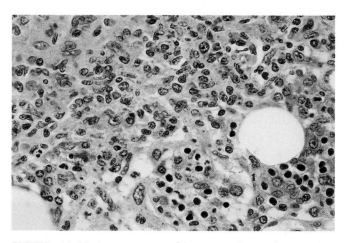

FIGURE 14-26. Bone marrow biopsy specimen, human immunodeficiency virus infection. Cellularity is increased owing to a diffuse increase in lymphocytes and plasma cells.

is characterized by anemia, thrombocytopenia, persistent CD4-positive T lymphopenia, and, in some cases, CD8-positive lymphocytosis. Myelodysplastic changes are present in the peripheral blood and bone marrow. In addition, the bone marrow often shows disruption of normal architecture, an increased number of denuded megakaryocytic nuclei, eosinophilia, plasmacytosis, granulomas, lymphohistiocytic aggregates, and fibrosis. Gelatinous transformation has been reported. Complications include acquired immunodeficiency syndrome and clonal hematolymphoid disease. The differential diagnosis includes idiopathic CD4-positive T lymphopenia (76–80).

Human immunodeficiency virus type 2 also causes CD4-positive T lymphopenia (81,82). Complications include acquired immunodeficiency syndrome and clonal hematolymphoid disease.

Human T lymphotropic virus type I becomes integrated into host hematolymphoid cells. Infection is associated with a range of hematolymphoid disorders, including CD8+ T lymphocytosis, clonal expansion of CD4+ and

CD8+ T cells, acute myeloid leukemia, and adult T-cell leukemia/lymphoma (83–87).

Human T lymphotropic virus type II is associated with peripheral lymphocytosis and clonal T-cell disorders (88–90). Little is known about the long-term hematologic complications of infection.

Influenza virus has been reported to cause hemophagocytic syndrome (1,91).

Measles virus infection is associated with peripheral cytopenias of CD4- and CD8-positive T cells, B cells, neutrophils, and monocytes; natural killer cell lymphocytosis; and T-cell apoptosis, which may persist for as long as 6 months after infection (92–96). Complications include death during the acute phase, especially in patients with prior immunosuppression, hemophagocytic syndrome, and possibly Paget disease of bone.

Parvovirus B19 infects erythroid precursors and causes serious disease primarily in fetuses, immunosuppressed patients, and patients with chronic hemolysis owing to thalassemia, hereditary spherocytosis, sickle cell anemia, or a prosthetic cardiac valve (97–110) (Figs. 14-27 through 14-30). Infection by Parvovirus B19 may be the first sign of underlying hereditary spherocytosis. The peripheral blood shows anemia and reticulocytopenia, sometimes accompanied by leukopenia and thrombocytopenia. In an immunocompetent patient, the bone marrow shows erythroid aplasia with rare giant pronormoblasts containing intranuclear viral inclusions (aplastic crisis). The inclusions appear as glassy, ill-defined intranuclear lucencies in Wright-stained smears and sharply defined cleared areas in histologic sections of the bone marrow. Erythropoietin therapy may produce a surge in erythroid precursors, with the appearance of the pathognomonic inclusions. Myelodysplastic changes may be present. In a fetus or immunocompromised patient, the bone marrow shows erythroid hyperplasia, with abundant viral inclusions at all stages of erythroid maturation. Recovery is accompanied by reticulocytosis and the reappearance of

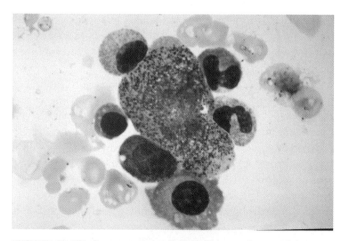

FIGURE 14-25. Bone marrow aspirate smear, human immunodeficiency virus infection. Dysgranulopoiesis is present.

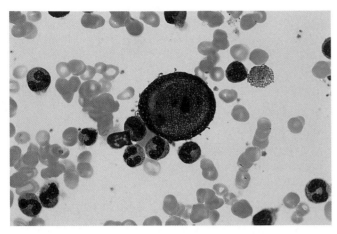

FIGURE 14-27. Bone marrow aspirate smear, Parvovirus B19 infection. A gigantic pronormoblast is seen, containing indistinct intranuclear inclusions.

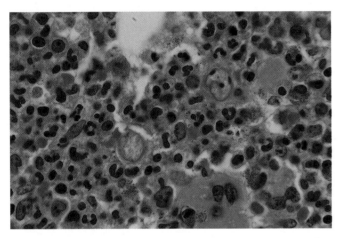

FIGURE 14-28. Bone marrow aspirate clot, Parvovirus B19 infection. Two very large pronormoblasts are present, showing cleared chromatin; other erythroid precursors are virtually absent and iron stores are increased.

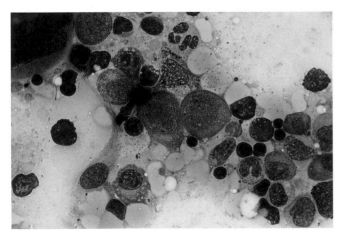

FIGURE 14-29. Bone marrow aspirate smear, Parvovirus B19 and human immunodeficiency virus infection. Two enlarged pronormoblasts are present as well as later normoblasts.

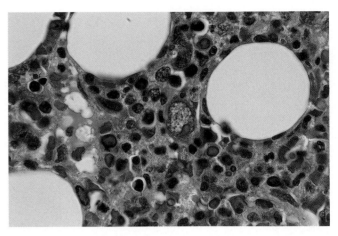

FIGURE 14-30. Bone marrow biopsy specimen, Parvovirus B19 and human immunodeficiency virus infection. A very large erythroid precursor and scattered later normoblasts are present, showing cleared chromatin and intranuclear inclusions.

normal erythropoiesis in the bone marrow. Complications include fetal hydrops and death attributable to anemia, hemophagocytic syndrome, chronic anemia and reticulocytopenia, and possibly acute leukemia. A second erythrovirus with similar pathogenicity was recently described (111).

Rubella virus has been associated with peripheral plasmacytosis and hemophagocytic syndrome (37,112,113).

Varicella-zoster virus is associated with peripheral monocytosis and atypical lymphocytosis (4,113–117). Lymphocyte apoptosis is present and may persist for as long as 6 months after infection. Complications include hemophagocytic syndrome and death caused by overwhelming visceral infection in which intranuclear viral inclusions may be found in bone marrow cells.

PROTOZOA

Babesia microti may cause overwhelming infection in immunosuppressed patients (1–3) (Fig. 14-31). The minute ring forms may occur singly or as several within a single red blood cell; formation of tetrads is characteristic. The small size of the ring form may lead to mistaken identification as *Plasmodium falciparum*. Hemophagocytic syndrome has been reported.

Leishmania spp cause disseminated infection, especially in children and immunosuppressed patients residing in endemic areas (4–7). The peripheral blood and marrow aspirate smears show intracellular amastigotes in phagocytic cells. Histologic sections of the bone marrow may show hematopoietic hypoplasia, fibrosis, reactive histiocytosis, and/or granulomas. Hemophagocytic syndrome is an important complication of leishmaniasis and may obscure the underlying pathogen. Dual infection with leishmania and atypical mycobacteria has been reported.

Plasmodium spp, the agents of malaria, cause numerous hematologic changes (8–13) (Figs. 14-32 through 14-35).

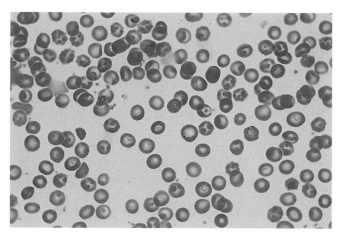

FIGURE 14-31. Peripheral blood smear, *Babesia microti* infection. Minute, delicate intraerythrocytic ring forms are present in this specimen from an experimentally infected mouse.

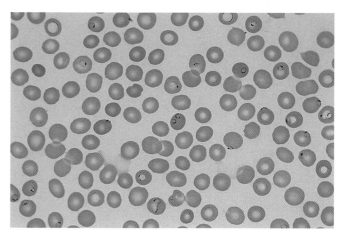

FIGURE 14-34. Peripheral blood smear, *Plasmodium falciparum* infection (falciparum malaria). Very small intraerythrocytic ring forms are present.

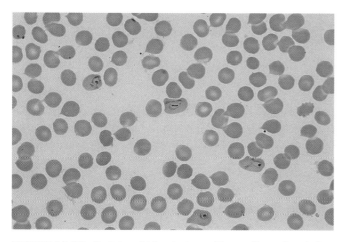

FIGURE 14-32. Peripheral blood smear, *Plasmodium vivax* infection (malaria). Large, irregular or ameboid intraerythrocytic ring forms are present.

P. falciparum causes anemia with erythrocyte parasitemia, neutrophilia, monocytosis, eosinopenia, and reactive lymphocytosis. The bone marrow shows trilineal hyperplasia, megaloblastic and dysplastic maturation, reactive eosinophilia and plasmacytosis, intracellular organisms in phagocytic cells, vascular obstruction by parasitized erythrocytes, increased hemophagocytosis, and lymphocytosis. *Plasmodium vivax* causes peripheral lymphopenia and eosinopenia. Hemophagocytic syndrome has been reported in patients infected with *P. falciparum* and with *P. vivax*.

Microsporidia of various types are emerging opportunistic pathogens that are occasionally found in the bone marrow (14,15).

Toxocara canis infection has been reported to cause marrow eosinophilia (16).

Toxoplasma gondii may cause disseminated infection in immunosuppressed patients (17–20). The peripheral blood may show an infectious mononucleosis-like syndrome. Bone marrow findings include interstitial edema, focal necrosis,

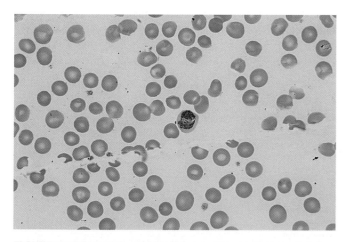

FIGURE 14-33. Peripheral blood smear, *Plasmodium ovale* infection (malaria). An intraerythrocytic gametocyte is present.

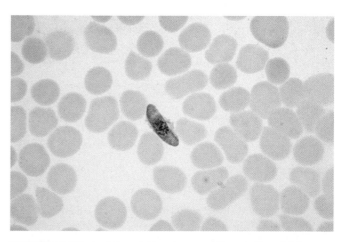

FIGURE 14-35. Peripheral blood smear, *Plasmodium falciparum* infection (falciparum malaria). A gametocyte is present.

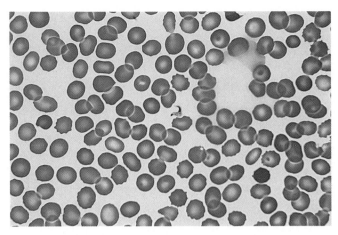

FIGURE 14-36. Peripheral blood smear, *Trypanosoma cruzi* infection (Chagas disease). A single, free-floating trypanosome is present in this specimen from a patient infected with human immunodeficiency virus.

granulomas, encysted and free parasites, and intracellular parasites in macrophages, granulocytes, and megakaryocytes.

Trypanosoma spp, including *Trypanosoma cruzi,* may appear in the peripheral blood, especially in patients with human immunodeficiency virus infection or other causes of immunodeficiency (21) (Fig. 14-36).

HELMINTHS

Microfilariae of *Mansonella perstans* and *Wuchereria bancrofti* have been described in bone marrow smears (1–5). Peripheral eosinophilia may also be present.

INFECTIOUS MONONUCLEOSIS

Infectious mononucleosis is a common condition of children and adults (1–19). The etiologic agents usually associated with infectious mononucleosis are Epstein-Barr virus and cytomegalovirus; however, many other agents cause infectious mononucleosis, including coxsackievirus, dengue virus, human herpesvirus 6, human immunodeficiency virus type 1, varicella-zoster virus, *T. gondii,* and other, as yet undescribed, agents (Table 14-2). Simultaneous infection with multiple agents occurs in some cases.

TABLE 14-2. INFECTIOUS AGENTS ASSOCIATED WITH INFECTIOUS MONONUCLEOSIS

Coxsackievirus
Cytomegalovirus
Epstein-Barr virus
Human herpesvirus 6
Human immunodeficiency virus type 1
Varicella-zoster virus
Toxoplasma gondii

The peripheral blood shows atypical lymphocytosis. Lymphocytes may exhibit a wide range of morphologic features. Some show large nuclei and abundant, pale-blue cytoplasm flowing among the surrounding red blood cells; others resemble immunoblasts, with an ovoid nucleus, prominent nucleolus, and deeply basophilic cytoplasm. Plasmacytoid lymphocytes and plasma cells may also be present. Apoptotic lymphocytes are frequently found. The combination of lymphocytosis, atypical lymphocytes, lymphocytes with cloverleaf nuclei, and smudge cells suggests Epstein-Barr virus infection. Genetic studies have rarely shown transient clonal T-cell proliferation (20).

The differential diagnosis includes atypical lymphocytosis occurring after transplantation and immunization, autoimmune disorders, drug hypersensitivity syndrome, Kikuchi disease and acute leukemia. Hypersensitivity syndrome and acute leukemia may coexist with viral infectious mononucleosis.

ACUTE INFECTIOUS LYMPHOCYTOSIS

Acute infectious lymphocytosis is an uncommon, self-limited disorder, usually affecting young children (1–8). Etiologic agents associated with acute infectious lymphocytosis include *Borrelia burgdorferi, Bordetella pertussis, Giardia lamblia, Blastocystis hominis,* coxsackievirus, echovirus, and enterovirus (Table 14-3). In some cases, no infectious agent has been identified. The peripheral blood shows marked lymphocytosis, composed primarily of small T cells and fewer B cells. Atypical lymphocytes, as seen in Epstein-Barr virus infection, are rare to absent. The bone marrow is normal. The differential diagnosis includes acute lymphocytic leukemia.

BONE MARROW GRANULOMAS

Bone marrow granulomas occur with a variety of infections and noninfectious conditions (Table 14-4). In some cases, no etiologic agent is found.

Infectious agents associated with bone marrow granulomas and/or foamy histiocytes include *Borrelia* spp, *Brucella*

TABLE 14-3. INFECTIOUS AGENTS ASSOCIATED WITH ACUTE INFECTIOUS LYMPHOCYTOSIS

Borrelia burgdorferi
Bordetella pertussis
Giardia lamblia
Blastocystis hominis
Coxsackievirus
Echovirus
Enterovirus

TABLE 14-4. CONDITIONS ASSOCIATED WITH GRANULOMAS OF BONE MARROW

Infectious Agents	Noninfectious Agents	Medical Conditions
Borrelia spp	Medications	Chronic granulomatous disease
Brucella spp	Prosthetic materials	Common variable immunodeficiency
Coxiella burnetii	Oxalate crystals	Connective tissue disease
Ehrlichia spp	Silica crystals	Farber lipogranulomatosis
Klebsiella rhinoscleromatis	Talc crystals	Sarcoidosis
Mycobacterium spp		Hematolymphoid disease
Salmonella typhi		Metastatic malignancies
Tropheryma whippelii		
Candida spp		
Cryptococcus neoformans		
Histoplasma capsulatum		
Paracoccidioides brasiliensis		
Penicillium marneffei		
Pneumocystis jiroveci (formerly *Pneumocystis carinii*)		
Cytomegalovirus		
Epstein-Barr virus		
Hepatitis viruses		
Leishmania spp		
Toxoplasma gondii		

spp, *C. burnetii, Ehrlichia* spp, *K. rhinoscleromatis, Mycobacteria* spp, *S. typhi, T. whippelii, C. neoformans, H. capsulatum, P. marneffei, P. jiroveci* (formerly *P. carinii*), cytomegalovirus, Epstein-Barr virus, hepatitis viruses, *Leishmania* spp, and *T. gondii.*

Medical conditions associated with bone marrow granulomas include chronic granulomatous disease, Farber lipogranulomatosis, sarcoidosis, common variable immunodeficiency, connective tissue disease, hematolymphoid disease (both clonal and nonclonal), and metastatic tumors (1–12) (Fig. 14-37).

Noninfectious agents associated with bone marrow granulomas include medications (13–19), materials released from worn prostheses (20), and oxalate, silica, and talc crystals (21–27). In the case of talc, the crystals appear to act synergistically with an infectious agent to produce widespread granulomatous inflammation.

Granuloma morphology, aside from visible organisms, does not indicate a specific etiology. Fibrin-ring granulomas have been reported in infection by *Borrelia* spp, *C. burnetii, Ehrlichia* spp, *Staphylococcus epidermidis,* cytomegalovirus, Epstein-Barr virus, hepatitis A virus, and *Leishmania* spp, and in drug hypersensitivity reactions and malignant lymphoma (28–33) (Fig. 14-38). Necrosis is an uncommon finding in bone marrow granulomas and may favor an infectious etiology.

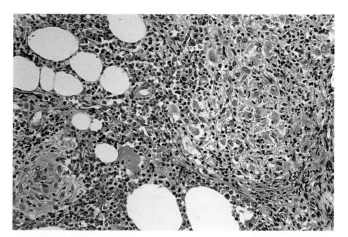

FIGURE 14-37. Bone marrow biopsy specimen, noninfectious granuloma. A well-formed granuloma is seen in this specimen from a patient with colon carcinoma.

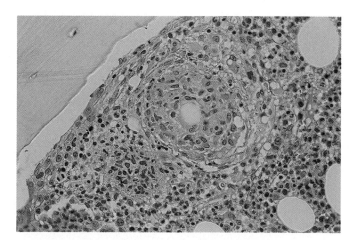

FIGURE 14-38. Bone marrow biopsy specimen, noninfectious fibrin-ring granuloma. A typical fibrin-ring granuloma is seen in this patient with fever of unknown origin.

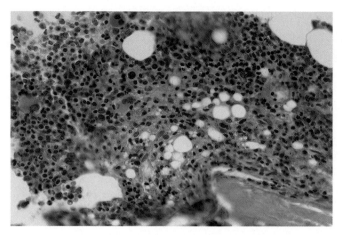

FIGURE 14-39. Bone marrow biopsy specimen, lipogranuloma. A poorly circumscribed collection of lymphocytes, histiocytes, and small fat droplets is present.

Lipogranulomas are small intratrabecular foci of lipid-containing histiocytes and lymphocytes and are of no clinical significance (Fig. 14-39).

REFERENCES

Bacteria

1. Ahsan N, Holman MJ, Riley TR, et al. Peliosis hepatis due to *Bartonella henselae* in transplantation: a hemato-hepato-renal syndrome. *Transplantation* 1998;65:1000–1003.
2. Fagan WA, Skinner SM, Ondo A, et al. Bacillary angiomatosis of the skin and bone marrow in a patient with HIV infection. *J Am Acad Dermatol* 1995;32:510–512.
3. LaRow JM, Wehbe P, Pascual AG. Cat-scratch disease in a child with unique magnetic resonance imaging findings. *Arch Pediatr Adolesc Med* 1998;152:394–396.
4. Hudnall SD, Molina CP. Marked increase in L-selectin-negative T cells in neonatal pertussis. The lymphocytosis explained? *Am J Clin Pathol* 2000;114:35–40.
5. Greig JR, Gunda SS, Kwan JTC. *Bordetella holmesii* bacteraemia in an individual on haemodialysis. *Scand J Infect Dis* 2001;33:716–717.
6. Hudnall SD, Molina CP. Marked increase in L-selectin-negative T cells in neonatal pertussis. The lymphocytosis explained? *Am J Clin Pathol* 2000;114:35–40.
7. Kubic VL, Kubic PT, Brunning RD. The morphologic and immunophenotypic assessment of the lymphocytosis accompanying Bordetella pertussis infection. *Am J Clin Pathol* 1991;95:809–815.
8. von Konig CH, Halperin S, Riffelmann M, et al. Pertussis of adults and infants. *Lancet Infect Dis* 2002;2:744–750.
9. Kvasnicka HM, Thiele J, Ahmadi T. Bone marrow manifestation of Lyme disease (Lyme borreliosis). *Br J Haematol* 2003;120:723.
10. Weinstein A, Britchkov M. Lyme arthritis and post-Lyme disease syndrome. *Curr Opin Rheumatol* 2002;14:383–387.
11. Yaramis A, Kervancioglu M, Yildirim I, et al. Severe microangiopathic hemolytic anemia and thrombocytopenia in a child with *Brucella* infection. *Ann Hematol* 2001;80:546–548.
12. Yildirmak Y, Palanduz A, Telhan L, et al. Bone marrow hypoplasia during *Brucella* infection. *J Pediatr Hematol Oncol* 2003;25:63–64.
13. Young EJ, Tarry A, Genta RM, et al. Thrombocytopenic purpura associated with brucellosis: report of 2 cases and literature review. *Clin Infect Dis* 2000;31:904–909.
14. Bottieau E, De Raeve H, Colebunders R, et al. Q fever after a journey in Syria: a diagnosis suggested by bone marrow biopsy. *Acta Clin Belg* 2000;55:30–33.
15. Hitchins R, Cobcroft RG, Hocker G. Transient severe hypoplastic anemia in Q fever. *Pathology* 1986;18:254–255.
16. Hufnagel M, Niemeyer C, Zimmerhackl LB, et al. Hemophagocytosis: a complication of acute Q fever in a child. *Clin Infect Dis* 1995;21:1029–1031.
17. Srigley JR, Vellend H, Palmer N, et al. Q-fever. The liver and bone marrow pathology. *Am J Surg Pathol* 1985;9:752–758.
18. Travis LB, Travis WD, Li CY, et al. Q fever. A clinicopathologic study of five cases. *Arch Pathol Lab Med* 1986;110:1017–1020.
19. Klein MB, Miller JS, Nelson CM, et al. Primary bone marrow progenitors of both granulocytic and monocytic lineages are susceptible to infection with the agent of human granulocytic ehrlichiosis. *J Infect Dis* 1997;176:1405–1409.
20. Lepidi H, Bunnell JE, Martin ME, et al. Comparative pathology, and immunohistology associated with clinical illness after *Ehrlichia phagocytophila*-group infections. *Am J Trop Med Hyg* 2000;62:29–37.
21. Trofe J, Reddy KS, Stratta RJ, et al. Human granulocytic ehrlichiosis in pancreas transplant recipients. *Transpl Infect Dis* 2001;3:34–39.
22. Walker DH, Dumler JS. Human monocytic and granulocytic ehrlichiosis. Discovery and diagnosis of emerging tick-borne infections and the critical role of the pathologist. *Arch Pathol Lab Med* 1997;121:785–791.
23. Porto R, Hevia O, Hensley GT, et al. Disseminated *Klebsiella rhinoscleromatis* infection. *Arch Pathol Lab Med* 1989;113:1381–1383.
24. Dederke B, Riecken EO, Weinke T. A case of BCG sepsis with bone marrow and liver involvement after intravesical BCG instillation. *Infection* 1998;26:54–57.
25. McKenzie RH, Roux P. Disseminated BCG infection following bone marrow transplantation for X-linked severe combined immunodeficiency. *Pediatr Dermatol* 2000;17:208–212.
26. Roesler J, Kofink B, Wendisch J, et al. *Listeria monocytogenes* and recurrent mycobacterial infections in a child with complete interferon-gamma-receptor (IFNgammaR1) deficiency: mutational analysis and evaluation of therapeutic options. *Exp Hematol* 1999;27:1368–1374.
27. Rosenfeldt V, Paerregaard A, Valerius NH. Disseminated infection with bacillus Calmette-Guerin in a child with advanced HIV disease. *Scand J Infect Dis* 1997;29:526–527.
28. Lapinsky SE, Baynes RD, Schulz EJ, et al. Anaemia, iron-related measurements and erythropoietin levels in untreated patients with active leprosy. *J Intern Med* 1992;232:273–278.
29. Sen R, Sehgal PK, Dixit V, et al. Lipid-laden macrophages in bone marrow of leprosy patients. *Lepr Rev* 1991;62:374–380.
30. Sen R, Yadav SS, Singh U, et al. Patterns of erythropoiesis and anaemia in leprosy. *Lepr Rev* 1991;62:158–170.
31. Suster S, Cabello-Inchausti B, Robinson MJ. Nongranulomatous involvement of the bone marrow in lepromatous leprosy. *Am J Clin Pathol* 1989;92:797–801.
32. Goto S, Aoike I, Shibasaki Y, et al. A successfully treated case of disseminated tuberculosis-associated hemophagocytic syndrome and multiple organ dysfunction syndrome. *Am J Kidney Dis* 2001;38:E19.
33. Karstaedt AS, Pantanowitz L, Omar T, et al. The utility of bone-marrow examination in HIV-infected adults in South Africa. *QJM* 2001;94:101–105.

34. Mert A, Bilir M, Tabak F, et al. Miliary tuberculosis: clinical manifestations, diagnosis and outcome in 38 adults. *Respirology* 2001;6:217–224.
35. Singh KJ, Ahluwalia G, Sharma SK, et al. Significance of haematological manifestations in patients with tuberculosis. *J Assoc Physicians India* 2001;49:788–794.
36. Akpek G, Lee SM, Gagnon DR, et al. Bone marrow aspiration, biopsy, and culture in the evaluation of HIV-infected patients for invasive *Mycobacteria* and *Histoplasma* infections. *Am J Hematol* 2001;67:100–106.
37. Farhi DC, Mason UG 3rd, Horsburgh CR Jr. The bone marrow in disseminated *Mycobacterium avium-intracellulare* infection. *Am J Clin Pathol* 1985;83:463–468.
38. Krebs T, Zimmerli S, Bodmer T, et al. *Mycobacterium genavense* infection in a patient with long-standing chronic lymphocytic leukaemia. *J Intern Med* 2000;248:343–348.
39. Torlakovic E, Clayton F, Ames ED. Refractile mycobacteria in Romanowsky-stained bone marrow smears. A comparison of acid-fast-stained tissue sections and Romanowsky-stained smears. *Am J Clin Pathol* 1991;97:318–321.
40. Chen YC, Chao TY, Chin JC. Scrub typhus-associated hemophagocytic syndrome. *Infection* 2000;28:178–179.
41. Iwasaki H, Ueda T, Uchida M, et al. Atypical lymphocytes with a multilobated nucleus from a patient with tsutsugamushi disease (scrub typhus) in Japan. *Am J Hematol* 1991;36:150–151.
42. James J, Dutta TK, Jayanthi S. Correlation of clinical and hematologic profiles with bone marrow responses in typhoid fever. *Am J Trop Med Hyg* 1997;57:313–316.
43. Mallouh AA, Sa'di AR. White blood cells and bone marrow in typhoid fever. *Pediatr Infect Dis J* 1987;6:527–529.
44. Sakhalkar VS, Rao SP, Gottessman SR, et al. Hemophagocytosis and granulomas in the bone marrow of a child with Down syndrome. *J Pediatr Hematol Oncol* 2001;23:623–625.
45. Serefhanoglu K, Kaya E, Sevinc A, et al. Isolated thrombocytopenia: the presenting finding of typhoid fever. *Clin Lab Haematol* 2003;25:63–65.
46. Sood R, Roy S, Kaushik P. Typhoid fever with severe pancytopenia. *Postgrad Med J* 1997;73:41–42.
47. Stephan JL, Kone-Paut I, Galambrun C, et al. Reactive haemophagocytic syndrome in children with inflammatory disorders. A retrospective study of 24 patients. *Rheumatology (Oxford)* 2001;40:1285–1292.
48. O'Connor HJ, O'Callaghan U. Fatal *Shigella sonnei* septicaemia in an adult complicated by marrow aplasia and intestinal perforation. *J Infect* 1981;3:277–279.
49. Prokocimer M, Matzner Y, Polliack A. Fatal *Shigella* dysentery complicated by toxic megacolon and bone marrow aplasia in a patient with chronic granulocytic leukemia in remission. *Hepatogastroenterology* 1980;27:401–406.
50. Dorfman DH, Glaser JH. Congenital syphilis presenting in infants after the newborn period. *N Engl J Med* 1990;323:1299–1302.
51. Karayalcin G, Khanijou A, Kim KY, et al. Monocytosis in congenital syphilis. *Am J Dis Child* 1977;131:782–783.
52. Levine Z, Sherer DM, Jacobs A, et al. Nonimmune hydrops fetalis due to congenital syphilis associated with negative intrapartum maternal serology screening. *Am J Perinatol* 1998;15:233–236.
53. Pohl M, Niemeyer CM, Hentschel R, et al. Haemophagocytosis in early congenital syphilis. *Eur J Pediatr* 1999;158:553–555.
54. James DG, Lipman MC. Whipple's disease: a granulomatous masquerader. *Clin Chest Med* 2002;23:513–519.
55. Jarolim DR, Parker GA, Sheehan WW. Bone marrow involvement by Whipple bacillus. *J Infect Dis* 1991;163:1169–1170.
56. Pron B, Poyart C, Abachin E, et al. Diagnosis and follow-up of Whipple's disease by amplification of the 16S rRNA gene of *Tropheryma whippelii*. *Eur J Clin Microbiol Infect Dis* 1999;18:62–65.
57. Walter R, Bachmann SP, Schaffner A, et al. Bone marrow involvement in Whipple's disease: rarely reported, but really rare? *Br J Haematol* 2001;112:677–679.

Fungi

1. Clark DM, Tringham VM. Candidal infection diagnosed on trephine biopsy sections. *Br J Haematol* 2003;120:175.
2. Korfel A, Menssen HD, Schwartz S, et al. Cryptococcosis in Hodgkin's disease: description of two cases and review of the literature. *Ann Hematol* 1998;76:283–286.
3. Numata K, Tsutsumi H, Wakai S, et al. A child case of haemophagocytic syndrome associated with cryptococcal meningoencephalitis. *J Infect* 1998;36:118–119.
4. Pantanowitz L, Omar T, Sonnendecker H, et al. Bone marrow cryptococcal infection in the acquired immunodeficiency syndrome. *J Infect* 2000;41:92–94.
5. Schiappa D, Gueyikian A, Kakar S, et al. An auxotrophic pigmented *Cryptococcus neoformans* strain causing infection of the bone marrow. *Med Mycol* 2002;40:1–5.
6. Akpek G, Lee SM, Gagnon DR, et al. Bone marrow aspiration, biopsy, and culture in the evaluation of HIV-infected patients for invasive mycobacteria and histoplasma infections. *Am J Hematol* 2001;67:100–106.
7. Hansen KE, St Clair EW. Disseminated histoplasmosis in systemic lupus erythematosus: case report and review of the literature. *Semin Arthritis Rheum* 1998;28:193–199.
8. Kumar N, Jain S, Singh ZN. Disseminated histoplasmosis with reactive hemophagocytosis: aspiration cytology findings in two cases. *Diagn Cytopathol* 2000;23:422–424.
9. Rao RD, Morice WG, Phyliky RL. Hemophagocytosis in a patient with chronic lymphocytic leukemia and histoplasmosis. *Mayo Clin Proc* 2002;77:287–290.
10. Roy V, Hammerschmidt DE. Disseminated histoplasmosis following prolonged low dose methotrexate therapy. *Am J Hematol* 2000;63:59–60.
11. Goldani LZ, Sugar AM. Paracoccidioidomycosis and AIDS: an overview. *Clin Infect Dis* 1995;21:1275–1281.
12. Ozaki KS, Munhoz Junior S, Pinheiro K, et al. The diagnosis of severe disseminated paracoccidioidomycosis in a bone marrow aspirate: a case report. *Rev Soc Bras Med Trop* 1996;29:363–366.
13. Hien TV, Loc PP, Hoa NT, et al. First cases of disseminated penicilliosis marneffei infection among patients with acquired immunodeficiency syndrome in Vietnam. *Clin Infect Dis* 2001;32:78–80.
14. Lin WC, Dai YS, Tsai MJ, et al. Systemic Penicillium marneffei infection in a child with common variable immunodeficiency. *J Formos Med Assoc* 1998;97:780–783.
15. Lo CY, Chan DT, Yuen KY, et al. *Penicillium marneffei* infection in a patient with SLE. *Lupus* 1995;4:229–231.
16. So CC, Wong KF. Bone marrow penicilliosis. *Br J Haematol* 2002;117:777.
17. Momose H, Lee S. *Pneumocystis carinii* as foamy exudate in bone marrow. *JAMA* 1991;265:1672.
18. Stephan JL, Kone-Paut I, Galambrun C, et al. Reactive haemophagocytic syndrome in children with inflammatory disorders. A retrospective study of 24 patients. *Rheumatology (Oxford)* 2001;40:1285–1292.
19. Stringer JR. *Pneumocystis*. *Int J Med Microbiol* 2002;292:391–404.
20. Stringer JR, Beard CB, Miller RF, et al. A new name (*Pneumocystis jiroveci*) for *Pneumocystis* from humans. *Emerg Infect Dis* 2002;8:891–896.

Viruses

1. Klein A, Corazza F, Demulder A, et al. Recurrent viral associated hemophagocytic syndrome in a child with Langerhans cell histiocytosis. *J Pediatr Hematol Oncol* 1999;21:554–556.

2. Arnez M, Cizman M, Jazbec J, et al. Acute infectious lymphocytosis caused by coxsackievirus B2. *Pediatr Infect Dis J* 1996; 15:1127–1128.

3. Begovac J, Puntaric V, Borcic D, et al. Mononucleosis-like syndrome associated with a multisystem coxsackievirus type B3 infection in adolescence. *Eur J Pediatr* 1988;147:426–427.

4. Stephan JL, Kone-Paut I, Galambrun C, et al. Reactive haemophagocytic syndrome in children with inflammatory disorders. A retrospective study of 24 patients. *Rheumatology (Oxford)* 2001; 40:1285–1292.

5. Bissinger AL, Sinzger C, Kaiserling E, et al. Human cytomegalovirus as a direct pathogen: correlation of multiorgan involvement and cell distribution with clinical and pathological findings in a case of congenital inclusion disease. *J Med Virol* 2002;67:200–206.

6. Fisgin T, Yarali N, Duru F, et al. CMV-induced immune thrombocytopenia and excessive hematogones mimicking an acute B-precursor lymphoblastic leukemia. *Leuk Res* 2003;27: 193–196.

7. Kronenberg A, Seebach JD, Bossart W, et al. Polyclonal proliferation of large granular lymphocytes during cytomegalovirus primary infection in a human immunodeficiency virus-infected patient receiving antiretroviral therapy. *Clin Infect Dis* 2001;33: E34–E36.

8. Mattes FM, McLaughlin JE, Emery VC, et al. Histopathological detection of owl's eye inclusions is still specific for cytomegalovirus in the era of human herpesviruses 6 and 7. *J Clin Pathol* 2000;53:612–614.

9. Miyahara M, Shimamoto Y, Yamada H, et al. Cytomegalovirus-associated myelodysplasia and thrombocytopenia in an immunocompetent adult. *Ann Hematol* 1997;74:99–101.

10. Pooley RJ Jr, Peterson L, Finn WG, et al. Cytomegalovirus-infected cells in routinely prepared peripheral blood films of immunosuppressed patients. *Am J Clin Pathol* 1999;112:108–112.

11. Randolph-Habecker J, Iwata M, Torok-Storb B. Cytomegalovirus mediated myelosuppression. *J Clin Virol* 2002;25: S51–S56.

12. Sakamoto O, Ando M, Yoshimatsu S, et al. Systemic lupus erythematosus complicated by cytomegalovirus-induced hemophagocytic syndrome and colitis. *Intern Med* 2002;41:151–155.

13. Young JF, Goulian M. Bone marrow fibrin ring granulomas and cytomegalovirus infection. *Am J Clin Pathol* 1993;99:65–68.

14. Liu CC, Huang KJ, Lin YS, et al. Transient CD4/CD8 ratio inversion and aberrant immune activation during dengue virus infection. *J Med Virol* 2002;68:241–252.

15. Playford EG, Phillips D, Looke DF, et al. Three cases of dengue 1 virus infection from islands in the Gulf of Thailand. *Commun Dis Intell* 1998;22:107–109.

16. Rothwell SW, Putnak R, La Russa VF. Dengue-2 virus infection of human bone marrow: characterization of dengue-2 antigen-positive stromal cells. *Am J Trop Med Hyg* 1996;54:503–510.

17. Hirst WJ, Layton DM, Singh S, et al. Haemophagocytic lymphohistiocytosis: experience at two U.K. centres. *Br J Haematol* 1994;88:731–739.

18. van der Sar A. Acute infectious lymphocytosis with Echo virus type 25. *West Indian Med J* 1979;28:185–188.

19. Grose C, Horwitz MS. Characterization of an enterovirus associated with acute infectious lymphocytosis. *J Gen Virol* 1976;30: 347–355.

20. Finlay J, Luft B, Yousem S, et al. Chronic infectious mononucleosis syndrome, pancytopenia, and polyclonal B-lymphoproliferation terminating in acute lymphoblastic leukemia. *Am J Pediatr Hematol Oncol* 1986;8:18–27.

21. Brigden ML, Au S, Thompson S, et al. Infectious mononucleosis in an outpatient population: diagnostic utility of 2 automated hematology analyzers and the sensitivity and specificity of Hoagland's criteria in heterophile-positive patients. *Arch Pathol Lab Med* 1999;123:875–881.

22. Imashuku S. Clinical features and treatment strategies of Epstein-Barr virus-associated hemophagocytic lymphohistiocytosis. *Crit Rev Oncol Hematol* 2002;44:259–272.

23. Kanegane H, Nomura K, Miyawaki T, et al. Biological aspects of Epstein-Barr virus (EBV)-infected lymphocytes in chronic active EBV infection and associated malignancies. *Crit Rev Oncol Hematol* 2002;44:239–249.

24. Kaptan K, Beyan C, Ural AU, et al. Successful treatment of severe aplastic anemia associated with human parvovirus B19 and Epstein-Barr virus in a healthy subject with allo-BMT. *Am J Hematol* 2001;67:252–255.

25. Koeppen H, Newell K, Baunoch DA, et al. Morphologic bone marrow changes in patients with posttransplantation lymphoproliferative disorders. *Am J Surg Pathol* 1998;22:208–214.

26. Krause JR, Kaplan SS. Bone marrow findings in infectious mononucleosis and mononucleosis-like diseases in the older adult. *Scand J Haematol* 1982;28:15–22.

27. Larochelle B, Flamand L, Gourde P, et al. Epstein-Barr virus infects and induces apoptosis in human neutrophils. *Blood* 1998; 92:291–299.

28. Mitterer M, Pescosta N, Fend F, et al. Chronic active Epstein-Barr virus disease in a case of persistent polyclonal B-cell lymphocytosis. *Br J Haematol* 1995;90:526–531.

29. Nakagawa A, Ito M, Saga S. Fatal cytotoxic T-cell proliferation in chronic active Epstein-Barr virus infection in childhood. *Am J Clin Pathol* 2002;117:283–290.

30. Pedersen PR, Gerber P, Sweeney G, et al. Infectious mononucleosis preceding acute myelomonocytic leukemia. *Am J Med Sci* 1975;269:131–135.

31. Sakajiri S, Mori K, Isobe Y, et al. Epstein-Barr virus-associated T-cell acute lymphoblastic leukaemia. *Br J Haematol* 2002; 117:127–129.

32. Walter RB, Hong TC, Bachli EB. Life-threatening thrombocytopenia associated with acute Epstein-Barr virus infection in an older adult. *Ann Hematol* 2002;81:672–675.

33. Avci Z, Turul T, Catal F, et al. Thrombocytopenia and emperipolesis in a patient with hepatitis A infection. *Pediatr Hematol Oncol* 2002;19:67–70.

34. Viallard JF, Boiron JM, Parrens M, et al. Severe pancytopenia triggered by recombinant hepatitis B vaccine. *Br J Haematol* 2000;110:230–233.

35. Faurschou M, Nielsen OJ, Hansen PB, et al. Fatal virus-associated hemophagocytic syndrome associated with coexistent chronic active hepatitis B and acute hepatitis C virus infection. *Am J Hematol* 1999;61:135–138.

36. Gasparotto D, De Re V, Boiocchi M. Hepatitis C virus, B-cell proliferation and lymphomas. *Leuk Lymphoma* 2002;43: 747–751.

37. Paquette RL, Kuramoto K, Tran L, et al. Hepatitis C virus infection in acquired aplastic anemia. *Am J Hematol* 1998;58: 122–126.

38. Itterbeek P, Vandenberghe P, Nevens F, et al. Aplastic anemia after transplantation for non-A, non-B, non-C fulminant hepatic failure: case report and review of the literature. *Transpl Int* 2002;15:117–123.

39. Nakamura Y, Yamamoto S, Tanaka S, et al. Herpes simplex viral infection in human neonates: an immunohistochemical and electron microscopic study. *Hum Pathol* 1985;16:1091–1097.

40. Akashi K, Eizuru Y, Sumiyoshi Y, et al. Brief report: severe

infectious mononucleosis-like syndrome and primary human herpesvirus 6 infection in an adult. *N Engl J Med* 1993;329: 168–171.

41. Clark DA. Human herpesvirus 6 and human herpesvirus 7: emerging pathogens in transplant patients. *Int J Hematol* 2002;76[Suppl 2]:246–252.

42. Descamps V, Bouscarat F, Laglenne S, et al. Human herpesvirus 6 infection associated with anticonvulsant hypersensitivity syndrome and reactive haemophagocytic syndrome. *Br J Dermatol* 1997;137:605–608.

43. Dockrell DH. Human herpesvirus 6: molecular biology and clinical features. *J Med Microbiol* 2003;52:5–18.

44. Fujino Y, Nakajima M, Inoue H, et al. Human herpesvirus 6 encephalitis associated with hypersensitivity syndrome. *Ann Neurol* 2002;51:771–774.

45. Hanukoglu A, Somekh E. Infectious mononucleosis-like illness in an infant with acute herpesvirus 6 infection. *Pediatr Infect Dis J* 1994;13:750–751.

46. Hashimoto H, Maruyama H, Fujimoto K, et al. Hematologic findings associated with thrombocytopenia during the acute phase of exanthem subitum confirmed by primary human herpesvirus-6 infection. *J Pediatr Hematol Oncol* 2002;24: 211–214.

47. Kanegane C, Katayama K, Kyoutani S, et al. Mononucleosis-like illness in an infant associated with human herpesvirus 6 infection. *Acta Paediatr Jpn* 1995;37:227–229.

48. Lorenzana A, Lyons H, Sawaf H, et al. Human herpesvirus 6 infection mimicking juvenile myelomonocytic leukemia in an infant. *J Pediatr Hematol Oncol* 2002;24:136–141.

49. Penchansky L, Jordan JA. Transient erythroblastopenia of childhood associated with human herpesvirus type 6, variant B. *Am J Clin Pathol* 1997;108:127–132.

50. Sumiyoshi Y, Kikuchi M, Ohshima K, et al. A case of human herpesvirus-6 lymphadenitis with infectious mononucleosis-like syndrome. *Pathol Int* 1995;45:947–951.

51. Tanaka H, Nishimura T, Hakui M, et al. Human herpesvirus 6-associated hemophagocytic syndrome in a healthy adult. *Emerg Infect Dis* 2002;8:87–88.

52. Yasukawa M, Inoue Y, Ohminami H, et al. Apoptosis of CD4+ T lymphocytes in human herpesvirus-6 infection. *J Gen Virol* 1998;79:143–147.

53. Yoshikawa T, Ihira M, Suzuki K, et al. Fatal acute myocarditis in an infant with human herpesvirus 6 infection. *J Clin Pathol* 2001;54:792–795.

54. Asano Y, Suga S, Yoshikawa T, et al. Clinical features and viral excretion in an infant with primary human herpesvirus 7 infection. *Pediatrics* 1995;95:187–190.

55. Clark DA. Human herpesvirus 6 and human herpesvirus 7: emerging pathogens in transplant patients. *Int J Hematol* 2002;76[Suppl 2]:246–252.

56. Suga S, Yoshikawa T, Nagai T, et al. Clinical features and virological findings in children with primary human herpesvirus 7 infection. *Pediatrics* 1997;99:E4.

57. Amin HM, Medeiros LJ, Manning JT, et al. Dissolution of the lymphoid follicle is a feature of the HHV8+ variant of plasma cell Castleman's disease. *Am J Surg Pathol* 2003;27: 91–100.

58. Costes V, Faumont N, Cesarman E, et al. Human herpesvirus-8-associated lymphoma of the bowel in human immunodeficiency virus-positive patients without history of primary effusion lymphoma. *Hum Pathol* 2002;33:846–849.

59. Du MQ, Diss TC, Liu H, et al. KSHV- and EBV-associated germinotropic lymphoproliferative disorder. *Blood* 2002;100: 3415–3418.

60. Hengge UR, Ruzicka T, Tyring SK, et al. Update on Kaposi's sarcoma and other HHV8 associated diseases. Part 2: pathogenesis, Castleman's disease, and pleural effusion lymphoma. *Lancet Infect Dis* 2002;2:344–352.

61. Huang Q, Chang KL, Gaal K, et al. Primary effusion lymphoma with subsequent development of a small bowel mass in an HIV-seropositive patient: a case report and literature review. *Am J Surg Pathol* 2002;26:1363–1367.

62. Luppi M, Barozzi P, Rasini V, et al. Severe pancytopenia and hemophagocytosis after HHV-8 primary infection in a renal transplant patient successfully treated with foscarnet. *Transplantation* 2002;74:131–132.

63. Maric I, Washington S, Schwartz A, et al. Human herpesvirus-8-positive body cavity-based lymphoma involving the atria of the heart: a case report. *Cardiovasc Pathol* 2002;11:244–247.

64. Oksenhendler E, Boulanger E, Galicier L, et al. High incidence of Kaposi sarcoma-associated herpesvirus-related non-Hodgkin lymphoma in patients with HIV infection and multicentric Castleman disease. *Blood* 2002;99:2331–2336.

65. Bain BJ. Pathogenesis and pathophysiology of anemia in HIV infection. *Curr Opin Hematol* 1999;6:89–93.

66. Cole JL, Marzec UM, Gunthel CJ, et al. Ineffective platelet production in thrombocytopenic human immunodeficiency virus-infected patients. *Blood* 1998;91:3239–3246.

67. Katsarou O, Terpos E, Patsouris E, et al. Myelodysplastic features in patients with long-term HIV infection and haemophilia. *Haemophilia* 2001;7:47–52.

68. Kobessho H, Matsushita A, Takahashi K, et al. Hepatic encephalopathy in primary human immunodeficiency virus type 1 (HIV-1) infection. *Intern Med* 2002;41:1069–1072.

69. McArthur CP, Subtil-DeOliveira A, Palmer D, et al. Characteristics of salivary diffuse infiltrative lymphocytosis syndrome in West Africa. *Arch Pathol Lab Med* 2000;124:1773–1779.

70. Mehta K, Gascon P, Robboy S. The gelatinous bone marrow (serous atrophy) in patients with acquired immunodeficiency syndrome. Evidence of excess sulfated glycosaminoglycan. *Arch Pathol Lab Med* 1992;116:504–508.

71. Ryu T, Ikeda M, Okazaki Y, et al. Myelodysplasia associated with acquired immunodeficiency syndrome. *Intern Med* 2001;40:795–801.

72. Smith PR, Cavenagh JD, Milne T, et al. Benign monoclonal expansion of CD8+ lymphocytes in HIV infection. *J Clin Pathol* 2000;53:177–181.

73. Steeper TA, Horwitz CA, Hanson M, et al. Heterophil-negative mononucleosis-like illnesses with atypical lymphocytosis in patients undergoing seroconversions to the human immunodeficiency virus. *Am J Clin Pathol* 1988;90:169–174.

74. Zaunders J, Carr A, McNally L, et al. Effects of primary HIV-1 infection on subsets of CD4+ and CD8+ T lymphocytes. *AIDS* 1995;9:561–566.

75. Zucker-Franklin D, Termin CS, Cooper MC. Structural changes in the megakaryocytes of patients infected with the human immune deficiency virus (HIV-1). *Am J Pathol* 1989;134:1295–1303.

76. Busse PJ, Cunningham-Rundles C. Primary leptomeningeal lymphoma in a patient with concomitant CD4+ lymphocytopenia. *Ann Allergy Asthma Immunol* 2002;88:339–342.

77. Gubinelli E, Posteraro P, Girolomoni G. Idiopathic CD4+ T lymphocytopenia associated with disseminated flat warts and alopecia areata. *J Dermatol* 2002;29:653–656.

78. Stetson CL, Rapini RP, Tyring SK, et al. CD4+ T lymphocytopenia with disseminated HPV. *J Cutan Pathol* 2002;29:502–505.

79. Von Bernuth H, Knochel B, Winkler U, et al. Immunodeficiency with recurrent panlymphocytopenia, impaired maturation of B lymphocytes, impaired interaction of T and B lymphocytes, and impaired integrity of epithelial tissue: A variant of idiopathic CD4+ T lymphocytopenia? *Pediatr Allergy Immunol* 2002;13:381–384.

80. Yamauchi PS, Nguyen NQ, Grimes PE. Idiopathic CD4+T-cell lymphocytopenia associated with vitiligo. *J Am Acad Dermatol* 2002;46:779–782.

81. Kempf W, Margolin DH, Dezube BJ, et al. Clinicopathological characterization of an HIV-2-infected individual with two clonally unrelated primary lymphomas. *Am J Hematol* 2000;65: 302–306.

82. Sousa AE, Carneiro J, Meier-Schellersheim M, et al. CD4 T cell depletion is linked directly to immune activation in the pathogenesis of HIV-1 and HIV-2 but only indirectly to the viral load. *J Immunol* 2002;169:3400–3406.

83. Eiraku N, Hingorani R, Ijichi S, et al. Clonal expansion within CD4+ and CD8+ T cell subsets in human T lymphotropic virus type I-infected individuals. *J Immunol* 1998;161:6674–6680.

84. Kojima K, Hara M, Sawada T, et al. Human T-lymphotropic virus type I provirus and T-cell prolymphocytic leukemia. *Leuk Lymphoma* 2000;38:381–386.

85. Mortreux F, Gabet AS, Wattel E. Molecular and cellular aspects of HTLV-1 associated leukemogenesis *in vivo*. *Leukemia* 2003;17:26–38.

86. Sakai R, Maruta A, Tomita N, et al. Improvement of quality of life after splenectomy in an HTLV-I carrier with T-cell prolymphocytic leukemia. *Leuk Lymphoma* 1999;35:607–611.

87. Tsukasaki K, Koeffler P, Tomonaga M. Human T-lymphotropic virus type 1 infection. *Baillieres Best Pract Res Clin Haematol* 2000;13:231–243.

88. Glynn SA, Murphy EL, Wright DJ, et al. Laboratory abnormalities in former blood donors seropositive for human T-lymphotropic virus types 1 and 2: a prospective analysis. *Arch Pathol Lab Med* 2000;124:550–555.

89. Love JL, Marchioli CC, Dube S, et al. Expansion of clonotypic T-cell populations in the peripheral blood of asymptomatic Gran Chaco Amerindians infected with HTLV-IIB. *J Acquir Immune Defic Syndr Hum Retrovirol* 1998;18:178–185.

90. Rosenblatt JD, Giorgi JV, Golde DW, et al. Integrated human T-cell leukemia virus II genome in CD8+ T cells from a patient with "atypical" hairy cell leukemia: evidence for distinct T and B cell lymphoproliferative disorders. *Blood* 1988;71: 363–369.

91. To KF, Chan PK, Chan KF, et al. Pathology of fatal human infection associated with avian influenza A H5N1 virus. *J Med Virol* 2001;63:242–246.

92. Moss WJ, Monze M, Ryon JJ, et al. Prospective study of measles in hospitalized, human immunodeficiency virus (HIV)-infected and HIV-uninfected children in Zambia. *Clin Infect Dis* 2002;35:189–196.

93. Okada H, Kobune F, Sato TA, et al. Extensive lymphopenia due to apoptosis of uninfected lymphocytes in acute measles patients. *Arch Virol* 2000;145:905–920.

94. Okada H, Sato TA, Katayama A, et al. Comparative analysis of host responses related to immunosuppression between measles patients and vaccine recipients with live attenuated measles vaccines. *Arch Virol* 2001;146:859–874.

95. Pignata C, Fiore M, de Filippo S, et al. Apoptosis as a mechanism of peripheral blood mononuclear cell death after measles and varicella-zoster virus infections in children. *Pediatr Res* 1998;43:77–83.

96. Reddy SV, Kurihara N, Menaa C, et al. Osteoclasts formed by measles virus-infected osteoclast precursors from hCD46 transgenic mice express characteristics of pagetic osteoclasts. *Endocrinology* 2001;142:2898–2905.

97. Borkowski J, Amrikachi M, Hudnall SD. Fulminant parvovirus infection following erythropoietin treatment in a patient with acquired immunodeficiency syndrome. *Arch Pathol Lab Med* 2000;124:441–445.

98. Crook TW, Rogers BB, McFarland RD, et al. Unusual bone marrow manifestations of Parvovirus B19 infection in immunocompromised patients. *Hum Pathol* 2000;31:161–168.

99. Geetha D, Zachary JB, Baldado HM, et al. Pure red cell aplasia caused by Parvovirus B19 infection in solid organ transplant recipients: a case report and review of literature. *Clin Transpl* 2000;14:586–591.

100. Heegaard ED, Brown KE. Human Parvovirus B19. *Clin Microbiol Rev* 2002;15:485–505.

101. Heegaard ED, Madsen HO, Schmiegelow K. Transient pancytopenia preceding acute lymphoblastic leukaemia (pre-ALL) precipitated by Parvovirus B19. *Br J Haematol* 2001;114: 810–813.

102. Kailasam C, Brennand J, Cameron AD. Congenital Parvovirus B19 infection: experience of a recent epidemic. *Fetal Diagn Ther* 2001;16:18–22.

103. Koduri PR, Kumapley R, Valladares J, et al. Chronic pure red cell aplasia caused by Parvovirus B19 in AIDS: use of intravenous immunoglobulin—a report of eight patients. *Am J Hematol* 1999;61:16–20.

104. Larroche C, Scieux C, Honderlick P, et al. Spontaneous resolution of hemophagocytic syndrome associated with acute parvovirus B19 infection and concomitant Epstein-Barr virus reactivation in an otherwise healthy adult. *Eur J Clin Microbiol Infect Dis* 2002;21:739–742.

105. Moreux N, Ranchin B, Calvet A, et al. Chronic Parvovirus B19 infection in a pediatric lung transplanted patient. *Transplantation* 2002;73:565–568.

106. Myers B, Dolan G. Parvovirus-induced pancytopenia in a child with acquired haemolytic anaemia. *Clin Lab Haematol* 1997;19:277–278.

107. Osaki M, Matsubara K, Iwasaki T, et al. Severe aplastic anemia associated with human Parvovirus B19 infection in a patient without underlying disease. *Ann Hematol* 1999;78: 83–86.

108. Serjeant BE, Hambleton IR, Kerr S, et al. Haematological response to Parvovirus B19 infection in homozygous sickle-cell disease. *Lancet* 2001;358:1779–1780.

109. Van Horn DK, Mortimer PP, Young N, et al. Human Parvovirus-associated red cell aplasia in the absence of underlying hemolytic anemia. *Am J Pediatr Hematol Oncol* 1986;8:235–239.

110. Yarali N, Duru F, Sipahi T, et al. Parvovirus B19 infection reminiscent of myelodysplastic syndrome in three children with chronic hemolytic anemia. *Pediatr Hematol Oncol* 2000;17: 475–482.

111. Nguyen QT, Wong S, Heegaard ED, et al. Identification and characterization of a second novel human erythrovirus variant, A6. *Virology* 2002;301:374–380.

112. Takenaka H, Kishimoto S, Ichikawa R, et al. Virus-associated haemophagocytic syndrome caused by rubella in an adult. *Br J Dermatol* 1998;139:877–880.

113. Takeoka Y, Hino M, Oiso N, et al. Virus-associated hemophagocytic syndrome due to rubella virus and varicella-zoster virus dual infection in patient with adult idiopathic thrombocytopenic purpura. *Ann Hematol* 2001;80:361–364.

114. Grant RM, Weitzman SS, Sherman CG, et al. Fulminant disseminated Varicella Zoster virus infection without skin involvement. *J Clin Virol* 2002;24:7–12.

115. Pignata C, Fiore M, de Filippo S, et al. Apoptosis as a mechanism of peripheral blood mononuclear cell death after measles and varicella-zoster virus infections in children. *Pediatr Res* 1998;43:77–83.

116. Tamayose K, Sugimoto K, Ando M, Oshimi K. Mononucleosis syndrome and acute monocytic leukemia. *Eur J Haematol* 2002;68:236–238.

117. Tsukahara T, Yaguchi A, Horiuchi Y. Significance of monocytosis in varicella and herpes zoster. *J Dermatol* 1992;19:94–98.

Protozoa

1. Krause PJ. Babesiosis. *Med Clin North Am* 2002;86:361–373.
2. Auerbach M, Haubenstock A, Soloman G. Systemic babesiosis. Another cause of the hemophagocytic syndrome. *Am J Med* 1986; 80:301–303.
3. Slovut DP, Benedetti E, Matas AJ. Babesiosis and hemophagocytic syndrome in an asplenic renal transplant recipient. *Transplantation* 1996;62:537–539.
4. Asensi V, Tricas L, Meana A, et al. Visceral leishmaniasis and other severe infections in an adult patient with p47-phox-deficient chronic granulomatous disease. *Infection* 2000;28:171–174.
5. Hofman V, Marty P, Perrin C, et al. The histological spectrum of visceral leishmaniasis caused by *Leishmania infantum* MON-1 in acquired immune deficiency syndrome. *Hum Pathol* 2000;31:75–84.
6. Marom D, Offer I, Tamary H, et al. Hemophagocytic lymphohistiocytosis associated with visceral leishmaniasis. *Pediatr Hematol Oncol* 2001;18:65–70.
7. Tunc B, Ayata A. Hemophagocytic syndrome: a rare life-threatening complication of visceral leishmaniasis in a young boy. *Pediatr Hematol Oncol* 2001;18:531–536.
8. Abdalla SH. Peripheral blood and bone marrow leucocytes in Gambian children with malaria: numerical changes and evaluation of phagocytosis. *Ann Trop Paediatr* 1988;8:250–258.
9. Aouba A, Noguera ME, Clauvel JP, et al. Haemophagocytic syndrome associated with plasmodium vivax infection. *Br J Haematol* 2000;108:832–833.
10. el-Shoura SM. Falciparum malaria in naturally infected human patients: IV—ultrastructural changes in peripheral white blood cells. *Ann Parasitol Hum Comp* 1993;68:169–175.
11. Lee HK, Lim J, Kim M, et al. Immunological alterations associated with *Plasmodium vivax* malaria in South Korea. *Ann Trop Med Parasitol* 2001;95:31–39.
12. Ohno T, Shirasaka A, Sugiyama T, et al. Hemophagocytic syndrome induced by *Plasmodium falciparum* malaria infection. *Int J Hematol* 1996;64:263–266.
13. Wickramasinghe SN, Abdalla SH. Blood and bone marrow changes in malaria. *Baillieres Best Pract Res Clin Haematol* 2000; 13:277–299.
14. Vavra J, Yachnis AT, Shadduck JA, et al. Microsporidia of the genus *Trachipleistophora*—causative agents of human microsporidiosis: description of *Trachipleistophora anthropophthera* n. sp. (Protozoa: Microsporidia). *J Eukaryot Microbiol* 1998;45: 273–283.
15. Yachnis AT, Berg J, Martinez-Salazar A, et al. Disseminated microsporidiosis especially infecting the brain, heart, and kidneys. Report of a newly recognized pansporoblastic species in two symptomatic AIDS patients. *Am J Clin Pathol* 1996;106: 535–543.
16. Rasmussen LN, Dirdal M, Birkebaek NH. "Covert toxocariasis" in a child treated with low-dose diethylcarbamazine. *Acta Paediatr* 1993;82:116–118.
17. Brouland JP, Audouin J, Hofman P, et al. Bone marrow involvement by disseminated toxoplasmosis in acquired immunodeficiency syndrome: the value of bone marrow trephine biopsy and immunohistochemistry for the diagnosis. *Hum Pathol* 1996; 27:302–306.
18. Guccion JG, Benator DA, Gibert CL, et al. Disseminated toxoplasmosis and acquired immunodeficiency syndrome: diagnosis by transmission electron microscopy. *Ultrastruct Pathol* 1995;19:95–99.
19. Soulier-Lauper M, Zulian G, Pizzolato G, et al. Disseminated toxoplasmosis in a severely immunodeficient patient: demonstration of cysts in bone marrow smears. *Am J Hematol* 1991;38: 324–326.
20. Tsaparas YF, Brigden ML, Mathias R, et al. Proportion positive for Epstein-Barr virus, cytomegalovirus, human herpesvirus 6, *Toxoplasma,* and human immunodeficiency virus types 1 and 2 in heterophile-negative patients with an absolute lymphocytosis or an instrument-generated atypical lymphocyte flag. *Arch Pathol Lab Med* 2000;124:1324–1330.
21. Sartori AM, Lopes MH, Benvenuti LA, et al. Reactivation of Chagas' disease in a human immunodeficiency virus-infected patient leading to severe heart disease with a late positive direct microscopic examination of the blood. *Am J Trop Med Hyg* 1998;59:784–786.

Helminths

1. Molina MA, Cabezas MT, Gimenez MJ. *Mansonella perstans* filariasis in a HIV patient: finding in bone marrow. *Haematologica* 1999;84:861.
2. Pradhan S, Lahiri VL, Elhence BR, et al. Microfilaria of *Wuchereria bancrofti* in bone marrow smear. *Am J Trop Med Hyg* 1976; 25:199–200.
3. Rani S, Beohar PC. Microfilaria in bone marrow aspirate: a case report. *Acta Cytol* 1981;25:425–429.
4. Shenoi U, Pai RR, Pai U, et al. Microfilariae in bone marrow aspiration smears. *Acta Cytol* 1998;42:815–816.
5. Singh T, Rani S, Ahuja P. Microfilaria in bone marrow aspirate. *J Assoc Physicians India* 1983;31:745.

Infectious Mononucleosis

1. Akashi K, Eizuru Y, Sumiyoshi Y, et al. Brief report: severe infectious mononucleosis-like syndrome and primary human herpesvirus 6 infection in an adult. *N Engl J Med* 1993;329: 168–171.
2. Begovac J, Puntaric V, Borcic D, et al. Mononucleosis-like syndrome associated with a multisystem coxsackievirus type B3 infection in adolescence. *Eur J Pediatr* 1988;147: 426–427.
3. Brigden ML, Au S, Thompson S, et al. Infectious mononucleosis in an outpatient population: diagnostic utility of 2 automated hematology analyzers and the sensitivity and specificity of Hoagland's criteria in heterophile-positive patients. *Arch Pathol Lab Med* 1999;123:875–881.
4. Descamps V, Bouscarat F, Laglenne S, et al. Human herpesvirus 6 infection associated with anticonvulsant hypersensitivity syndrome and reactive haemophagocytic syndrome. *Br J Dermatol* 1997;137:605–608.
5. Felsenstein D, Carney WP, Iacoviello VR, et al. Phenotypic properties of atypical lymphocytes in cytomegalovirus-induced mononucleosis. *J Infect Dis* 1985;152:198–203.
6. Fisher MS Jr, Guerra CG, Hickman JR, et al. Peripheral blood lymphocyte apoptosis: a clue to the diagnosis of acute infectious mononucleosis. *Arch Pathol Lab Med* 1996;120:951–955.
7. Fujino Y, Nakajima M, Inoue H, et al. Human herpesvirus 6 encephalitis associated with hypersensitivity syndrome. *Ann Neurol* 2002;51:771–774.
8. Kanegane C, Katayama K, Kyoutani S, et al. Mononucleosis-like illness in an infant associated with human herpesvirus 6 infection. *Acta Paediatr Jpn* 1995;37:227–229.
9. Kobessho H, Matsushita A, Takahashi K, et al. Hepatic encephalopathy in primary human immunodeficiency virus type 1 (HIV-1) infection. *Intern Med* 2002;41:1069–1072.
10. Lach-Szyrma V, Brito-Babapulle F. The clinical significance of apoptotic cells in peripheral blood smears. *Clin Lab Haematol* 1999;21:277–280.
11. Nakahara K, Utsunomiya A, Hanada S, et al. Transient

appearance of CD3+ CD8+ T lymphocytes with monoclonal gene rearrangement of T-cell receptor beta locus. *Br J Haematol* 1998;100:411–414.

12. Playford EG, Phillips D, Looke DF, et al. Three cases of dengue 1 virus infection from islands in the Gulf of Thailand. *Commun Dis Intell* 1998;22:107–109.

13. Shiftan TA, Mendelsohn J. The circulating "atypical" lymphocyte. *Hum Pathol* 1978;9:51–61.

14. Steeper TA, Horwitz CA, Ablashi DV, et al. The spectrum of clinical and laboratory findings resulting from human herpesvirus-6 (HHV-6) in patients with mononucleosis-like illnesses not resulting from Epstein-Barr virus or cytomegalovirus. *Am J Clin Pathol* 1990;93:776–783.

15. Steeper TA, Horwitz CA, Hanson M, et al. Heterophil-negative mononucleosis-like illnesses with atypical lymphocytosis in patients undergoing seroconversions to the human immunodeficiency virus. *Am J Clin Pathol* 1988;90:169–174.

16. Sumiyoshi Y, Kikuchi M, Ohshima K, et al. A case of human herpesvirus-6 lymphadenitis with infectious mononucleosis-like syndrome. *Pathol Int* 1995;45:947–951.

17. Tamayose K, Sugimoto K, Ando M, et al. Mononucleosis syndrome and acute monocytic leukemia. *Eur J Haematol* 2002;68:236–238.

18. Tsaparas YF, Brigden ML, Mathias R, et al. Proportion positive for Epstein-Barr virus, cytomegalovirus, human herpesvirus 6, *Toxoplasma,* and human immunodeficiency virus types 1 and 2 in heterophile-negative patients with an absolute lymphocytosis or an instrument-generated atypical lymphocyte flag. *Arch Pathol Lab Med* 2000;124:1324–1330.

19. Crowley B, Dempsey J, Olujohungbe A, et al. Unusual manifestations of primary cytomegalovirus infection in patients without HIV infection and without organ transplants. *J Med Virol* 2002;68:237–240.

20. Malik UR, Oleksowicz L, Dutcher JP, et al. Atypical clonal T-cell proliferation in infectious mononucleosis. *Med Oncol* 1996;13:207–213.

Acute Infectious Lymphocytosis

1. Arribas JM, Fernandez GH, Escalera GI, et al. Acute infectious lymphocytosis associated to Giardia lamblia and Blastocystis hominis coinfection. *An Esp Pediatr* 2001;54:518–520.

2. Arnez M, Cizman M, Jazbec J, et al. Acute infectious lymphocytosis caused by coxsackievirus B2. *Pediatr Infect Dis J* 1996;15:1127–1128.

3. Bertotto A, de Felicis Arcangeli C, Spinozzi F, et al. Acute infectious lymphocytosis: phenotype of the proliferating cell. *Acta Paediatr Scand* 1985;74:633–635.

4. Grose C, Horwitz MS. Characterization of an enterovirus associated with acute infectious lymphocytosis. *J Gen Virol* 1976;30:347–355.

5. Kvasnicka HM, Thiele J, Ahmadi T. Bone marrow manifestation of Lyme disease (Lyme borreliosis). *Br J Haematol* 2003;120:723.

6. van der Sar A. Acute infectious lymphocytosis with Echo virus type 25. *West Indian Med J* 1979;28:185–188.

7. Ward PC. The lymphoid leukocytoses. *Postgrad Med* 1980;67:217–223.

8. Yalaburgi SB. Infectious lymphocytosis in a black girl. A case report. *S Afr Med J* 1984;65:219–220.

Bone Marrow Granulomas

1. Bhargava V, Farhi DC. Bone marrow granulomas: clinicopathologic findings in 72 cases and review of the literature. *Hematol Pathol* 1988;2:43–50.

2. Bodem CR, Hamory BH, Taylor HM, et al. Granulomatous bone marrow disease. A review of the literature and clinicopathologic analysis of 58 cases. *Medicine (Baltimore)* 1983;62:372–383.

3. Vilalta-Castel E, Valdes-Sanchez MD, Guerra-Vales JM, et al. Significance of granulomas in bone marrow: a study of 40 cases. *Eur J Haematol* 1988;41:12–16.

4. Johnston RB Jr. Clinical aspects of chronic granulomatous disease. *Curr Opin Hematol* 2001;8:17–22.

5. Nowaczyk MJ, Feigenbaum A, Silver MM, et al. Bone marrow involvement and obstructive jaundice in Farber lipogranulomatosis: clinical and autopsy report of a new case. *J Inherit Metab Dis* 1996;19:655–660.

6. Baughman RP, Teirstein AS, Judson MA, et al. Clinical characteristics of patients in a case control study of sarcoidosis. *Am J Respir Crit Care Med* 2001;164:1885–1889.

7. Mitarnun W. Granulomatous reaction in peripheral T-cell proliferative disease: a case report. *J Med Assoc Thai* 1997;80:795–798.

8. Ng T, Yeghen T, Pagliuca A, et al. Non-caseating granulomata associated with hypocellular myelodysplastic syndrome. *Leuk Lymphoma* 2000;39:397–403.

9. Tangen JM, Naess A, Aasen T, et al. Non-caseating granulomas in patients with hematologic malignancies. *Acta Med Scand* 1988;223:83–87.

10. Tefferi A, Li CY. Bone marrow granulomas associated with chronic natural killer cell lymphopoiesis. *Am J Hematol* 1997;54:258–262.

11. Kettle P, Allen DC. Bone marrow granulomas in infiltrating lobular breast cancer. *J Clin Pathol* 1997;50:166–168.

12. Stather D, Ford S, Kisilevsky R. Sarcoid, amyloid, and acute myocardial failure. *Mod Pathol* 1998;11:901–904.

13. Andersson DE, Langworth S, Newman HC, et al. Reversible bone marrow granulomas-adverse effect of oxyphenbutazone therapy. *Acta Med Scand* 1980;207:131–133.

14. Ben-Yehuda A, Bloom A, Lijovetzky G, et al. Chlorpromazine-induced liver and bone marrow granulomas associated with agranulocytosis. *Isr J Med Sci* 1990;26:449–451.

15. Kettaneh A, Fain O, Ziol M, et al. Minocycline-induced systemic adverse reaction with liver and bone marrow granulomas and Sezary-like cells. *Am J Med* 2000;108:353–354.

16. Rigberg LA, Robinson MJ, Espiritu CR. Chlorpropamide-induced granulomas. A probable hypersensitivity reaction in liver and bone marrow. *JAMA* 1976;235:409–410.

17. Siboni A, Mourits-Andersen T, Moesner J. Granulomatous bone marrow inflammation during treatment of chronic myeloid leukaemia with interferon alpha-2b. *J Clin Pathol* 1995;48:878–880.

18. Varkel Y, Braester A, Nusem D, et al. Methyldopa-induced syndrome of inappropriate antidiuretic hormone secretion and bone marrow granulomatosis. *Drug Intell Clin Pharm* 1988;22:700–701.

19. Yamreudeewong W, McIntyre WW, Sun TJ, et al. Bone marrow granulomas possibly associated with amiodarone. *Pharmacotherapy* 2000;20:855–859.

20. Dannenmaier WC, Haynes DW, Nelson CL. Granulomatous reaction and cystic bony destruction associated with high wear rate in a total knee prosthesis. *Clin Orthop* 1985;198:224–230.

21. Bianco P, Silvestrini G, Ballanti P, et al. Paramyxovirus-like nuclear inclusions identical to those of Paget's disease of bone detected in giant cells of primary oxalosis. *Virchows Arch A Pathol Anat Histopathol* 1992;421:427–433.

22. Schnitzler CM, Kok JA, Jacobs DW, et al. Skeletal manifestations of primary oxalosis. *Pediatr Nephrol* 1991;5:193–199.

23. Fide J, Gylseth B, Skaug V. Silicotic lesions of the bone marrow: histopathology and microanalysis. *Histopathology* 1984;8:693–703.

24. Pelstring RJ, Kim CK, Lower EE, et al. Marrow granulomas in coal workers' pneumoconiosis. A histologic study with elemental analysis. *Am J Clin Pathol* 1988;89:553–556.

25. Lewis JH, Sundeen JT, Simon GL, et al. Disseminated talc granulomatosis. An unusual finding in a patient with acquired immunodeficiency syndrome and fatal cytomegalovirus infection. *Arch Pathol Lab Med* 1985;109:147–150.

26. Mariani-Costantini R, Jannotta FS, Johnson FB. Systemic visceral talc granulomatosis associated with miliary tuberculosis in a drug addict. *Am J Clin Pathol* 1982;78:785–789.

27. Racela LS, Papasian CJ, Watanabe I, et al. Systemic talc granulomatosis associated with disseminated histoplasmosis in a drug abuser. *Arch Pathol Lab Med* 1988;112:557–560.

28. Grant AC, Hunter S, Partin WC. A case of acute monocytic ehrlichiosis with prominent neurologic signs. *Neurology* 1997;48:1619–1623.

29. Kvasnicka HM, Thiele J, Ahmadi T. Bone marrow manifestation of Lyme disease (Lyme borreliosis). *Br J Haematol* 2003;120:723.

30. Ruel M, Sevestre H, Henry-Biabaud E, et al. Fibrin ring granulomas in hepatitis A. *Dig Dis Sci* 1992;37:1915–1917.

31. Raya Sanchez JM, Arguelles HA, Brito Barroso ML, et al. Bone marrow fibrin-ring (doughnut) granulomas and peripheral T-cell lymphoma: an exceptional association. *Haematologica* 2001;86:112.

32. Srigley JR, Vellend H, Palmer N, et al. Q-fever. The liver and bone marrow pathology. *Am J Surg Pathol* 1985;9:752–758.

33. Young JF, Goulian M. Bone marrow fibrin ring granulomas and cytomegalovirus infection. *Am J Clin Pathol* 1993;99:65–68.

SYSTEMIC DISEASE

ENDOCRINE DISORDERS

Hyperthyroidism

Hyperthyroidism has been associated with diverse hematologic effects (1–5). The peripheral blood may show erythrocytosis, anemia, or pancytopenia. The bone marrow may show hypercellularity, arrested hematopoiesis, ringed sideroblasts, and/or osteoporosis. Concomitant pernicious anemia may be present (6). Complications of antithyroid medications include agranulocytosis, granulocytic maturation arrest and aplasia, sideroblastic anemia, aplastic anemia, and reactive bone marrow plasmacytosis (7–10).

Hypothyroidism

Hypothyroidism has been associated with decreased red blood cell mass and plasma volume (1,11–13). The peripheral blood characteristically shows macrocytic anemia with acanthocytes; however, the red blood cells are normocytic or microcytic in some cases. Severe hypothyroidism may be accompanied by pancytopenia, marrow hypoplasia, and myxedema or gelatinous transformation of the marrow (Fig. 15-1).

Hyperparathyroidism

Hyperparathyroidism, whether primary or secondary, produces effects on the bone marrow (14–19). Primary hyperparathyroidism is associated with anemia, marrow fibrosis, and osteosclerosis. Secondary hyperparathyroidism, usually seen in chronic renal failure, is associated with anemia and osteomalacia (renal osteodystrophy), directly proportional to the degree and duration of renal failure. Uremic serum contains cytokines and other factors that inhibit erythropoiesis. The anemia is normocytic and normochromic, with a mean hemoglobin level of 6.1 g/dL. The bone marrow shows mild to moderate hypocellularity owing to decreased erythropoiesis. Iron stores are typically increased. Erythropoietin therapy increases the serum hemoglobin level, erythropoiesis, and megakaryopoiesis and restores the myeloid:erythroid ratio and iron stores to normal levels.

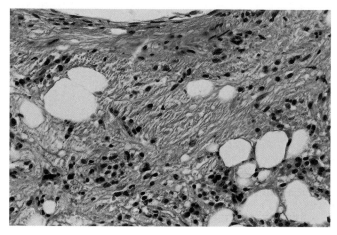

FIGURE 15-1. Bone marrow biopsy specimen, hypothyroidism and multiple myeloma. The stroma shows diffuse, amphophilic deposits of extracellular material. Although multiple myeloma may also be accompanied by stromal changes, in this case, the stromal findings are probably attributable to hypothyroidism.

IMMUNOLOGIC AND RELATED DISORDERS

Chronic Granulomatous Disease

Chronic granulomatous disease is a constitutional disorder of neutrophils in which production of superoxide dismutase is impaired (1–3) (Figs. 15-2 and 15-3). Bactericidal activity is therefore compromised, and characteristic granulomas are formed in numerous organs in response to infection. The bone marrow may show reactive neutrophilia, reactive histiocytosis, sea-blue histiocytes, and granulomas. In some cases, the histiocytes contain faint brownish pigment, probably lipofuscin or other oxidative product.

Common Variable Immunodeficiency

Common variable immunodeficiency is associated with anemia, cyclic thrombocytopenia, γ/δ T lymphocytosis, myelokathexis, and bone marrow granulomas (4–10). Complications include opportunistic infection and clonal lymphoproliferative disease.

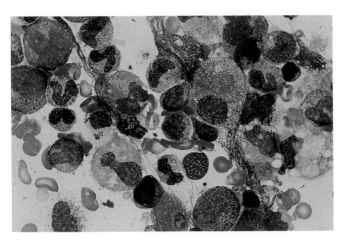

FIGURE 15-2. Bone marrow aspirate smear, chronic granulomatous disease. Neutrophils and histiocytes are increased. Faint pigment may be seen in the histiocytes.

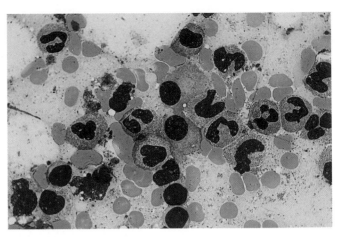

FIGURE 15-4. Bone marrow aspirate smear, systemic lupus erythematosus. Reactive plasmacytosis is present.

amyloidosis, opportunistic infections, osteoporosis, and clonal hematolymphoid disease (32–34).

Connective Tissue Disease

Connective tissue disease (systemic lupus erythematosus, rheumatoid arthritis, Sjögren syndrome, and other disorders) is accompanied by numerous hematologic changes (11–31) (Figs. 15-4 and 15-5). The peripheral blood may show iron deficiency anemia, immune-mediated cytopenias, anemia of chronic disease, T-cell large granular lymphocytosis, and/or hyperviscosity syndrome.

The bone marrow may show myelodysplastic changes, granulocytic maturation arrest, erythroid aplasia, increased apoptosis, alterations in blast count, benign lymphoid aggregates, reactive lymphocytosis, reactive plasmacytosis, storage histiocytosis, increased hemophagocytic activity, overt hemophagocytic syndrome, fibrosis, vasculitis, and gelatinous transformation. Complications include drug-induced cytopenias and hematopoietic hypoplasia, reactive and clonal

Necrotizing Lymphadenitis

Necrotizing lymphadenitis, or Kikuchi (-Fujimoto) disease, may be accompanied by hematologic abnormalities (35–42). The peripheral blood often shows cytopenias. The bone marrow may show granulocytic maturation arrest, erythroid hyperplasia, activated T lymphocytosis resembling malignant lymphoma, increased monocytes and histiocytes, and increased hemophagocytic activity or frank hemophagocytic syndrome. The differential diagnosis includes necrotizing lymphadenitis caused by an adverse drug reaction (39,42).

Sarcoidosis

Sarcoidosis is a disorder of unknown etiology that appears to be transmissible through stem cell transplantation (43–51) (Figs. 15-6 through 15-8). The peripheral blood may show

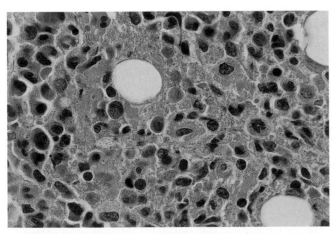

FIGURE 15-3. Bone marrow biopsy specimen, chronic granulomatous disease. Granulocytes and histiocytes are increased, and a granuloma is present. Faint pigment may be seen in the histiocytes.

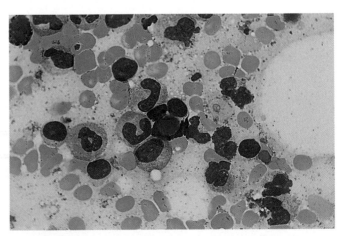

FIGURE 15-5. Bone marrow aspirate smear, systemic lupus erythematosus. An LE cell formed *in vivo* is present, compressing a neutrophil nucleus.

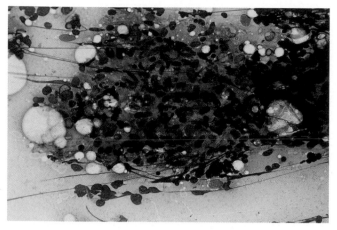

FIGURE 15-6. Bone marrow aspirate smear, sarcoidosis. A granuloma is present, composed of a tight cluster of histiocytes.

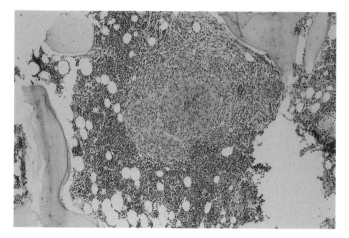

FIGURE 15-7. Bone marrow biopsy specimen, sarcoidosis. A well-formed granuloma is present in the intratrabecular space.

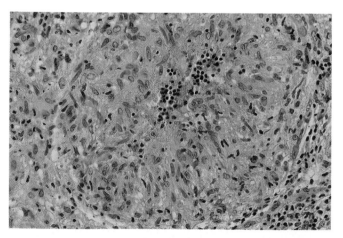

FIGURE 15-8. Bone marrow biopsy specimen, sarcoidosis. The granuloma is typical of sarcoidosis, composed of epithelioid histiocytes and a central aggregate of small lymphocytes.

anemia. When involved, the bone marrow contains well-formed granulomas composed of epithelioid histiocytes and lymphocytes. Other findings include vasculitis, increased hemophagocytosis, reactive and clonal amyloidosis, malignant lymphoma, and multiple myeloma. Clonal disease may obscure coexistent sarcoidosis, and vice versa.

BODY WEIGHT DISORDERS

Excess Body Weight

Excess body weight (obesity) affects hematopoiesis via leptin, a product of fat cells, and the leptin receptor, a protein expressed in hematopoietic stem cells (1). Leptin stimulates hematopoiesis, and obesity has been implicated as a risk factor for myelodysplastic syndromes and acute myeloid leukemia (2–5).

Low Body Weight

Low body weight, as seen in anorexia nervosa and other forms of starvation, is associated with numerous hematopoietic effects proportional to the degree of underweight (6–9). The peripheral blood shows acanthocytosis and decreased white blood cell, neutrophil, monocyte, and platelet counts. The hemoglobin and hematocrit may remain within the normal range until fat stores are severely depleted. The bone marrow shows trilineal hypoplasia or aplasia, shrunken or absent fat cells (serous fat atrophy), and gelatinous transformation, beginning in the distal skeleton and eventually involving the proximal femur (10,11). Hematopoietic cell necrosis and lymphocytic infiltration have been reported (12,13). Concomitant iron deficiency may be present (14). The hematologic changes are rapidly reversible with nutritional support. In some cases, granulocyte colony-stimulating factor and erythropoietin have been used to speed recovery.

SUBSTANCE ABUSE

Ethanol Abuse

Ethanol abuse, defined as the regular daily intake of more than 80 g of ethanol, is a common cause of hematologic abnormalities, usually reversible within days to weeks of discontinuing alcohol intake (1–7) (Table 15-1). The peripheral blood typically shows macrocytosis, often without anemia, and increased red cell distribution width. Aniso- and poikilocytosis are present in alcohol-induced sideroblastic anemia (Figs. 15-9 through 15-11). Lymphocytosis and thrombocytopenia may be present. The bone marrow characteristically shows dyserythropoiesis, vacuolation of erythroid and granulocytic precursors, and ringed sideroblasts. Megaloblastic hematopoiesis caused by dietary folate deficiency may be present. Other findings associated with alcoholism include

TABLE 15-1. EFFECTS OF ETHANOL ABUSE ON THE PERIPHERAL BLOOD AND BONE MARROW

Peripheral Blood	Bone Marrow
Macrocytosis	Dyserythropoiesis
Increased red cell distribution width	Erythroid and granulocytic precursor vacuolation
Anemia	Ringed sideroblasts
Lymphocytosis	Megaloblastic change caused by folate deficiency
Thrombocytopenia	Absent iron stores owing to hemorrhage
	Amegakaryocytic thrombocytopenia
	Hematopoietic hypoplasia
	Iron-containing plasma cells
	Gelatinous transformation
	Osteoporosis
	Osteonecrosis
	Fat necrosis attributable to alcohol-related pancreatitis

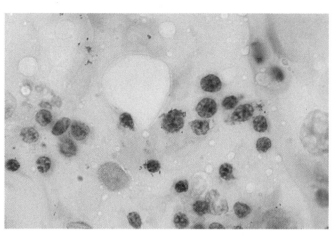

FIGURE 15-11. Bone marrow aspirate, ethanol abuse. Abundant ringed sideroblasts are seen in this specimen from a patient with sideroblastic anemia attributable to alcoholism (Prussian blue).

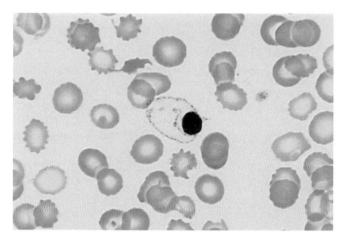

FIGURE 15-9. Peripheral blood smear, ethanol abuse. Striking red blood cell abnormalities are seen in this specimen from a patient with sideroblastic anemia attributable to alcoholism.

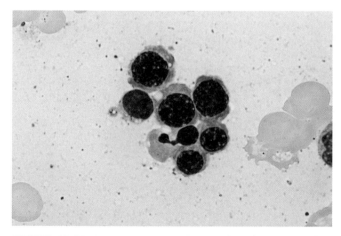

FIGURE 15-10. Bone marrow aspirate, ethanol abuse. A cluster of erythroid precursors, one showing a dysplastic nucleus, is seen in this specimen from a patient with sideroblastic anemia attributable to alcoholism.

absent histiocytic iron stores because of hemorrhage, vitamin B_6 (pyridoxine) deficiency, amegakaryocytic thrombocytopenia, trilineal hypoplasia, iron-containing plasma cells, gelatinous transformation, osteoporosis, osteonecrosis, and fat necrosis owing to alcohol-induced pancreatitis (8–14). Alcoholism is a risk factor for acute myeloid leukemia (15).

Cigarette Smoking

Cigarette smoking causes hematologic changes directly proportional to the number of pack-years smoked, cigarettes smoked per day, and years elapsed since cessation (4,16–19). Smoking-induced changes regress slowly after cessation, persisting for 5 years or more. The peripheral blood shows erythrocytosis caused by carbon monoxide–induced hypoxia. The absolute neutrophil, band, T-cell, B-cell, monocyte, and eosinophil counts are increased, with a more pronounced increase in neutrophils and a corresponding shift in the white blood cell differential count. Circulating neutrophils show phenotypic changes, including increased myeloperoxidase content. The bone marrow shows increased granulopoiesis with a shift toward mature segmented neutrophils, increased macrophages with phagocytic activity, and a higher percentage of dyserythropoietic cells and blasts. Smoking is a risk factor for acute myeloid and lymphoid leukemia and multiple myeloma and is associated with early onset of blast crisis and reduced survival in patients with chronic myeloid leukemia (20–23).

Drug Abuse

Drug abuse, both intravenous and nonintravenous, may cause bone marrow abnormalities. Intravenous drug abuse is associated with marrow eosinophilia, reactive plasmacytosis, and granulomatous inflammation (24–28). Granulomas may be attributable to infectious disease, talc (magnesium silicate), or both. Concomitant infection with human immunodeficiency virus, *Mycobacterium tuberculosis*, histoplasma capsulatum, and other organisms is relatively frequent in intravenous drug users and may produce additional abnormalities of the peripheral blood and bone marrow. Talc, a common contaminant of illicit intravenous drugs, appears in the bone marrow as intracellular, birefringent crystalline material, with or without a granulomatous reaction. Nonintravenous drug abuse has been reported to cause bone marrow necrosis and aplastic anemia (29,30).

REFERENCES

Endocrine Disorders

1. Das KC, Mukherjee M, Sarkar TK, et al. Erythropoiesis and erythropoietin in hypo- and hyperthyroidism. *J Clin Endocrinol Metab* 1975;40:211–220.
2. Justo Firvida E, Maceda Vilarino S, et al. Hyperthyroidism as a cause of chronic anemia. *An Med Interna* 1995;12:442–444.
3. Soeki T, Tamura Y, Kondo N, et al. A case of thyrotoxicosis with pancytopenia. *Endocr J* 2001;48:385–389.
4. Lahtinen R. Sideroblasts and haemosiderin in thyrotoxicosis. *Scand J Haematol* 1980;25:237–243.
5. Kelepouris N, Harper KD, Gannon F, et al. Severe osteoporosis in men. *Ann Intern Med* 1995;123:452–460.
6. Burns RW, Burns TW. Pancytopenia due to vitamin B12 deficiency associated with Graves' disease. *Mo Med* 1996;93:368–372.
7. Adorf D, Grajer KH, Kaboth W, et al. Agranulocytosis induced by antithyroid therapy: effects of treatment with granulocyte colony stimulating factor. *Clin Investig* 1994;72:390–392.
8. Breier DV, Rendo P, Gonzalez J, et al. Massive plasmocytosis due to methimazole-induced bone marrow toxicity. *Am J Hematol* 2001;67:259–261.
9. Mamianetti A, Munoz A, Ronchetti RD, et al. Acquired sideroblastic anemia and cholestasis in a hyperthyroid patient treated with methimazole and atenolol. *Medicina (B Aires)* 1995;55:693–696.
10. Mezquita P, Luna V, Munoz-Torres M, et al. Methimazole-induced aplastic anemia in third exposure: successful treatment with recombinant human granulocyte colony-stimulating factor. *Thyroid* 1998;8:791–794.
11. Horton L, Coburn RJ, England JM, et al. The haematology of hypothyroidism. *QJM* 1976;45:101–123.
12. Savage RA, Sipple C. Marrow myxedema. Gelatinous transformation of marrow ground substance in a patient with severe hypothyroidism. *Arch Pathol Lab Med* 1987;111:375–377.
13. Song SH, McCallum CJ, Campbell IW. Hypoplastic anaemia complicating myxoedema coma. *Scott Med J* 1998;43:149–150.
14. Boxer M, Ellman L, Geller R, et al. Anemia in primary hyperparathyroidism. *Arch Intern Med* 1977;137:588–593.
15. Boechat MI, Westra SJ, Van Dop C, et al. Decreased cortical and increased cancellous bone in two children with primary hyperparathyroidism. *Metabolism* 1996;45:76–81.
16. Allen DA, Breen C, Yaqoob MM, et al. Inhibition of CFU-E colony formation in uremic patients with inflammatory disease: role of IFN-gamma and TNF-alpha. *J Investig Med* 1999;47:204–211.
17. Alm JH, Yoon KS, Lee WI, et al. Bone marrow findings before and after treatment with recombinant human erythropoietin in chronic hemodialyzed patients. *Clin Nephrol* 1995;43:189–195.
18. Biljanovic-Paunovic L, Djukanovic L, Lezaic V, et al. *In vivo* effects of recombinant human erythropoietin on bone marrow hematopoiesis in patients with chronic renal failure. *Eur J Med Res* 1998;3:564–570.
19. Sikole A, Stojanovic A, Polenakovic M, et al. How erythropoietin affects bone marrow of uremic patients. *Am J Nephrol* 1997;17:128–136.

Immunologic and Related Disorders

1. Gahr M, Jendrossek V, Peters AM, et al. Sea blue histiocytes in the bone marrow of variant chronic granulomatous disease with residual monocyte NADPH-oxidase activity. *Br J Haematol* 1991;78:278–280.
2. Johnston RB Jr. Clinical aspects of chronic granulomatous disease. *Curr Opin Hematol* 2001;8:17–22.
3. Kottilil S, Malech HL, Gill VJ, et al. Infections with Haemophilus species in chronic granulomatous disease: insights into the interaction of bacterial catalase and H_2O_2 production. *Clin Immunol* 2003;106:226–230.
4. Christopoulos C, Papadaki T, Vlavianos P, et al. Hodgkin's disease in a patient with common variable immunodeficiency. *J Clin Pathol* 1995;48:871–873.
5. Fakhouri F, Robino C, Lemaire M, et al. Granulomatous renal disease in a patient with common variable immunodeficiency. *Am J Kidney Dis* 2001;38:E7.
6. Gottesman SR, Haas D, Ladanyi M, et al. Peripheral T cell lymphoma in a patient with common variable immunodeficiency disease: case report and literature review. *Leuk Lymphoma* 1999;32:589–595.
7. Gur H, Koldanov R, Segal A, et al. Common variable immunodeficiency associated with myelocathexis and altered membrane sodium-proton antiport. *Pathobiology* 1997;65:46–50.
8. Katial RK, Lieberman MM, Muehlbauer SL, et al. Gamma delta T lymphocytosis associated with common variable immunodeficiency. *J Clin Immunol* 1997;17:34–42.
9. Kubota M, Nakamura K, Watanabe K, et al. A case of common variable immunodeficiency associated with cyclic thrombocytopenia. *Acta Paediatr Jpn* 1994;36:690–692.
10. Lin WC, Dai YS, Tsai MJ, et al. Systemic Penicillium marneffei infection in a child with common variable immunodeficiency. *J Formos Med Assoc* 1998;97:780–783.
11. Bowman SJ. Hematological manifestations of rheumatoid arthritis. *Scand J Rheumatol* 2002;31:251–259.
12. Coakley G, Brooks D, Iqbal M, et al. Major histocompatibility complex haplotypic associations in Felty's syndrome and large granular lymphocyte syndrome are secondary to allelic association with HLA-DRB1 *0401. *Rheumatology (Oxford)* 2000;39:393–398.
13. Friedman J, Klepfish A, Miller EB, et al. Agranulocytosis in Sjogren's syndrome: two case reports and analysis of 11 additional reported cases. *Semin Arthritis Rheum* 2002;31:338–345.
14. Funato K, Kuriyama Y, Uchida Y, et al. Myelodysplastic syndrome accompanied by Addison's disease and multiple autoimmune phenomena: steroid therapy resolved cytopenias and all immune disorders. *Intern Med* 2001;40:1041–1044.
15. Hellmich B, Csernok E, Schatz H, et al. Autoantibodies against granulocyte colony-stimulating factor in Felty's syndrome and neutropenic systemic lupus erythematosus. *Arthritis Rheum* 2002;46:2384–2391.
16. Kokori SI, Ioannidis JP, Voulgarelis M, et al. Autoimmune hemolytic anemia in patients with systemic lupus erythematosus. *Am J Med* 2000;108:198–204.

17. Kumakura S, Kobayashi S, Ishikura H. Neutrophil phagocytosis in Felty's syndrome. *Am J Med* 2001;111:579–580.

18. La Montagna G, Baruffo A, Abbadessa A, et al. Pure red cell aplasia in Felty's syndrome: a case report of successful reversal after cyclosporin A treatment. *Clin Rheumatol* 1999;18:244–247.

19. Lin SJ, Jaing TH. Thrombocytopenia in systemic-onset juvenile chronic arthritis: report of two cases with unusual bone marrow features. *Clin Rheumatol* 1999;18:241–243.

20. Min JK, Cho CS, Kim HY, et al. Bone marrow findings in patients with adult Still's disease. *Scand J Rheumatol* 2003;32:119–121.

21. Papadaki HA, Boumpas DT, Gibson FM, et al. Increased apoptosis of bone marrow CD34(+) cells and impaired function of bone marrow stromal cells in patients with systemic lupus erythematosus. *Br J Haematol* 2001;115:167–174.

22. Papadaki HA, Kritikos HD, Valatas V, et al. Anemia of chronic disease in rheumatoid arthritis is associated with increased apoptosis of bone marrow erythroid cells: improvement following anti-tumor necrosis factor-alpha antibody therapy. *Blood* 2002; 100:474–482.

23. Paquette RL, Meshkinpour A, Rosen PJ. Autoimmune myelofibrosis. A steroid-responsive cause of bone marrow fibrosis associated with systemic lupus erythematosus. *Medicine (Baltimore)* 1994;73:145–152.

24. Pereira RM, Velloso ER, Menezes Y, et al. Bone marrow findings in systemic lupus erythematosus patients with peripheral cytopenias. *Clin Rheumatol* 1998;17:219–222.

25. Sawhney S, Woo P, Murray KJ. Macrophage activation syndrome: a potentially fatal complication of rheumatic disorders. *Arch Dis Child* 2001;85:421–426.

26. Starkebaum G, Loughran TP Jr, Gaur LK, et al. Immunogenetic similarities between patients with Felty's syndrome and those with clonal expansions of large granular lymphocytes in rheumatoid arthritis. *Arthritis Rheum* 1997;40:624–626.

27. Stephan JL, Kone-Paut I, Galambrun C, et al. Reactive haemophagocytic syndrome in children with inflammatory disorders. A retrospective study of 24 patients. *Rheumatology (Oxford)* 2001;40:1285–1292.

28. Takahashi K, Kumakura S, Ishikura H, et al. Reactive hemophagocytosis in systemic lupus erythematosus. *Intern Med* 1998;37: 550–553.

29. Tanvetyanon T, Leighton JC. Severe anemia and marrow plasmacytosis as presentation of Sjogren's syndrome. *Am J Hematol* 2002;69:233.

30. Voulgarelis M, Kokori SI, Ioannidis JP, et al. Anaemia in systemic lupus erythematosus: aetiological profile and the role of erythropoietin. *Ann Rheum Dis* 2000;59:217–222.

31. Zakzook SI, Yunus MB, Mulconrey DS. Hyperviscosity syndrome in rheumatoid arthritis with Felty's syndrome: case report and review of the literature. *Clin Rheumatol* 2002;21:82–85.

32. Delevaux I, Andre M, Amoura Z, et al. Concomitant diagnosis of primary Sjogren's syndrome and systemic AL amyloidosis. *Ann Rheum Dis* 2001;60:694–695.

33. Kolte B, Baer AN, Sait SN, et al. Acute myeloid leukemia in the setting of low dose weekly methotrexate therapy for rheumatoid arthritis. *Leuk Lymphoma* 2001;42:371–378.

34. McCarthy CJ, Sheldon S, Ross CW, et al. Cytogenetic abnormalities and therapy-related myelodysplastic syndromes in rheumatic disease. *Arthritis Rheum* 1998;41:1493–1496.

35. Chmait RH, Meimin DL, Koo CH, et al. Hemophagocytic syndrome in pregnancy. *Obstet Gynecol* 2000;95:1022–1024.

36. Hussein A, Hellquist HB. Necrotizing lymphadenitis of the neck (Kikuchi's disease). *APMIS* 1994;102:633–637.

37. Kelly J, Kelleher K, Khan MK, et al. A case of haemophagocytic syndrome and Kikuchi-Fujimoto disease occurring concurrently in a 17-year-old female. *Int J Clin Pract* 2000;54:547–549.

38. Lima M, Silvestre F, Correia J, et al. Kikuchi's disease: a case report with emphasis on flow cytometric studies. *Sangre (Barc)* 1996;41: 383–386.

39. Lorand-Metze I, Vassallo J, Mori S. Histiocytic necrotizing lymphadenitis in Brazil: report of a case and review of the literature. *Pathol Int* 1994;44:548–550.

40. Mahadeva U, Allport T, Bain B, et al. Haemophagocytic syndrome and histiocytic necrotising lymphadenitis (Kikuchi's disease). *J Clin Pathol* 2000;53:636–638.

41. Sumiyoshi Y, Kikuchi M, Ohshima K, et al. A case of histiocytic necrotizing lymphadenitis with bone marrow and skin involvement. *Virchows Arch A Pathol Anat Histopathol* 1992;420: 275–279.

42. Lau G, Kwan C, Chong SM. The 3-week sulphasalazine syndrome strikes again. *Forensic Sci Int* 2001;122:79–84.

43. Baughman RP, Teirstein AS, Judson MA, et al. Clinical characteristics of patients in a case control study of sarcoidosis. *Am J Respir Crit Care Med* 2001;164:1885–1889.

44. Fernandes SR, Singsen BH, Hoffman GS. Sarcoidosis and systemic vasculitis. *Semin Arthritis Rheum* 2000;30:33–46.

45. Haran MZ, Feldberg E, Berrebi A. Lymphoma masking sarcoidosis. *Leuk Lymphoma* 2002;43:1709–1710.

46. Kobayashi H, Kato Y, Hakamada M, et al. Malignant lymphoma of the bone associated with systemic sarcoidosis. *Intern Med* 2001;40:435–438.

47. Lower EE, Smith JT, Martelo OJ, et al. The anemia of sarcoidosis. *Sarcoidosis* 1988;5:51–55.

48. Padilla ML, Schilero GJ, Teirstein AS. Donor-acquired sarcoidosis. *Sarcoidosis Vasc Diffuse Lung Dis* 2002;19:18–24.

49. Sen F, Mann KP, Medeiros LJ. Multiple myeloma in association with sarcoidosis. *Arch Pathol Lab Med* 2002;126:365–368.

50. Stather D, Ford S, Kisilevsky R. Sarcoid, amyloid, and acute myocardial failure. *Mod Pathol* 1998;11:901–904.

51. Taylor HG, Berenberg JL. Bone marrow phagocytosis in sarcoidosis. *Arch Intern Med* 1982;142:479–480.

Body Weight Disorders

1. Fantuzzi G, Faggioni R. Leptin in the regulation of immunity, inflammation, and hematopoiesis. *J Leukoc Biol* 2000;68: 437–446.

2. Estey E, Thall P, Kantarjian H, et al. Association between increased body mass index and a diagnosis of acute promyelocytic leukemia in patients with acute myeloid leukemia. *Leukemia* 1997;11:1661–1664.

3. Hino M, Nakao T, Yamane T, et al. Leptin receptor and leukemia. *Leuk Lymphoma* 2000;36:457–461.

4. Konopleva M, Mikhail A, Estrov Z, et al. Expression and function of leptin receptor isoforms in myeloid leukemia and myelodysplastic syndromes: proliferative and anti-apoptotic activities. *Blood* 1999;93:1668–1676.

5. Laharrague P, Oppert JM, Brousset P, et al. High concentration of leptin stimulates myeloid differentiation from human bone marrow CD34+ progenitors: potential involvement in leukocytosis of obese subjects. *Int J Obes Relat Metab Disord* 2000;24:1212–1216.

6. Abella E, Feliu E, Granada I, et al. Bone marrow changes in anorexia nervosa are correlated with the amount of weight loss and not with other clinical findings. *Am J Clin Pathol* 2002;118: 582–588.

7. Lambert M, Hubert C, Depresseux G, et al. Hematological changes in anorexia nervosa are correlated with total body fat mass depletion. *Int J Eat Disord* 1997;21:329–334.

8. Orlandi E, Boselli P, Covezzi R, et al. Reversal of bone marrow hypoplasia in anorexia nervosa: case report. *Int J Eat Disord* 2000;27:480–482.

9. Saito S, Kita K, Morioka CY, Watanabe A. Rapid recovery from anorexia nervosa after a life-threatening episode with severe thrombocytopenia: report of three cases. *Int J Eat Disord* 1999;25:113–118.

10. Geiser F, Murtz P, Lutterbey G, et al. Magnetic resonance spectroscopic and relaxometric determination of bone marrow changes in anorexia nervosa. *Psychosom Med* 2001;63:631–637.

11. Vande Berg BC, Malghem J, Lecouvet FE, et al. Distribution of serouslike bone marrow changes in the lower limbs of patients with anorexia nervosa: predominant involvement of the distal extremities. *AJR Am J Roentgenol* 1996;166:621–625.

12. Smith RR, Spivak JL. Marrow cell necrosis in anorexia nervosa and involuntary starvation. *Br J Haematol* 1985;60:525–530.

13. Fukudo S, Tanaka A, Muranaka M, et al. Case report: reversal of severe leukopenia by granulocyte colony-stimulating factor in anorexia nervosa. *Am J Med Sci* 1993;305:314–317.

14. Nonaka D, Tanaka M, Takaki K, et al. Gelatinous bone marrow transformation complicated by self-induced malnutrition. *Acta Haematol* 1998;100:88–90.

Substance Abuse

1. Budde R, Hellerich U. Alcohol dyshaematopoiesis: morphological features of alcohol-induced bone marrow damage in biopsy sections compared with aspiration smears. *Acta Haematol* 1995;94:74–77.

2. Fink A, Hays RD, Moore AA, et al. Alcohol-related problems in older persons. Determinants, consequences, and screening. *Arch Intern Med* 1996;156:1150–1156.

3. Maruyama S, Hirayama C, Yamamoto S, et al. Red blood cell status in alcoholic and non-alcoholic liver disease. *J Lab Clin Med* 2001;138:332–337.

4. Michot F, Gut J. Alcohol-induced bone marrow damage. A bone marrow study in alcohol-dependent individuals. *Acta Haematol* 1987;78:252–257.

5. Parry H, Cohen S, Schlarb JE, et al. Smoking, alcohol consumption, and leukocyte counts. *Am J Clin Pathol* 1997;107:64–67.

6. Savage DG, Ogundipe A, Allen RH, et al. Etiology and diagnostic evaluation of macrocytosis. *Am J Med Sci* 2000;319:343–352.

7. Seppa K, Sillanaukee P, Saarni M. Blood count and hematologic morphology in nonanemic macrocytosis: differences between alcohol abuse and pernicious anemia. *Alcohol* 1993;10:343–347.

8. Gewirtz AM, Hoffman R. Transitory hypomegakaryocytic thrombocytopenia: aetiological association with ethanol abuse and implications regarding regulation of human megakaryocytopoiesis. *Br J Haematol* 1986;62:333–344.

9. Nakao S, Harada M, Kondo K, et al. Reversible bone marrow hypoplasia induced by alcohol. *Am J Hematol* 1991;37:120–123.

10. Wulfhekel U, Dullmann J. Storage of iron in bone marrow plasma cells. Ultrastructural characterization, mobilization, and diagnostic significance. *Acta Haematol* 1999;101:7–15.

11. Bohm J. Gelatinous transformation of the bone marrow: the spectrum of underlying diseases. *Am J Surg Pathol* 2000;24:56–65.

12. Kelepouris N, Harper KD, Gannon F, et al. Severe osteoporosis in men. *Ann Intern Med* 1995;123:452–460.

13. Hernigou P, Beaujean F. Abnormalities in the bone marrow of the iliac crest in patients who have osteonecrosis secondary to corticosteroid therapy or alcohol abuse. *J Bone Joint Surg Am* 1997;79:1047–1053.

14. Ahn BC, Lee J, Suh KJ, et al. Intramedullary fat necrosis of multiple bones associated with pancreatitis. *J Nucl Med* 1998;39:1401–1404.

15. Crane MM, Strom SS, Halabi S, et al. Correlation between selected environmental exposures and karyotype in acute myelocytic leukemia. *Cancer Epidemiol Biomarkers Prev* 1996;5:639–644.

16. Budde R, Schaefer HE. Smokers' dysmyelopoiesis—bone marrow alterations associated with cigarette smoking. *Pathol Res Pract* 1989;185:347–350.

17. Fernandez-Ferrero S, Ramos F. Dyshaemopoietic bone marrow features in healthy subjects are related to age. *Leuk Res* 2001;25:187–189.

18. Schwartz J, Weiss ST. Cigarette smoking and peripheral blood leukocyte differentials. *Ann Epidemiol* 1994;4:236–4242.

19. van Eeden SF, Hogg JC. The response of human bone marrow to chronic cigarette smoking. *Eur Respir J* 2000;15:915–921.

20. Crane MM, Strom SS, Halabi S, et al. Correlation between selected environmental exposures and karyotype in acute myelocytic leukemia. *Cancer Epidemiol Biomarkers Prev* 1996;5:639–644.

21. Mills PK, Newell GR, Beeson WL, et al. History of cigarette smoking and risk of leukemia and myeloma: results from the Adventist health study. *J Natl Cancer Inst* 1990;82:1832–1836.

22. Sandler DP, Shore DL, Anderson JR, et al. Cigarette smoking and risk of acute leukemia: associations with morphology and cytogenetic abnormalities in bone marrow. *J Natl Cancer Inst* 1993;85:1994–2003.

23. Archimbaud E, Maupas J, Lecluze-Palazzolo C, et al. Influence of cigarette smoking on the presentation and course of chronic myelogenous leukemia. *Cancer* 1989;63:2060–2065.

24. Gonzalez Aza C, Grilo Reina A, Lopez Martin JC, et al. Changes in bone marrow among HIV-positive and HIV-negative parenteral drug addicts. *Med Clin (Barc)* 1995;104:89–91.

25. Kringsholm B, Christoffersen P. The nature and the occurrence of birefringent material in different organs in fatal drug addiction. *Forensic Sci Int* 1987;34:53–62.

26. Lewis JH, Sundeen JT, Simon GL, et al. Disseminated talc granulomatosis. An unusual finding in a patient with acquired immunodeficiency syndrome and fatal cytomegalovirus infection. *Arch Pathol Lab Med* 1985;109:147–150.

27. Mariani-Costantini R, Jannotta FS, Johnson FB. Systemic visceral talc granulomatosis associated with miliary tuberculosis in a drug addict. *Am J Clin Pathol* 1982;78:785–789.

28. Racela LS, Papasian CJ, Watanabe I, et al. Systemic talc granulomatosis associated with disseminated histoplasmosis in a drug abuser. *Arch Pathol Lab Med* 1988;112:557–560.

29. Marsh JC, Abboudi ZH, Gibson FM, et al. Aplastic anaemia following exposure to 3,4-methylenedioxymethamphetamine ('Ecstasy'). *Br J Haematol* 1994;88:281–285.

30. Moore J, Ma DD, Concannon A. Non-malignant bone marrow necrosis: a report of two cases. *Pathology* 1998;30:318–320.

16

EFFECTS OF THERAPY

Numerous therapeutic agents are used in treating hematolymphoid disorders, and their effects are diverse. This section focuses on morphologic changes observed in the peripheral blood and bone marrow as a result of these agents.

CYTOTOXIC CHEMOTHERAPY

Cytotoxic chemotherapy usually entails a combination of several different agents, with the goal of reducing or eliminating tumor cells (Figs. 16-1 through 16-4). Normal hematopoietic and stromal cells are also affected.

This type of therapy produces three morphologic stages in the bone marrow: cell death within the first week, hypocellularity at 1 to 2 weeks, and regeneration at approximately 2 weeks and thereafter (1–4). The first posttherapy marrow biopsy specimen is usually taken at 2 weeks (14 days), and thus the initial stages of cell death are often missed. At 10 to 14 days, the marrow is usually depleted of hematopoietic cells. Aspirate smears may show eosinophilic ground substance and mucoid strands between particles. Sections show the absence of hematopoietic cells, with a relative sparing of or increase in lymphocytes and plasma cells. The marrow sinusoids are dilated. The intersinusoidal area is filled with

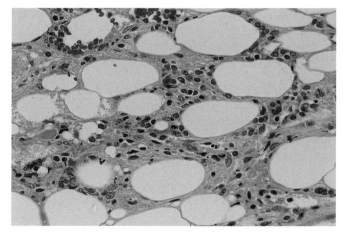

FIGURE 16-2. Bone marrow biopsy specimen, hypoplasia after cytotoxic chemotherapy. Hematopoietic tissue is virtually absent, leaving stromal cells, lymphocytes, plasma cells, and histiocytes.

loose fibrinous material, hemorrhage, and foamy histiocytes. Fat cells are shrunken and surrounded by eosinophilic material. The persistence of leukemic blasts at this point is a poor prognostic sign.

Regeneration begins with the appearance of small erythroid colonies in the interstitial space (sometimes as early as

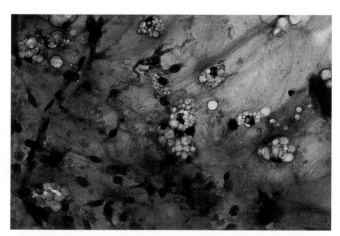

FIGURE 16-1. Bone marrow aspirate, hypoplasia after combination chemotherapy. A particle consists almost entirely of stromal cells and foamy histiocytes.

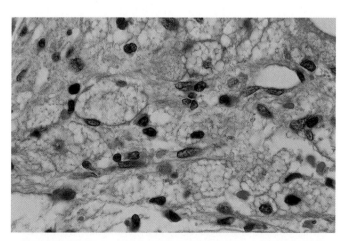

FIGURE 16-3. Bone marrow biopsy specimen, hypoplasia after cytotoxic chemotherapy. Foamy histiocytes are prominent.

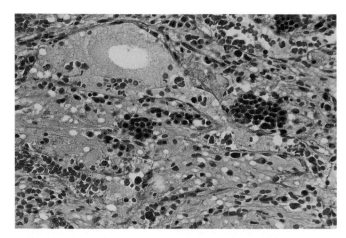

FIGURE 16-4. Bone marrow biopsy specimen, regeneration after cytotoxic chemotherapy. Erythroid islands are seen in a background of stromal collapse and dilated sinusoids.

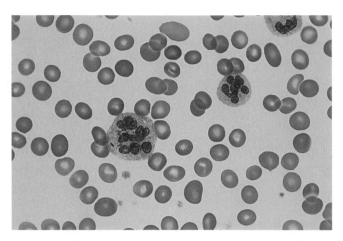

FIGURE 16-6. Peripheral blood smear, methotrexate effect. A segmented neutrophil shows megaloblastic change.

5 days), followed by scattered myeloid precursors, and finally by megakaryocytes. Hematopoietic dysplasia may be present during regeneration, which should not necessarily be taken as evidence of recurrent disease. During this phase, it may be difficult to differentiate normal precursors from leukemic blasts. Immunophenotyping and cytogenetic studies may be helpful in this regard. Ultimately, repeat biopsy after the passage of time is the most reliable way to ascertain whether tumor is present. Concomitant with marrow regrowth is a recovery in peripheral blood cell counts.

Specific bone marrow changes are difficult to link with specific agents because most cases are treated with multiagent chemotherapy. Dysplastic changes, both transient and permanent (clonal), occur with many of the commonly used drugs. Megaloblastic change is particularly associated with hydroxyurea and methotrexate (Figs. 16-5 and 16-6).

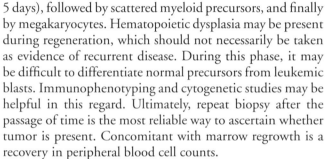

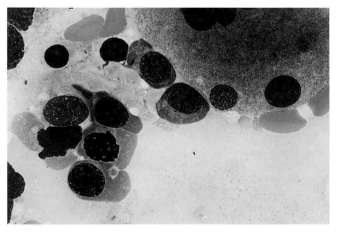

FIGURE 16-5. Peripheral blood smear, hydroxyurea effect. Erythroid precursors show megaloblastic change in this specimen from a patient with essential thrombocythemia treated with hydroxyurea.

DIFFERENTIATION THERAPY

Differentiation therapy is used in the treatment of granulocytic malignancies, primarily acute promyelocytic leukemia (Table 16-1). It not only induces maturation in the malignant cells but in many instances eliminates the malignant clone without affecting normal hematopoietic cells. Differentiation therapy is frequently combined with cytotoxic therapy for greater efficacy.

All-*trans*-Retinoic Acid

All-*trans* retinoic acid (ATRA) has been successfully used in the treatment of acute promyelocytic leukemia and promyelocytic blast crisis of chronic myeloid leukemia, with both the standard t(15;17) and variant translocations (1–13). ATRA initially produces peripheral leukocytosis, followed by morphologic, cytochemical, and functional maturation of malignant promyelocytes to segmented neutrophils. Maturation is evident in the peripheral blood, bone marrow, and extramedullary sites. Although the cells mature, they retain the t(15;17) or variant translocation. The neutrophils may show retained Auer rods, nuclear filaments and blebs, and a paucity of secondary granules. Eventually, normal segmented neutrophils replace those derived from the clonal cells.

Adverse bone marrow effects of ATRA therapy include necrosis and fibrosis, reversible with cessation of therapy (12,13).

TABLE 16-1. DIFFERENTIATION THERAPY ASSOCIATED WITH HEMATOPOIETIC CHANGES

All-trans retinoic acid
Arsenic trioxide

Arsenic Trioxide

Arsenic trioxide has also been used in acute promyelocytic leukemia to promote granulocytic differentiation and induce remission (14–22). Arsenic trioxide initially induces leukopenia, followed in 15 to 20 days by leukocytosis, with maturing granulocytes. At the same time, the marrow blast count decreases, granulocytic progenitors mature, and apoptosis may be observed. Maturation is seen in both peripheral blood and marrow granulocytic precursors. Adverse effects are similar to those seen with the use of ATRA, including retinoic acid syndrome during the phase of leukocytosis and marrow necrosis.

HEMATOPOIETIC GROWTH FACTORS

Hematopoietic growth factors are used primarily to promote recovery of peripheral cell counts after chemotherapy and radiotherapy but have also, on occasion, helped to produce clinical remission of clonal hematopoietic disease (Table 16-2).

Erythropoietin

Erythropoietin (EPO) has been successfully used to promote erythropoiesis in anemic patients with chronic renal failure, myelodysplastic syndrome, recovery from cytotoxic chemotherapy, and normal marrow donors (1–6) (Fig. 16-7).

In patients with chronic renal failure treated with EPO, the peripheral blood shows an increase in hemoglobin from an average of 6 to 10 gm/dL. The bone marrow shows increased cellularity, increased erythropoiesis with a concomitant reduction in the myeloid:erythroid ratio, and decreased intracellular iron stores.

Hematopoietic complications of EPO therapy include rapid iron utilization, requiring concomitant iron therapy. Neutralizing antibodies to EPO may develop, resulting in intractable pure red cell aplasia (7,8). In myelodysplastic syndrome, EPO may produce accelerated disease or apparent conversion to acute leukemia, reversible on discontinuation of the drug (9). In patients with erythroid hypoplasia caused by Parvovirus B19 infection, the administration of EPO may unmask characteristic pathologic changes (10).

TABLE 16-2. GROWTH FACTORS ASSOCIATED WITH HEMATOPOIETIC CHANGES

Erythropoietin
Granulocyte and granulocyte/macrophage colony-stimulating factors
Thrombopoietin

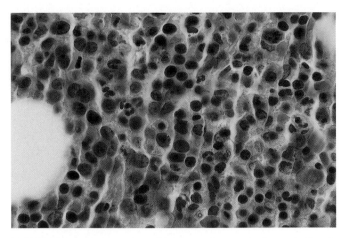

FIGURE 16-7. Bone marrow biopsy specimen, erythropoietin effect. The bone marrow is hypercellular, predominantly owing to proliferating erythroid precursors.

Granulocyte and Granulocyte-Macrophage Colony-Stimulating Factors

Granulocyte and granulocyte-macrophage colony-stimulating factors (G/GM-CSFs) are used to ameliorate neutropenia and prevent infection (11) (Figs. 16-8 through 16-10). In myelodysplastic syndromes, G-CSF reduces ineffective hematopoiesis, possibly by inducing neutrophil differentiation (12). This effect may underlie the G/GM-CSF–induced remissions reported in myelodysplastic syndrome, chronic myeloid leukemia, and acute promyelocytic leukemia (13,14).

After therapy, the peripheral blood shows a rapid, transient increase in the white blood cell count, consisting predominantly of neutrophils and immature neutrophilic precursors (15,16). The white blood cell count may reach nearly 90×10^9 cells/L. Monocytes, lymphocytes, eosinophils, basophils, and nucleated red blood cells are often increased.

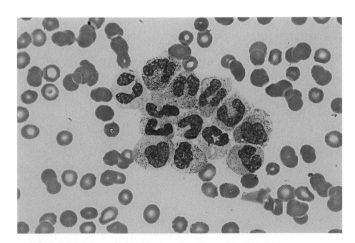

FIGURE 16-8. Peripheral blood smear, granulocyte colony-stimulating factor effect. Neutrophils, including segmented and band forms, are increased and show prominent granularity.

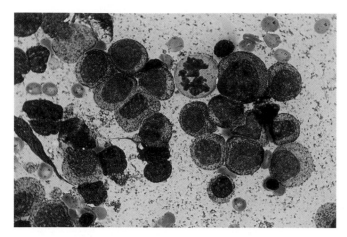

FIGURE 16-9. Bone marrow aspirate, granulocyte colony-stimulating factor effect. Heavily granulated promyelocytes and myelocytes show synchronous regeneration, with features reminiscent of acute promyelocytic leukemia.

Rare blasts may be seen. The neutrophils show intense granularity, vacuolation, Döhle bodies, and increased leukocyte (neutrophil) alkaline phosphatase. Neutrophils may also display abnormal nuclear lobation, double nuclei, and ring nuclei. The bone marrow shows increased granulocytopoiesis, sometimes accompanied by increased erythropoiesis and increased megakaryocytes. The predominant cells are promyelocytes and myelocytes that show heavy granularity and prominent Golgi zones. These findings may be mistaken for acute promyelocytic leukemia in specimens examined without obtaining a clinical history of G/GM-CSF therapy. The reactive promyelocytes induced by G-CSF differ from neoplastic promyelocytes in their uniform morphology, round to ovoid nuclei, prominent Golgi zones, and lack of Auer rods.

Two unusual bone marrow effects of G/GM-CSF have been reported: systemic, polyclonal plasmacytosis, possibly mediated by G/GM-CSF stimulation of interleukin-6

(17,18), and diffuse proliferation of foamy histiocytes in patients failing to recover hematopoietic function after stem cell transplantation (SCT) (19,20).

Adverse hematopoietic effects of therapy have been reported. G/GM-CSFs may accelerate the clinicopathologic findings in myeloproliferative and myelodysplastic disorders (21–23). These changes are often reversible on discontinuation of therapy. Bone marrow necrosis has also been reported (24,25). G-CSF may precipitate fatal sickle cell crisis in patients with sickling disorders (26). Concern persists regarding the clonogenic potential of prolonged G/GM-CSF therapy [see Chapter 18 (Risk Factors for Hematopoietic Neoplasia)].

Thrombopoietin

Thrombopoietin, or human megakaryocyte growth and development factor, has been used for increasing platelet counts in patients with chronic thrombocytopenia, those recovering from cytotoxic chemotherapy, and normal platelet donors (27–29).

The peripheral blood shows increased platelets, increased progenitors of all hematopoietic lineages, and circulating megakaryocytes. The bone marrow shows increased megakaryopoiesis, with atypical megakaryocytes and, in some cases, reticulin fibrosis. These changes are reversible after discontinuation of therapy and should not be mistaken for a myeloproliferative disorder (30).

Adverse hematopoietic effects include the development of neutralizing antibodies to thrombopoietin, with resultant amegakaryocytosis or aplastic anemia (31,32).

RADIOTHERAPY

The effects of therapeutic radiation on the bone marrow are derived from both histologic examination and imaging studies of the bone marrow (Figs. 16-11 and 16-12).

The earliest effects of radiotherapy, occurring during the first 2 weeks after initiation of therapy, are marrow edema

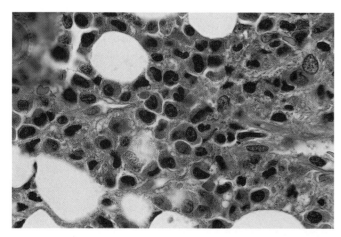

FIGURE 16-10. Bone marrow biopsy specimen, granulocyte colony-stimulating factor effect. The bone marrow contains large irregular islands of regenerating neutrophils and precursors.

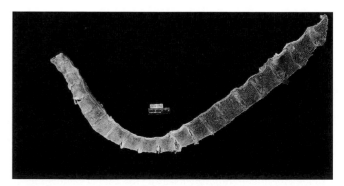

FIGURE 16-11. Bone marrow, radiation effect. A marked difference is seen between the irradiated bone marrow, which is pale yellow-white owing to hypoplasia, and residual nonirradiated tissue, which is deep red owing to normal cellularity.

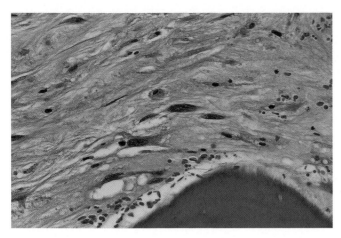

FIGURE 16-12. Bone marrow biopsy specimen, radiation effect. The bone marrow is fibrotic, and radiation-induced changes are seen in the stromal cells.

and necrosis (1–6). Other effects of radiotherapy include osteopenia, osteosclerosis, and disorganization and coarsening of trabecular architecture. Focal fibrosis and inflammatory infiltrates may radiographically resemble metastatic disease. At 2 to 3 months, hematopoietic tissue is usually replaced by adipose tissue in the irradiated areas. Fatty replacement and low peripheral blood counts may persist for years. Persistent macrophage activation and neutrophilic infiltration may contribute to posttherapeutic genetic damage (7).

OTHER THERAPEUTIC AGENTS

Many other agents have been used in the treatment of hematolymphoid disease and more will undoubtedly become rapidly available (Table 16-3).

Anti-CD20

Anti-CD20 antibody (rituximab) is used in the treatment of disorders caused by CD20-expressing B cells (1–8). After therapy, B cells are usually undetectable in the peripheral blood and bone marrow. In bone marrow foci previously involved by B-cell lymphoma, T-cell aggregates may persist, preserving the outlines of the original malignancy. It is important not to interpret such areas as foci of persistent lymphoma (9). Adverse hematopoietic effects reported after anti-CD20 therapy include agranulocytosis and thrombocytopenia.

TABLE 16-3. OTHER THERAPEUTIC AGENTS ASSOCIATED WITH HEMATOPOIETIC CHANGES

Anti-CD20
Azathioprine
Cyclosporin A
Interferons
Interleukins
Tyrosine kinase inhibitors

Azathioprine

Azathioprine has been used alone and in combination with other agents primarily to induce immunosuppression in organ transplant recipients but also to treat hematopoietic disorders, including pure red cell aplasia, neutrophil aplasia, and cyclic thrombocytopenia (10–12). Paradoxically, adverse hematologic effects attributable to azathioprine include severe megaloblastic anemia, pure red cell aplasia, agranulocytosis, and aplastic anemia (13–16). Various hematopoietic and lymphoid neoplasms have been reported after long-term azathioprine therapy (17–21).

Cyclosporin A

Cyclosporin A has been used alone and with other agents for the treatment of various cytopenias and hematopoietic disorders (22–28). Adverse hematopoietic effects include bone marrow edema, a hemolytic uremia-like syndrome, and clonal expansion in myelodysplastic syndrome and malignant lymphoma (29–31). Many of these changes are reversible after cessation of therapy.

Interferons

Interferon (IFN) alpha (IFN-α) has been used primarily to treat myeloproliferative and lymphoid neoplasms, especially chronic myeloid leukemia and hairy cell leukemia (32–41). After treatment, the peripheral blood and bone marrow usually show morphologic improvement, even to the point of complete hematologic and cytogenetic remission. IFN-α has a variable effect on marrow fibrosis, with some cases showing increased fibrosis and persistent osteosclerosis. Adverse effects of IFN-α include cytopenias, pure red cell aplasia, aplastic anemia, drug-related granulomas, and sarcoidosis (42–44). Bone marrow necrosis has been reported (45). Some patients on long-term therapy with IFN-α have developed blast crisis and new hematolymphoid malignancies (46–49).

IFN gamma has been used successfully in congenital osteopetrosis to decrease trabecular bone volume and increase hematopoiesis, with a corresponding increase in peripheral blood cell counts and improved leukocyte function (50).

Interleukins

Interleukin-3 and interleukin-11 have occasionally been used in the treatment of hematopoietic disease to increase peripheral blood cell counts (51,52). Marked erythrophagocytosis has been reported after therapy with interleukin-3 (53).

Tyrosine Kinase Inhibitors

Tyrosine kinase inhibitors are designed for use in diseases characterized by constitutive activation of tyrosine kinase, such as chronic myeloid leukemia and systemic mastocytosis (54–60). In most cases of chronic myeloid leukemia, therapy with a tyrosine kinase inhibitor produces near-normalization of cell counts and morphology, sometimes with slight basophilia remaining. The bone marrow shows dramatic changes, with the virtual disappearance of the morphologic characteristics of chronic myeloid leukemia. Reticulin fibrosis often regresses. Cytogenetic response may or may not accompany the morphologic normalization of the marrow. No significant adverse hematologic effects have been reported.

STEM CELL TRANSPLANTATION

Stem cell transplantation is the infusion of hematopoietic stem cells, performed to repopulate bone marrow incapable of sustaining adequate hematopoiesis. The stem cells may be derived from the peripheral blood or bone marrow of the patient him- or herself (autologous transplantation), an identical twin (syngeneic transplantation), or another individual (allogeneic transplantation).

After SCT, the peripheral blood shows cytopenias and the bone marrow is hypoplastic (1–6) (Figs. 16-13 and 16-14). The bone marrow shows focal erythroid regeneration at 1 to 2 weeks, followed by scattered early granulocytic precursors, and eventually by megakaryocytes, typically the last lineage to recover. The bone marrow may remain hypoplastic for years because of hematopoietic stem cell and stromal cell damage. Myelodysplasia and clonal karyotypic abnormalities have been reported after SCT but should not necessarily be interpreted as myelodysplastic syndrome because regression eventually occurs in some cases.

Adverse hematopoietic effects seen after SCT include therapy-related myelodysplastic syndrome and acute

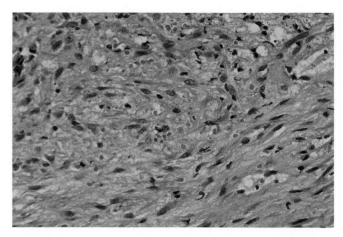

FIGURE 16-14. Bone marrow biopsy specimen, late hematopoietic stem cell graft failure. The bone marrow shows no hematopoietic cells and is replaced by dense fibrous connective tissue, fibroblasts, and histiocytes.

leukemia attributable to the accumulated burden of cytotoxic therapies given to patients before undergoing SCT (7–9).

REFERENCES

Cytotoxic Chemotherapy

1. Dick FR, Burns CP, Weiner GJ, et al. Bone marrow morphology during induction phase of therapy for acute myeloid leukemia (AML). *Hematol Pathol* 1995;9:95–106.
2. Feng CS. A variant of gelatinous transformation of marrow in leukemic patients post-chemotherapy. *Pathology* 1993;25:294–296.
3. Liso V, Albano F, Pastore D, et al. Bone marrow aspirate on the 14th day of induction treatment as a prognostic tool in de novo adult acute myeloid leukemia. *Haematologica* 2000;85:1285–1290.
4. Sandlund JT, Harrison PL, Rivera G, et al. Persistence of lymphoblasts in bone marrow on day 15 and days 22 to 25 of remission induction predicts a dismal treatment outcome in children with acute lymphoblastic leukemia. *Blood* 2002;100:43–47.

Differentiation Therapy

1. Advani SH, Nair R, Bapna A, et al. Acute promyelocytic leukemia: all-trans retinoic acid (ATRA) along with chemotherapy is superior to ATRA alone. *Am J Hematol* 1999;60:87–93.
2. Bapna A, Nair R, Tapan KS, et al. All-trans-retinoic acid (ATRA): pediatric acute promyelocytic leukemia. *Pediatr Hematol Oncol* 1998;15:243–248.
3. Colovic MD, Jankovic GM, Elezovic I, et al. Effect of all-trans-retinoic acid alone or in combination with chemotherapy in newly diagnosed acute promyelocytic leukaemia. *Med Oncol* 1997;14:65–72.
4. Fenaux P, Chastang C, Chevret S, et al. A randomized comparison of all transretinoic acid (ATRA) followed by chemotherapy and ATRA plus chemotherapy and the role of maintenance therapy in newly diagnosed acute promyelocytic leukemia. *Blood* 1999;94:1192–2000.

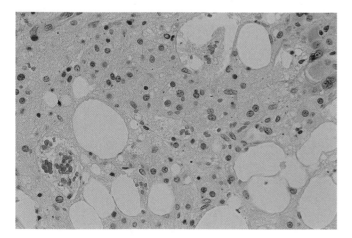

FIGURE 16-13. Bone marrow biopsy specimen, early hematopoietic stem cell graft failure. The bone marrow is hypoplastic, with almost no residual hematopoietic cells. The stroma is edematous and stromal cells are increased.

5. Hara T, Tsurumi H, Yamada T, et al. Detection of acute promyelocytic leukemia (APL) cells intermediately differentiated by all-trans retinoic acid in the cerebrospinal fluid: central nervous system involvement in APL. *Leuk Lymphoma* 2000;39: 213–215.

6. Lim LC, Vellupillai M, Ghafar AA. Clinico-biological features of 30 patients with acute promyelocytic leukemia and response to combination induction chemotherapy with all-trans retinoic acid and anthracycline. *Med Oncol* 2000;17:301–306.

7. Mandelli F, Diverio D, Avvisati G, et al. Molecular remission in PML/RAR alpha-positive acute promyelocytic leukemia by combined all-trans retinoic acid and idarubicin (AIDA) therapy. *Blood* 1997;90:1014–1021.

8. Miyauchi J, Ohyashiki K, Inatomi Y, et al. Neutrophil secondary-granule deficiency as a hallmark of all-trans retinoic acid-induced differentiation of acute promyelocytic leukemia cells. *Blood* 1997; 90:803–813.

9. Redner RL, Corey SJ, Rush EA. Differentiation of t(5;17) variant acute promyelocytic leukemic blasts by all-trans retinoic acid. *Leukemia* 1997;11:1014–1016.

10. Tallman MS. Differentiating therapy in acute myeloid leukemia. *Leukemia* 1996;10[Suppl 2]:S33–S38.

11. Vyas RC, Frankel SR, Agbor P, et al. Probing the pathobiology of response to all-trans retinoic acid in acute promyelocytic leukemia: premature chromosome condensation/fluorescence in situ hybridization analysis. *Blood* 1996;87:218–226.

12. Cull GM, Eikelboom JW, Cannell PK. Exacerbation of coagulopathy with concurrent bone marrow necrosis, hepatic and renal dysfunction secondary to all-trans retinoic acid therapy for acute promyelocytic leukemia. *Hematol Oncol* 1997;15:13–17.

13. Hatake K, Ohtsuki T, Uwai M, et al. Tretinoin induces bone marrow collagenous fibrosis in acute promyelocytic leukaemia: new adverse, but reversible effect. *Br J Haematol* 1996;93: 646–649.

14. Agis H, Weltermann A, Mitterbauer G, et al. Successful treatment with arsenic trioxide of a patient with ATRA-resistant relapse of acute promyelocytic leukemia. *Ann Hematol* 1999;78: 329–332.

15. Che-Pin Lin, Huang MJ, Chang IY, et al. Retinoic acid syndrome induced by arsenic trioxide in treating recurrent all-trans retinoic acid resistant acute promyelocytic leukemia. *Leuk Lymphoma* 2000;38:195–198.

16. Chim CS, Lam CC, Wong KF, et al. Atypical blasts and bone marrow necrosis associated with near-triploid relapse of acute promyelocytic leukemia after arsenic trioxide treatment. *Hum Pathol* 2002;33:849–851.

17. Kwong YL, Au WY, Chim CS, et al. Arsenic trioxide- and idarubicin-induced remissions in relapsed acute promyelocytic leukaemia: clinicopathological and molecular features of a pilot study. *Am J Hematol* 2001;66:274–279.

18. Ohnishi K, Yoshida H, Shigeno K, et al. Arsenic trioxide therapy for relapsed or refractory Japanese patients with acute promyelocytic leukemia: need for careful electrocardiogram monitoring. *Leukemia* 2002;16:617–622.

19. Shen Y, Shen ZX, Yan H, et al. Studies on the clinical efficacy and pharmacokinetics of low-dose arsenic trioxide in the treatment of relapsed acute promyelocytic leukemia: a comparison with conventional dosage. *Leukemia* 2001;15:735–741.

20. Soignet SL, Frankel SR, Douer D, et al. United States multicenter study of arsenic trioxide in relapsed acute promyelocytic leukemia. *J Clin Oncol* 2001;19:3852–3860.

21. Soignet SL, Maslak P, Wang ZG, et al. Complete remission after treatment of acute promyelocytic leukemia with arsenic trioxide. *N Engl J Med* 1998;339:1341–1348.

22. Zhang T, Westervelt P, Hess JL. Pathologic, cytogenetic and molecular assessment of acute promyelocytic leukemia patients treated with arsenic trioxide (As_2O_3). *Mol Pathol* 2000;13:954–961.

Hematopoietic Growth Factors

1. Biljanovic-Paunovic L, Djukanovic L, Lezaic V, et al. In vivo effects of recombinant human erythropoietin on bone marrow hematopoiesis in patients with chronic renal failure. *Eur J Med Res* 1998;3:564–570.

2. Hellstrom-Lindberg E, Kanter-Lewensohn L, Ost A. Morphological changes and apoptosis in bone marrow from patients with myelodysplastic syndromes treated with granulocyte-CSF and erythropoietin. *Leuk Res* 1997;21:415–425.

3. Martinez AM, Sastre A, Munoz A, et al. Recombinant human erythropoietin (rh-Epo) administration to normal child bone marrow donors. *Bone Marrow Transplant* 1998;22:137–138.

4. Osterbor A. The role of recombinant human erythropoietin in the management of anaemic cancer patients: focus on haematological malignancies. *Med Oncol* 2000;17:S17–S22.

5. Sikole A, Stojanovic A, Polenakovic M, et al. How erythropoietin affects bone marrow of uremic patients. *Am J Nephrol* 1997;17: 128–136.

6. Stasi R, Brunetti M, Bussa S, et al. Response to recombinant human erythropoietin in patients with myelodysplastic syndromes. *Clin Cancer Res* 1997;3:733–739.

7. Casadevall N, Nataf J, Viron B, et al. Pure red-cell aplasia and antierythropoietin antibodies in patients treated with recombinant erythropoietin. *N Engl J Med* 2002;346:469–475.

8. Viron B, Kolta A, Kiladjian JJ, et al. Antibodies against human recombinant erythropoietin: an unusual cause of erythropoietin resistance. *Nephrologie* 2002;23:19–22.

9. Bunworasate U, Arnouk H, Minderman H, et al. Erythropoietin-dependent transformation of myelodysplastic syndrome to acute monoblastic leukemia. *Blood* 2001;98:3492–3494.

10. Borkowski J, Amrikachi M, Hudnall SD. Fulminant parvovirus infection following erythropoietin treatment in a patient with acquired immunodeficiency syndrome. *Arch Pathol Lab Med* 2000;124:441–445.

11. Heussner P, Haase D, Kanz L, et al. G-CSF in the long-term treatment of cyclic neutropenia and chronic idiopathic neutropenia in adult patients. *Int J Hematol* 1998;62:225–234.

12. Hellstrom-Lindberg E, Kanter-Lewensohn L, Ost A. Morphological changes and apoptosis in bone marrow from patients with myelodysplastic syndromes treated with granulocyte-CSF and erythropoietin. *Leuk Res* 1997;21:415–425.

13. Carlo-Stella C, Regazzi E, Andrizzi C, et al. Use of granulocyte-macrophage colony-stimulating factor (GM-CSF) in combination with hydroxyurea as post-transplant therapy in chronic myelogenous leukemia patients autografted with unmanipulated hematopoietic cells. *Haematologica* 1997;82:291–296.

14. Kondo H, Kasahara Y, Mori A. Remission induction of refractory anaemia with excess blasts in transformation by sole treatment with granulocyte colony-stimulating factor with persistent chromosomal abnormality. *Acta Haematol* 2002;107: 177–181.

15. Harris AC, Todd WM, Hackney MH, et al. Bone marrow changes associated with recombinant granulocyte-macrophage and granulocyte colony-stimulating factors. Discrimination of granulocytic regeneration. *Arch Pathol Lab Med* 1994;118:624–629.

16. Schmitz LL, McClure JS, Litz CE, et al. Morphologic and quantitative changes in blood and marrow cells following growth factor therapy. *Am J Clin Pathol* 1994;101:67–75.

17. Csaki C, Ferencz T, Sipos G, et al. Diffuse plasmacytosis in a child with brainstem glioma following multiagent chemotherapy

and intensive growth factor support. *Med Pediatr Oncol* 1996;26: 367–371.

18. Jego G, Avet-Loiseau H, Robillard N, et al. Reactive plasmacytoses in multiple myeloma during hematopoietic recovery with G- or GM-CSF. *Leuk Res* 2000;24:627–630.

19. Al-Homaidhi A, Prince HM, Al-Zahrani H, et al. Granulocyte-macrophage colony-stimulating factor-associated histiocytosis and capillary-leak syndrome following autologous bone marrow transplantation: two case reports and a review of the literature. *Bone Marrow Transplant* 1998;21:209–214.

20. Rosenthal NS, Farhi DC. Failure to engraft after bone marrow transplantation: bone marrow morphologic findings. *Am J Clin Pathol* 1994;102:821–824.

21. Meyerson HJ, Farhi DC, Rosenthal NS. Transient increase in blasts mimicking acute leukemia and progressing myelodysplasia in patients receiving growth factor. *Am J Clin Pathol* 1998;109:675–681.

22. Vasef MA, Neiman RS, Meletiou SD, et al. Marked granulocytic proliferation induced by granulocyte colony-stimulating factor in the spleen simulating a myeloid leukemia infiltrate. *Mod Pathol* 1998;11:1138–1141.

23. Zuberbier T, Welker P, Grabbe J, et al. Effect of granulocyte macrophage colony-stimulating factor in a patient with benign systemic mastocytosis. *Br J Dermatol* 2001;145:661–666.

24. Katayama Y, Deguchi S, Shinagawa K, et al. Bone marrow necrosis in a patient with acute myeloblastic leukemia during administration of G-CSF and rapid hematologic recovery after allotransplantation of peripheral blood stem cells. *Am J Hematol* 1998;57:238–240.

25. Seki Y, Koike T, Yano M, et al. Bone marrow necrosis with dyspnea in a patient with malignant lymphoma and plasma levels of thrombomodulin, tumor necrosis factor-alpha, and D-dimer. *Am J Hematol* 2002;70:250–253.

26. Adler BK, Salzman DE, Carabasi MH, et al. Fatal sickle cell crisis after granulocyte colony-stimulating factor administration. *Blood* 2001;97:3313–3314.

27. Geddis AE, Linden HM, Kaushansky K. Thrombopoietin: a pan-hematopoietic cytokine. *Cytokine Growth Factor Rev* 2002;13: 61–73.

28. Kaushansky K. Use of thrombopoietic growth factors in acute leukemia. *Leukemia* 2000;14:505–508.

29. Nash RA, Kurzrock R, DiPersio J, et al. A phase I trial of recombinant human thrombopoietin in patients with delayed platelet recovery after hematopoietic stem cell transplantation. *Biol Blood Marrow Transplant* 2000;6:25–34.

30. Douglas VK, Tallman MS, Cripe LD, et al. Thrombopoietin administered during induction chemotherapy to patients with acute myeloid leukemia induces transient morphologic changes that may resemble chronic myeloproliferative disorders. *Am J Clin Pathol* 2002;117:844–850.

31. Basser RL, O'Flaherty E, Green M, et al. Development of pancytopenia with neutralizing antibodies to thrombopoietin after multicycle chemotherapy supported by megakaryocyte growth and development factor. *Blood* 2002;99:2599–2602.

32. Li J, Yang C, Xia Y, et al. Thrombocytopenia caused by the development of antibodies to thrombopoietin. *Blood* 2001;98:3241–3248.

Radiotherapy

1. Argiris A, Maris T, Papavasiliou G, et al. Radiotherapy effects on vertebral bone marrow: easily recognizable changes in T2 relaxation times. *Magn Reson Imaging* 1996;14:633–638.

2. Banfi A, Bianchi G, Galotto M, et al. Bone marrow stromal damage after chemo/radiotherapy: occurrence, consequences and possibilities of treatment. *Leuk Lymphoma* 2001;42:863–870.

3. Ha CS, Tucker SL, Blanco AI, et al. Hematologic recovery after central lymphatic irradiation for patients with stage I-III follicular lymphoma. *Cancer* 2001;92:1074–1079.

4. Kanberoglu K, Mihmanli I, Kurugoglu S, et al. Bone marrow changes adjacent to the sacroiliac joints after pelvic radiotherapy mimicking metastases on MRI. *Eur Radiol* 2001;11:1748–1752.

5. Mitchell MJ, Logan PM. Radiation-induced changes in bone. *Radiographics* 1998;18:1125–1136.

6. Onu M, Savu M, Lungu-Solomonescu C, et al. Early MR changes in vertebral bone marrow for patients following radiotherapy. *Eur Radiol* 2001;11:1463–1469.

7. Lorimore SA, Coates PJ, Scobie GE, et al. Inflammatory-type responses after exposure to ionizing radiation in vivo: a mechanism for radiation-induced bystander effects? *Oncogene* 2001;20:7085–7095.

Other Therapeutic Agents

1. Auner HW, Wolfler A, Beham-Schmid C, et al. Restoration of erythropoiesis by rituximab in an adult patient with primary acquired pure red cell aplasia refractory to conventional treatment. *Br J Haematol* 2002;116:727–728.

2. Egerer G, Sauerland K, Ho AD. Remarkable response to rituximab in a 72-year-old patient with refractory non-Hodgkin's lymphoma and marrow aplasia. *Leuk Lymphoma* 2001;42:551–553.

3. Ghielmini M, Schmitz SF, Burki K, et al. The effect of Rituximab on patients with follicular and mantle-cell lymphoma. Swiss Group for Clinical Cancer Research (SAKK). *Ann Oncol* 2000;11:123–126.

4. Igarashi T, Kobayashi Y, Ogura M, et al. Factors affecting toxicity, response and progression-free survival in relapsed patients with indolent B-cell lymphoma and mantle cell lymphoma treated with rituximab: a Japanese phase II study. *Ann Oncol* 2002;13: 928–943.

5. Jandula BM, Nomdedeu J, Marin P, et al. Rituximab can be useful as treatment for minimal residual disease in bcr-abl-positive acute lymphoblastic leukemia. *Bone Marrow Transplant* 2001;27: 225–227.

6. Milpied N, Vasseur B, Parquet N, et al. Humanized anti-CD20 monoclonal antibody (Rituximab) in post transplant B-lymphoproliferative disorder: a retrospective analysis on 32 patients. *Ann Oncol* 2000;11:113–116.

7. Seipelt G, Bohme A, Koschmieder S, et al. Effective treatment with rituximab in a patient with refractory prolymphocytoid transformed B-chronic lymphocytic leukemia and Evans syndrome. *Ann Hematol* 2001;80:170–173.

8. Treon SP, Agus TB, Link B, et al. CD20-directed antibody-mediated immunotherapy induces responses and facilitates hematologic recovery in patients with Waldenstrom's macroglobulinemia. *J Immunother* 2001;24:272–279.

9. Douglas VK, Gordon LI, Goolsby CL, et al. Lymphoid aggregates in bone marrow mimic residual lymphoma after rituximab therapy for non-Hodgkin lymphoma. *Am J Clin Pathol* 1999;112: 844–853.

10. Dan K, Inokuchi K, An E, et al. Cell-mediated cyclic thrombocytopenia treated with azathioprine. *Br J Haematol* 1991;77: 365–370.

11. Mathieson PW, O'Neill JH, Durrant ST, et al. Antibody-mediated pure neutrophil aplasia, recurrent myasthenia gravis and previous thymoma: case report and literature review. *QJM* 1990;74: 57–61.

12. Tohda S, Nara N, Tanikawa S, et al. Pure red cell aplasia following autoimmune haemolytic anaemia. Cell-mediated suppression of erythropoiesis as a possible pathogenesis of pure red cell aplasia. *Acta Haematol* 1992;87:98–102.

13. Bacon BR, Treuhaft WH, Goodman AM. Azathioprine-induced pancytopenia. Occurrence in two patients with connective-tissue diseases. *Arch Intern Med* 1981;141:223–226.

14. Kim CJ, Park KI, Inoue H, et al. Azathioprine-induced megaloblastic anemia with pancytopenia 22 years after living-related renal transplantation. *Int J Urol* 1998;5:100–102.

15. McGrath BP, Ibels LS, Raik E, et al. Erythroid toxicity of azathioprine. Macrocytosis and selective marrow hypoplasia. *QJM* 1975;44:57–63.

16. Sebbag L, Boucher P, Davelu P, et al. Thiopurine S-methyl-transferase gene polymorphism is predictive of azathioprine-induced myelosuppression in heart transplant recipients. *Transplantation* 2000;69:1524–1527.

17. Morrison VA, Dunn DL, Manivel JC, et al. Clinical characteristics of post-transplant lymphoproliferative disorders. *Am J Med* 1994;97:14–24.

18. Myllykangas-Luosujarvi R, Aho K, Isomaki H. Death attributed to antirheumatic medication in a nationwide series of 1666 patients with rheumatoid arthritis who have died. *J Rheumatol* 1995;22:2214–2217.

19. Oertel SH, Riess H. Immunosurveillance, immunodeficiency and lymphoproliferations. *Recent Results Cancer Res* 2002;159:1–8.

20. Silvergleid AJ, Schrier SL. Acute myelogenous leukemia in two patients treated with azathioprine for nonmalignant diseases. *Am J Med* 1974;57:885–888.

21. Vismans JJ, Briet E, Meijer K, et al. Azathioprine and subacute myelomonocytic leukemia. *Acta Med Scand* 1980;207:315–319.

22. Azuno Y, Yaga K. Successful cyclosporin A therapy for acquired amegakaryocytic thrombocytopenic purpura. *Am J Hematol* 2002;69:298–299.

23. Bangerter M, Griesshammer M, Tirpitz C, et al. Myelodysplastic syndrome with monosomy 7 after immunosuppressive therapy in Behcet's disease. *Scand J Rheumatol* 1999;28.117–119.

24. Catalano L, Selleri C, Califano C, et al. Prolonged response to cyclosporin-A in hypoplastic refractory anemia and correlation with in vitro studies. *Haematologica* 2000;85:133–138.

25. Kondo H, Narita K, Iwasaki H, et al. Effectiveness of cyclosporin A in a patient with pure red cell aplasia associated with T cell-lineage granular lymphocyte proliferative disorders resistant to cyclophosphamide therapy. *Eur J Haematol* 2000;64:206–207.

26. La Montagna G, Baruffo A, Abbadessa A, et al. Pure red cell aplasia in Felty's syndrome: a case report of successful reversal after cyclosporin A treatment. *Clin Rheumatol* 1999;18:244–247.

27. Leach JW, Hussein KK, George JN. Acquired pure megakaryocytic aplasia report of two cases with long-term responses to antithymocyte globulin and cyclosporine. *Am J Hematol* 1999;62:115–117.

28. Zeng W, Nakao S, Takamatsu H, et al. Characterization of T-cell repertoire of the bone marrow in immune-mediated aplastic anemia: evidence for the involvement of antigen-driven T-cell response in cyclosporine-dependent aplastic anemia. *Blood* 1999;93:3008–3016.

29. Hetzel GR, Malms J, May P, et al. Post-transplant distal-limb bone-marrow oedema: MR imaging and therapeutic considerations. *Nephrol Dial Transplant* 2000;15:1859–1864.

30. Itoh M, Yago K, Shimada H, et al. Reversible acceleration of disease progression following cyclosporin A treatment in a patient with myelodysplastic syndrome. *Int J Hematol* 2002;75:302–304.

31. Pielop JA, Jones D, Duvic M. Transient CD30+ nodal transformation of cutaneous T-cell lymphoma associated with cyclosporine treatment. *Int J Dermatol* 2001;40:505–511.

32. Damasio EE, Clavio M, Masoudi B, et al. Alpha-interferon as induction and maintenance therapy in hairy cell leukemia: a long-term follow-up analysis. *Eur J Haematol* 2000;64:47–52.

33. Frassoni F, Podesta M, Piaggio G, et al. Interferon-alpha protects Philadelphia-negative progenitors from exhaustion in chronic myeloid leukemia patients with cytogenetic response. *Hematol J* 2001;2:26–32.

34. Martinelli G, Testoni N, Amabile M, et al. Quantification of BCR-ABL transcripts in CML patients in cytogenetic remission after interferon-alpha-based therapy. *Bone Marrow Transplant* 2000;25:729–736.

35. Millot F, Brice P, Philippe N, et al. Alpha-interferon in combination with cytarabine in children with Philadelphia chromosome-positive chronic myeloid leukemia. *J Pediatr Hematol Oncol* 2002;24:18–22.

36. Schoffski P, Ganser A, Pascheberg U, et al. Complete haematological and cytogenetic response to interferon alpha-2a of a myeloproliferative disorder with eosinophilia associated with a unique t(4;7) aberration. *Ann Hematol* 2000;79:95–98.

37. Shamseddine A, Taher A, Jaafar H, et al. Interferon alpha is an effective therapy for congenital dyserythropoietic anaemia type I. *Eur J Haematol* 2000;65:207–209.

38. Sick C, Schultheis B, Pasternak G, et al. Predominantly BCR-ABL negative myeloid precursors in interferon-alpha treated chronic myelogenous leukemia: a follow-up study of peripheral blood colony-forming cells with fluorescence in situ hybridization. *Ann Hematol* 2001;80:9–16.

39. Tefferi A, Elliot MA, Yoon SY, et al. Clinical and bone marrow effects of interferon alfa therapy in myelofibrosis with myeloid metaplasia. *Blood* 2001;97:1896.

40. Thiele J, Kvasnicka HM. Comparative effects of interferon and hydroxyurea on bone marrow fibrosis in chronic myelogenous leukemia. *Leuk Lymphoma* 2001;42:855–862.

41. Thiele J, Kvasnicka HM, Schmitt-Graeff A, et al. Effects of chemotherapy (busulfan-hydroxyurea) and interferon-alfa on bone marrow morphologic features in chronic myelogenous leukemia. Histochemical and morphometric study on sequential trephine biopsy specimens with special emphasis on dynamic features. *Am J Clin Pathol* 2000;114:57–65.

42. Fiegl M, Chott A, Seewann HL, et al. Persisting bone marrow aplasia following interferon-alpha combined with ara-C for chronic myelogenous leukemia. *Leuk Lymphoma* 1999;34:191–195.

43. Frankova H, Gaja A, Hejlova N. Pulmonary sarcoidosis in a patient with essential thrombocythemia treated with interferon alpha: a short case report. *Med Sci Monit* 2000;6:380–382.

44. Hirri HM, Green PJ. Pure red cell aplasia in a patient with chronic granulocytic leukaemia treated with interferon-alpha. *Clin Lab Haematol* 2000;22:53–54.

45. Chim CS, Ma SK, Lam CK. Bone marrow necrosis masquerading as interferon toxicity in chronic myeloid leukemia. *Leuk Lymphoma* 1999;33:385–388.

46. Beedassy A, Topolsky D, Styler M, et al. Extramedullary blast crisis in a patient with chronic myelogenous leukemia in complete cytogenetic and molecular remission on interferon-alpha therapy. *Leuk Res* 2000;24:733–735.

47. Bose S, Chowdhry VP, Saxena R, et al. Lymphoid blast crisis during complete cytogenetic remission following interferon-alpha and hydroxyurea therapy. *Acta Haematol* 1997;98:155–159.

48. Goto H, Tsurumi H, Hara T, et al. Lymphoid blast crisis during interferon-alpha therapy in a patient with chronic myelogenous leukemia in myeloid blast crisis. *Int J Hematol* 2000;72:474–476.

49. Zamecnikova A, Krizana P, Gyarfas J, et al. Philadelphia-positive chronic myelogenous leukemia with a 5q-abnormality in a patient following interferon-alpha therapy. *Cancer Genet Cytogenet* 2001;127:134–139.

50. Key LL Jr, Rodriguiz RM, Willi SM, et al. Long-term treatment of osteopetrosis with recombinant human interferon gamma. *N Engl J Med* 1995;332:1594–1599.

51. Bastion Y, Campos L, Roubi N, et al. IL-3 increases marrow and peripheral erythroid precursors in chronic pure red cell aplasia presenting in childhood. *Br J Haematol* 1995;89:413–416.

52. Schwertschlag US, Trepicchio WL, Dykstra KH, et al. Hematopoietic, immunomodulatory and epithelial effects of interleukin-11. *Leukemia* 1999;13:1307–1315.

53. Hurwitz N, Probst A, Zufferey G, et al. Fatal vascular leak syndrome with extensive hemorrhage, peripheral neuropathy and reactive erythrophagocytosis: an unusual complication of recombinant IL-3 therapy. *Leuk Lymphoma* 1996;20:337–340.

54. Apperley JF, Gardembas M, Melo JV, et al. Response to imatinib mesylate in patients with chronic myeloproliferative diseases with rearrangements of the platelet-derived growth factor receptor beta. *N Engl J Med* 2002;347:481–487.

55. Beham-Schmid C, Apfelbeck U, Sill H, et al. Treatment of chronic myelogenous leukemia with the tyrosine kinase inhibitor STI571 results in marked regression of bone marrow fibrosis. *Blood* 2002;99:381–383.

56. Cross NC, Reiter A. Tyrosine kinase fusion genes in chronic myeloproliferative diseases. *Leukemia* 2002;16:1207–1212.

57. Hasserjian RP, Boecklin F, Parker S, et al. ST1571 (imatinib mesylate) reduces bone marrow cellularity and normalizes morphologic features irrespective of cytogenetic response. *Am J Clin Pathol* 2002;117:360–367.

58. Heinrich MC, Blanke CD, Druker BJ, et al. Inhibition of KIT tyrosine kinase activity: a novel molecular approach to the treatment of KIT-positive malignancies. *J Clin Oncol* 2002;20:1692–1703.

59. Liao AT, Chien MB, Shenoy N, et al. Inhibition of constitutively active forms of mutant kit by multitargeted indolinone tyrosine kinase inhibitors. *Blood* 2002;100:585–593.

60. Talpaz M, Silver RT, Druker BJ, et al. Imatinib induces durable hematologic and cytogenetic responses in patients with accelerated phase chronic myeloid leukemia: results of a phase 2 study. *Blood* 2002;99:1928–1937.

Stem Cell Transplantation

1. Amigo ML, del Canizo MC, Rios A, et al. Diagnosis of secondary myelodysplastic syndromes (MDS) following autologous transplantation should not be based only on morphological criteria used for diagnosis of de novo MDS. *Bone Marrow Transplant* 1999;23:997–1002.

2. Annaloro C, Oriani A, Pozzoli E, et al. Histological alterations in bone marrow in patients with late engraftment after autologous bone marrow transplantation. *Bone Marrow Transplant* 2000;25:837–841.

3. del Canizo C, Lopez N, Caballero D, et al. Haematopoietic damage persists 1 year after autologous peripheral blood stem cell transplantation. *Bone Marrow Transplant* 1999;23:901–905.

4. Galotto M, Berisso G, Delfino L, et al. Stromal damage as consequence of high-dose chemo/radiotherapy in bone marrow transplant recipients. *Exp Hematol* 1999;27:1460–1466.

5. Martinez-Climent JA, Comes AM, Vizcarra E, et al. Chromosomal abnormalities in women with breast cancer after autologous stem cell transplantation are infrequent and may not predict development of therapy-related leukemia or myelodysplastic syndrome. *Bone Marrow Transplant* 2000;25:1203–1208.

6. Okamoto T, Kanamaru A, Okada M, et al. Myelodysplastic changes in three cases within 100 days after allogeneic bone marrow transplantation. *Int J Hematol* 1996;63:155–160.

7. Milligan DW. Secondary leukaemia and myelodysplasia after autografting for lymphoma: is the transplant to blame? *Leuk Lymphoma* 2000;39:223–228.

8. Pedersen-Bjergaard J, Andersen MK, Christiansen DꞮ I. Therapy-related acute myeloid leukemia and myelodysplasia after high-dose chemotherapy and autologous stem cell transplantation. *Blood* 2000;95:3273–3279.

9. Sevilla J, Rodriguez A, Hernandez-Maraver D, et al. Secondary acute myeloid leukemia and myelodysplasia after autologous peripheral blood progenitor cell transplantation. *Ann Hematol* 2002;81:11–15.

17

OTHER NONNEOPLASTIC CONDITIONS

ACQUIRED NONCLONAL MYELODYSPLASIA

Acquired nonclonal myelodysplasia (MD) is undoubtedly underrecognized. It closely mimics constitutional hematopoietic disorders and clonal myelodysplastic syndromes and may easily be mistaken for them. Nonclonal MD is frequently reversible with time and appropriate therapy. A wide array of underlying conditions is associated with nonclonal MD (Table 17-1) (Figs. 17-1 through 17-3).

Aromatic hydrocarbons found in the work environment may produce dyshematopoiesis (1). Age is directly associated with an increase in dyserythropoiesis and dysgranulopoiesis, findings that are more common in the elderly (2). Cigarette smoking is associated with dyserythropoiesis and a slight increase in bone marrow blasts (2). Erythroid hyperplasia and/or ineffective erythropoiesis is a relatively common cause of dyserythropoiesis. Heavy metal intoxication causes MD proportionate to the amount and duration of ingestion. In arsenic poisoning, the peripheral blood may show anemia with coarse basophilic stippling and macroovalocytes, leukopenia, granulocytopenia, eosinophilia, and reticulocytopenia; the bone marrow is hypercellular with megaloblastic change, trilineal MD, and increased karyorrhexis (3–10). In lead poisoning, the peripheral blood shows karyorrhectic nucleated red blood cells; the bone marrow shows marked dyserythropoiesis and increased karyorrhexis (3).

Carcinoma has been associated with acquired myelokathexis (11). The differential diagnosis includes constitutional myelokathexis (see Chapter 5) and myelodysplastic

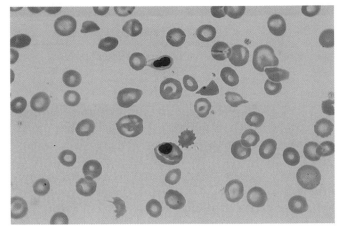

FIGURE 17-1. Peripheral blood smear, acquired nonclonal myelodysplasia. Dyserythropoietic nucleated red blood cells are seen in this specimen from a patient with sickle cell anemia.

syndrome with myelokathexis (12,13). Copper deficiency, whether primary or secondary to increased zinc, causes dyshematopoiesis with ringed sideroblasts (14). Ethanol abuse, defined as the regular daily intake of more than 80 g of ethanol per day, can cause bone marrow hypocellularity,

TABLE 17-1. CONDITIONS ASSOCIATED WITH ACQUIRED NONCLONAL MYELODYSPLASIA

Advanced age	Heavy metal intoxication
Advanced liver disease	Hemophagocytic syndrome
Aromatic hydrocarbon exposure	Hereditary disorders of metabolism
Carcinoma	Increased age
Cigarette smoking	Infectious agents
Copper deficiency	Medications
Erythroid hyperplasia and/or ineffective erythropoiesis	Solid organ transplantation
Ethanol abuse	

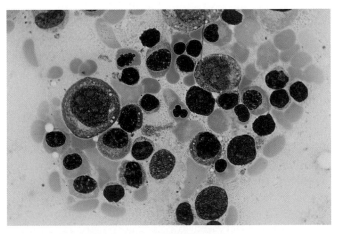

FIGURE 17-2. Bone marrow aspirate smear, acquired nonclonal myelodysplasia. Dyserythropoietic nucleated red blood cell precursors are present in this specimen from a patient with erythroid hyperplasia caused by cigarette smoking.

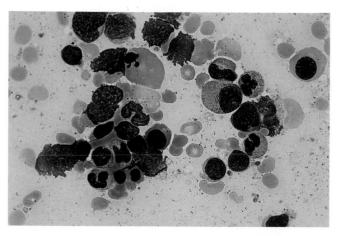

FIGURE 17-3. Bone marrow aspirate, acquired nonclonal myelodysplasia. A dysplastic erythroid precursor in seen in this specimen from a patient with human immunodeficiency virus infection.

TABLE 17-2. CONDITIONS ASSOCIATED WITH ACQUIRED NONCLONAL DYSERYTHROPOIESIS

Autoimmune hemolytic anemia	Iron deficiency
	Malaria
Congenital Fas deficiency	Necrotic bone marrow
Erythroblastic synartesis	metastasis
Hairy cell leukemia	Systemic lupus
Hemoglobinopathy	erythematosus
Hemophagocytic syndrome	Turner syndrome
Hyperosmolarity	Toxic reactions to drugs and other substances
	Vitamin B_{12} deficiency

megaloblastic change, vacuolation of erythroid and granulocytic precursors, multinuclearity of erythroid precursors, ringed sideroblasts, and impaired granulocyte maturation (15–22).

Infectious agents causing hematopoietic dysplasia include cytomegalovirus, human herpesvirus 6, and parvovirus B19 (23–26). Human immunodeficiency virus infection is associated with dysplastic and megaloblastic hematopoiesis (human immunodeficiency virus myelopathy), attributable to both the direct effects of human immunodeficiency virus infection and antiretroviral therapy (27–30). *Plasmodium falciparum* infection (malaria) has been associated with numerous bone marrow changes, including myeloid and erythroid hyperplasia, megaloblastosis, dyserythropoiesis, erythroid karyorrhexis, and giant metamyelocytes (31–34). Visceral leishmaniasis is associated with dyserythropoiesis and dysgranulopoiesis (35).

Medications can cause MD. Valproic acid causes Pelger-Hüet anomaly of neutrophils, thrombocytopenia, macrocytic anemia, macrocytosis, MD, aplastic anemia, and marrow changes resembling acute promyelocytic leukemia (36–38). Ganciclovir can produce intracytoplasmic and intranuclear inclusions in neutrophils and monocytes (39). Colchicine produces, in addition to marked bone marrow suppression, unusual mitotic figures arrested in metaphase (attributable to microtubular dysfunction) and striking dyserythropoiesis and dysgranulopoiesis (40). Tetracycline analogues may cause sideroblastic anemia (41).

Other conditions associated with acquired MD include hereditary disorders of metabolism (42,43), solid organ transplantation (44), advanced liver disease (45), hemophagocytic syndrome (46), and other inflammatory conditions characterized by increased cytokine production (47–49).

Dyserythropoiesis may be the predominant finding, especially in cases of increased and/or ineffective erythropoiesis

(Table 17-2). Underlying disorders include congenital Fas deficiency, hemoglobinopathy, iron and vitamin B_{12} deficiencies, malaria, autoimmune hemolytic anemia, systemic lupus erythematosus, toxic reactions to drugs and other substances, hemophagocytic syndrome, and necrotic bone marrow metastasis (50–62). Turner syndrome may be accompanied by macrocytic anemia, dyserythropoiesis, and multinuclearity of erythroid precursors (63). Hairy cell leukemia may be accompanied by marked abnormalities in erythroid precursors, including megaloblastic change, abnormal nuclear lobation, multinuclearity, and ringed sideroblasts (64,65). Hyperosmolarity is an unusual cause of erythroblast vacuolation (66). Erythroblastic synartesis is a rare disorder in which erythroid precursors are linked by tight interdigitating membranes; it appears to be caused by an antimembrane immunoglobulin, which may account for its occurrence with monoclonal gammopathy (52,67). The differential diagnosis includes artifactual changes in erythroid precursors owing to storage in ethylenediaminetetraacetic acid (68).

Acquired (pseudo-) Pelger-Hüet anomaly (PHA) is the appearance of hypolobated neutrophil nuclei, usually in adult life (Table 17-3). It may be the only sign of acquired nonclonal MD and is typically reversible with elimination of the underlying condition. Disorders and agents associated with acquired PHA include tuberculosis, *Mycoplasma* pneumonia, some medications, chronic lymphocytic leukemia, malignant lymphoma, multiple myeloma, and Hodgkin lymphoma (38,69–80). The differential diagnosis includes constitutional PHA (see Chapter 5) and acquired clonal PHA, a frequent finding in hematopoietic neoplasia with chromosome 17p deletion.

TABLE 17-3. CONDITIONS ASSOCIATED WITH ACQUIRED NONCLONAL PELGER-HÜET ANOMALY

Chronic lymphocytic leukemia	Medications
Malignant lymphoma	Mycoplasma pneumonia
Multiple myeloma	Tuberculosis
Hodgkin lymphoma	

TABLE 17-4. CONDITIONS ASSOCIATED WITH BONE MARROW NECROSIS

Alcoholism	Infectious disease
Anorexia nervosa	Malignancy
Coagulopathy	Myelotoxins
Dysbarism	Pancreatic fat necrosis
Erdheim-Chester disease	Pregnancy
Gaucher disease	Sickling hemoglobinopathies
Hyperparathyroidism	Therapeutic agents

NECROSIS

Bone marrow necrosis is an uncommon finding (1) (Table 17-4). The underlying condition, not necrosis *per se*, determines the clinical course (Figs. 17-4 through 17-6). Reported conditions associated with bone marrow necrosis include coagulopathies (1–3), infectious disease (4–15), hematolymphoid neoplasms and other malignancies (15–29), Gaucher disease (30), Erdheim-Chester disease (31), myelotoxic exposure (32–34), pancreatic fat necrosis (35,36), sickling hemoglobinopathies (8,11,37–39), corticosteroids and other therapeutic agents (21,32,40–49), graft-versus-host disease (50), dysbarism (51), pregnancy (52), anorexia nervosa (53), and hyperparathyroidism (54). In developed countries, malignancy underlies more than 90% of cases.

Proposed mechanisms of bone marrow necrosis include hypoxemia, vascular insufficiency, CD8+ T-cell activation, and local cytokine release (55).

Patients may be asymptomatic or present with bone pain, cytopenias, hypercalcemia, and increased serum lactate dehydrogenase levels. Imaging studies may show evidence of bone marrow edema or osteonecrosis (56). The bone marrow aspirate may appear viscous or granular and may be yellow-brown to dark brown instead of red (57). Biopsy specimens may be pale and crumbly, instead of the usual firm red marrow core.

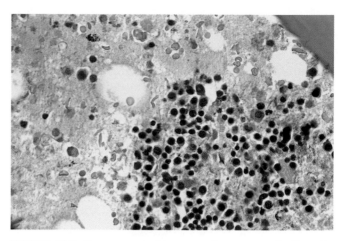

FIGURE 17-5. Bone marrow biopsy specimen, necrosis. Necrotic tissue contrasts with viable tissue showing erythroid hyperplasia in this specimen from a patient with hemoglobin SC disease. A few sickled red blood cells are visible.

Peripheral blood smears often show leukoerythroblastosis. Bone marrow aspirate smears show clumped, smeared, and smudged cells. The cardinal finding is the lack of clear nuclear and cytoplasmic architecture. It is important not to interpret clumped necrotic cells as tumor cells. Histologic sections of the bone marrow show smudged, eosinophilic tissue with pyknotic nuclear remnants, involving some or all of the marrow space. The trabecular bone may be viable or necrotic. Residual viable tissue may reveal an underlying sickling disorder or malignancy. In cases without viable tissue, the remaining architecture should be examined for indications of preexisting normal to hyperplastic hematopoietic tissue or marrow replacement by malignancy.

The differential diagnosis includes overstaining with eosin caused by prolonged decalcification; however, this artifact does not cause loss of cellular definition.

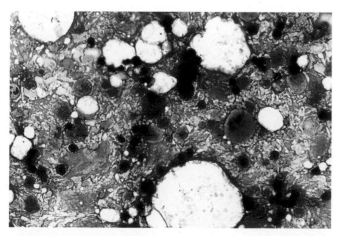

FIGURE 17-4. Bone marrow aspirate smear, necrosis. Smudged cellular remnants are seen in a background of dense amorphous material in this specimen from a patient with hemoglobin SC disease.

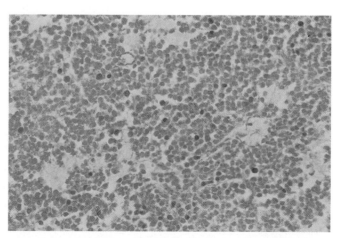

FIGURE 17-6. Bone marrow biopsy specimen, necrosis. The bone marrow is completely necrotic; however, the cellular remnants show that the tissue was composed of a monomorphous population of small round tumor cells. The underlying disease was acute lymphoblastic leukemia.

ORGANIC CRYSTALS

Organic crystals are rarely found in the bone marrow, where they may be found within cells or lying free (Table 17-5). Definite identification can often be made based on morphologic findings and other clinical and laboratory data.

Auer rods are familiar needle-shaped crystals of primary granules found in myclodysplastic syndromes and acute myeloid leukemia (1,2). They are considered pathognomonic of clonal myeloid disease, although they have also been reported in immature fetal myeloid precursors (3).

Charcot-Leyden crystals are rarely found in the bone marrow and other tissues, in association with eosinophilic differentiation of chronic myeloid leukemia, myclodysplastic syndromes, and acute myeloid leukemia (4–8). The differential diagnosis includes Charcot-Leyden crystals deposited as a result of reactive eosinophilia (8–11).

Cholesterol crystals from atherosclerotic plaques are occasionally found as emboli in the bone marrow.

Cholesteryl ester crystals are the hallmark of cholesteryl ester storage disease, a rare inherited metabolic disorder (12,13). The peripheral blood may show anemia. The bone marrow shows sea-blue histiocytes containing intracellular crystals.

Cystine crystals are found in hereditary cystinosis, a rare autosomal recessive disorder of lysosomal cystine transport in which cystine crystals accumulate in renal tubular epithelial cells and histiocytes (14–17) (Figs. 17-7 and 17-8). The bone marrow is hypocellular, with prominent crystal-containing histiocytes, renal osteodystrophy, and markedly increased iron stores. Cystine crystals are hexagonal, tubular, and rectangular and are birefringent with polarized light.

Gaucher-like histiocytes in chronic myeloid leukemia and other disorders may contain crystalline or crystal-like inclusions (18).

Immunoglobulin crystals are rarely deposited in tissues as a side effect of clonal lymphoplasmacytic disorders (19–30). The crystals may be located within neoplastic cells, hematopoietic cells, lymphocytes, histiocytes, and/or renal tubular epithelial cells. Prominent involvement of histiocytes is termed crystal-storing histiocytosis. The crystals may be composed of immunoglobulin heavy and light chains or light chains only and may show the properties of a cryoglobulin.

TABLE 17-5. ORGANIC CRYSTALS FOUND IN THE BONE MARROW

Auer rods
Charcot-Leyden crystals
Cholesteryl ester crystals
Cystine crystals
Crystals in Gaucher-like histiocytes
Immunoglobulin crystals
Oxalate crystals

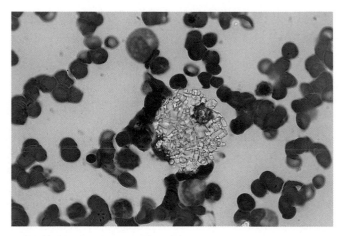

FIGURE 17-7. Bone marrow aspirate smear, cystinosis. A histiocyte is filled with brightly refractile short quadrilateral crystals.

Their morphology is variable, in some cases resembling Auer rods. The bone marrow may show crystal deposition in a variety of cell types, renal osteodystrophy, and evidence of the underlying lymphoplasmacytic disorder. The differential diagnosis includes storage disease, acute myeloid leukemia with Auer rods, and sarcoma. Immunoglobulin crystals are not a pathognomonic sign of clonality because they have also been reported in polyclonal inflammatory infiltrates (31,32).

Oxalate crystals occur in oxalosis, a rare autosomal recessive disorder (33–40) (Fig. 17-9). After the onset of renal failure, rosette-shaped arrays of intrahistiocytic needle-shaped, birefringent calcium oxalate crystals are deposited in the bone marrow and other tissues, surrounded by a brisk foreign-body giant cell reaction. The peripheral blood shows pancytopenia and a leukoerythroblastic reaction. The bone marrow shows replacement of hematopoietic tissue by granulomas, foreign-body giant cells, fibrosis, and increased

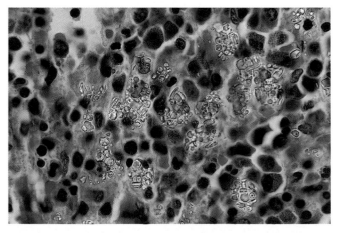

FIGURE 17-8. Bone marrow biopsy specimen, cystinosis. Histiocytes are increased and filled with brightly refractile crystals.

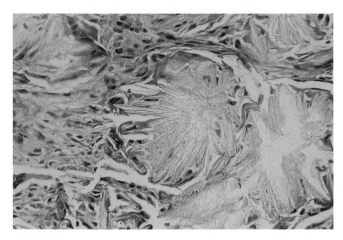

FIGURE 17-9. Bone marrow biopsy specimen, oxalosis. The bone marrow is replaced by massive crystal deposits in the form of a starburst, surrounded by foreign body giant cells and fibrosis.

bone resorption. Paramyxovirus-like intranuclear inclusions in bone marrow histiocytes have also been reported.

MINERAL DEPOSITS

Mineral deposits occur in the bone marrow as crystals and granules (Table 17-6). Radiographic microanalysis and other techniques may be required for secure identification.

Barium sulfate has been reported in the bone marrow after inadvertent introduction of barium into body cavities (1). The bone marrow shows histiocytes filled with electron-dense granules.

Gold salts are used in the therapy of rheumatoid arthritis, and deposits may be found in the bone marrow by electron microscopy (2–5). Other hematopoietic effects of gold salts are impaired HLA-DR expression in monocytes and aplastic anemia.

Silica crystals may be deposited in the bone marrow in pneumoconiosis (6,7). The bone marrow shows birefringent intrahistiocytic silica crystals, free silica, lymphocytosis and plasmacytosis, granulomas, and fibrosis.

Talc crystals are birefringent silicate particles, found within bone marrow histiocytes in specimens from intravenous drug abusers (8–11). Talc deposits alone do not necessarily elicit a granulomatous reaction. However, extensive talc deposition and bone marrow granulomas have been

TABLE 17-6. MINERAL DEPOSITS FOUND IN THE BONE MARROW

Barium sulfate
Gold salts
Silica
Talc
Thorium dioxide

TABLE 17-7. EMBOLIZED TISSUES AND SUBSTANCES FOUND IN THE BONE MARROW

Carcinoma
Cardiac myxoma
Cholesterol from atherosclerotic plaques
Gas (during episodes of hyperbarism)
Vegetations from noninfectious (marantic) thrombotic
  endocarditis
Nucleus pulposus

reported in association with *Histoplasma capsulatum*, *Mycobacterium tuberculosis*, human immunodeficiency virus, and cytomegalovirus infections.

Thorium dioxide was administered intraarterially to patients from 1928 to 1955 as a radioactive contrast material (12–15). It is sequestered in bone marrow histiocytes where it is visible microscopically as a brownish refractile material and emits alpha particles, which are visible on radiography. In addition to mineral deposits, the bone marrow may show fibrosis, aplastic anemia, myelodysplastic syndromes, acute leukemia, and sarcomas.

EMBOLI

Emboli to the bone marrow have rarely been reported (Table 17-7). They may be composed of a variety of tissues and substances, including carcinoma, especially of the digestive tract (1), cardiac myxoma (2), cholesterol from atherosclerotic plaques (3–5), gas during episodes of hyperbarism (6,7), vegetations originating from noninfectious (marantic) thrombotic endocarditis (8,9), and nucleus pulposus (10). In some cases, associated bone marrow necrosis, fractures, and new bone formation are also found. Gas bubbles and bone marrow necrosis associated with hyperbarism should be distinguished from the bone marrow gas and necrosis reported with *Escherichia coli* sepsis (11).

REFERENCES

Acquired Nonclonal Myelodysplasia

1. Hristeva-Mirtcheva V. Changes in the peripheral blood of workers with occupational exposure to aromatic hydrocarbons. *Int Arch Occup Environ Health* 1998;71[Suppl]:S81–S83.
2. Fernandez-Ferrero S, Ramos F. Dyshaemopoietic bone marrow features in healthy subjects are related to age. *Leuk Res* 2001;25:187–189.
3. Eichner ER. Erythroid karyorrhexis in the peripheral blood smear in severe arsenic poisoning: a comparison with lead poisoning. *Am J Clin Pathol* 1984;81:533–537.
4. Feussner JR, Shelburne JD, Bredehoeft S, et al. Arsenic-induced bone marrow toxicity: ultrastructural and electron-probe analysis. *Blood* 1979;53:820–827.

5. Franzblau A, Lilis R. Acute arsenic intoxication from environmental arsenic exposure. *Arch Environ Health* 1989;44:385–390.

6. Hall AH. Chronic arsenic poisoning. *Toxicol Lett* 2002;128: 69–72.

7. Lerman BB, Ali N, Green D. Megaloblastic, dyserythropoietic anemia following arsenic ingestion. *Ann Clin Lab Sci* 1980;10: 515–517.

8. Pralle H, Manz F. Influence of chronic arsenic poisoning on bone marrow morphology. A case report. *Blut* 1985;50:51–54.

9. Rezuke WN, Anderson C, Pastuszak WT, et al. Arsenic intoxication presenting as a myelodysplastic syndrome: a case report. *Am J Hematol* 1991;36:291–293.

10. Westhoff DD, Samaha RJ, Barnes A Jr. Arsenic intoxication as a cause of megaloblastic anemia. *Blood* 1975;45:241–246.

11. Maran R, Mittelman M, Cohen AM, et al. Myelokathexis and monocytosis in a patient with gastric cancer. *Acta Haematol* 1992; 87:210–212.

12. Rassam SM, Roderick P, al-Hakim I, et al. A myelokathexis-like variant of myelodysplasia. *Eur J Haematol* 1989;42:99–102.

13. Sheridan BL, Pinkerton PH, Curtis JE, et al. The myelokathexis-like variant of the myelodysplastic syndrome—a second example. *Clin Lab Haematol* 1991;13:81–85.

14. Gregg XT, Reddy V, Prchal JT. Copper deficiency masquerading as myelodysplastic syndrome. *Blood* 2002;100:1493–1495.

15. Ballard HS. Alcohol-associated pancytopenia with hypocellular bone marrow. *Am J Clin Pathol* 1980;73:830–834.

16. Budde R, Hellerich U. Alcohol dyshaematopoiesis: morphological features of alcohol-induced bone marrow damage in biopsy sections compared with aspiration smears. *Acta Haematol* 1995; 94:74–77.

17. Casagrande G, Michot F. Alcohol-induced bone marrow damage: status before and after a 4-week period of abstinence from alcohol with or without disulfiram. A randomized bone marrow study in alcohol-dependent individuals. *Blut* 1989;59:231–236.

18. Liu YK. Effects of alcohol on granulocytes and lymphocytes. *Semin Hematol* 1980;17:130–136.

19. Michot F, Gut J. Alcohol-induced bone marrow damage. A bone marrow study in alcohol-dependent individuals. *Acta Haematol* 1987;78:252–257.

20. Nakao S, Harada M, Kondo K, et al. Reversible bone marrow hypoplasia induced by alcohol. *Am J Hematol* 1991;37: 120–123.

21. Savage D, Lindenbaum J. Anemia in alcoholics. *Medicine (Baltimore)* 1986;65:322–338.

22. Seppa K, Laippala P, Saarni M. Macrocytosis as a consequence of alcohol abuse among patients in general practice. *Alcohol Clin Exp Res* 1991;15:871–876.

23. Miyahara M, Shimamoto Y, Yamada H, et al. Cytomegalovirus-associated myelodysplasia and thrombocytopenia in an immunocompetent adult. *Ann Hematol* 1997;74:99–101.

24. Lorenzana A, Lyons H, Sawaf H, et al. Human herpesvirus 6 infection mimicking juvenile myelomonocytic leukemia in an infant. *J Pediatr Hematol Oncol* 2002;24:136–141.

25. Hasle H, Kerndrup G, Jacobsen BB, et al. Chronic parvovirus infection mimicking myelodysplastic syndrome in a child with subclinical immunodeficiency. *Am J Pediatr Hematol Oncol* 1994; 16:329–333.

26. Yarali N, Duru F, Sipahi T, et al. Parvovirus B19 infection reminiscent of myelodysplastic syndrome in three children with chronic hemolytic anemia. *Pediatr Hematol Oncol* 2000;17:475–482.

27. Calenda V, Chermann JC. The effects of HIV on hematopoiesis. *Eur J Haematol* 1992;48:181–186.

28. Katsarou O, Terpos E, Patsouris E, et al. Myelodysplastic features in patients with long-term HIV infection and haemophilia. *Haemophilia* 2001;7:47–52.

29. Ryu T, Ikeda M, Okazaki Y, et al. Myelodysplasia associated with acquired immunodeficiency syndrome. *Intern Med* 2001;40: 795–801.

30. Treacy M, Lai L, Costello C, et al. Peripheral blood and bone marrow abnormalities in patients with HIV related disease. *Br J Haematol* 1987;65:289–294.

31. Abdalla SH. Hematopoiesis in human malaria. *Blood Cells* 1990; 16:401–416.

32. Das BS, Nanda NK, Rath PK, et al. Anaemia in acute, *Plasmodium falciparum* malaria in children from Orissa state, India. *Ann Trop Med Parasitol* 1999;93:109–118.

33. Gandapur AS, Malik SA, Raziq F. Bone marrow changes in human malaria: a retrospective study. *J Pak Med Assoc* 1997;47: 137–139.

34. Wickramasinghe SN, Abdalla SH. Blood and bone marrow changes in malaria. *Baillieres Best Pract Res Clin Haematol* 2000; 13:277–299.

35. Shahriar D, Reza MP, Reza AM, et al. Cytological clues of bone marrow findings in Kala-Azar. *Diagn Cytopathol* 1999;20: 208–211.

36. Acharya S, Bussel JB. Hematologic toxicity of sodium valproate. *J Pediatr Hematol Oncol* 2000;22:62–65.

37. Brichard B, Vermylen C, Scheiff JM, et al. Haematological disturbances during long-term valproate therapy. *Eur J Pediatr* 1994;153:378–380.

38. Ganick DJ, Sunder T, Finley JL. Severe hematologic toxicity of valproic acid. A report of four patients. *Am J Pediatr Hematol Oncol* 1990;12:80–85.

39. Ghosh K, Muirhead D, Christie B, et al. Ultrastructural changes in peripheral blood neutrophils in a patient receiving ganciclovir for CMV pneumonitis following allogenic bone marrow transplantation. *Bone Marrow Transplant* 1999;24:429–431.

40. Finklestein M, Goldman L, Grace ND, et al. Granulocytopenia complicating colchicine therapy for primary biliary cirrhosis. *Gastroenterology* 1987;93:1231–1235.

41. Rudek MA, Horne M, Figg WD, et al. Reversible sideroblastic anemia associated with the tetracycline analogue COL-3. *Am J Hematol* 2001;67:51–53.

42. Gilbert-Barness E, Barness LA. Isovaleric acidemia with promyelocytic myeloproliferative syndrome. *Pediatr Dev Pathol* 1999; 2:286–291.

43. Hinson DD, Rogers ZR, Hoffmann GF, et al. Hematological abnormalities and cholestatic liver disease in two patients with mevalonate kinase deficiency. *Am J Med Genet* 1998;78: 408–412.

44. Castello A, Dal Bello B, Klersy C, et al. Bone marrow changes in heart transplant recipients with peripheral cytopenia. *Transplantation* 1999;67:840–846.

45. Keung YK, Morgan D, Hodges D, et al. Myelodysplasia-like syndrome and end-stage liver disease: report of 2 cases. *Acta Haematol* 2001;105:100–102.

46. Imashuku S, Kitazawa K, Ishii M, et al. Bone marrow changes mimicking myelodysplasia in patients with hemophagocytic lymphohistiocytosis. *Int J Hematol* 2000;72:353–357.

47. Murata H, Yoshimoto H, Ryu T, et al. High fever, renal failure, disseminated intravascular coagulation and myelodysplasia accompanied with enhanced angiogenesis possibly due to overexpression of vascular endothelial growth factor. *Intern Med* 2000;39: 570–575.

48. Shimamoto T, Hayashi S, Ando K, et al. Anaplastic large-cell lymphoma which showed severe inflammatory status and myelodysplasia with increased VEGF and IL-6 serum levels after long-term immunosuppressive therapy. *Am J Hematol* 2001;66:49–52.

49. Yetgin S, Ozen S, Yenicesu I, et al. Myelodysplastic features in polyarteritis nodosa. *Pediatr Hematol Oncol* 2001;18:157–160.

50. Bader-Meunier B, Rieux-Laucat F, Croisille L, et al. Dyserythropoiesis associated with a fas-deficient condition in childhood. *Br J Haematol* 2000;108:300–304.

51. Chintagumpala MM, Dreyer ZA, Steuber CP, et al. Pancytopenia with chromosomal fragility: vitamin B12 deficiency. *J Pediatr Hematol Oncol* 1996;18:166–170.

52. Croisille L, Tchernia G, Casadevall N. Autoimmune disorders of erythropoiesis. *Curr Opin Hematol* 2001;8:68–73.

53. Feng CS, Ng MH, Szeto RS, et al. Bone marrow findings in lupus patients with pancytopenia. *Pathology* 1991;23:5–7.

54. Keefer MJ, Solanki DL. Dyserythropoiesis and erythroblast-phagocytosis preceding pure red cell aplasia. *Am J Hematol* 1988;27:132–135.

55. Lombardi SM, Girelli DG, Corrocher R. Severe multisystemic hypersensitivity reaction to carbamazepine including dyserythropoietic anemia. *Ann Pharmacother* 1999;33:571–575.

56. Macheta M, Will AM, Houghton JB, et al. Prominent dyserythropoiesis in four cases of haemophagocytic lymphohistiocytosis. *J Clin Pathol* 2001;54:961–963.

57. Mills AE, Meyer JH, Karabus CD, et al. Transient dyserythropoiesis occurring during the involutionary phase of stage IV-S neuroblastoma. *Am J Pediatr Hematol Oncol* 1989;11:23–27.

58. Mohan K, Stevenson MM. Dyserythropoiesis and severe anaemia associated with malaria correlate with deficient interleukin-12 production. *Br J Haematol* 1998;103:942–949.

59. Rebar AH. General responses of the bone marrow to injury. *Toxicol Pathol* 1993;21:118–129.

60. Roush GR, Rosenthal NS, Gerson SL, et al. An unusual case of autoimmune hemolytic anemia with reticulocytopenia, erythroid dysplasia, and an IgG2 autoanti-U. *Transfusion* 1996;36:575–580.

61. Rozman M, Masat T, Feliu E, et al. Dyserythropoiesis in iron-deficiency anemia: ultrastructural reassessment. *Am J Hematol* 1992;41:147–150.

62. Zago MA, Costa FF, Bottura C. Dyserythropoiesis in iron deficiency and in beta-thalassemia. *Braz J Med Biol Res* 1984;17:135–142.

63. Foster LA, Abboud MR, Taylor AB, et al. Myelodysplasia associated with Turner syndrome. *J Pediatr Hematol Oncol* 1996;18:299–301.

64. Pangalis GA, Kittas C, Viniou N, et al. Hairy cell leukemia: bone marrow changes following splenectomy and alpha-interferon therapy. *Leukemia* 1987;1:343–346.

65. Zak P, Chrobak L, Podzimek K, et al. Dyserythropoietic changes and sideroblastic anemia in patients with hairy cell leukemia before and after therapy with 2-chlorodeoxyadenosine. *Neoplasma* 1998;45:261–265.

66. Lehane DE. Vacuolated erythroblasts in hyperosmolar coma. *Arch Intern Med* 1974;134:763–765.

67. Cramer EM, Garcia I, Masse JM, et al. Erythroblastic synartesis: an auto-immune dyserythropoiesis. *Blood* 1999;94:3683–3693.

68. Wang LJ, Glasser L. Spurious dyserythropoiesis. *Am J Clin Pathol* 2002;117:57–59.

69. Cicchitto G, Parravicini M, De Lorenzo S, et al. Tuberculosis and Pelger-Hüet anomaly. Case report. *Panminerva Med* 1999;41:367–369.

70. Deutsch PH, Mandell GL. Reversible Pelger-Hüet anomaly associated with ibuprofen therapy. *Arch Intern Med* 1985;145:166.

71. Ganick DJ, Sunder T, Finley JL. Severe hematologic toxicity of valproic acid. A report of four patients. *Am J Pediatr Hematol Oncol* 1990;12:80–85.

72. Gondo H, Okamura C, Osaki K, et al. Acquired Pelger-Hüet anomaly in association with concomitant tacrolimus and fluconazole therapy following allogeneic bone marrow transplantation. *Bone Marrow Transplant* 2000;26:1255–1257.

73. Juneja SK, Matthews JP, Luzinat R, et al. Association of acquired Pelger-Hüet anomaly with taxoid therapy. *Br J Haematol* 1996;93:139–141.

74. Kennedy GA, Kay TD, Johnson DW, et al. Neutrophil dysplasia characterised by a pseudo-Pelger-Hüet anomaly occurring with the use of mycophenolate mofetil and ganciclovir following renal transplantation: a report of five cases. *Pathology* 2002;34:263–266.

75. Kornberg A, Goldfarb A, Shalev O. Pseudo-Pelger-Hüet anomaly in chronic lymphocytic leukemia. *Acta Haematol* 1981;66:127–128.

76. Liesveld J, Smith BD. Acquired Pelger-Hüet anomaly in a case of non-Hodgkin's lymphoma. *Acta Haematol* 1988;79:46–49.

77. May RB, Sunder TR. Hematologic manifestations of long-term valproate therapy. *Epilepsia* 1993;34:1098–1101.

78. Savage PJ, Dellinger RP, Barnes JV, et al. Pelger-Hüet anomaly of granulocytes in a patient with tuberculosis. *Chest* 1984;85:131–132.

79. Shenkenberg TD, Rice L, Waddell CC. Acquired Pelger-Hüet nuclear anomaly with tuberculosis. *Arch Intern Med* 1982;142:153–154.

80. van Hook L, Spivack C, Duncanson FP. Acquired Pelger-Hüet anomaly associated with *Mycoplasma pneumoniae* pneumonia. *Am J Clin Pathol* 1985;84:248–251.

Necrosis

1. Paydas S, Ergin M, Baslamisli F, et al. Bone marrow necrosis: clinicopathologic analysis of 20 cases and review of the literature. *Am J Hematol* 2002;70:300–305.

2. Murphy PT, Sivakumaran M, Casey MC, et al. Lymphoma associated bone marrow necrosis with raised anticardiolipin antibody. *J Clin Pathol* 1998;51:407–409.

3. Gonzalez N, Rios E, Martin-Noya A, et al. Thrombotic thrombocytopenic purpura and bone marrow necrosis as a complication of gastric neoplasm. *Haematologica* 2002;87:ECR01.

4. Brada M, Bellingham AJ. Bone-marrow necrosis and Q fever. *BMJ* 1980;281:1108–1109.

5. Brouland JP, Audouin J, Hofman P, et al. Bone marrow involvement by disseminated toxoplasmosis in acquired immunodeficiency syndrome: the value of bone marrow trephine biopsy and immunohistochemistry for the diagnosis. *Hum Pathol* 1996;27:302–306.

6. Cagnoni PJ, Zangari M, Seremetis S. Air in the bone in a case of bone marrow necrosis associated with *Escherichia coli* septicemia. *Am J Hematol* 1995;48:58–60.

7. Caraveo J, Trowbridge AA, Amaral BW, et al. Bone marrow necrosis associated with a Mucor infection. *Am J Med* 1977;62:404–408.

8. Eichhorn RF, Buurke EJ, Blok P, et al. Sickle cell-like crisis and bone marrow necrosis associated with parvovirus B19 infection and heterozygosity for haemoglobins S and E. *J Intern Med* 1999;245:103–106.

9. Gupta RK. Extensive fatal bone marrow necrosis in typhoid fever. *Indian J Pathol Microbiol* 1992;35:66–68.

10. Katzen H, Spagnolo SV. Bone marrow necrosis from miliary tuberculosis. *JAMA* 1980;244:2438–2439.

11. Kolquist KA, Vnencak-Jones CL, Swift L, et al. Fatal fat embolism syndrome in a child with undiagnosed hemoglobin S/beta+ thalassemia: a complication of acute Parvovirus B19 infection. *Pediatr Pathol Lab Med* 1996;16:71–82.

12. Nakamura Y, Yamamoto S, Tanaka S, et al. Herpes simplex viral infection in human neonates: an immunohistochemical and electron microscopic study. *Hum Pathol* 1985;16:1091–1097.

13. Rustgi VK, Sacher RA, O'Brien P, et al. Fatal disseminated cytomegalovirus infection in an apparently normal adult. *Arch Intern Med* 1983;143:372–373.

14. Terheggen HG, Lampert F. Acute bone marrow necrosis caused by streptococcal infection. *Eur J Pediatr* 1979;130:53–58.

15. O'Carroll DI, McKenna RW, Brunning RD. Bone marrow manifestations of Hodgkin's disease. *Cancer* 1976;38:1717–1728.

16. Chim CS, Ma SK, Lam CK. Bone marrow necrosis masquerading as interferon toxicity in chronic myeloid leukemia. *Leuk Lymphoma* 1999;33:385–388.

17. Kendra JR, Pickens S, Singh AK, et al. Bone marrow necrosis at transformation of chronic granulocytic leukaemia treated with interferon. *J Clin Pathol* 1992;45:830–831.

18. Abbas AA, Husain AH, Abdelaal MA, et al. Acute lymphoblastic leukemia presenting with extensive skeletal lesions and bone marrow necrosis. *Med Pediatr Oncol* 2001;37:64–66.

19. Lazda EJ, Berry PJ. Bone marrow metastasis in Ewing's sarcoma and peripheral primitive neuroectodermal tumor: an immunohistochemical study. *Pediatr Dev Pathol* 1998;1:125–130.

20. Forrest DL, Mack BJ, Nevill TJ, et al. Bone marrow necrosis in adult acute leukemia and non-Hodgkin's lymphoma. *Leuk Lymphoma* 2000;38:627–632.

21. Hudson J, Cobby M, Yates P, et al. Extensive infiltration of bone with marrow necrosis in a case of hairy cell leukaemia. *Skeletal Radiol* 1995;24:228–231.

22. Kwong YL, Pollock A, Wei D, et al. Philadelphia chromosome positive acute lymphoblastic leukemia masquerading as persistent asymptomatic bone marrow necrosis. *Pathology* 1994;26:183–185.

23. Majumdar G. Massive bone marrow necrosis as the presenting feature in a case of primary bone marrow high grade non-Hodgkin's lymphoma. *Leuk Lymphoma* 1997;26:409–412.

24. Majumdar G, Phillips JK, Pearson TC. Massive bone marrow necrosis and postnecrotic myelofibrosis in a patient with primary thrombocythaemia. *J Clin Pathol* 1994;47:674–676.

25. Markovic SN, Phyliky RL, Li CY. Pancytopenia due to bone marrow necrosis in acute myelogenous leukemia: role of reactive CD8 cells. *Am J Hematol* 1998;59:74–78.

26. Nakayama T, Kabe K, Nakamoto R, et al. Bone marrow necrosis associated with medulloblastoma. *Acta Paediatr Jpn* 1988;30:723–727.

27. Paterlini P, Venturoni L, Cretara G, et al. Bone marrow necrosis: an unusual presenting feature of small cell lung carcinoma. *Tumori* 1985;71:403–406.

28. Pui CH, Stass S, Green A. Bone marrow necrosis in children with malignant disease. *Cancer* 1985;56:1522–1525.

29. Zhu AX, Niesvizky R, Hedrick E, et al. Extensive bone marrow necrosis associated with multiple myeloma. *Leukemia* 1999;13:2118–2120.

30. Blocklet D, Abramowicz M, Schoutens A. Bone, bone marrow, and MIBI scintigraphic findings in Gaucher's disease "bone crisis." *Clin Nucl Med* 2001;26:765–769.

31. Kim NR, Ko YH, Choe YH, et al. Erdheim-Chester disease with extensive marrow necrosis: a case report and literature review. *Int J Surg Pathol* 2001;9:73–79.

32. Hernigou P, Beaujean F. Abnormalities in the bone marrow of the iliac crest in patients who have osteonecrosis secondary to corticosteroid therapy or alcohol abuse. *J Bone Joint Surg Am* 1997;79:1047–1053.

33. Moore J, Ma DD, Concannon A. Non-malignant bone marrow necrosis: a report of two cases. *Pathology* 1998;30:318–320.

34. Ruiz MA, Augusto LG, Vassallo J, et al. Bone marrow morphology in patients with neutropenia due to chronic exposure to organic solvents (benzene): early lesions. *Pathol Res Pract* 1994;190:151–154.

35. Ahn BC, Lee J, Suh KJ, et al. Intramedullary fat necrosis of multiple bones associated with pancreatitis. *J Nucl Med* 1998;39:1401–1404.

36. Good AE, Schnitzer B, Kawanishi H, et al. Acinar pancreatic tumor with metastatic fat necrosis: report of a case and review of rheumatic manifestations. *Am J Dig Dis* 1976;21:978–987.

37. Ataga KI, Orringer EP. Bone marrow necrosis in sickle cell disease: a description of three cases and a review of the literature. *Am J Med Sci* 2000;320:342–347.

38. Ballas SK, Pindzola A, Chang CD, et al. Postmortem diagnosis of hemoglobin SC disease complicated by fat embolism. *Ann Clin Lab Sci* 1998;28:144–149.

39. Johnson K, Stastny JF, Rucknagel DL. Fat embolism syndrome associated with asthma and sickle cell-beta(+)-thalassemia. *Am J Hematol* 1994;46:354–357.

40. Aboulafia DM, Demirer T. Fatal bone marrow necrosis following fludarabine administration in a patient with indolent lymphoma. *Leuk Lymphoma* 1995;19:181–184.

41. Chernetsky SG, Mont MA, LaPorte DM, et al. Pathologic features in steroid and nonsteroid associated osteonecrosis. *Clin Orthop* 1999;368:149–161.

42. Chim CS, Ooi C, Ma SK, et al. Bone marrow necrosis in bone marrow transplantation: the role of MR imaging. *Bone Marrow Transplant* 1998;22:1125–1128.

43. Cull GM, Eikelboom JW, Cannell PK. Exacerbation of coagulopathy with concurrent bone marrow necrosis, hepatic and renal dysfunction secondary to all-trans retinoic acid therapy for acute promyelocytic leukemia. *Hematol Oncol* 1997;15:13–17.

44. Katayama Y, Deguchi S, Shinagawa K, et al. Bone marrow necrosis in a patient with acute myeloblastic leukemia during administration of G-CSF and rapid hematologic recovery after allotransplantation of peripheral blood stem cells. *Am J Hematol* 1998;57:238–240.

45. Seki Y, Koike T, Yano M, et al. Bone marrow necrosis with dyspnea in a patient with malignant lymphoma and plasma levels of thrombomodulin, tumor necrosis factor-alpha, and D-dimer. *Am J Hematol* 2002;70:250–253.

46. Kumakura S, Ishikura H, Kobayashi S. Bone marrow necrosis and the Lambert-Eaton syndrome associated with interferon alfa treatment. *N Engl J Med* 1998;338:199–200.

47. Lau G, Kwan C, Chong SM. The 3-week sulphasalazine syndrome strikes again. *Forensic Sci Int* 2001;122:79–84.

48. Ojala AE, Paakko E, Lanning FP, et al. Osteonecrosis during the treatment of childhood acute lymphoblastic leukemia: a prospective MRI study. *Med Pediatr Oncol* 1999;32:11–17.

49. Zhang T, Westervelt P, Hess JL. Pathologic, cytogenetic and molecular assessment of acute promyelocytic leukemia patients treated with arsenic trioxide (As2O3). *Mod Pathol* 2000;13:954–961.

50. Mori A, Hashino S, Kobayashi S, et al. Avascular necrosis in the femoral head secondary to bone marrow infarction in a patient with graft-versus-host disease after unrelated bone marrow transplantation. *Ann Hematol* 2001;80:238–242.

51. Jones JP Jr, Ramirez S, Doty SB. The pathophysiologic role of fat in dysbaric osteonecrosis. *Clin Orthop* 1993;296:256–264.

52. Knickerbocker WJ, Quenville NF. Widespread marrow necrosis during pregnancy. *Skeletal Radiol* 1982;9:37–40.

53. Smith RR, Spivak JL. Marrow cell necrosis in anorexia nervosa and involuntary starvation. *Br J Haematol* 1985;60:525–530.

54. Tavassoli M. Bone marrow necrosis secondary to hyperparathyroidism. *J Miss State Med Assoc* 1983;24:39–41.

55. Janssens AM, Offner FC, Van Hove WZ. Bone marrow necrosis. *Cancer* 2000;88:1769–1780.

56. Iida S, Harada Y, Shimizu K, et al. Correlation between bone marrow edema and collapse of the femoral head in steroid-induced osteonecrosis. *AJR Am J Roentgenol* 2000;174:735–743.

57. Leyssen MH, Verwilghen RL. Diagnosis of bone marrow necrosis. *Clin Lab Haematol* 1979;1:197–202.

Organic Crystals

1. Ritter J, Vormoor J, Creutzig U, et al. Prognostic significance of Auer rods in childhood acute myelogenous leukemia: results of the studies AML-BFM-78 and -83. *Med Pediatr Oncol* 1989;17: 202–209.
2. Wong KF, So CC. Hypoplastic myelodysplastic syndrome-a clinical, morphologic, or genetic diagnosis? *Cancer Genet Cytogenet* 2002;138:85–88.
3. Newburger PE, Novak TJ, McCaffrey RP. Eosinophilic cytoplasmic inclusions in fetal leukocytes: are Auer bodies a recapitulation of fetal morphology? *Blood* 1983;61:593–595.
4. Healey JH, Lane JM, Erlandson RA, et al. Solid leukemic tumor. An uncommon presentation of a common disease. *Clin Orthop* 1985;194:248–251.
5. Kuto F, Nagaoka T, Watanabe Y, et al. Chronic myelocytic leukemia: ultrastructural histopathology of bone marrow from patients in the chronic phase. *Ultrastruct Pathol* 1984;6: 307–317.
6. Ma SK, Wong KF, Chan JK, et al. Refractory cytopenia with t(1;7),+8 abnormality and dysplastic eosinophils showing intranuclear Charcot-Leyden crystals: a fluorescence in situ hybridization study. *Br J Haematol* 1995;90:216–218.
7. Strauchen JA, Gordon RE. Crystalline inclusions in granulocytic sarcoma. *Arch Pathol Lab Med* 2002;126:85–86.
8. Arora VK, Singh N, Bhatia A. Charcot-Leyden crystals in fine needle aspiration cytology. *Acta Cytol* 1997;41:409–412.
9. Kanner RE, Hammar SP. Chronic eosinophilic pneumonia. Ultrastructural evidence of marked immunoglobulin production plus macrophagic ingestion of eosinophils and eosinophilic lysosomes leading to intracytoplasmic Charcot-Leyden crystals. *Chest* 1977;71:95–98.
10. Kumar PV, Mousavi A, Karimi M, et al. Fine needle aspiration of Langerhans cell histiocytosis of the lymph nodes. A report of six cases. *Acta Cytol* 2002;46:753–756.
11. Pinto GM, Lamarao P, Vale T. Captopril-induced pemphigus vegetans with Charcot-Leyden crystals. *J Am Acad Dermatol* 1992;27:281–284.
12. Elleder M, Chlumska A, Ledvinova J, et al. Testis—a novel storage site in human cholesteryl ester storage disease. Autopsy report of an adult case with a long-standing subclinical course complicated by accelerated atherosclerosis and liver carcinoma. *Virchows Arch* 2000;436:82–87.
13. vom Dahl S, Harzer K, Rolfs A, et al. Hepatosplenomegalic lipidosis: what unless Gaucher? Adult cholesteryl ester storage disease (CESD) with anemia, mesenteric lipodystrophy, increased plasma chitotriosidase activity and a homozygous lysosomal acid lipase -1 exon 8 splice junction mutation. *J Hepatol* 1999;31: 741–746.
14. Busuttil DP, Liu Yin JA. The bone marrow in hereditary cystinosis. *Br J Haematol* 2000;111:385.
15. Gahl WA, Thoene JG, Schneider JA. Cystinosis. *N Engl J Med* 2002;347:111–121.
16. Gebrail F, Knapp M, Perrotta G, et al. Crystalline histiocytosis in hereditary cystinosis. *Arch Pathol Lab Med* 2002;126:1135.
17. Kalatzis V, Cohen-Solal L, Cordier B, et al. Identification of 14 novel CTNS mutations and characterization of seven splice site mutations associated with cystinosis. *Hum Mutat* 2002;20: 439–446.
18. Hayhoe FG, Flemans RJ, Cowling DC. Acquired lipidosis of marrow macrophages: birefringent blue crystals and Gaucher-like cells, sea-blue histiocytes, and grey-green crystals. *J Clin Pathol* 1979;32:420–428.
19. Castoldi G, Piva N, Tomasi P. Multiple myeloma with Auer-rod-like inclusions. *Haematologica* 1999;84:859–860.
20. Florensa L, Larriba I, Woessner S. Unique intranuclear inclusion in an IgG kappa multiple myeloma. *Haematologica* 2000;85: 1323.
21. Gabriel L, Escribano L, Perales J, et al. Multiple myeloma with crystalline inclusions in most hemopoietic cells. *Am J Hematol* 1985;18:405–411.
22. Gardais J, Genevieve F, Foussard C, et al. Is there any significance for intracellular crystals in plasma cells from patients with monoclonal gammopathies? *Eur J Haematol* 2001;67:119–122.
23. Goteri G, Lorenzini P, Morroni M, et al. Bone marrow extracellular large geometric crystals in IgG/lambda MGUS. *Pathol Res Pract* 2002;198:299–302.
24. Gruszecki AC, Vishnu VVB. Plasma cell crystalline inclusions. *Arch Pathol Lab Med* 2002;126:755.
25. Jones D, Bhatia VK, Krausz T, et al. Crystal-storing histiocytosis: a disorder occurring in plasmacytic tumors expressing immunoglobulin kappa light chain. *Hum Pathol* 1999;30:1441–1448.
26. Kapadia SB, Enzinger FM, Heffner DK, et al. Crystal-storing histiocytosis associated with lymphoplasmacytic neoplasms. Report of three cases mimicking adult rhabdomyoma. *Am J Surg Pathol* 1993;17:461–467.
27. Lebeau A, Zeindl-Eberhart E, Muller EC, et al. Generalized crystal-storing histiocytosis associated with monoclonal gammopathy: molecular analysis of a disorder with rapid clinical course and review of the literature. *Blood* 2002;100:1817–1827.
28. Martin AW, Carstens PH, Yam LT. Crystalline deposits in ascites in a case of cryoglobulinemia. *Acta Cytol* 1987;31:631–636.
29. Pillay GS, Jacobs P. Crystalline cytoplasmic inclusions in myeloma. *Arch Pathol Lab Med* 1994;118:1169–1170.
30. Stavem P, Forre O. The same type of crystalline inclusions in T-lymphocytes as in plasma cells and B-lymphocytes in multiple myeloma. A pathological clone originating from a common lymphocyte stem cell? *Scand J Haematol* 1981;26:265–271.
31. Magalhaes R, Gehrke T, Souto-Carneiro MM, et al. Extensive plasma cell infiltration with crystal IgG inclusions and mutated IgV(H) gene in an osteoarthritis patient with lymphoplasmacellular synovitis. A case report. *Pathol Res Pract* 2002;198: 45–50.
32. Rao NA, Font RL. Plasmacytic conjunctivitis with crystalline inclusions. Immunohistochemical and ultrastructural studies. *Arch Ophthalmol* 1980;98:836–841.
33. Bianco P, Silvestrini G, Ballanti P, et al. Paramyxovirus-like nuclear inclusions identical to those of Paget's disease of bone detected in giant cells of primary oxalosis. *Virchows Arch A Pathol Anat Histopathol* 1992;421:427–433.
34. Emile JF, Shouval D, Samuel D. Images in hepatology. Bone marrow deposits of oxalate crystals. *J Hepatol* 2000;33:167.
35. Gherardi G, Poggi A, Sisca S, et al. Bone oxalosis and renal osteodystrophy. *Arch Pathol Lab Med* 1980;104:105–111.
36. Hricik DE, Hussain R. Pancytopenia and hepatosplenomegaly in oxalosis. *Arch Intern Med* 1984;144:167–168.
37. McKenna RW, Dehner LP. Oxalosis. An unusual cause of myelophthisis in childhood. *Am J Clin Pathol* 1976;66: 991–997.
38. Schnitzler CM, Kok JA, Jacobs DW, et al. Skeletal manifestations of primary oxalosis. *Pediatr Nephrol* 1991;5:193–199.
39. Walter MJ, Dang CV. Pancytopenia secondary to oxalosis in a 23-year-old woman. *Blood* 1998;91:4394.
40. Yamaguchi K, Grant J, Noble-Jamieson G, et al. Hypercalcaemia in primary oxalosis: role of increased bone resorption and effects of treatment with pamidronate. *Bone* 1995;16:61–67.

Mineral Deposits

1. David R, Berezesky IK, Bohlman M, et al. Fatal barium embolization due to incorrect vaginal rather than colonic insertion. An ultrastructural and x-ray microanalysis study. *Arch Pathol Lab Med* 1983;107:548–551.
2. Cheson BD, Clegg DO, Moatamed F. Ultrastructural evidence for persistent gold in the bone marrow of a patient with aplastic anemia. *Arthritis Rheum* 1986;29:128–132.
3. Hansen RM, Csuka ME, McCarty DJ, et al. Gold induced aplastic anemia. Complete response to corticosteroids, plasmapheresis, and N-acetylcysteine infusion. *J Rheumatol* 1985;12: 794–797.
4. Hirohata S, Yanagida T, Hashimoto H, et al. Differential influences of gold sodium thiomalate and bucillamine on the generation of CD14+ monocyte-lineage cells from bone marrow of rheumatoid arthritis patients. *Clin Immunol Immunopathol* 1997;84:290–295.
5. McKendry RJ, Huebsch L, Leclair B. Progression of rheumatoid arthritis following bone marrow transplantation. A case report with a 13-year followup. *Arthritis Rheum* 1996;39:1246–1253.
6. Eide J, Gylseth B, Skaug V. Silicotic lesions of the bone marrow: histopathology and microanalysis. *Histopathology* 1984;8: 693–703.
7. Pelstring RJ, Kim CK, Lower EE, et al. Marrow granulomas in coal workers' pneumoconiosis. A histologic study with elemental analysis. *Am J Clin Pathol* 1988;89:553–556.
8. Kringsholm B, Christoffersen P. The nature and the occurrence of birefringent material in different organs in fatal drug addiction. *Forensic Sci Int* 1987;34:53–62.
9. Lewis JH, Sundeen JT, Simon GL, et al. Disseminated talc granulomatosis. An unusual finding in a patient with acquired immunodeficiency syndrome and fatal cytomegalovirus infection. *Arch Pathol Lab Med* 1985;109:147–150.
10. Mariani-Costantini R, Jannotta FS, Johnson FB. Systemic visceral talc granulomatosis associated with miliary tuberculosis in a drug addict. *Am J Clin Pathol* 1982;78:785–789.
11. Racela LS, Papasian CJ, Watanabe I, et al. Systemic talc granulomatosis associated with disseminated histoplasmosis in a drug abuser. *Arch Pathol Lab Med* 1988;112:557–560.
12. Graham SJ, Heaton RB, Garvin DF, et al. Whole-body pathologic analysis of a patient with Thorotrast-induced myelodysplasia. *Health Phys* 1992;63:20–26.
13. Harrist TJ, Schiller AL, Trelstad RL, et al. Thorotrast-associated sarcoma of bone: a case report and review of the literature. *Cancer* 1979;44:2049–2058.
14. Hirose Y, Konda S, Sasaki K, et al. Erythroleukemia and gastric cancer following thorotrast injection. *Jpn J Med* 1991;30:43–46.
15. Kamiyama R, Ishikawa Y, Hatakeyama S, et al. Clinicopathological study of hematological disorders after Thorotrast administration in Japan. *Blut* 1988;56:153–160.

Emboli

1. dos Santos VM, Rodrigues DB, Castro EC, et al. Widespread hematogenous metastases and Trousseau's syndrome in gastric adenocarcinoma. *Rev Hosp Clin Fac Med Sao Paulo* 2001;56:91–96.
2. Kamata S, Kawada T, Kikuchi K, et al. Clinical analysis of embolism with left atrial myxomas. *Kyobu Geka* 1996;49:297–300.
3. Muretto P, Carnevali A, Ansini AL. Cholesterol embolism of bone marrow clinically masquerading as systemic or metastatic tumor. *Haematologica* 1991;76:248–250.
4. Pierce JR Jr, Wren MV, Cousar JB Jr. Cholesterol embolism: diagnosis antemortem by bone marrow biopsy. *Ann Intern Med* 1978;89:937–938.
5. Rywlin AM. Cholesterol embolism in bone marrow. *Ann Intern Med* 1979;90:443–444.
6. Gregg PJ, Walder DN. Caisson disease of bone. *Clin Orthop* 1986; 210:43–54.
7. Jones JP Jr, Ramirez S, Doty SB. The pathophysiologic role of fat in dysbaric osteonecrosis. *Clin Orthop* 1993;296:256–264.
8. Garcia I, Fainstein V, Rios A, et al. Nonbacterial thrombotic endocarditis in a male homosexual with Kaposi's sarcoma. *Arch Intern Med* 1983;143:1243–1244.
9. Vega R. Systemic embolization from a thrombotic noninfectious endocarditis. *Clin Transpl* 1989:313.
10. Schreck RI, Manion WL, Kambin P, et al. Nucleus pulposus pulmonary embolism. A case report. *Spine* 1995;20:2463–2466.
11. Cagnoni PJ, Zangari M, Seremetis S. Air in the bone in a case of bone marrow necrosis associated with *Escherichia coli* septicemia. *Am J Hematol* 1995;48:58–60.

18

RISK FACTORS FOR HEMATOPOIETIC NEOPLASIA

Acute leukemia and other hematopoietic disorders result from a complex series of genetic events. Circumstances favoring these events are risk factors. These fall into two broad groups: constitutional factors, which are present at conception, and acquired factors, which appear after conception (Tables 18-1 and 18-2). Significant progress has been made recently in elucidating both inherited and environmental causes of hematopoietic neoplasia. In many cases, a common element can be found between acute leukemia and other disorders in the same patient. In some instances, the presence of acute leukemia is the first sign of an underlying genetic disorder.

This section is included to enable the clinician and pathologist to recognize the underlying risk factors in myeloproliferative disorders, myelodysplastic syndromes, and acute leukemia and to suggest further appropriate studies in affected patients.

CONSTITUTIONAL RISK FACTORS

Population-Based Factors

Population-based factors predisposing to hematopoietic neoplasia are recognized, but in most cases, the underlying mechanisms remain obscure.

Gender is an important risk factor. Females are over-represented among neonates and infants with acute leukemia, especially leukemia with *MLL* rearrangement (1,2). Males predominate among all patients with acute leukemia (3).

TABLE 18-1. CONSTITUTIONAL RISK FACTORS FOR HEMATOPOIETIC NEOPLASIA

Population-based factors
Genetic factors
Chromosomal instability and bone marrow failure
  syndromes
Dysmorphic syndromes
Other constitutional hematopoietic disorders

TABLE 18-2. ACQUIRED RISK FACTORS FOR HEMATOPOIETIC NEOPLASIA

Environmental factors
Acquired hematopoietic disease and blood donation
Infectious and immune-related factors
Medical interventions
Pregnancy and birth-related factors
Other acquired risk factors

Some ethnic groups, such as Ashkenazi Jews, show a high incidence of myeloproliferative disease, possibly attributable to transmission of HLA type or an unknown genetic factor (4). Particular HLA variants predispose to or protect against hematologic malignancy (5–7).

Some kindreds have been described with an unusually high incidence of myeloproliferative disorders, Langerhans cell histiocytosis, myclodysplastic syndrome, and acute leukemia (8–18). Most kindreds show a predisposition for one type of neoplasia; some show multiple types. Familial disease may show a progressively earlier age at onset and an unusually rapid course, especially when acquired risk factors are superimposed (19).

True ethnic or familial risk factors may be difficult to distinguish from case clustering of hematologic neoplasia caused by common exposure to environmental agents, either in a geographic area or *in utero*.

Genetic Factors

Constitutional autosomal anomalies are known to predispose to hematopoietic neoplasia. They are especially relevant in therapy-induced neoplasia, in which constitutional and acquired risk factors act synergistically. Interestingly, many resemble the genetic anomalies commonly seen as acquired anomalies in hematopoietic malignancy.

Many karyotypic abnormalities are associated with hematopoietic malignancy, involving almost one-half of the somatic chromosomes and both sex chromosomes (20–40). In many cases, inheritance of the anomaly does not in itself predict acute leukemia, suggesting that the anomaly acts as an initial genetic aberration or "hit," followed by one or more additional hits in the patient eventually diagnosed with a clonal hematopoietic disease. In cases of mosaicism, hematopoietic malignancy may arise in either a karyotypically normal or abnormal cell.

Inherited mutations and polymorphisms of several genes are known to confer an increased risk of hematopoietic malignancy (41–63). The involved genes include those encoding *N*-acetyl transferase, DNA ligase IV, glutathione-S-transferase, NAD(P)H quinone oxidoreductase, thiopurine methyltransferase, the Ikaros gene, *AML1*, *CYP1A1*, *ERBB*, *NF1*, *p53*, and others.

Chromosomal Instability and Bone Marrow Failure Syndromes

These disorders are similar, often presenting with cytopenias and skeletal malformations and carrying an increased risk of acute leukemia, especially therapy-related leukemia. In some cases, the onset of acute leukemia is the first sign of an underlying constitutional disorder.

The chromosomal instability syndromes are characterized by an inability to synthesize and/or repair DNA correctly, with a consequently high incidence of disease attributable to common environmental factors such as sunlight (63–66). Pathologic changes typically occur in many tissues, including the skeleton, heart, kidney, and skin in addition to the bone marrow. Ataxia telangiectasia is associated with a high risk of T-cell and, to a lesser extent, B-cell and myeloid malignancy (67–69). Fanconi anemia carries an increased risk of clonal myeloid and lymphoid disease as well as therapy-related malignancy (70–72). Bloom syndrome, dyskeratosis congenita, Griscelli syndrome, and Werner syndrome are other rare chromosomal instability disorders with a propensity to develop acute leukemia (73–76).

The bone marrow failure syndromes are characterized by the early onset of cytopenias and an increased risk of acute leukemia. In some cases, the underlying genetic defect has been discovered. These disorders include congenital hypoplastic (Diamond-Blackfan) anemia (77), familial sideroblastic anemia (78), severe congenital neutropenia (Kostmann syndrome) (79,80), marrow-pancreas (Shwachman-Diamond) syndrome (81–84), and thrombocytopenia-absent radii (TAR) syndrome (85,86).

Dysmorphic Syndromes

Dysmorphism or congenital anomalies, which may be attributable to either constitutional or acquired factors, are associated with an increased incidence of hematopoietic malignancy (87–89).

Specific dysmorphic disorders reported with hematologic neoplasia include Adams-Oliver syndrome, cardiofaciocutaneous syndrome and other cardiac anomalies, cleft lip and palate, DiGeorge syndrome, Dubowitz syndrome, Ehlers-Danlos syndrome, familial microcephaly, gonadal dysgenesis, Grönblad-Strandberg syndrome, lamellar ichthyosis, Marfan syndrome, Marinesco-Sjögren syndrome, neuroectodermal dysplasia (CHIME syndrome), Noonan syndrome, Poland syndrome, Seckel syndrome, Sipple syndrome, and Sotos syndrome (87–113).

Other Constitutional Hematopoietic Disorders

Preexisting constitutional hematopoietic disorders are present in some patients with hematopoietic neoplasia. It is tempting to speculate that chronic stimulation of hematopoiesis is the unifying characteristic in these disorders. Possibly the constant demand for stem cell renewal creates an increased opportunity for the genetic aberrations that initiate clonal disease.

Hemoglobinopathies reported in patients with hematopoietic neoplasia include β thalassemia, hemoglobin C, hemoglobin D, hemoglobin Lepore, hemoglobin S, and others (114–121).

Other hematopoietic disorders reported with hematologic neoplasia include glucose-6-phosphatase deficiency, hemophilia, hereditary spherocytosis, myeloperoxidase deficiency, platelet storage pool deficiency, porphyria, and pyruvate kinase deficiency (122–132). Cystic fibrosis also may also predispose patients to acute leukemia (133–135).

ACQUIRED FACTORS

Environmental Factors

The environment contains numerous risk factors for hematologic neoplasia. These act synergistically with constitutional risk factors to produce hematopoietic disease at an earlier age and higher frequency than might otherwise occur. Substances in the environment act directly on the exposed individual and indirectly on those exposed to that individual, especially family members (see Pregnancy and Birth-Related Factors section). Many of these substances are found in the workplace and others in the general environment. Those found in the workplace contribute to an increased risk of leukemia in some occupations.

Environmental agents and substances implicated in hematopoietic oncogenesis include arsenic, cadmium, trihalomethanes, chloroform, and zinc, all found in drinking water; asbestos and related minerals; benzene, paints, petroleum products, and other organic solvents; electromagnetic fields; pesticides and other agricultural chemicals; radiation from solar and earth sources, nuclear reactors and weapons, and therapeutic devices; ethanol; and tobacco (1–20).

Acquired Hematopoietic Disease and Blood Donation

Preexisting hematopoietic disease may be present years before the onset of hematopoietic neoplasia; in such cases, it likely acts as a risk factor. As in the case of constitutional hematopoietic disease, it is tempting to speculate that acquired hematopoietic diseases require an increased, long-term demand for hematopoietic stem cells and thus increase the chance of a genetic event leading to neoplasia. In some cases, an increase in hematopoietic stem cells and clonal emergence caused by increased cell cycling have been documented (21–23).

Hematopoietic disorders, which appear to carry increased risk of leukemia, include aplastic anemia, pure red cell aplasia, immune-mediated thrombocytopenia, and pernicious anemia (23–29). Coexistent pernicious anemia may mask a myeloproliferative disorder, and vice versa (30,31).

Frequent blood donation appears to confer an increased risk of polycythemia vera and essential thrombocythemia (32–34). Blood donation and familial predisposition may combine to increase the risk of polycythemia vera in some individuals.

Infectious and Immune-Related Factors

Infectious and immune disorders have long been implicated in leukemogenesis. General evidence in support of this hypothesis comes from demonstration of increased risk with population mixing and exposure to siblings and clustering of leukemia cases in space and time (35–39).

Infectious agents associated with an increased risk of hematologic neoplasia include cytomegalovirus (40), Epstein-Barr virus (40–42), dengue virus (43), hepatitis viruses (44,45), human herpesvirus 6 (46,47), human immunodeficiency virus (48,49), human T lymphotropic virus type I (50–52), influenza virus (53–55), measles virus (56), Parvovirus B19 (57,58), rubella virus (59–61), and varicella virus (62,63).

Hypoimmune states are associated with an increased risk of leukemia and other hematopoietic neoplasms. Such states include congenital immunodeficiency (64), common variable immunodeficiency (65), Kawasaki disease (66), idiopathic CD4+ lymphocytopenia (67,68), human immunodeficiency virus infection, and prior appendectomy and tonsillectomy (69).

Medical Interventions

Medical interventions have become an increasingly important cause of hematopoietic neoplasia (70,71). Iatrogenic etiologies currently account for at least 30% of myelodysplastic syndrome and acute leukemia cases, a figure that may be expected to rise as the population of cancer and stem cell transplantation survivors increases. Populations at especially high risk are patients with underlying constitutional risk factors and those treated for prior malignancies. Numerous different therapies have been implicated in leukemogenesis.

Antibiotics and antiinflammatory agents have occasionally been implicated in leukemogenesis (72–76). In most cases, these drugs are no longer commonly used.

Antineoplastic agents are well-known leukemogens and are especially potent when used in patients with constitutional risk factors and those with leukemia and lymphoma (77–88). Increased risk exists even for single agents administered briefly and/or in low doses.

Granulocyte and granulocyte-monocyte colony-stimulating factors are associated with the onset and rapid progression of leukemia (89,90). The relative contribution to leukemia risk is difficult to evaluate because these agents are typically used in patients with underlying constitutional or acquired risk factors. Caution must be used in making a diagnosis of high-grade myelodysplastic syndrome or acute leukemia in patients on growth factors because clonal expansion may reverse on drug withdrawal.

Immunosuppressive agents are strongly implicated in the onset and progression of hematologic neoplasia (91–94). As with patients on granulocyte colony-stimulating factor, caution must be used before making a diagnosis of myelodysplastic syndrome or acute leukemia because regression of disease has been reported after drug withdrawal (95).

Psoralen and ultraviolet light therapy have been associated with the onset and acceleration of hematologic malignancy, possibly acting synergistically with psoriasis as a risk factor in some patients (96).

Radiotherapy is a well-known risk factor for the development of myelodysplastic syndrome and acute leukemia (97–103). Its effect is potentiated by constitutional risk factors (104) and the administration of antineoplastic drugs.

Splenectomy has been associated with an increased incidence of blast transformation in patients with myelofibrosis with myeloid metaplasia (105).

Stem cell transplantation is the setting for increasing numbers of leukemia cases (106–113). In such cases, underlying constitutional risk factors and/or prior antineoplastic therapy are virtually always present. After transplantation, leukemia usually arises in host cells but may occur in donor cells (114–116). Caution should be exercised in making the diagnosis of acute leukemia after stem cell transplantation because dysplastic changes and even clonal proliferations may regress over time.

The differential diagnosis of therapy-induced hematologic malignancy includes relapse or blast transformation of the original disease (117,118) and, rarely, inadvertent transmission of donor leukemia (119).

Pregnancy and Birth-Related Factors

Abundant evidence indicates that childhood leukemia arises *in utero,* likely from intrauterine exposure to environmental risk factors (120–124). It is often difficult to separate intrauterine from other risk factors; in the case of multiple affected siblings, the possibility of constitutional factors cannot be excluded.

After a clone arises, it may remain confined to the fetus or to one of a set of twins or spread from mother to fetus or between fetuses, regardless of zygosity. Thus, genetically identical hematologic malignancies have occurred in mother and fetus and in twins (125–129). The maximal latency period between the appearance of a clone *in utero* and overt leukemia is unknown, although it is clearly more than 10 years (130). In some cases, spontaneous remission of overt leukemia occurs (131,132). These findings indicate that additional factors are required to transform a clone into persistent acute leukemia.

Risk factors related to pregnancy and birth may be parental or nonparental in origin. Parental risk factors for childhood leukemia include exposure to environmental carcinogens, maternal age younger than 21 or older than 40 years, and maternal consumption of dietary bioflavonoids (133–141). Dietary bioflavonoids are naturally occurring DNA topoisomerase II inhibitors that cleave sites on *MLL*; maternal ingestion may account for the high rate of *MLL* translocation seen in infant leukemia.

Nonparental risk factors include birth weight less than 2,500 or more than 4,000 g, delivery by cesarean section, multiple birth, and low neonatal serum thyroid-stimulating hormone level (142–144). Birth order affects the risk of childhood leukemia. The risk of acute lymphoblastic is highest for a firstborn child and decreases thereafter; the risk of acute myeloid leukemia is lowest for a firstborn child and increases thereafter.

Other Acquired Risk Factors

Age is directly correlated with the incidence of hematopoietic neoplasia, likely attributable to the combined effect of constitutional and acquired factors over time (145,146). Myelodysplastic syndrome and acute leukemia in the elderly resembles that seen in patients with therapy- and toxin-induced disease.

Increased body weight may be directly related to the risk of acute leukemia in adults as it is in newborns (147).

Connective tissue diseases associated with hematologic neoplasia include systemic lupus erythematosus, rheumatoid arthritis, polymyositis and dermatomyositis, systemic sclerosis, and Behçet disease (148–151). Such cases are not to be confused with those in which patients with connective tissue disease have been treated with leukemogenic agents. Connective tissue disease also occurs in patients with myelodysplastic syndrome as a result of clonal differentiation to self-reactive B cells.

Endocrine disorders associated with hematopoietic neoplasia include hyperparathyroidism, acromegaly, and a wide variety of biologically active endocrine neoplasms (152–

159). Hormones are potent hematopoietic growth factors. Interestingly, in some cases, resection of the affected gland has produced hematologic remission.

Inflammatory bowel disease appears to be a risk factor for hematopoietic malignancy (160,161). As with connective tissue diseases, confounding factors include prior cytotoxic therapy and the occurrence of bowel disease as a paraneoplastic phenomenon in myelodysplastic syndrome.

Germ cell tumors (GCTs) are strongly associated with hematopoietic neoplasia (162–168). The GCT is usually malignant and located in the mediastinum. The hematopoietic disease often shows myeloid, mast cell, or histiocytic differentiation. Klinefelter syndrome is frequently present. Hematopoietic neoplasia appears to arise within the GCTs, a hypothesis supported by the observation of hematopoietic tissue within GCT and the frequent finding of isochromosome 12p, a GCT-associated anomaly, in clonal hematopoietic cells.

Other tumors, especially those of blastic origin, are associated with an increased risk of hematopoietic neoplasia (169–173). Underlying genetic risk factors may be present in many cases.

Psoriasis is associated with hematopoietic neoplasia (174–177). Therapy likely acts synergistically to increase the risk of onset or acceleration of disease.

Renal disorders of many types are associated with an increased risk of polycythemia vera and, to a lesser degree, other hematopoietic diseases (174–184). The underlying mechanism is likely related to renal production of erythropoietin, a hematopoietic growth factor. Cytotoxic and immunosuppressive therapy potentiate the risk in some patients.

REFERENCES

Constitutional Risk Factors

1. Ross JA, Potter JD, Shu XO, et al. Evaluating the relationships among maternal reproductive history, birth characteristics, and infant leukemia: a report from the Children's Cancer Group. *Ann Epidemiol* 1997;7:172–179.
2. Ross JA, Robison LL. MLL rearrangements in infant leukemia: is there a higher frequency in females? *Leuk Res* 1997;21:793–795.
3. Jackson N, Menon BS, Zarina W, et al. Why is acute leukemia more common in males? A possible sex-determined risk linked to the ABO blood group genes. *Ann Hematol* 1999;78:233–236.
4. Najean Y, Rain JD, Billotey C. Epidemiological data in polycythaemia vera: a study of 842 cases. *Hematol Cell Ther* 1998;40:159–165.
5. Dorak MT, Burnett AK, Worwood M. Hemochromatosis gene in leukemia and lymphoma. *Leuk Lymphoma* 2002;43:467–477.
6. Posthuma EF, Falkenburg JH, Apperley JF, et al. HLA-DR4 is associated with a diminished risk of the development of chronic myeloid leukemia (CML). Chronic Leukemia Working Party of the European Blood and Marrow Transplant Registry. *Leukemia* 2000;14:859–862.
7. Posthuma EF, Falkenburg JH, Apperley JF, et al. HLA-B8 and HLA-A3 coexpressed with HLA-B8 are associated with a

reduced risk of the development of chronic myeloid leukemia. The Chronic Leukemia Working Party of the EBMT. *Blood* 1999;93:3863–3865.

8. Arico M, Nichols K, Whitlock JA, et al. Familial clustering of Langerhans cell histiocytosis. *Br J Haematol* 1999;107:883–888.

9. Brubaker LH, Wasserman LR, Goldberg JD, et al. Increased prevalence of polycythemia vera in parents of patients on Polycythemia Vera Study Group protocols. *Am J Hematol* 1984;16:367–373.

10. de Chadarevian JP, Pawel BR. Hereditary Langerhans cell histiocytosis: instances of apparent vertical transmission. *Med Pediatr Oncol* 1998;31:559.

11. Gilbert HS. Familial myeloproliferative disease. *Baillieres Clin Haematol* 1998;11:849–858.

12. Horwitz M, Sabath DE, Smithson WA, et al. A family inheriting different subtypes of acute myelogenous leukemia. *Am J Hematol* 1996;52:295–304.

13. Kumar T, Mandla SG, Greer WL. Familial myelodysplastic syndrome with early age of onset. *Am J Hematol* 2000;64:53–58.

14. Mandla SG, Goobie S, Kumar RT, et al. Genetic analysis of familial myelodysplastic syndrome: absence of linkage to chromosomes 5q31 and 7q22. *Cancer Genet Cytogenet* 1998;105:113–118.

15. Marsden K, Challis D, Kimber R. Familial myelodysplastic syndrome with onset late in life. *Am J Hematol* 1995;49:153–156.

16. Novik Y, Marino P, Makower DF, et al. Familial erythroleukemia: a distinct clinical and genetic type of familial leukemias. *Leuk Lymphoma* 1998;30:395–401.

17. Rosbotham JL, Malik NM, Syrris P, et al. Lack of c-kit mutation in familial urticaria pigmentosa. *Br J Dermatol* 1999;140:849–852.

18. Siebert R, Jhanwar S, Brown K, et al. Familial acute myeloid leukemia and DiGuglielmo syndrome. *Leukemia* 1995;9:1091–1094.

19. Horwitz M, Goode EL, Jarvik GP. Anticipation in familial leukemia. *Am J Hum Genet* 1996;59:990–998.

20. Mozziconacci MJ, Sobol H, Philip N, et al. Constitutional balanced pericentric inversions of chromosomes X, 2, and 5 in myeloid malignancies. *Cancer Genet Cytogenet* 1998;107:28–31.

21. Olopade OI, Roulston D, Baker T, et al. Familial myeloid leukemia associated with loss of the long arm of chromosome 5. *Leukemia* 1996;10:669–674.

22. Kwong YL, Ng MH, Ma SK. Familial acute myeloid leukemia with monosomy 7: late onset and involvement of a multipotential progenitor cell. *Cancer Genet Cytogenet* 2000;116:170–173.

23. Stanley WS, Burkett SS, Segel B, et al. Constitutional inversion of chromosome 7 and hematologic cancers. *Cancer Genet Cytogenet* 1997;96:46–49.

24. Egesten A, Hagerstrand I, Kristoffersson U, et al. Hypereosinophilic syndrome in a child mosaic for a congenital triplication of the short arm of chromosome 8. *Br J Haematol* 1997;96:369–373.

25. Martin Ramos ML, Barreiro E, Lopez-Perez J, et al. Acute megakaryoblastic leukemia in a patient with a familial pericentric inversion of chromosome 8, inv(8)(p23.1q13). *Cancer Genet Cytogenet* 1998;105:74–78.

26. Seghezzi L, Maserati E, Minelli A, et al. Constitutional trisomy 8 as first mutation in multistep carcinogenesis: clinical, cytogenetic, and molecular data on three cases. *Genes Chromosomes Cancer* 1996;17:94–101.

27. Goi K, Sugita K, Nakamura M, et al. Development of acute lymphoblastic leukemia with translocation (4;11) in a young girl with familial pericentric inversion 12. *Cancer Genet Cytogenet* 1999;110:124–127.

28. Frost JD, Wiersma SR. Progressive Langerhans cell histiocytosis in an infant with Klinefelter syndrome successfully treated with allogeneic bone marrow transplantation. *J Pediatr Hematol Oncol* 1996;18:396–400.

29. Milunsky JM, Wyandt HE, Milunsky A. Familial supernumerary chromosome and malignancy. *Cancer Genet Cytogenet* 1996;89:170–172.

30. Gao Q, Horwitz M, Roulston D, et al. Susceptibility gene for familial acute myeloid leukemia associated with loss of 5q and/or 7q is not localized to the commonly deleted portion of 5q. *Genes Chromosomes Cancer* 2000;28:164–172.

31. Hasle H, Clemmensen IH, Mikkelsen M. Risks of leukaemia and solid tumours in individuals with Down's syndrome. *Lancet* 2000;355:165–169.

32. Foster LA, Abboud MR, Taylor AB, et al. Myelodysplasia associated with Turner syndrome. *J Pediatr Hematol Oncol* 1996;18:299–301.

33. Takeshita A, Shinjo K, Yamashita M, et al. Extensive cytogenetic studies of clonality following interferon-alpha therapy in chronic myeloid leukemia occurring in monosomic cells in a patient with Turner syndrome mosaic. *Leukemia* 1999;13:1749–1753.

34. Garcia JL, Hernandez JM, Gonzalez M, et al. Translocation (15;17)(q22;q21) in a patient with Klinefelter syndrome. *Cancer Genet Cytogenet* 1996;86:86.

35. Yano T, Yuzurio S, Kimura K, et al. Ph-positive acute lymphocytic leukemia in a man with Klinefelter syndrome. *Cancer Genet Cytogenet* 2000;118:83–84.

36. Govender D, Pillay SV. Mediastinal immature teratoma with yolk sac tumor and myelomonocytic leukemia associated with Klinefelter's syndrome. *Int J Surg Pathol* 2002;10:157–162.

37. Okada H, Imai T, Itoh S, et al. XYY male with essential thrombocythemia in childhood. *Int J Hematol* 2000;71:55–58.

38. Palanduz S, Aktan M, Ozturk S, et al. 47,XYY karyotype in acute myeloid leukemia. *Cancer Genet Cytogenet* 1998;106:76–77.

39. Sandlund JT, Krance R, Pui CH, et al. XYY syndrome in children with acute lymphoblastic leukemia. *Med Pediatr Oncol* 1997;28:6–8.

40. Mozziconacci MJ, Sobol H, Costello R, et al. Askin tumor and acute myeloid leukemia in a patient with constitutional partial Y disomy. *Cancer Genet Cytogenet* 1998;103:11–14.

41. Krajinovic M, Labuda D, Sinnett D. Childhood acute lymphoblastic leukemia: genetic determinants of susceptibility and disease outcome. *Rev Environ Health* 2001;16:263–279.

42. Krajinovic M, Richer C, Sinnett H, et al. Genetic polymorphisms of N-acetyltransferases 1 and 2 and gene–gene interaction in the susceptibility to childhood acute lymphoblastic leukemia. *Cancer Epidemiol Biomarkers Prev* 2000;9:557–562.

43. Riballo E, Critchlow SE, Teo SH, et al. Identification of a defect in DNA ligase IV in a radiosensitive leukaemia patient. *Curr Biol* 1999;9:699–702.

44. Song WJ, Sullivan MG, Legare RD, et al. Haploinsufficiency of CBFA2 causes familial thrombocytopenia with propensity to develop acute myelogenous leukemia. *Nat Genet* 1999;23:166–175.

45. Feng B, Lei J, Lin Z, et al. Genetic studies on a family with acute myelogenous leukemia. *Cancer Genet Cytogenet* 1999;112:134–137.

46. Bowen DT, Frew ME, Rollinson S, et al. CYP1A1 *2B (Val) allele is overrepresented in a subgroup of acute myeloid leukemia patients with poor-risk karyotype associated with NRAS mutation, but not associated with FLT3 internal tandem duplication. *Blood* 2003;101(7):2770–2774.

47. Papageorgio C, Seiter K, Feldman EJ. Therapy-related myelodysplastic syndrome in adults with neurofibromatosis. *Leuk Lymphoma* 1999;32:605–608.

48. Side LE, Emanuel PD, Taylor B, et al. Mutations of the *NF1* gene in children with juvenile myelomonocytic leukemia without

clinical evidence of neurofibromatosis, type 1. *Blood* 1998;92: 267–272.

49. Wiemels JL, Smith RN, Taylor GM, et al. Methylenetetrahydrofolate reductase (MTHFR) polymorphisms and risk of molecularly defined subtypes of childhood acute leukemia. *Proc Natl Acad Sci U S A* 2001;98:4004–4009.

50. Felix CA, Megonigal MD, Chervinsky DS, et al. Association of germline p53 mutation with MLL segmental jumping translocation in treatment-related leukemia. *Blood* 1998;91:4451–4456.

51. Kleihues P, Schauble B, zur Hausen A, et al. Tumors associated with p53 germline mutations: a synopsis of 91 families. *Am J Pathol* 1997;150:1–13.

52. Infante-Rivard C, Krajinovic M, Labuda D, et al. Parental smoking, CYP1A1 genetic polymorphisms and childhood leukemia. *Cancer Causes Control* 2000;11:547–553.

53. Davies SM, Robison LL, Buckley JD, et al. Glutathione S-transferase polymorphisms in children with myeloid leukemia: a Children's Cancer Group study. *Cancer Epidemiol Biomarkers Prev* 2000;9:563–566.

54. Rollinson S, Roddam P, Kane E, et al. Polymorphic variation within the glutathione S-transferase genes and risk of adult acute leukaemia. *Carcinogenesis* 2000;21:43–47.

55. Sasai Y, Horiike S, Misawa S, et al. Genotype of glutathione S-transferase and other genetic configurations in myelodysplasia. *Leuk Res* 1999;23:975–981.

56. Stanulla M, Schrappe M, Brechlin AM, et al. Polymorphisms within glutathione S-transferase genes (GSTM1, GSTT1, GSTP1) and risk of relapse in childhood B-cell precursor acute lymphoblastic leukemia: a case-control study. *Blood* 2000;95:1222–1228.

57. Woo MH, Shuster JJ, Chen C, et al. Glutathione S-transferase genotypes in children who develop treatment-related acute myeloid malignancies. *Leukemia* 2000;14:232–237.

58. Sun L, Goodman PA, Wood CM, et al. Expression of aberrantly spliced oncogenic ikaros isoforms in childhood acute lymphoblastic leukemia. *J Clin Oncol* 1999;17:3753–3766.

59. Yagi T, Hibi S, Takanashi M, et al. High frequency of Ikaros isoform 6 expression in acute myelomonocytic and monocytic leukemias: implications for up-regulation of the antiapoptotic protein Bcl-XL in leukemogenesis. *Blood* 2002;99:1350–1355.

60. Naoe T, Takeyama K, Yokozawa T, et al. Analysis of genetic polymorphism in NQO1, GST-M1, GST-T1, and CYP3A4 in 469 Japanese patients with therapy-related leukemia/myelodysplastic syndrome and de novo acute myeloid leukemia. *Clin Cancer Res* 2000;6:4091–4095.

61. Bo J, Schroder H, Kristinsson J, et al. Possible carcinogenic effect of 6-mercaptopurine on bone marrow stem cells: relation to thiopurine metabolism. *Cancer* 1999;86:1080–1086.

62. McLeod HL, Krynetski EY, Relling MV, et al. Genetic polymorphism of thiopurine methyltransferase and its clinical relevance for childhood acute lymphoblastic leukemia. *Leukemia* 2000;14:567–572.

63. Di Rocco M, Arslanian A, Romanengo M, et al. Ataxia, ocular telangiectasia, chromosome instability, and Langerhans cell histiocytosis in a patient with an unknown breakage syndrome. *J Med Genet* 1999;36:159–160.

64. Infante-Rivard C, Mathonnet G, Sinnett D. Risk of childhood leukemia associated with diagnostic irradiation and polymorphisms in DNA repair genes. *Environ Health Perspect* 2000;108:495–498.

65. Kolialexi A, Mavrou A, Tsenghi C, et al. Chromosome fragility and predisposition to childhood malignancies. *Anticancer Res* 1998;18:2359–2364.

66. Vessey CJ, Norbury CJ, Hickson ID. Genetic disorders associated with cancer predisposition and genomic instability. *Prog Nucleic Acid Res Mol Biol* 1999;63:189–221.

67. Khanna KK. Cancer risk and the ATM gene: a continuing debate. *J Natl Cancer Inst* 2000;92:795–802.

68. Stankovic T, Kidd AM, Sutcliffe A, et al. ATM mutations and phenotypes in ataxia-telangiectasia families in the British Isles: expression of mutant ATM and the risk of leukemia, lymphoma, and breast cancer. *Am J Hum Genet* 1998;62:334–345.

69. Takeuchi S, Koike M, Park S, et al. The ATM gene and susceptibility to childhood T-cell acute lymphoblastic leukaemia. *Br J Haematol* 1998;103:536–538.

70. Alter BP, Caruso JP, Drachtman RA, et al. Fanconi anemia: myelodysplasia as a predictor of outcome. *Cancer Genet Cytogenet* 2000;117:125–131.

71. Sugita K, Taki T, Hayashi Y, et al. MLL-CBP fusion transcript in a therapy-related acute myeloid leukemia with the t(11;16)(q23;p13) which developed in an acute lymphoblastic leukemia patient with Fanconi anemia. *Genes Chromosomes Cancer* 2000;27:264–269.

72. Thurston VC, Ceperich TM, Vance GH, et al. Detection of monosomy 7 in bone marrow by fluorescence in situ hybridization. A study of Fanconi anemia patients and review of the literature. *Cancer Genet Cytogenet* 1999;109:154–160.

73. Aktas D, Koc A, Boduroglu K, et al. Myelodysplastic syndrome associated with monosomy 7 in a child with Bloom syndrome. *Cancer Genet Cytogenet* 2000;116:44–46.

74. Knight S, Vulliamy T, Copplestone A, et al. Dyskeratosis Congenita (DC) Registry: identification of new features of DC. *Br J Haematol* 1998;103:990–996.

75. Cetin M, Hicsonmez G, Gogus S. Myelodysplastic syndrome associated with Griscelli syndrome. *Leuk Res* 1998;22:859–862.

76. Moser MJ, Bigbee WL, Grant SG, et al. Genetic instability and hematologic disease risk in Werner syndrome patients and heterozygotes. *Cancer Res* 2000;60:2492–2496.

77. Willig TN, Gazda H, Sieff CA. Diamond-Blackfan anemia. *Curr Opin Hematol* 2000;7:85–94.

78. Kardos G, Veerman AJ, de Waal FC, et al. Familial sideroblastic anemia with emergence of monosomy 5 and myelodysplastic syndrome. *Med Pediatr Oncol* 1996;26:54–56.

79. Hunter MG, Avalos BR. Deletion of a critical internalization domain in the G-CSFR in acute myelogenous leukemia preceded by severe congenital neutropenia. *Blood* 1999;93:440–446.

80. Ward AC, van Aesch YM, Schelen AM, et al. Defective internalization and sustained activation of truncated granulocyte colony-stimulating factor receptor found in severe congenital neutropenia/acute myeloid leukemia. *Blood* 1999;93:447–458.

81. Dokal I, Rule S, Chen F, et al. Adult onset of acute myeloid leukaemia (M6) in patients with Shwachman-Diamond syndrome. *Br J Haematol* 1999;99:171–173.

82. Faber J, Lauener R, Wick F, et al. Shwachman-Diamond syndrome: early bone marrow transplantation in a high risk patient and new clues to pathogenesis. *Eur J Pediatr* 1999;158:995–1000.

83. Sokolic RA, Ferguson W, Mark HF. Discordant detection of monosomy 7 by GTG-banding and FISH in a patient with Shwachman-Diamond syndrome without evidence of myelodysplastic syndrome or acute myelogenous leukemia. *Cancer Genet Cytogenet* 1999;115:106–113.

84. Spirito FR, Crescenzi B, Matteucci C, et al. Cytogenetic characterization of acute myeloid leukemia in Shwachman's syndrome. A case report. *Haematologica* 2000;85:1207–1210.

85. Camitta BM, Rock A. Acute lymphoidic leukemia in a patient with thrombocytopenia/absent radii (TAR) syndrome. *Am J Pediatr Hematol Oncol* 1993;15:335–337.

86. Rao VS, Shenoi UD, Krishnamurthy PN. Acute myeloid leukemia in TAR syndrome. *Indian J Pediatr* 1997;64:563–565.

87. Mehes K, Kajtar P, Sandor G, et al. Excess of mild errors of morphogenesis in childhood lymphoblastic leukemia. *Am J Med Genet* 1998;75:22–27.

88. Mertens AC, Wen W, Davies SM, et al. Congenital abnormalities in children with acute leukemia: a report from the Children's Cancer Group. *J Pediatr* 1998;133:617–623.

89. Nishi M, Miyake H, Takeda T, et al. Congenital malformations and childhood cancer. *Med Pediatr Oncol* 2000;34:250–254.

90. Farrell SA, Warda LJ, LaFlair P, et al. Adams-Oliver syndrome: a case with juvenile chronic myelogenous leukemia and chylothorax. *Am J Med Genet* 1993;47:1175–1179.

91. van Den Berg H, Hennekam RC. Acute lymphoblastic leukaemia in a patient with cardiofaciocutaneous syndrome. *J Med Genet* 1999;36:799–800.

92. Lin CH, Lo LJ, Wang ML, et al. Major hematological diseases associated with cleft lip and palate. *Cleft Palate Craniofac J* 2000;37: 512–515.

93. Levendoglu-Tugal O, Noto R, Juster F, et al. Langerhans cell histiocytosis associated with partial DiGeorge syndrome in a newborn. *J Pediatr Hematol Oncol* 1996;18:401–404.

94. Moller KT, Gorlin RJ. The Dubowitz syndrome: a retrospective. *J Craniofac Genet Dev Biol Suppl* 1985;1:283–286.

95. Asano T, Yamamoto M. Acute lymphoblastic leukemia in Ehlers-Danlos syndrome. *Int J Hematol* 1996;64:283–285.

96. Heney D, Mueller R, Turner G, et al. Familial microcephaly with normal intelligence in a patient with acute lymphoblastic leukemia. *Cancer* 1992;69:962–965.

97. Kaplan SS, Bornstein SG, Christopherson WA, et al. Associated leukemia and mixed germ cell tumor in a patient with gonadal dysgenesis. *Int J Gynaecol Obstet* 1991;35:83–88.

98. Koo CH, Reifel J, Kogut N, et al. True histiocytic malignancy associated with a malignant teratoma in a patient with 46XY gonadal dysgenesis. *Am J Surg Pathol* 1992;16:175–183.

99. Tasaka T, Nagai M, Kubota Y, et al. Acute myelocytic leukemia associated with thrombocytosis and inv 3(q21.3; q26.2) in a case of Gronbland-Strandberg syndrome. *Leuk Res* 1992;16:1187–1190.

100. al-Sheyyab M, el Shanti H, Todd D, et al. Autosomal recessive lamellar ichthyosis and acute lymphoblastic leukemia. *Eur J Hum Genet* 1996;4:105–107.

101. Lee JJ, Kim HJ, Chung IJ, et al. A case of Marfan syndrome with acute monoblastic leukemia. *Korean J Intern Med* 1998;13: 140–142.

102. Fukuda S, Yamada Y, Nishimura M, et al. Marinesco-Sjogren syndrome associated with acute myeloblastic leukemia. *Clin Genet* 1997;51:278–280.

103. Schnur RE, Greenbaum BH, Heymann WR, et al. Acute lymphoblastic leukemia in a child with the CHIME neuroectodermal dysplasia syndrome. *Am J Med Genet* 1997;72:24–29.

104. Bader-Meunier B, Tchernia G, Mielot F, et al. Occurrence of myeloproliferative disorder in patients with Noonan syndrome. *J Pediatr* 1997;130:885–889.

105. Choong K, Freedman MH, Chitayat D, et al. Juvenile myelomonocytic leukemia and Noonan syndrome. *J Pediatr Hematol Oncol* 1999;21:523–527

106. Johannes JM, Garcia ER, De Vaan GA, et al. Noonan's syndrome in association with acute leukemia. *Pediatr Hematol Oncol* 1995;12:571–575.

107. Costa R, Afonso E, Benedito M, et al. Poland's syndrome associated with chronic granulocytic leukemia. *Sangre (Barc)* 1991;36: 417–418.

108. Esquembre C, Ferris J, Verdeguer A, et al. Poland syndrome and leukaemia. *Eur J Pediatr* 1987;146:444.

109. Parikh PM, Karandikar SM, Koppikar S, et al. Poland's syndrome with acute lymphoblastic leukemia in an adult. *Med Pediatr Oncol* 1988;16:290–292.

110. Arnold SR, Spicer D, Kouseff B, et al. Seckel-like syndrome in three siblings. *Pediatr Dev Pathol* 1999;2:180–187.

111. Hayani A, Suarez CR, Molnar Z, et al. Acute myeloid leukaemia in a patient with Seckel syndrome. *J Med Genet* 1994;31: 148–149.

112. Bergevin PR, Blom J. Sipple syndrome and acute lymphoblastic leukemia. *JAMA* 1975;231:390.

113. Yule SM. Cancer in Sotos syndrome. *Arch Dis Child* 1999; 80:493.

114. Chatterjee R, Kottaridis PD, McGarrigle HH, et al. Hypogonadotrophism fails to prevent severe testicular damage induced by total body irradiation in a patient with beta-thalassaemia major and acute lymphoblastic leukaemia. *Bone Marrow Transplant* 2001;28:989–991.

115. Voskaridou E, Terpos E, Komninaka V, et al. Chronic myeloid leukaemia with marked thrombocytosis in a patient with thalassaemia major: complete haematological remission under the combination of hydroxyurea and anagrelide. *Br J Haematol* 2002;116:155–157.

116. Lacan P, Francina A, Souillet G, et al. Two new alpha chain variants: Hb Boghe [alpha58(E7)His—>Gln, alpha2], a variant on the distal histidine, and Hb CHarolles [alpha103(G10)His-Tyr, alpha1]. *Hemoglobin* 1999;23:345–352.

117. Votaw ML, Spannuth C Jr, Krish G, et al. Acute renal failure in a patient with essential thrombocythemia, diabetes mellitus, and heterozygous hemoglobin C disease. *South Med J* 1990;83: 57–59.

118. Dash S, Kumar S, Dash RJ. Hematological malignancy in hemoglobin D disease. *Am J Hematol* 1988;27:305.

119. Quattrin N, Luzzatto L, Quattrin S Jr. New clinical and biochemical findings from 235 patients with hemoglobin Lepore. *Ann N Y Acad Sci* 1980;344:364–374.

120. Sotomayor EA, Glasser L. Acute lymphoblastic leukemia in sickle cell disease. *Arch Pathol Lab Med* 1999;123:745–746.

121. Wilson S. Acute leukemia in a patient with sickle-cell anemia treated with hydroxyurea. *Ann Intern Med* 2000;133: 925–926.

122. Ferraris AM, Broccia G, Meloni T, et al. Glucose 6-phosphate dehydrogenase deficiency and incidence of hematologic malignancy. *Am J Hum Genet* 1988;42:516–520.

123. Altay C, Hicsonmez G, Zamani VP, et al. Acute leukemia in two patients with hemophilia. *Cancer* 1985;55:510–511.

124. Kawakami K, Takezaki T, Nakazono S, et al. Acute childhood leukemia in a patient with hemophilia: first report in Japan. *Acta Paediatr Jpn* 1994;36:91–94.

125. Conti JA, Howard LM. Hereditary spherocytosis and hematologic malignancy. *N J Med* 1994;91:95–97.

126. Martinez-Climent JA, Lopez-Andreu JA, Ferris-Tortajada J, et al. Acute lymphoblastic leukaemia in a child with hereditary spherocytosis. *Eur J Pediatr* 1995;154:753–754.

127. Hunh D, Belohradsky BH, Haas R. Familial peroxidase-deficiency and acute myeloic leukemia. *Acta Haematol* 1978;59: 129–143.

128. Gerrard JM, McNicol A. Platelet storage pool deficiency, leukemia, and myelodysplastic syndromes. *Leuk Lymphoma* 1992;8:277–281.

129. Au WY, Tam SC, Ho KM, et al. Hypertrichosis due to porphyria cutanea tarda associated with blastic transformation of myelofibrosis. *Br J Dermatol* 1999;141:932.

130. McKenna DB, Browne M, O'Donnell R, et al. Porphyria cutanea tarda and hematologic malignancy—a report of 4 cases. *Photodermatol Photoimmunol Photomed* 1997;13:143–146.

131. Wooten MD, Scott JW, Miller AM, et al. Chronic myelogenous leukemia and porphyria cutanea tarda in a patient with limited systemic sclerosis. *South Med J* 1998;91:493–495.

132. Ieki R, Miwa S, Fujii H, et al. Patient with pyruvate kinase deficiency developed acute myelogenous leukemia. *Am J Hematol* 1990;34:64–68.

133. al-Jader LN, West RR, Holmes JA, et al. Leukaemia mortality among relatives of cystic fibrosis patients. *Arch Dis Child* 1991;66:317–319.

134. Biggs BG, Vaughan W, Colombo JL, et al. Cystic fibrosis complicated by acute leukemia. *Cancer* 1986;57:2441–2443.

135. Rizzari C, Conter V, Jankovic M, et al. Acute lymphoblastic leukaemia in a child with cystic fibrosis. *Haematologica* 1992;77:427–429.

Acquired Risk Factors

1. Baris B, Demir AU, Shehu V, et al. Environmental fibrous zeolite (erionite) exposure and malignant tumors other than mesothelioma. *J Environ Pathol Toxicol Oncol* 1996;15:183–189.

2. Colt JS, Blair A. Parental occupational exposures and risk of childhood cancer. *Environ Health Perspect* 1998;106[Suppl 3]:909–925.

3. Crane MM, Strom SS, Halabi S, et al. Correlation between selected environmental exposures and karyotype in acute myelocytic leukemia. *Cancer Epidemiol Biomarkers Prev* 1996;5:639–644.

4. Daniels JL, Olshan AF, Savitz DA. Pesticides and childhood cancers. *Environ Health Perspect* 1997;105:1068–1077.

5. Davico L, Sacerdote C, Ciccone G, et al. Chromosome 8, occupational exposures, smoking, and acute nonlymphocytic leukemias: a population-based study. *Cancer Epidemiol Biomarkers Prev* 1998;7:1123–1125.

6. Gluzman DF, Abramenko IV, Sklyarenko LM, et al. Acute leukemias in children from the city of Kiev and Kiev region after the Chernobyl NPP catastrophe. *Pediatr Hematol Oncol* 1999;16:355–360.

7. Gundestrup M, Storm HH. Radiation-induced acute myeloid leukaemia and other cancers in commercial jet cockpit crew: a population-based cohort study. *Lancet* 1999;354:2029–2031.

8. Hromas R, Shopnick R, Jumean HG, et al. A novel syndrome of radiation-associated acute myeloid leukemia involving AML1 gene translocations. *Blood* 2000;95:4011–4013.

9. Infante-Rivard C, Krajinovic M, Labuda D, et al. Parental smoking, CYP1A1 genetic polymorphisms and childhood leukemia. *Cancer Causes Control* 2000;11:547–553.

10. Infante-Rivard C, Labuda D, Krajinovic M, et al. Risk of childhood leukemia associated with exposure to pesticides and with gene polymorphisms. *Epidemiology* 1999;10:481–487.

11. Bloemen LJ, Youk A, Bradley TD, et al. Lymphohaematopoienic cancer risk among chemical workers exposed to benzene *Occup Environ Med* 2004;61:270–274.

12. Infante-Rivard C, Olson E, Jacques L, et al. Drinking water contaminants and childhood leukemia. *Epidemiology* 2001;12:13–19.

13. Jarvholm B, Mellblom B, Norrman R, et al. Cancer incidence of workers in the Swedish petroleum industry. *Occup Environ Med* 1997;54:686–691.

14. Kane EV, Roman E, Cartwright R, et al. Tobacco and the risk of acute leukaemia in adults. *Br J Cancer* 1999;81:1228–1233.

15. Little MP, Weiss HA, Boice JD Jr, et al. Risks of leukemia in Japanese atomic bomb survivors, in women treated for cervical cancer, and in patients treated for ankylosing spondylitis. *Radiat Res* 1999;152:280–292.

16. Meinert R, Schuz J, Kaletsch U, et al. Leukemia and non-Hodgkin's lymphoma in childhood and exposure to pesticides: results of a register-based case-control study in Germany. *Am J Epidemiol* 2000;151:639–646.

17. Nilsson RI, Nordlinder R, Horte LG, et al. Leukaemia, lymphoma, and multiple myeloma in seamen on tankers. *Occup Environ Med* 1998;55:517–521.

18. Nordlinder R, Jarvholm B. Environmental exposure to gasoline and leukemia in children and young adults—an ecology study. *Int Arch Occup Environ Health* 1997;70:57–60.

19. Rigolin GM, Cuneo A, Roberti MG, et al. Exposure to myelotoxic agents and myelodysplasia: case-control study and correlation with clinicobiological findings. *Br J Haematol* 1998;103:189–197.

20. Rinsky RA, Hornung RW, Silver SR, et al. Benzene exposure and hematopoietic mortality: A long-term epidemiologic risk assessment. *Am J Ind Med* 2002;42:474–480.

21. Callea V, Comis M, Iaria G, et al. Clinical significance of HLA-DR+, CD19+, CD10+ immature B-cell phenotype and CD34+ cell detection in bone marrow lymphocytes from children affected with immune thrombocytopenic purpura. *Haematologica* 1997;82:471–473.

22. Mizutani K, Azuma E, Komada Y, et al. An infantile case of cytomegalovirus induced idiopathic thrombocytopenic purpura with predominant proliferation of CD10 positive lymphoblast in bone marrow. *Acta Paediatr Jpn* 1995;37:71–74.

23. Nissen C, Genitsch A, Sendelov S, et al. Cell cycling stress in the monocyte line as a risk factor for progression of the aplastic anaemia/paroxysmal nocturnal haemoglobinuria syndrome to myelodysplastic syndrome. *Acta Haematol* 2000;103:33–40.

24. Mortazavi Y, Tooze JA, Gordon-Smith EC, et al. N-RAS gene mutation in patients with aplastic anemia and aplastic anemia/paroxysmal nocturnal hemoglobinuria during evolution to clonal disease. *Blood* 2000;95:646–650.

25. Socie G, Rosenfeld S, Frickhofen N, et al. Late clonal diseases of treated aplastic anemia. *Semin Hematol* 2000;37:91–101.

26. Suvajdzic N, Marisavljevic D, Jovanovic V, et al. Pure red cell aplasia evolving through the hyperfibrotic myelodysplastic syndrome to the acute myeloid leukemia: some pathogenetic aspects. *Hematol Cell Ther* 1999;41:27–29.

27. Gondo H, Hamasaki Y, Nakayama H, et al. Acute leukemia during pregnancy. Association with immune-mediated thrombocytopenia in mother and infant. *Acta Haematol* 1990;83:140–144.

28. Drabick JJ, Davis BJ, Byrd JC. Concurrent pernicious anemia and myelodysplastic syndrome. *Ann Hematol* 2001;80:243–245.

29. Hsing AW, Hansson LE, McLaughlin JK, et al. Pernicious anemia and subsequent cancer. A population-based cohort study. *Cancer* 1993;71:745–750.

30. Remacha A, Souto JC, Ortuno F, et al. Pernicious anemias with subtle or atypical presentation. *Sangre (Barc)* 1992;37:109–113.

31. Britt RP, Rose DP. Pernicious anemia with a normal serum vitamin B-12 level in a case of chronic granulocytic leukemia. *Arch Intern Med* 1966;117:32–33.

32. Merk K, Mattsson B, Mattsson A, et al. The incidence of cancer among blood donors. *Int J Epidemiol* 1990;19:505–509.

33. Najean Y, Rain JD, Billotey C. Epidemiological data in polycythaemia vera: a study of 842 cases. *Hematol Cell Ther* 1998;40:159–165.

34. Randi ML, Rossi C, Barbone E, et al. Myeloproliferative disease in patients with a history of multiple blood donations: a report of 8 cases. *Haematologica* 1994;79:137–140.

35. Birch JM, Alexander FE, Blair V, et al. Space-time clustering patterns in childhood leukaemia support a role for infection. *Br J Cancer* 2000;82:1571–1576.

36. Kinlen LJ, Balkwill A. Infective cause of childhood leukaemia and wartime population mixing in Orkney and Shetland, UK. *Lancet* 2001;357:858.

37. McNally RJ, Alexander FE, Birch JM. Space-time clustering analyses of childhood acute lymphoblastic leukaemia by immunophenotype. *Br J Cancer* 2002;87:513–515.

38. Wen WQ, Shu XO, Steinbuch M, et al. Paternal military service and risk for childhood leukemia in offspring. *Am J Epidemiol* 2000;151:231–240.

39. Westergaard T, Andersen PK, Pedersen JB, et al. Birth characteristics, sibling patterns, and acute leukemia risk in childhood: a population-based cohort study. *J Natl Cancer Inst* 1997;89:939–947.

40. Hermouet S, Sutton CA, Rose TM, et al. Qualitative and quantitative analysis of human herpesviruses in chronic and acute B cell lymphocytic leukemia and in multiple myeloma. *Leukemia* 2003;17:185–195.

41. Ariad S, Argov S, Manor E, et al. Acute blast crisis with EBV-infected blasts, in a patient with chronic myeloid leukemia, and vasculitis. *Leuk Lymphoma* 2000;37:431–435.

42. Sakajiri S, Mori K, Isobe Y, et al. Epstein-Barr virus-associated T-cell acute lymphoblastic leukaemia. *Br J Haematol* 2002;117:127–129.

43. Au WY, Ma ES, Kwong YL. Acute myeloid leukemia precipitated by dengue virus infection in a patient with hemoglobin H disease. *Haematologica* 2001;86:E17.

44. Gentile G, Mele A, Monarco B, et al. Hepatitis B and C viruses, human T-cell lymphotropic virus types I and II, and leukemias: a case-control study. The Italian Leukemia Study Group. *Cancer Epidemiol Biomarkers Prev* 1996;5:227–230.

45. Pavlova BG, Heinz R, Selim U, et al. Association of GB virus C (GBV-C)/hepatitis G virus (HGV) with haematological diseases of different malignant potential. *J Med Virol* 1999;57:361–366.

46. Salonen MJ, Siimes MA, Salonen EM, et al. Antibody status to HHV-6 in children with leukaemia. *Leukemia* 2002;16:716–719.

47. Yoshikawa T, Kobayashi I, Asano Y, et al. Clinical features of primary human herpesvirus-6 infection in an infant with acute lymphoblastic leukemia. *Am J Pediatr Hematol Oncol* 1993;15:424–426.

48. Granovsky MO, Mueller BU, Nicholson HS, et al. Cancer in human immunodeficiency virus-infected children: a case series from the Children's Cancer Group and the National Cancer Institute. *J Clin Oncol* 1998;16:1729–1735.

49. Hentrich M, Rockstroh J, Sandner R, et al. Acute myelogenous leukaemia and myelomonocytic blast crisis following polycythemia vera in HIV positive patients: report of cases and review of the literature. *Ann Oncol* 2000;11:195–200.

50. Karlic H, Mostl M, Mucke H, et al. Association of human T-cell leukemia virus and myelodysplastic syndrome in a central European population. *Cancer Res* 1997;57:4718–4721.

51. Kawachi Y, Watanabe A, Sakamoto Y, et al. Acute myeloblastic leukemia associated with an intermediate state between the healthy carrier state and adult T-cell leukemia. *Leuk Lymphoma* 1995;16:505–509.

52. Tsukasaki K, Koba T, Iwanaga M, et al. Possible association between adult T-cell leukemia/lymphoma and acute myeloid leukemia. *Cancer* 1998;82:488–494.

53. Austin DF, Karp S, Dworsky R, et al. Excess leukemia in cohorts of children born following influenza epidemics. *Am J Epidemiol* 1975;101:77–83.

54. Dockerty JD, Skegg DC, Elwood JM, et al. Infections, vaccinations, and the risk of childhood leukaemia. *Br J Cancer* 1999;80:1483–1489.

55. Timonen TT. A hypothesis concerning deficiency of sunlight, cold temperature, and influenza epidemics associated with the onset of acute lymphoblastic leukemia in northern Finland. *Ann Hematol* 1999;78:408–414.

56. Cooper GS, Kamel F, Sandler DP, et al. Risk of adult acute leukemia in relation to prior immune-related conditions. *Cancer Epidemiol Biomarkers Prev* 1996;5:867–872.

57. Heegaard ED, Madsen HO, Schmiegelow K. Transient pancytopenia preceding acute lymphoblastic leukaemia (pre-ALL) precipitated by Parvovirus B19. *Br J Haematol* 2001;114:810–813.

58. Sitar G, Balduini CL, Manenti L, et al. Possible evolution of human parvovirus B19 infection into erythroleukemia. *Haematologica* 1999;84:957–959.

59. Ashby MA, Williams CJ, Buchanan RB, et al. Mediastinal germ cell tumour associated with malignant histiocytosis and high rubella titres. *Hematol Oncol* 1986;4:183–194.

60. Kelly SJ, Gibbs T, Cheetham CH. Acute myelomonocytic leukaemia following atypical congenital rubella. *J Clin Pathol* 1993;46:764–765.

61. Matamoros N, Matutes E, Hernandez M, et al. Neonatal mixed lineage acute leukaemia. *Leukemia* 1994;8:1236–1242.

62. Blot WJ, Draper G, Kinlen L, et al. Childhood cancer in relation to prenatal exposure to chickenpox. *Br J Cancer* 1980;42:342–344.

63. Vianna NJ, Polan AK. Childhood lymphatic leukemia: prenatal seasonality and possible association with congenital varicella. *Am J Epidemiol* 1976;103:321–332.

64. Kitahama S, Iitaka M, Shimizu T, et al. Thyroid involvement by malignant histiocytosis of Langerhans' cell type. *Clin Endocrinol (Oxf)* 1996;45:357–363.

65. Belickova M, Schroeder HW Jr, Guan YL, et al. Clonal hematopoiesis and acquired thalassemia in common variable immunodeficiency. *Mol Med* 1994;1:56–61.

66. Murray JC, Bomgaars LR, Carcamo B, et al. Lymphoid malignancies following Kawasaki disease. *Am J Hematol* 1995;50:299–300.

67. Manna A, Porcellini A, Marelli A, et al. A case of Langerhans histiocytosis with HIV-like immunodeficiency. *Haematologica* 1992;77:73–75.

68. Weemaes CM, Preijers F, de Vaan GA, et al. CD4 deficiency in myelodysplastic syndrome with monosomy 7. *Eur J Pediatr* 1996;155:96–98.

69. Schuz J, Kaletsch U, Meinert R, et al. Association of childhood leukaemia with factors related to the immune system. *Br J Cancer* 1999;80:585–590.

70. Leone G, Mele L, Pulsoni A, et al. The incidence of secondary leukemias. *Haematologica* 1999;84:937–945.

71. Karp JE, Sarkodee-Adoo CB. Therapy-related acute leukemia. *Clin Lab Med* 2000;20:71–81.

72. Abbas Z, Malik I, Khan A. Sequential induction of aplastic anemia and acute leukemia by chloramphenicol. *J Pak Med Assoc* 1993;43:58–59.

73. Nagaratnam N, Chetiyawardana AD, Rajiyah S. Aplasia and leukaemia following chloroquine therapy. *Postgrad Med J* 1978;54:108–112.

74. Mitarnun W, Peerabool R. Blood dyscrasia evolving into acute lymphoblastic leukemia following ingestion of phenylbutazone, indomethacin, dexamethasone and prednisolone. *J Med Assoc Thai* 1983;66:649–654.

75. Ohyashiki K, Ohyashiki JH, Raza A, et al. Phenylbutazone-induced myelodysplastic syndrome with Philadelphia translocation. *Cancer Genet Cytogenet* 1987;26:213–216.

76. Witwer MW, Schmid FR, Tesar JT. Acute myelomonocytic leukaemia and multiple myeloma after sulphinpyrazone and colchicine treatment of gout. *BMJ* 1976;2:89.

77. Hudson MM, Poquette CA, Lee J, et al. Increased mortality

after successful treatment for Hodgkin's disease. *J Clin Oncol* 1998;16:3592–3600.

78. Kollmannsberger C, Beyer J, Droz JP, et al. Secondary leukemia following high cumulative doses of etoposide in patients treated for advanced germ cell tumors. *J Clin Oncol* 1998;16:3386–3391.

79. Kolte B, Baer AN, Sait SN, et al. Acute myeloid leukemia in the setting of low dose weekly methotrexate therapy for rheumatoid arthritis. *Leuk Lymphoma* 2001;42:371–378.

80. Kushner BH, Heller G, Cheung NK, et al. High risk of leukemia after short-term dose-intensive chemotherapy in young patients with solid tumors. *J Clin Oncol* 1998;16:3016–3020.

81. Loning L, Zimmermann M, Reiter A, et al. Secondary neoplasms subsequent to Berlin-Frankfurt-Munster therapy of acute lymphoblastic leukemia in childhood: significantly lower risk without cranial radiotherapy. *Blood* 2000;95:2770–2775.

82. Orchard JA, Bolam S, Oscier DG. Association of myelodysplastic changes with purine analogues. *Br J Haematol* 1998;100:677–679.

83. Pagano L, Annino L, Ferrari A, et al. Secondary haematological neoplasm after treatment of adult acute lymphoblastic leukemia: analysis of 1170 adult ALL patients enrolled in the GIMEMA trials. Gruppo Italiano Malattie Ematologiche Maligne dell'Adulto. *Br J Haematol* 1998;100:669–676.

84. Rigolin GM, Cuneo A, Roberti MG, et al. Exposure to myelotoxic agents and myelodysplasia: case-control study and correlation with clinicobiological findings. *Br J Haematol* 1998;103:189–197.

85. Schneider DT, Hilgenfeld E, Schwabe D, et al. Acute myelogenous leukemia after treatment for malignant germ cell tumors in children. *J Clin Oncol* 1999;17:3226–3233.

86. Smith MA, Rubinstein L, Anderson JR, et al. Secondary leukemia or myelodysplastic syndrome after treatment with epipodophyllotoxins. *J Clin Oncol* 1999;17:569–577

87. Turker A, Guler N. Therapy related acute myeloid leukemia after exposure to 5-fluorouracil: a case report. *Hematol Cell Ther* 1999;41:195–196.

88. Zompi S, Legrand O, Bouscary D, et al. Therapy-related acute myeloid leukaemia after successful therapy for acute promyelocytic leukaemia with t(15;17): a report of two cases and a review of the literature. *Br J Haematol* 2000;110:610–613.

89. Kaito K, Kobayashi M, Katayama T, et al. Long-term administration of G-CSF for aplastic anaemia is closely related to the early evolution of monosomy 7 MDS in adults. *Br J Haematol* 1998;103:297–303.

90. Nishimura M, Yamada T, Andoh T, et al. Granulocyte colony-stimulating factor (G-CSF) dependent hematopoiesis with monosomy 7 in a patient with severe aplastic anemia after ATG/CsA/G-CSF combined therapy. *Int J Hematol* 1998;68:203–211.

91. Arnold JA, Ranson SA, Abdalla SH. Azathioprine-associated acute myeloid leukaemia with trilineage dysplasia and complex karyotype: a case report and review of the literature. *Clin Lab Haematol* 1999;21:289–292

92. Arican A, Ozbek N, Baltaci V, et al. Philadelphia chromosome (+) T-cell acute lymphoblastic leukemia after renal transplantation. *Transplant Proc* 1999;31:3242–3243.

93. Huebner G, Karthaus M, Pethig K, et al. Myelodysplastic syndrome and acute myelogenous leukemia secondary to heart transplantation. *Transplantation* 2000;70:688–690.

94. Robak T, Kasznicki M, Strzelecka B, et al. Atypical chronic myelogenous leukemia following immunosuppressive therapy for severe aplastic anemia. *Leuk Lymphoma* 1999;35:193–199.

95. Thalhammer-Scherrer R, Wieselthaler G, Knoebl P, et al. Post-

96. Kwong YL, Au WY, Ng MH, et al. Acute myeloid leukemia following psoralen with ultraviolet A therapy: a fluorescence in situ hybridization study. *Cancer Genet Cytogenet* 1997;99:11–13.

97. van Kaick G, Dalheimer A, Hornik S, et al. The German thorotrast study: recent results and assessment of risks. *Radiat Res* 1999;152:S64–S71.

98. Balan KK, Critchley M. Outcome of 259 patients with primary proliferative polycythaemia (PPP) and idiopathic thrombocythaemia (IT) treated in a regional nuclear medicine department with phosphorus-32—a 15 year review. *Br J Radiol* 1997;70:1169–1173.

99. Kossman SE, Weiss MA. Acute myelogenous leukemia after exposure to strontium-89 for the treatment of adenocarcinoma of the prostate. *Cancer* 2000;88:620–624.

100. Laurenti L, Salutari P, Sica S, et al. Acute myeloid leukemia after iodine-131 treatment for thyroid disorders. *Ann Hematol* 1998;76:271–272.

101. Little MP, Weiss HA, Boice JD Jr, et al. Risks of leukemia in Japanese atomic bomb survivors, in women treated for cervical cancer, and in patients treated for ankylosing spondylitis. *Radiat Res* 1999;152:280–292.

102. Najean Y, Rain JD. Treatment of polycythemia vera: use of 32P alone or in combination with maintenance therapy using hydroxyurea in 461 patients greater than 65 years of age. The French Polycythemia Study Group. *Blood* 1997;89:2319–2327.

103. Roldan Schilling V, Fernandez Abellan P, Dominguez Escribano JR, et al. Acute leukemias after treatment with radioiodine for thyroid cancer. *Haematologica* 1998;83:767–768.

104. Infante-Rivard C, Mathonnet G, Sinnett D. Risk of childhood leukemia associated with diagnostic irradiation and polymorphisms in DNA repair genes. *Environ Health Perspect* 2000;108:495–498.

105. Barosi G, Ambrosetti A, Centra A, et al. Splenectomy and risk of blast transformation in myelofibrosis with myeloid metaplasia. Italian Cooperative Study Group on Myeloid with Myeloid Metaplasia. *Blood* 1998;91:3630–3636.

106. Abruzzese E, Radford JE, Miller JS, et al. Detection of abnormal pretransplant clones in progenitor cells of patients who developed myelodysplasia after autologous transplantation. *Blood* 1999;94:1814–1819.

107. Friedberg JW, Neuberg D, Stone RM, et al. Outcome in patients with myelodysplastic syndrome after autologous bone marrow transplantation for non-Hodgkin's lymphoma. *J Clin Oncol* 1999;17:3128–3135.

108. Krishnan A, Bhatia S, Slovak ML, et al. Predictors of therapy-related leukemia and myelodysplasia following autologous transplantation for lymphoma: an assessment of risk factors. *Blood* 2000;95:1588–1593.

109. Lambertenghi Deliliers G, Annaloro C, Pozzoli E, et al. Cytogenetic and myelodysplastic alterations after autologous hemopoietic stem cell transplantation. *Leuk Res* 1999;23:291–297.

110. Laughlin MJ, McGaughey DS, Crews JR, et al. Secondary myelodysplasia and acute leukemia in breast cancer patients after autologous bone marrow transplant. *J Clin Oncol* 1998;16:1008–1012.

111. Micallef IN, Lillington DM, Apostolidis J, et al. Therapy-related myelodysplasia and secondary acute myelogenous leukemia after high-dose therapy with autologous hematopoietic progenitor-cell support for lymphoid malignancies. *J Clin Oncol* 2000;18:947–955.

112. Sobecks RM, Le Beau MM, Anastasi J, et al. Myelodysplasia and acute leukemia following a high-dose chemotherapy and

autologous bone marrow or peripheral blood stem cell transplantation. *Bone Marrow Transplant* 1999;23:1161–1165.

113. Toren A, Rechavi G, Nagler A. Early fulminant leukaemia post autologous bone marrow transplantation in non-Hodgkin's lymphoma patients. *Med Oncol* 1998;15:109–112.

114. Cooley LD, Sears DA, Udden MM, et al. Donor cell leukemia: report of a case occurring 11 years after allogeneic bone marrow transplantation and review of the literature. *Am J Hematol* 2000;63:46–53.

115. Hambach L, Eder M, Dammann E, et al. Donor cell-derived acute myeloid leukemia developing 14 months after matched unrelated bone marrow transplantation for chronic myeloid leukemia. *Bone Marrow Transplant* 2001;28:705–707.

116. Saito Y, Uzuka Y, Sakai N, et al. A Philadelphia chromosome positive acute lymphoblastic leukemia of donor origin after allogeneic bone marrow transplantation for chronic myelogenous leukemia in chronic phase. *Bone Marrow Transplant* 2000;25:1209–1211.

117. Dawson L, Slater R, Hagemeijer A, et al. Secondary T-acute lymphoblastic leukaemia mimicking blast crisis in chronic myeloid leukaemia. *Br J Haematol* 1999;106:104–106.

118. Manley R, Cochrane J, McDonald M, et al. Clonally unrelated BCR-ABL-negative acute myeloblastic leukemia masquerading as blast crisis after busulphan and interferon therapy for BCR-ABL-positive chronic myeloid leukemia. *Leukemia* 1999;13:126–129.

119. Niederwieser DW, Appelbaum FR, Gastl G, et al. Inadvertent transmission of a donor's acute myeloid leukemia in bone marrow transplantation for chronic myelocytic leukemia. *N Engl J Med* 1990;322:1794–1796.

120. Alexander FE, Patheal SL, Biondi A, et al. Transplacental chemical exposure and risk of infant leukemia with MLL gene fusion. *Cancer Res* 2001;61:2542–2546.

121. Fasching K, Panzer S, Haas OA, et al. Presence of clone-specific antigen receptor gene rearrangements at birth indicates an in utero origin of diverse types of early childhood acute lymphoblastic leukemia. *Blood* 2000;95:2722–2724.

122. McHale CM, Wiemels JL, Zhang L, et al. Prenatal origin of TEL-AML1-positive acute lymphoblastic leukemia in children born in California. *Genes Chromosomes Cancer* 2003;37:36–43.

123. Taub JW, Konrad MA, Ge Y, et al. High frequency of leukemic clones in newborn screening blood samples of children with B-precursor acute lymphoblastic leukemia. *Blood* 2002;99:2992–2996.

124. Yagi T, Hibi S, Tabata Y, et al. Detection of clonotypic IGH and TCR rearrangements in the neonatal blood spots of infants and children with B-cell precursor acute lymphoblastic leukemia. *Blood* 2000;96:264–268.

125. Chin YM, Wan Ariffin A, Lin HP, et al. Concordant childhood acute lymphoblastic leukemia in monozygotic twins. *Med J Malaysia* 1996;51:145–148.

126. Ford AM, Pombo-de-Oliveira MS, McCarthy KP, et al. Monoclonal origin of concordant T-cell malignancy in identical twins. *Blood* 1997;89:281–285.

127. Olah E, Stenszky V, Kiss A, et al. Familial leukemia: Ph1 positive acute lymphoid leukemia of a mother and her infant. *Blut* 1981;43:265–272.

128. Richkind KE, Loew T, Meisner L, et al. Identical cytogenetic clones and clonal evolution in pediatric monozygotic twins with acute myeloid leukemia: presymptomatic disease detection by interphase fluorescence *in situ* hybridization and review of the literature. *J Pediatr Hematol Oncol* 1998;20:264–267.

129. Sato-Matsumura KC, Matsumura T, Koizumi H, et al. Analysis of c-kit exon 11 and exon 17 of urticaria pigmentosa that occurred in monozygotic twin sisters. *Br J Dermatol* 1999;140:1130–1132.

130. Wiemels JL, Ford AM, Van Wering ER, et al. Protracted and variable latency of acute lymphoblastic leukemia after TEL-AML1 gene fusion *in utero*. *Blood* 1999;94:1057–1062.

131. Mora J, Dobrenis AM, Bussel JB, et al. Spontaneous remission of congenital acute nonlymphoblastic leukemia with normal karyotype in twins. *Med Pediatr Oncol* 2000;35:110–113.

132. van der Velden VH, Willemse MJ, Mulder MF, et al. Clearance of maternal leukaemic cells in a neonate. *Br J Haematol* 2001;114:104–106.

133. Infante-Rivard C, Krajinovic M, Labuda D, et al. Parental smoking, CYP1A1 genetic polymorphisms and childhood leukemia. *Cancer Causes Control* 2000;11:547–553.

134. Reynolds P, Von Behren J, Elkin EP. Birth characteristics and leukemia in young children. *Am J Epidemiol* 2002;155:603–613.

135. Roman E, Doyle P, Maconochie N, et al. Cancer in children of nuclear industry employees: report on children aged under 25 years from nuclear industry family study. *BMJ* 1999;318:1443–1450.

136. Schuz J, Kaletsch U, Meinert R, et al. Risk of childhood leukemia and parental self-reported occupational exposure to chemicals, dusts, and fumes: results from pooled analyses of German population-based case-control studies. *Cancer Epidemiol Biomarkers Prev* 2000;9:835–838.

137. Severson RK, Ross JA. The causes of acute leukemia. *Curr Opin Oncol* 1999;11:20–24.

138. Shu XO, Stewart P, Wen WQ, et al. Parental occupational exposure to hydrocarbons and risk of acute lymphocytic leukemia in offspring. *Cancer Epidemiol Biomarkers Prev* 1999;8:783–791.

139. Smulevich VB, Solionova LG, Belyakova SV. Parental occupation and other factors and cancer risk in children: I. Study methodology and non-occupational factors. *Int J Cancer* 1999;83:712–717.

140. Strick R, Strissel PL, Borgers S, et al. Dietary bioflavonoids induce cleavage in the MLL gene and may contribute to infant leukemia. *Proc Natl Acad Sci U S A* 2000;97:4790–4795.

141. Wen WQ, Shu XO, Steinbuch M, et al. Paternal military service and risk for childhood leukemia in offspring. *Am J Epidemiol* 2000;151:231–240.

142. Lei U, Wohlfahrt J, Hjalgrim H, et al. Neonatal level of thyroid-stimulating hormone and acute childhood leukemia. *Int J Cancer* 2000;88:486–488.

143. Ross JA, Potter JD, Shu XO, et al. Evaluating the relationships among maternal reproductive history, birth characteristics, and infant leukemia: a report from the Children's Cancer Group. *Ann Epidemiol* 1997;7:172–179.

144. Westergaard T, Andersen PK, Pedersen JB, et al. Birth characteristics, sibling patterns, and acute leukemia risk in childhood: a population-based cohort study. *J Natl Cancer Inst* 1997;89:939–947.

145. Nagura E, Minami S, Nagata K, et al. Acute myeloid leukemia in the elderly: 159 Nagoya case studies—Nagoya Cooperative Study Group for Elderly Leukemia. *Nagoya J Med Sci* 1999;62:135–144.

146. Rossi G, Pelizzari AM, Bellotti D, et al. Cytogenetic analogy between myelodysplastic syndrome and acute myeloid leukemia of elderly patients. *Leukemia* 2000;14:636–641.

147. Estey E, Thall P, Kantarjian H, et al. Association between increased body mass index and a diagnosis of acute promyelocytic leukemia in patients with acute myeloid leukemia. *Leukemia* 1997;11:1661–1664.

148. Colovic M, Jankovic G, Lazarevic V, et al. Acute megakaryoblastic leukaemia in a patient with systemic lupus erythematosus. *Med Oncol* 1997;14:31–34.

149. Della Rossa A, Tavoni A, Tognetti A, et al. Behcet's disease with gastrointestinal involvement associated with myelodysplasia in a patient with congenital panhypopituitarism. *Clin Rheumatol* 1998;17:515–517.

150. Ogawa H, Kuroda T, Inada M, et al. Intestinal Behcet's disease associated with myelodysplastic syndrome with chromosomal trisomy 8—a report of two cases and a review of the literature. *Hepatogastroenterology* 2001;48:416–420.

151. Wooten MD, Scott JW, Miller AM, et al. Chronic myelogenous leukemia and porphyria cutanea tarda in a patient with limited systemic sclerosis. *South Med J* 1998;91:493–495.

152. Godeau P, Bletry O, Brochard C, et al. Polycythemia vera and primary hyperparathyroidism. *Arch Intern Med* 1981;141:951–953.

153. Grellier P, Chanson P, Casadevall N, et al. Remission of polycythemia vera after surgical cure of acromegaly. *Ann Intern Med* 1996;124:495–496.

154. Lara JF, Rosen PP. Extramedullary hematopoiesis in a bronchial carcinoid tumor. An unusual complication of agnogenic myeloid metaplasia. *Arch Pathol Lab Med* 1990;114:1283–1285.

155. Pizzolito S, Barbone F, Rizzi C, et al. Parathyroid adenomas and malignant neoplasms: coincidence or etiological association? *Adv Clin Pathol* 1997;1:275–280.

156. Sham RL, von Doenhoff L, Dipoala J, et al. Polycythemia vera associated with metastatic carcinoid. *Cancer Invest* 1996;14:120–123.

157. Teramoto S, Ouchi V. Polycythemia vera in acromegaly. *Ann Intern Med* 1997;126:87.

158. Weinstein RS. Parathyroid carcinoma associated with polycythemia vera. *Bone* 1991;12:237–239.

159. Yeh SP, Wang JS, Wu H, et al. Nesidioblastosis, myelodysplastic syndrome and nodular diabetic glomerulosclerosis in an elderly nondiabetic woman: an autopsy report. *Diabetes Med* 1999;16:437–441.

160. Harewood GC, Loftus EV Jr, Tefferi A, et al. Concurrent inflammatory bowel disease and myelodysplastic syndromes. *Inflamm Bowel Dis* 1999;5:98–103.

161. Perard L, Thomas X, Jaumain H, et al. T-cell lineage acute lymphoblastic leukemia with chromosome 5 abnormality in a patient with Crohn's disease and lipoid nephrosis. *Ann Hematol* 2000;79:222–225.

162. Drut R. Mast cell disease and malignant germ cell tumors. *Hum Pathol* 1999;30:727.

163. Hale GA, Greenwood MF, Geil JD, et al. Langerhans cell histiocytosis after therapy for a malignant germ cell tumor of the central nervous system. *J Pediatr Hematol Oncol* 2000;22:355–357.

164. Lin JT, Lachmann E, Nagler W. Low back pain and myalgias in acute and relapsed mast cell leukemia: a case report. *Arch Phys Med Rehabil* 2002;83:860–863.

165. Miyagawa S, Hirota S, Park YD, et al. Cutaneous mastocytosis associated with a mixed germ cell tumour of the ovary: report of a case and review of the literature. *Br J Dermatol* 2001;145:309–312.

166. Murty VV, Chaganti RS. A genetic perspective of male germ cell tumors. *Semin Oncol* 1998;25:133–144.

167. Saito A, Watanabe K, Kusakabe T, et al. Mediastinal mature teratoma with coexistence of angiosarcoma, granulocytic sarcoma and a hematopoietic region in the tumor: a rare case of association between hematological malignancy and mediastinal germ cell tumor. *Pathol Int* 1998;48:749–753.

168. Sasou S, Nakamura SI, Habano W, et al. True malignant histiocytosis developed during chemotherapy for mediastinal immature teratoma. *Hum Pathol* 1996;27:1099–1103.

169. Fischer A, Jones L, Lowis SP. Concurrent Langerhans cell histiocytosis and neuroblastoma. *Med Pediatr Oncol* 1999;32:223–224.

170. Ishida Y, Kato K, Kigasawa H, et al. Synchronous occurrence of pleuropulmonary blastoma and cystic nephroma: possible genetic link in cystic lesions of the lung and the kidney. *Med Pediatr Oncol* 2000;35:85–87.

171. Kiratli H, Bilgic S, Ozerdem U. Retinoblastoma with acute lymphoblastic leukemia, polyposis coli, and multiple hamartomas. *J AAPOS* 1998;2:385–386.

172. Mozziconacci MJ, Sobol H, Costello R, et al. Askin tumor and acute myeloid leukemia in a patient with constitutional partial Y disomy. *Cancer Genet Cytogenet* 1998;103:11–14.

173. Priest JR, Watterson J, Strong L, et al. Pleuropulmonary blastoma: a marker for familial disease. *J Pediatr* 1996;128:220–224.

174. Cooper GS, Kamel F, Sandler DP, et al. Risk of adult acute leukemia in relation to prior immune-related conditions. *Cancer Epidemiol Biomarkers Prev* 1996;5:867–872.

175. Kishimoto Y, Yamamoto Y, Ito T, et al. Transfer of autoimmune thyroiditis and resolution of palmoplantar pustular psoriasis following allogeneic bone marrow transplantation. *Bone Marrow Transplant* 1997;19:1041–1043.

176. Metzler G, Cerroni L, Schmidt H, et al. Leukemic cells within skin lesions of psoriasis in a patient with acute myelogenous leukemia. *J Cutan Pathol* 1997;24:445–448.

177. van der Kerkhof PC, Steijlen PM, Raymakers RA. Acrodermatitis continua of Hallopeau in a patient with myelodysplastic syndrome. *Br J Dermatol* 1996;134:754–757.

178. Fernandez-Escribano M, Junquera JM, Santos I. Chronic myelomonocytic leukemia and renal carcinoma: a rare association. *Sangre (Barc)* 1997;42:88–89.

179. Kasuno K, Ono T, Kamata T, et al. IgA nephropathy associated with polycythaemia vera: accelerated course. *Nephrol Dial Transplant* 1997;12:212–215.

180. Nishikubo CY, Kunkel LA, Figlin R, et al. An association between renal cell carcinoma and lymphoid malignancies. A case series of eight patients. *Cancer* 1996;78:2421–2426.

181. Noguchi Y, Goto T, Yufu Y, et al. Gene expression of erythropoietin in renal cell carcinoma. *Intern Med* 1999;38:991–994.

182. Okamoto T, Okada M, Itoh T, et al. Myelodysplastic syndrome with B cell clonality in a patient five years after renal transplantation. *Int J Hematol* 1998;68:61–65.

183. Shih LY, Wang ML, Fu JF. Simultaneous occurrence of multiple aetiologies of polycythaemia: renal cell carcinoma, sleep apnoea syndrome, and relative polycythaemia in a smoker with masked polycythaemia rubra vera. *J Clin Pathol* 2000;53:561–564.

184. Subar M, Gucalp R, Benstein J, et al. Acute leukaemia following renal transplantation. *Med Oncol* 1996;13:9–13.

ACUTE MYELOID LEUKEMIA

GENERAL FEATURES

Classification

Acute myeloid (myelocytic, myeloblastic) leukemia (AML) is classified according to morphologic, immunophenotypic, and genetic characteristics. The most recent classification of AML is that used by the World Health Organization (WHO) (1,2) (Table 19-1). The earlier French-American-British (FAB) classification is also still widely used (3–6). The classification used in this chapter adheres to the WHO classification, with slight modifications (Table 19-2). In the WHO classification, the acute leukemias of ambiguous lineage consists of two subtypes: cases with no apparent differentiation (acute undifferentiated leukemia) and cases with mixed differentiation [acute biphenotypic leukemia (ABiL)] (Table 19-3). These are discussed individually.

AML is currently diagnosed at a peripheral blood or bone marrow blast percentage of at least 20%. This definition may be expected to change because methods of blast enumeration and quantitative criteria continue to evolve.

Clinical Course

AML pursues a generally downward course, complicated by bone marrow failure caused by the disease and the therapy. Combination chemotherapy induces remission in more than one-half of patients but is followed eventually by relapse in most. Stem cell transplantation offers the best chance of long-term remission or cure.

Spontaneous (or nearly spontaneous) remission occasionally occurs in AML. In infants, spontaneous remission is

TABLE 19-1. CLASSIFICATION OF ACUTE MYELOID LEUKEMIA ACCORDING TO THE WORLD HEALTH ORGANIZATION

AML with recurrent cytogenetic abnormalities
  AML with t(8;21)(q22;q22) (*AML1/ETO*)
  AML with inv(16)(p13q22) or t(16;16) (*CBFβ/MYH11*)
  Acute promyelocytic leukemia [AML with t(15;17)(q22;q12)
    (*PML/RARα*) and variants]
  AML with 11q23 (*MLL*) abnormalities
AML with multilineage dysplasia
AML and myelodysplastic syndrome, therapy-related
  Alkylating agent related
  Topoisomerase II inhibitor related
AML not otherwise categorized
  AML, minimally differentiated
  AML without maturation
  AML with maturation
  AML
  Acute monoblastic and monocytic leukemia
  Acute erythroid leukemia
  Acute megakaryoblastic leukemia
  Acute basophilic leukemia
  Acute panmyelosis with myelofibrosis
  Myeloid sarcoma
  Acute leukemias of ambiguous lineage

AML, acute myeloid leukemia.

TABLE 19-2. ORGANIZATION OF ACUTE MYELOID LEUKEMIA IN THIS CHAPTER

Morphologic and immunophenotypic subtypes
  AML with minimal differentiation (FAB M0)
  AML without maturation (FAB M1)
  AML with maturation (FAB M2)
  Acute promyelocytic leukemia (FAB M3)
  Acute myelomonocytic leukemia (FAB M4 and M4Eo)
  Acute monocytic leukemia (FAB M5)
  Acute erythroid leukemia (FAB M6)
  Acute megakaryocytic leukemia (FAB M7)
  Acute eosinophilic leukemia
  Acute basophilic leukemia
  AML with multilineage dysplasia
  Acute leukemia and myelodysplastic syndrome,
    therapy-related
  Acute panmyelosis with myelofibrosis
  Acute undifferentiated leukemia
  Acute biphenotypic leukemia

Genotypic subtypes
  AML with t(1;22)(p13;q13)
  AML with translocations of chromosome 3q21 and/or 3q26
  AML with t(6;9)(p23;q34)
  AML with t(8;16)(p11;p13) (*MOZ/CBP*)
  AML with t(8;21)(q22;q22) (*AML1/ETO*)
  AML with t(9;22)(q34;q11) (*BCR/ABL*)
  AML with anomalies of chromosome 11q23 and/or *MLL*
  AML with t(15;17)(q22;q12) (*PML/RARα*)
  AML with inv(16)(p13q22) or t(16;16) (*CBFβ/MYH11*)
  AML with t(16;21)(p11;q22) (*TLS/ERG*)
  AML with loss of chromosome 17p
  AML with constitutional trisomy 21

AML, acute myeloid leukemia.

TABLE 19-3. ACUTE LEUKEMIAS OF AMBIGUOUS LINEAGE ACCORDING TO THE WORLD HEALTH ORGANIZATION

Acute undifferentiated leukemia
Acute biphenotypic leukemia

associated with monocytic differentiation and skin involvement (7–12) and with constitutional trisomy 21 (see later). In older patients, spontaneous remission is associated with conditions affecting immunity and granulocyte production, such as severe infection, hypergammaglobulinemia, blood transfusion, corticosteroid therapy, and both administration and withdrawal of granulocyte colony-stimulating factor (13–20). Spontaneous remission may be either transient or permanent.

Peripheral Blood

The peripheral blood usually shows anemia and thrombocytopenia. The red blood cells may show aniso- and poikilocytosis. Platelets may be of abnormal size and show hypogranularity. The white blood cell count and blast percentage are highly variable. A peripheral blood blast percentage of 20% warrants a diagnosis of acute leukemia, even if the bone marrow blast percentage is lower (21). In cases of pancytopenia, the peripheral blood smear should be carefully searched for blasts. Dysplastic neutrophils, monocytes, and nucleated red blood cells often appear in the peripheral blood in AML and are clues to the diagnosis. The peripheral blood may show other hematologic abnormalities, such as autoimmune hemolytic anemia (22).

Bone Marrow

Bone marrow aspirate smears typically show 20% or more blasts, admixed with other hematopoietic cells, lymphocytes, and plasma cells. The myeloid:erythroid ratio may be unevaluable because of blast infiltration. Differentiated hematopoietic cells often show dysplastic features, especially in AML arising from myelotoxic exposure or preexisting hematopoietic disease (see Acute Myeloid Leukemia with Multilineage Dysplasia section).

Histologic sections of the marrow show hypercellularity for site and age. Hypoplastic or hypocellular AML refers to cases with cellularity of 30% or less (23). Use of this arbitrary criterion does not take into account normal site- and age-specific cellularity and does not appear to define a clinicopathologic entity (24).

Other bone marrow findings in AML include reactive plasmacytosis, granulomas, fibrosis, osteosclerosis, osteoporosis, and hyperplasia of precursor B-cells (25).

Other diseases reported with AML include sarcoidosis (26,27) and clonal histiocytic, B-cell, plasma cell, and T-cell disorders (28–35). Coexistent neoplasms may be either clonally related or unrelated to the AML.

Blast Morphology

Blast morphology is highly variable in AML and is discussed in greater detail with the morphologic subtypes. In general, blasts range from approximately 15 to 30 μm in diameter. The nucleus is round to elongated, often showing folds or other nuclear membrane irregularities. The chromatin is finely divided, and nucleoli are usually visible. The cytoplasm ranges from scant to abundant and usually contains small primary (azurophilic or reddish) granules. In approximately 20% of cases, the primary granules coalesce into needle-like Auer rods, irregular Auer bodies, or Chediak-Higashi–like inclusions (36–38).

Blast size occasionally provides a clue to the karyotype. Small blast size and hand-mirror morphology have been described in AML with trisomy 13 (39). Huge blast size and bizarre morphology have been reported in AML with polyploidy (40–45).

Blasts occasionally show hemophagocytosis, especially in AML with t(8;16) (45–47).

Cytochemistry

Cytochemistry is less important than it once was in the diagnosis of AML (48,49). In brief, granulocytic differentiation is revealed by cytoplasmic positivity for Sudan black B and myeloperoxidase (MPO) and, in more differentiated blasts, chloroacetate esterase. Monocytic differentiation is revealed by cytoplasmic positivity for nonspecific esterase (NSE), inhibitable by sodium fluoride.

Flow Cytometry

Immunophenotyping by flow cytometry is essential for the accurate diagnosis and classification of acute leukemia and for monitoring minimal residual disease.

AML commonly shows surface antigens CD13, CD14, CD15, CD33, and CD117, and the intracellular antigen myeloperoxidase (MPO) (50–60). CD45 is expressed in more than 95% of cases. HLA-DR is expressed in 85% of cases, and CD34 in 35% to 60% of cases. CD13 and MPO, the most sensitive myeloid-specific antigens, are each expressed in 75% to 95% of cases. CD33 expression is seen in 65% to 95% of cases. CD117 expression, seen in approximately 70% of cases, is virtually specific for a diagnosis of AML.

Compared with their normal counterparts, leukemic myeloblasts show cross-lineage and asynchronous antigen expression in almost 90% of cases. CD4 is expressed in 60% of cases; CD7, CD19, and CD20 in 10% to 20%; and CD2, CD3, CD5, and CD10 in 5% to 10%. CD2 expression is characteristic of acute promyelocytic leukemia (APL) and acute myelomonocytic leukemia (AMML) with eosinophilia. Coexpression of CD7 with the early hematopoietic antigens CD34, CD117, and terminal deoxynucleotidyl transferase (TdT) reproduces a stem cell immunophenotype and augurs a poor prognosis (61).

Other antigens that may be expressed in AML are CD11b, CD11c, CD14, CD15, CD34, CD56, and TdT. CD14 and CD15 expression is typically found in cases with monocytic differentiation. CD56, expressed in 24% of cases, appears to predict a poor prognosis (62).

Immunophenotype changes occur in more than 90% of AML cases over time (63,64). Relapses may show gain of CD13, CD33, and CD34 expression and/or loss of CD14, CD19, and CD56 expression. Immunophenotype switching from myeloid to lymphoid immunophenotype has been reported (see Acute Biphenotypic Leukemia section). Immunophenotype is further discussed with each subtype of AML.

Immunohistochemistry

Immunophenotyping by immunohistochemistry may be used for classification of AML. This method is especially useful for the diagnosis of extramedullary disease, when no tissue may have been submitted for immunophenotyping by flow cytometry (65). Immunohistochemistry may be more sensitive than flow cytometry for MPO detection and less sensitive for CD15 and CD117 detection (66).

Genetic Analysis

Genetic analysis is invaluable in AML to assess clonality and to detect the important translocation (15;17), and other abnormalities defining clinicopathologic entities and prognosis (53,67–74). Clonal karyotypic abnormalities are found in approximately 90% of childhood and 60% of adult disease; the figure is higher when more sensitive molecular methods are used. The most common karyotypic findings are loss of a sex chromosome; deletions of 5, 5q, 7, and 7q; trisomy 8; rearrangements of 3q21-26, 11q23, and 12q13; translocations (8;21), (1;22), (6;9), (8;21), (9;22), and (15;17); and inversion of chromosome 16. Rare cases of AML are multiclonal (75).

Immunoglobulin heavy chain (IgH) and/or T-cell receptor (TCR) gene rearrangements are found in approximately 35% to 45% of cases expressing B-cell antigens, and 10% of cases expressing T-cell antigens (76–78). Rearrangements are rarely found in cases lacking these antigens and are not predictive of genotype or prognosis.

Genotype is further discussed with each subtype of AML.

Extramedullary Disease

Extramedullary disease has been variously reported as granulocytic sarcoma, myeloid sarcoma, and extramedullary hematopoietic tumor (Figs. 19-1 and 19-2). It may occur at any point in the disease and has been reported in all AML subtypes. Any body organ or cavity may be affected. Molec-

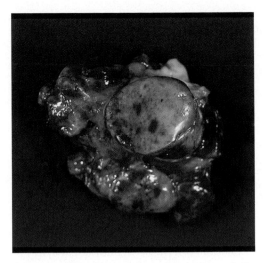

FIGURE 19-1. Perithoracic lymph nodes, extramedullary acute myeloid leukemia (granulocytic sarcoma). The freshly cut surface shows the characteristic greenish color, which is the origin of the term chloroma.

ular testing reveals bone marrow involvement in virtually all cases (79).

Extramedullary disease is particularly associated with monocytic differentiation (especially in neonates), CD56 expression, t(8;21), and translocations involving 11q23 (80–85). Involvement of multiple extramedullary sites is characteristic of relapse after stem cell transplantation (86). The differential diagnosis includes malignant lymphoma and, especially in cases of megakaryocytic differentiation, nonhematolymphoid malignancies (87–89).

Differential Diagnosis

The differential diagnosis of AML includes nonneoplastic and neoplastic conditions (Table 19-4).

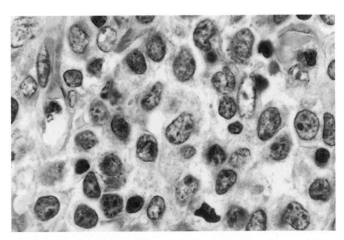

FIGURE 19-2. Lymph node, extramedullary acute myeloid leukemia (granulocytic sarcoma). A diffuse infiltrate of blasts is present. Without ancillary studies such as cytochemistry and/or flow cytometry, this infiltrate may be mistaken for malignant lymphoma.

TABLE 19-4. DIFFERENTIAL DIAGNOSIS OF ACUTE MYELOID LEUKEMIA

Nonneoplastic conditions
   Leukemoid reactions
   Infectious mononucleosis
   Hematopoietic growth factor therapy
   Florid megaloblastic change
   Precursor B-cell hyperplasia
Neoplastic conditions
   Acute lymphoid leukemia
   Malignant lymphoma with leukemic phase
   Malignant histiocytosis
   Neuroblastoma
   Embryonal rhabdomyosarcoma

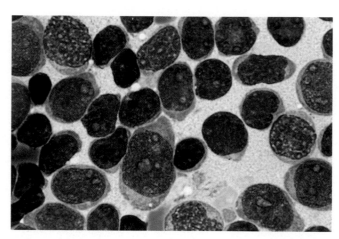

FIGURE 19-3. Bone marrow aspirate smear, acute myeloid leukemia with minimal differentiation (FAB M0). Numerous blasts are present, showing no cytoplasmic granules or Auer rods.

Nonneoplastic conditions resembling AML are a heterogeneous group. Many of these disorders have been reported to coexist with myelodysplastic syndromes (MDSs) and AML. When occurring in MDSs, they may result in a mistaken or premature diagnosis of AML.

Leukemoid reactions may consist predominantly of blasts, promyelocytes, or monocytes and thus be mistaken for AML or acute promyelocytic or monocytic leukemia (90–102). Patients presenting with sore throat and atypical circulating cells have been mistakenly diagnosed with infectious mononucleosis instead of acute monocytic leukemia; rarely, infectious mononucleosis and AML occur together (103). Hematopoietic growth factor therapy may cause a transient increase in peripheral blood and bone marrow monocytes or blasts (104–108). Florid folate- or vitamin B$_{12}$–related megaloblastic change is characterized by pancytopenia, bone marrow hyperplasia, increased early erythroid precursors with fine blastlike chromatin, and numerous mitotic figures arrested in metaphase (109). These findings are easily misinterpreted as acute leukemia if histologic sections are examined without corresponding bone marrow aspirate smears. Precursor B-cell hyperplasia has been reported in AML and must be distinguished from a myeloid-to-lymphoid immunophenotype switch and from therapy-related acute lymphoid leukemia (ALL) (25).

Neoplastic conditions resembling AML include malignant lymphoma, malignant histiocytosis, and nonhematolymphoid tumors, especially neuroblastoma and embryonal rhabdomyosarcoma (110). These disorders may present with a leukemic phase and/or massive bone marrow involvement. It should be kept in mind that AML has been reported with other hematolymphoid neoplasms (see previously) and with neuroblastoma (111).

MORPHOLOGIC AND IMMUNOPHENOTYPIC SUBTYPES

AML typically shows differentiation along a predominant lineage, evident by morphologic and/or immunopheno-

typic analysis. Notable exceptions are acute megakaryocytic and erythroid leukemias, which show considerable overlap.

Acute Myeloid Leukemia with Minimal Differentiation (FAB M0)

AML with minimal differentiation (FAB M0) accounts for approximately 5% of AML cases (1–8) (Figs. 19-3 and 19-4). It is concentrated in children younger than 3 years old and adults (especially men) older than 60 years of age. The majority of blasts lack cytoplasmic granules, Auer rods, and cytochemical markers of myeloid differentiation. The peripheral white blood cell count may be low. Myelodysplasia is often present. Flow cytometry shows variable expression of CD13 and CD33. The stem cell markers CD7, CD34, HLA-DR, and TdT are frequently expressed. MPO

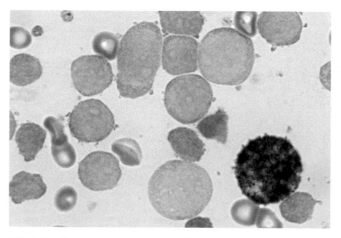

FIGURE 19-4. Bone marrow aspirate smear, acute myeloid leukemia with minimal differentiation (FAB M0). A granulocytic precursor contains myeloperoxidase, but the blasts are myeloperoxidase negative (myeloperoxidase stain). Flow cytometry showed myeloid antigen expression.

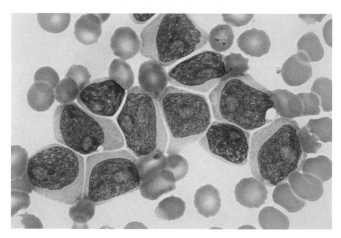

FIGURE 19-5. Bone marrow aspirate smear, acute myeloid leukemia without maturation (FAB M1). Numerous blasts are present.

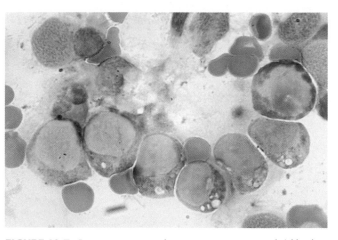

FIGURE 19-7. Bone marrow aspirate smear, acute myeloid leukemia without maturation (FAB M1). The blasts show prominent myeloperoxidase positivity.

expression is consistently found. The genotype resembles that found in myelotoxin- and therapy-related AML, with multiple and/or complex anomalies and nonspecific rearrangements of IgH and TCR genes. The prognosis is poor.

Acute Myeloid Leukemia without Maturation (FAB M1)

This is the most common type of AML (9) (Figs. 19-5 through 19-8). Many blasts show primary granules and cytochemical positivity for Sudan black B and/or MPO. Auer rods are often present. Flow cytometry shows consistent expression of CD13, CD33, CD34, and HLA-DR, and variable expression of CD7 and TdT. Genetic studies show a relatively high incidence of t(9;22), 11q23 anomalies, and *MLL* rearrangement.

Acute Myeloid Leukemia with Maturation (FAB M2)

This type of AML shows a mixture of blasts, dysplastic neutrophil precursors, and dysplastic segmented neutrophils (Figs. 19-9 through 19-12). Auer rods are often present in blasts and may even be seen in segmented neutrophils and bands (10). Some cases show eosinophilic, basophilic, and/or mast cell differentiation; these are discussed as acute eosinophilic leukemia, acute basophilic leukemia, and mast cell leukemia, respectively. Flow cytometry shows expression of myeloid antigens. Translocation (8;21), found in approximately 33% of cases, is associated with CD13 negativity and has a good prognosis. Cases with translocation of 11q23 tend not to show dysgranulopoiesis or Auer rods (11).

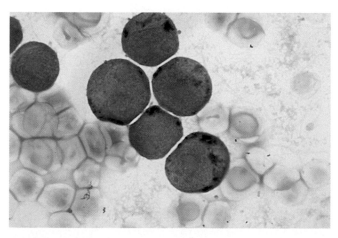

FIGURE 19-6. Bone marrow aspirate smear, acute myeloid leukemia without maturation (FAB M1). The blasts show prominent Sudan black B positivity.

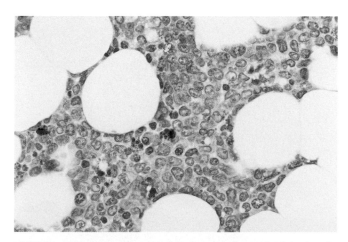

FIGURE 19-8. Bone marrow biopsy, acute myeloid leukemia without maturation (FAB M2). Blasts replace hematopoietic cells but do not completely fill the marrow; iron stores are increased because of the lack of erythroid precursors.

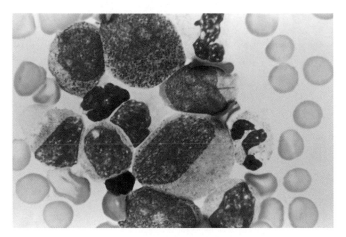

FIGURE 19-9. Bone marrow aspirate smear, acute myeloid leukemia with maturation (FAB M2). Blasts are admixed with abnormal maturing granulocytes; one blast contains an Auer rod.

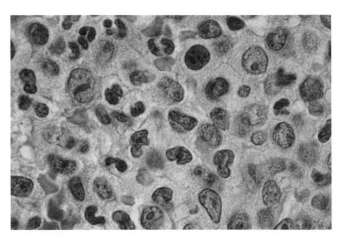

FIGURE 19-12. Bone marrow biopsy specimen, acute myeloid leukemia with maturation (FAB M2). A diffuse infiltrate of blasts and abnormal maturing granulocytes is present.

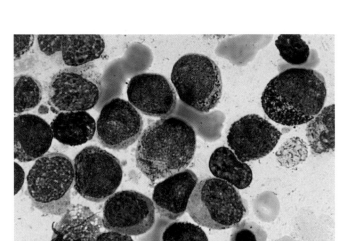

FIGURE 19-10. Bone marrow aspirate smear, acute myeloid leukemia with maturation (FAB M2). Blasts show prominent cytoplasmic granularity (compare with acute promyelocytic leukemia).

Acute Promyelocytic Leukemia (FAB M3)

APL accounts for 10% to 15% of AML cases in most published reports (12–29) (Figs. 19-13 through 19-16). This subtype is complicated by disseminated fibrinolysis owing to the release of granule contents from the neoplastic cells. The peripheral white blood cell count and blast percentage may be low, and the diagnosis therefore missed initially.

APL is morphologically variable. The hypergranular blast predominates in most cases. The nucleus is large and lobated, and the cytoplasm is abundant and heavily granulated. Auer rods are typically (but not always) present and may be multiple within a single cell. The smaller microgranular blast predominates in 15% to 20% of cases (FAB M3v). The nucleus is bilobed or folded, and the cytoplasm is moderately abundant, with fine dustlike or submicroscopic granules. The cytoplasm may appear hypo- or agranular with Wright

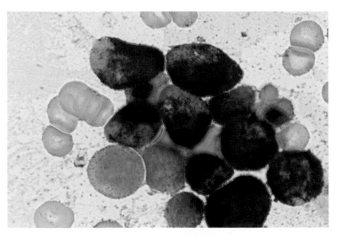

FIGURE 19-11. Bone marrow aspirate smear, acute myeloid leukemia with maturation (FAB M2). Blasts and other early granulocytic precursors show intense chloroacetate esterase positivity.

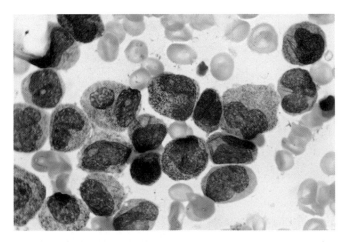

FIGURE 19-13. Bone marrow aspirate smear, acute promyelocytic leukemia (FAB M3). Numerous blasts are present, showing folded and lobated nuclei and abundant cytoplasm containing Auer rods and granules. Karyotyping showed t(15;17).

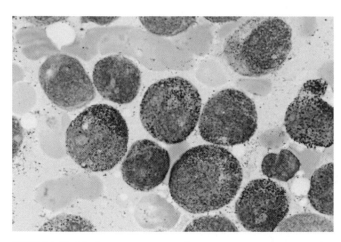

FIGURE 19-14. Bone marrow aspirate smear, acute promyelocytic leukemia (FAB M3). The blasts are relatively monomorphous and show heavily granulated cytoplasm without Auer rods (compare with acute myeloid leukemia with maturation). Karyotyping showed t(15;17).

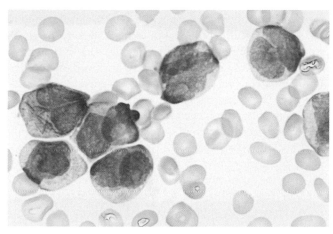

FIGURE 19-15. Bone marrow aspirate smear, acute promyelocytic leukemia (FAB M3). The blasts are very large, with lobated nuclei, fine dustlike cytoplasmic granules, and numerous Auer rods. Karyotyping showed t(15;17).

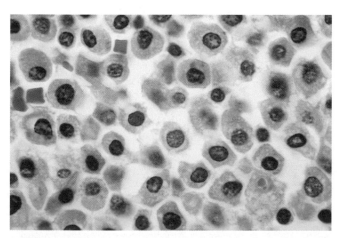

FIGURE 19-16. Bone marrow clot, acute promyelocytic leukemia (FAB M3). The marrow is replaced by a diffuse infiltrate of blasts with abundant, heavily granulated cytoplasm.

stain because of the small granule size. The lobated nucleus and apparently agranular cytoplasm may prompt an erroneous diagnosis of acute monocytic leukemia. Basophilic APL is a rare variant associated with hyperhistaminemia. The blasts show scant, basophilic cytoplasm with large, deep violet granules and vacuoles. The granules may be scarce. Like basophil granules, they stain metachromatic (pink) with toluidine blue stain. Some cases of APL show predominantly promyelocyte-like cells but few blasts, thus resembling AML with maturation. In some cases, the predominant blast is a promyelocyte-like cell with innumerable large, dark granules but no Auer rods. In other cases, blasts with a few small primary granules predominate, thus resembling AML without maturation. Histologic sections of APL show marrow replacement by cells with reniform or lobated nuclei surrounded by faintly eosinophilic, abundant cytoplasm, creating a distinctive "fried-egg" appearance. Marked fibrosis has been reported.

Cytochemical staining of hypergranular blasts shows strong reactions for Sudan black B, MPO, and chloroacetate esterase, and, in some cases, fluoride-sensitive NSE; microgranular blasts show weaker reactions. Basophilic APL shows weaker MPO staining and may be NSE positive.

Flow cytometry shows antigen expression corresponding to the degree of morphologic maturation. Hypergranular blasts show a mature myeloid phenotype, with expression of CD13 and/or CD33; they usually lack expression of CD2, CD4, CD7, CD14, CD15, CD19, CD34, and HLA-DR. Microgranular blasts show a more immature phenotype, with coexpression of CD2 and CD19, CD34, and, in some cases, CD56 and HLA-DR. Rare cases show an even more primitive phenotype, with expression of CD2, CD13, CD33, CD34, CD117, and TdT. Although APL may show expression of either CD34 or HLA-DR, it does not show expression of both (8).

Genetic studies show t(15;17) in more than 90%, but not all, APL cases. APL and AML with t(15;17) are not identical. Some cases show promyelocytic morphology but lack t(15;17); others show t(15;17) but lack promyelocytic morphology. The presence or absence of t(15;17), not morphology, is the determining prognostic and therapeutic factor.

The differential diagnosis includes—depending on blast morphology—granulocytic maturation arrest, AML with or without maturation, acute monocytic leukemia, acute basophilic leukemia, and mast cell leukemia (30). Recovery from acute agranulocytosis may be distinguished from APL by CD117, which is expressed in APL, and CD11b, which is expressed in promyelocytes in recovery (31).

Acute Myelomonocytic Leukemia (FAB M4 and M4Eo)

AMML has two peaks in incidence: one in infancy and one in adulthood (32,33) (Figs. 19-17 through 19-20). Extramedullary disease is common. Peripheral blood and

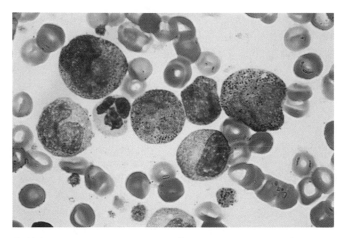

FIGURE 19-17. Bone marrow aspirate smear, acute myelomonocytic leukemia (FAB M4). Abnormal cells are present, showing a mixture of granulocytic and monocytic features.

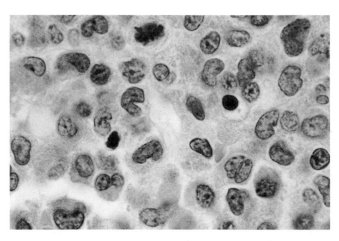

FIGURE 19-20. Bone marrow clot, acute myelomonocytic leukemia (FAB M4). The marrow is filled with blasts showing indented and irregular nuclei.

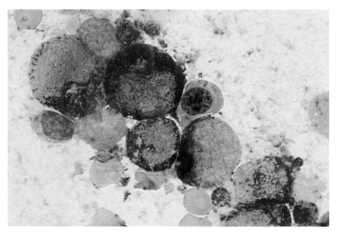

FIGURE 19-18. Bone marrow aspirate smear, acute myelomonocytic leukemia (FAB M4). The blasts show prominent cytoplasmic positivity for chloroacetate esterase.

marrow aspirate smears show a heterogeneous population of blasts and myeloid precursors with a mixture of granulocytic and monocytic characteristics. The peripheral blood often shows more differentiated cells than the bone marrow. Cytochemical staining for MPO and fluoride-inhibitable NSE is positive. In rare cases, the blasts are morphologically undifferentiated but cytochemically positive. Histologic sections of the bone marrow show a mixed population of pleomorphic blasts and myeloid precursors. Flow cytometry shows expression of myeloid antigens (CD13, CD33) and monocytic antigens (usually CD14). Genetic studies show t(11)(q23) and/or *MLL* rearrangement in approximately 20% of cases. Both genetic lesions are associated with onset in infancy, leukocytosis, and *IgH* rearrangement.

AMML with eosinophilia (FAB M4Eo) is a distinctive subset of AMML (34–36) (Figs. 19-21 through 19-23). Peripheral blood and marrow aspirate smears show large cells

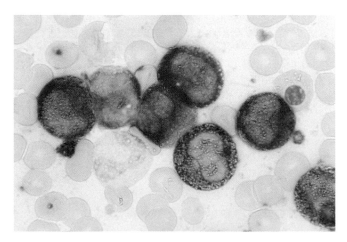

FIGURE 19-19. Bone marrow aspirate smear, acute myelomonocytic leukemia (FAB M4). The blasts also show prominent cytoplasmic positivity for nonspecific esterase, inhibitable with the addition of sodium fluoride.

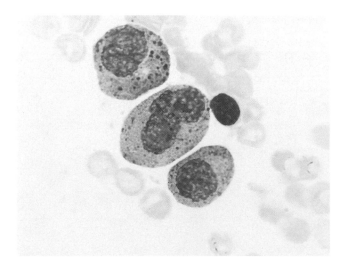

FIGURE 19-21. Bone marrow aspirate smear, acute myelomonocytic leukemia with eosinophilia (FAB M4Eo). Abnormal myeloid precursors show large eosinophilic granules. Karyotyping showed inv(16).

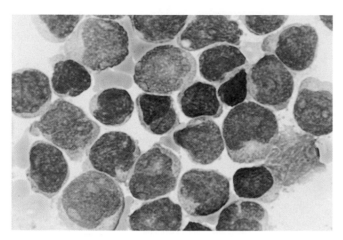

FIGURE 19-22. Bone marrow aspirate smear, acute myelomonocytic leukemia with inv(16) (FAB M4Eo). Undifferentiated blasts are present, without evidence of eosinophilia. Karyotyping showed inv(16).

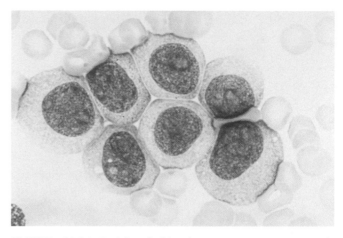

FIGURE 19-24. Peripheral blood smear, acute monocytic leukemia (FAB M5). The blasts show round nuclei and abundant agranular cytoplasm; little evidence of monocytic differentiation is present.

with notably large, eosinophilic, and sometimes basophilic, cytoplasmic granules. Charcot-Leyden crystals may be found in aspirate smears, lying free or within macrophages. Cytochemical staining is positive for both MPO and NSE. Histologic sections show a mixed population of blasts, neutrophilic and eosinophilic precursors, and dysplastic eosinophils. Flow cytometry shows expression of CD13, CD33, CD34, and/or CD36. Genetic studies show inv(16), sometimes masked, in more than 90% of cases; various other anomalies have been reported in the remainder. The prognosis is relatively good in cases with inv(16).

Acute Monocytic Leukemia (FAB M5)

Acute monocytic (or monoblastic) leukemia is similar to AMML, with a peak in infancy and frequent extramedullary disease (37–39) (Figs. 19-24 through 19-27). It is morphologically heterogeneous. Peripheral blood and marrow

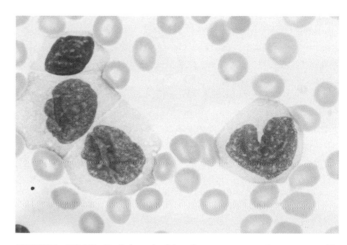

FIGURE 19-25. Peripheral blood smear, acute monocytic leukemia (FAB M5). The blasts show indented and reniform nuclei, consistent with monocytic differentiation.

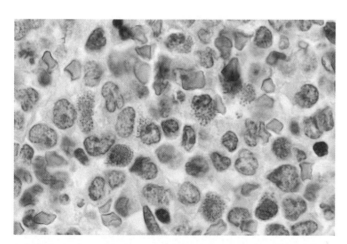

FIGURE 19-23. Bone marrow biopsy specimen, acute myelomonocytic leukemia with eosinophilia (FAB M4Eo). The marrow is filled with blasts, many containing eosinophilic granules.

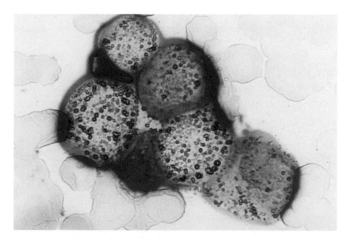

FIGURE 19-26. Peripheral blood smear, acute monocytic leukemia (FAB M5). The blasts show marked nonspecific esterase positivity, indicative of monocytic differentiation. Positivity was abolished with sodium fluoride.

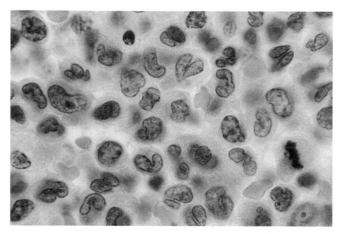

FIGURE 19-27. Bone marrow clot, acute monocytic leukemia (FAB M5). The blasts show prominent nuclear indentations, consistent with monocytic differentiation.

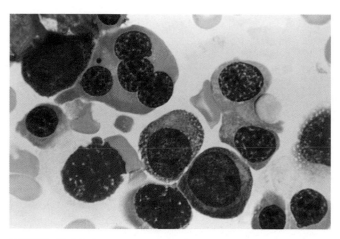

FIGURE 19-28. Bone marrow aspirate smear, acute erythroid leukemia (FAB M6). Erythroid precursors show marked abnormalities, including multilobation.

aspirate smears may show a monomorphous population of undifferentiated blasts (FAB M5a) or a heterogeneous population of monocytoid cells (FAB M5b). A third, more differentiated subtype of acute monocytic leukemia has been reported, which is likely indistinguishable from malignant histiocytosis (FAB M5c) (49,50).

The peripheral blood in acute monocytic leukemia, as in AMML, often shows more differentiated cells than the marrow, a phenomenon that may be misinterpreted as atypical lymphocytosis or infectious mononucleosis. Although occasional reddish cytoplasmic granules may be found in the neoplastic cells, Auer rods are typically absent. Histologic sections of the bone marrow show blasts with reniform and folded nuclei and moderately abundant cytoplasm.

Flow cytometry shows expression of CD4, CD11b, CD11c, CD13, CD14, CD15, CD33, CD34, and/or CD117. Morphologic differentiation and immunophenotypic differentiation tend to parallel one another, with undifferentiated blasts expressing CD34 and CD117 and monocytoid cells expressing CD4, CD13, CD14, CD15, and CD33.

Genetic studies show translocation involving chromosome 11q23 in 25 to 35% of cases. *MLL* rearrangement is present in more than 90% of acute monocytic leukemia occurring in infants. A distinctive subset of cases shows t(8;16) (see later).

Acute Erythroid Leukemia (FAB M6)

Acute erythroid leukemia (AEL) has two peaks in incidence: one in children with constitutional trisomy 21 and one in adults with exposure to myelotoxins and/or a preexisting MDS (40–52) (Figs. 19-28 through 19-30). MDS with prominent erythroid differentiation (previously known as Di Guglielmo disease or syndrome) and AEL form a continuum and may be difficult to distinguish.

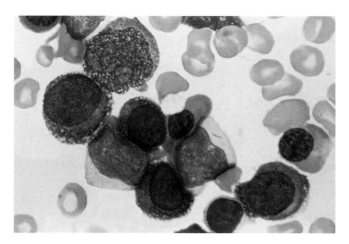

FIGURE 19-29. Bone marrow aspirate smear, acute erythroid leukemia (FAB M6). Admixed with abnormal erythroid precursors are myeloblasts, one containing an Auer rod.

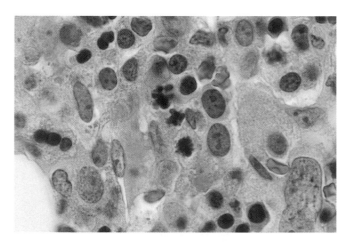

FIGURE 19-30. Bone marrow biopsy, acute erythroid leukemia (FAB M6). The marrow is filled with abnormal erythroid precursors, dysplastic megakaryocytes, and blasts.

AEL is morphologically heterogeneous. The most common form shows prominent erythroid hyperplasia, dyserythropoiesis, numerous early erythroid precursors, dysplastic megakaryocytes, and a relatively low marrow blast percentage (10% to 20%). The blasts tend to show a large, round nucleus with slightly condensed chromatin, surrounded by a rim of basophilic cytoplasm. Prominent findings include myelodysplasia, ringed sideroblasts, and periodic acid–Schiff-positive cytoplasmic inclusions of glycogen within erythroid precursors. Myeloid blasts containing cytoplasmic granules and/or Auer rods are often present. This type of AEL shows both myeloid and erythroid characteristics and may evolve over time to a more usual type of AML (FAB M0, M1, or M2). A second and uncommon form of AEL shows little or no morphologic evidence of erythroid lineage and thus resembles AML with minimal differentiation (FAB M0). A third and rare form of AEL presents with pancytopenia and massive organ infiltration but lacks overt leukemia (erythremic myelosis).

Flow cytometry shows expression of erythroid antigens (glycophorin A, ABO antigens, erythropoietin receptor, spectrin) as well as variable expression of megakaryocytic (CD41, CD61, thrombopoietin receptor) and myeloid (CD13, CD15, CD33) antigens. Erythroid differentiation is also indicated by the presence of cytoplasmic α-globin mRNA and megakaryocytic differentiation by cytoplasmic glycoprotein II mRNA.

Genetic studies reveal karyotypic anomalies in most cases. Findings associated with AEL include t(3;5) and constitutional trisomy 21.

Acute Megakaryocytic Leukemia (FAB M7)

Acute megakaryocytic (or megakaryoblastic) leukemia (AMegL) accounts for less than 2% of AML cases overall (53–64) (Figs. 19-31 through 19-35). Like AEL, AMegL has two peaks in incidence: one in infancy and one in adulthood. In infants, AMegL is associated with t(1;22) and constitutional trisomy 21. In adults, AMegL occurs as a *de novo* disease and as a transformation of preexisting AML and myeloproliferative disorders. AMegL may be the initial manifestation of chronic myeloid leukemia. Whether primary or secondary, AMegL often presents with extramedullary disease and bony abnormalities. Spontaneous remission has often been reported, especially in infants with constitutional trisomy 21; many of these cases subsequently relapse.

The peripheral blood smear shows a variable percentage of dysplastic megakaryocytic and erythroid precursors and blasts. The neoplastic cells have a highly variable morphology. They range from medium-sized cells, with round to folded nuclei and scant cytoplasm, to very large cells, with complex nuclei and cytoplasmic blebs and protrusions. A constant feature is condensed, dark-staining chromatin, unlike that of blasts seen in other types of AML. Nuclear

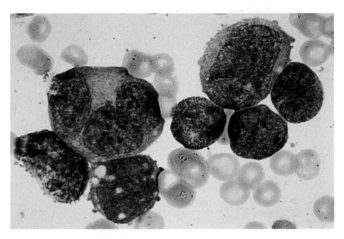

FIGURE 19-31. Bone marrow aspirate smear, acute megakaryocytic leukemia (FAB M7). Numerous abnormal megakaryocytes are present, ranging from small blastlike forms to large multinucleated cells.

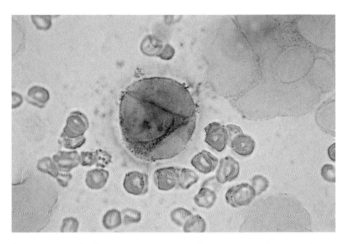

FIGURE 19-32. Bone marrow aspirate smear, acute megakaryocytic leukemia (FAB M7). An abnormal megakaryocyte shows positivity for platelet glycoprotein (anti-glycoprotein II/III stain).

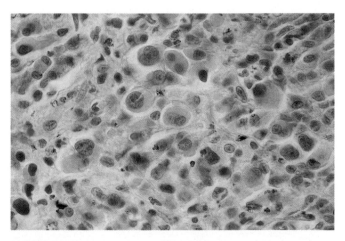

FIGURE 19-33. Bone marrow biopsy specimen, acute megakaryocytic leukemia (FAB M7). The marrow is filled with atypical megakaryocytes and smaller cells; the presence of increased reticulin is indicated by the single-file arrangement of the neoplastic cells.

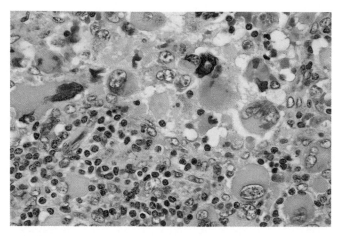

FIGURE 19-34. Lymph node, acute megakaryocytic leukemia (FAB M7). A focus of large, pleomorphic and multinucleated cells is present, which may be mistaken for a nonhematolymphoid neoplasm. This type of infiltrate has also been termed megakaryocytic myelosis.

pleomorphism, condensed chromatin, and bizarre cytoplasmic contours create diagnostic difficulties. Thus, AMegL is more likely than other types of acute leukemia to be misdiagnosed as nonhematopoietic malignancy.

Bone marrow aspiration is frequently unsuccessful because of fibrosis. Histologic sections of the marrow show fibrosis, thickened and irregular trabecular bone, and a heterogeneous population of dysplastic megakaryocytes, erythroid precursors, and blasts. Enumeration of cell types, including blasts, is often difficult owing to compression by fibrous tissue. In some cases, the diagnosis of acute leukemia has been made based on the blast percentage in the peripheral blood rather than the bone marrow.

Flow cytometry shows expression of megakaryocytic antigens and variable expression of erythroid and myeloid markers, as in AEL.

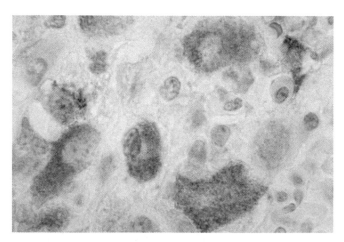

FIGURE 19-35. Bone marrow biopsy specimen, acute megakaryocytic leukemia (FAB M7). Small, atypical megakaryocytes show factor VIII positivity, confirming megakaryocytic differentiation (anti–factor VIII stain).

Genetic studies often show karyotypic anomalies, including t(1;22), inv(3) and other chromosome 3 anomalies, t(16;21), constitutional trisomy 21, and acquired extra copies of chromosome 21.

Acute Eosinophilic Leukemia

Acute eosinophilic leukemia is a rare variant of AML with maturation (65–73). This type of AML may be difficult to distinguish from chronic eosinophilic leukemia, the eosinophilic variant of APL, and AMML with eosinophilic differentiation.

Peripheral blood and marrow aspirate smears show dysplastic eosinophilic precursors and blasts. In acute eosinophilic leukemia with t(8;21), Auer rods may be found within neoplastic eosinophils. Flow cytometry shows expression of CD4, CD13, CD33, and/or MPO. Genetic studies have revealed t(2;5), t(5;12), t(5;14), t(6;9), t(8;21), t(10;11), and t(15;17).

Acute Basophilic Leukemia

ABL is a rare variant of AML with maturation (74–85) (Figs. 19-36 through 19-39). The clinical presentation may include coagulopathy and hyperhistaminic syndrome caused by degranulation of neoplastic cells containing basophilic granules. Most cases present with leukemia, but a few have been reported in which tissue infiltrates are present, without an overt leukemic phase. This type of AML may be difficult to distinguish from chronic basophilic leukemia, the basophilic variant of APL, and acute monocytic leukemia with basophilia.

The peripheral blood and bone marrow show blasts with basophilic characteristics. These consist of large, dark, toluidine blue–positive cytoplasmic granules and cytoplasmic vacuoles, representing emptied granules. Granules and vacuoles may be scarce and easily overlooked. The granules stain

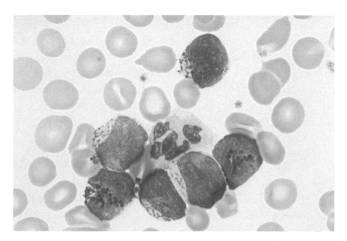

FIGURE 19-36. Bone marrow aspirate smear, acute basophilic leukemia. The blasts show large basophilic granules.

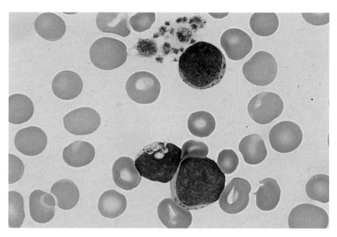

FIGURE 19-37. Peripheral blood smear, acute basophilic leukemia. The blasts show a few dark-staining granules and characteristic vacuoles, which are basophilic granules devoid of contents.

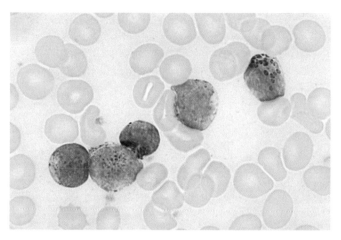

FIGURE 19-38. Peripheral blood smear, acute basophilic leukemia. The large granules show metachromatic (i.e., pink) staining with toluidine blue, confirming basophilic differentiation.

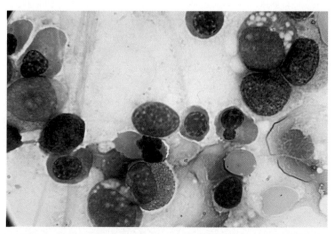

FIGURE 19-39. Bone marrow aspirate smear, acute myeloid leukemia with multilineage dysplasia. Blasts and dysplastic erythroid precursors are present in this specimen classified as acute myeloid leukemia with maturation (FAB M2).

metachromatically (pink) with toluidine blue. Histologic sections of the bone marrow show a diffuse infiltrate of blasts with round nuclei; granules may not be apparent. Electron microscopy may demonstrate theta granules, characteristic of basophils. Flow cytometry shows expression of myeloid markers (CD13, CD22, CD33, CD117, MPO). Surface antigens more specific for basophilic differentiation (CDw17, CD88, and FcεRI) may or may not be present. Genetic studies have demonstrated t(2;6), t(5;12), t(6;9), monosomy 7, t(9;22), trisomy 21, and other anomalies.

Acute Myeloid Leukemia with Multilineage Dysplasia

AML with multilineage (or trilineage) dysplasia is listed as a distinct entity in the WHO classification; however, many morphologic subtypes of AML show dysplastic maturation (86–90) (Fig. 19-39). Marked myelodysplasia may be a clue to AML resulting from a myelotoxic exposure or a preexisting MDS. Although dysplastic features have been associated with poor prognosis, outcome appears to be determined more by the number and type of cytogenetic abnormalities than dysplasia *per se.*

Acute Leukemia and Myelodysplastic Syndrome, Therapy-Related

MDS, AML, and ALL may arise after cytotoxic therapy for aggressive clinical conditions, including acute leukemia itself (91–105). Thus, therapy-related acute leukemia may mimic a relapse of primary acute leukemia. The risk of therapy-related disease is in part determined by the presence of particular genetic polymorphisms. Two main categories of therapy-related MDS and acute leukemia have been described: cases related to alkylating agents and cases related to topoisomerase II inhibitors.

Alkylator-related disease is characterized by older patient age, onset of MDS or AML 5 to 7 years after therapy, unbalanced translocations (especially involving chromosomes 5 and 7), and balanced translocations involving 1p36 and 3q26-27 (106–108). Alkylator-related disease is clinically and genetically similar to cases of MDS and acute leukemia arising in patients with prior exposure to other known myelotoxins (e.g., insecticides and organic solvents) and in the elderly.

Topoisomerase II inhibitor–related disease is characterized by younger patient age, onset of AML or ALL within 2 years of therapy, and balanced reciprocal translocations involving *MLL* at 11q23, *AML1* at 21q22, and other genes (109–113). Topoisomerase-related disease is clinically and genetically indistinguishable from *de novo* AML and ALL with identical translocations. Apparent *de novo* infantile acute leukemia with *MLL* rearrangement may, in fact, be related to the ingestion of naturally occurring topoisomerase II inhibitors in the maternal diet (114–117).

Acute Panmyelosis with Myelofibrosis

This disorder typically shows less than 20% peripheral blood or bone marrow blasts but prominent myelodysplasia. It has most often been reported as acute or malignant myelosclerosis or myelofibrosis. An early and accurate name coined for this disease is acute myelodysplasia with fibrosis, and it is discussed as such with the other myelodysplastic syndromes (see Chapter 21).

Acute Undifferentiated Leukemia

Acute undifferentiated leukemia is classified by the WHO as acute leukemia of ambiguous lineage (Table 19-3). Acute undifferentiated, or stem cell, leukemia accounts for less than 1% of all cases of acute leukemia (118–121). The blasts lack granules and Auer rods and show no significant cytochemical positivity. Flow cytometry often shows a pattern reminiscent of the multipotential hematopoietic stem cell, with expression of CD2, CD7, CD34, CD56, HLA-DR, and TdT, but not CD3, CD13, CD19, CD20, CD33, or MPO. Genetic studies may show del(5)(q), t(6;9), t(9;22), t(11)(q23), trisomy 13, del(17)(p), and immunoglobulin and/or TCR gene rearrangements. The prognosis is very poor.

Acute Biphenotypic Leukemia

ABiL is classified by the WHO as acute leukemia of ambiguous lineage (Table 19-3). ABiL accounts for approximately 1% to 2% of all acute leukemias (122–124). The definition of biphenotypism remains imprecise. Theoretically, ABiL may take the form of (a) AML with differentiation along multiple myeloid lineages, (b) ALL with differentiation along multiple lymphoid lineages, or (c) acute leukemia with differentiation along both myeloid and lymphoid lineages (Table 19-5). These possibilities are not always separable.

AML with differentiation along multiple myeloid lineages is common and is not usually interpreted as biphenotypic.

ALL with differentiation along multiple lymphoid lineages is rare. Blasts may express T-cell and B-cell antigens

TABLE 19-5. DIFFERENT TYPES OF ACUTE BIPHENOTYPIC LEUKEMIA

Acute myeloid leukemia with multiple myeloid lineages[a]
Acute lymphoid leukemia with multiple lymphoid lineages
Acute T-cell/B-cell leukemia
Acute T-cell/natural killer cell leukemia
Acute leukemia with both myeloid and lymphoid lineages
Acute leukemia (either acute myeloid leukemia or acute lymphoid leukemia) with t(9;22)
Acute myeloid/natural killer cell leukemia

[a]Not usually diagnosed as biphenotypic.

TABLE 19-6. DIFFERENTIAL DIAGNOSIS OF ACUTE BIPHENOTYPIC LEUKEMIA

Acute leukemia with aberrant antigen expression
AML with CD2, CD4, CD7, and/or terminal deoxynucleotidyl transferase expression
ALL with CD13, CD33, and/or CD56 expression
Acute leukemia with immunophenotype switch at relapse
AML switching to ALL
ALL switching to AML
Acute leukemia followed by therapy-related acute leukemia
AML followed by therapy-related ALL
ALL followed by therapy-related AML

AML, acute myeloid leukemia; ALL, acute lymphoid leukemia.

(125,126) or T-cell and natural killer (NK) cell antigens (127,128). ALL with CD56 expression may fall into the latter category (129,130).

Acute leukemia with differentiation along both myeloid and lymphoid lineages is often interpreted as ABiL. One disease in this category is acute leukemia (either AML or ALL) with t(9;22) and production of both p190 and p210 BCR/ABL fusion proteins. Another is acute myeloid/NK cell leukemia, a distinctive type of leukemia with a notably poor prognosis (131–140). Acute myeloid/NK leukemia occurs *de novo* and as a blast crisis of myeloproliferative disease. Flow cytometry shows expression of the NK antigens CD7 (bright) and CD56, and the myeloid antigens CD13 and CD33.

The differential diagnosis of ABiL includes several entities (Table 19-6). Acute leukemia may show aberrant or cross-lineage antigen expression, as in AML with CD4, CD7, and/or TdT expression and ALL with CD13, CD33, and/or CD56 expression (141). Genotype does not always clarify the diagnosis because AML and ALL may show identical *MLL, IgH,* and *TCR* gene rearrangements. Acute leukemia may also show immunophenotype switching, either from myeloid to lymphoid (142–144) or vice versa (145–150). Multiple switches may occur within a single case (151). Acute leukemia may be succeeded, after treatment, by a second, therapy-related AML or ALL. Genetic analysis, including molecular studies of *IgH* and *TCR* gene rearrangement patterns, is helpful in distinguishing this event from relapse of the original acute leukemia.

GENOTYPIC SUBTYPES

Acute Myeloid Leukemia with t(1;22)(p13;q13)

AML with t(1;22)(p13;q13) is invariably megakaryocytic and accounts for more than 65% of AMegL occurring in neonates and infants (1–5). Visceral infiltrates are prominent and may be mistaken for nonhematopoietic tumors. The prognosis is poor. This translocation should be distinguished from other translocations of t(1;22) involving different genes and breakpoints (6,7).

Acute Myeloid Leukemia with Translocations of Chromosome 3q21 and/or 3q26

AML with translocations involving chromosome 3q21 and/or 3q26 is associated with prior mutagenic exposure, treated myeloproliferative disorders, and myelodysplastic syndromes (8–11). Characteristic findings include thrombocytosis, dyserythropoiesis, and dysmegakaryopoiesis. The morphology is variable, comprising all types of AML except APL. The prognosis is poor.

Acute Myeloid Leukemia with t(6;9)(p23;q34) Involving *DEK/CAN* and *DEK/SET*

This type of AML consists of two clinically and genetically different entities, involving *DEK* at chromosome band 6p23 and either *CAN* or *SET* at chromosome band 9q34 (12–17). AML with *DEK/CAN* rearrangement is associated with eosinophilic and/or basophilic differentiation. AML with *DEK/SET* rearrangement is associated with lack of differentiation (acute undifferentiated leukemia). The prognosis is poor.

Acute Myeloid Leukemia with t(8;16)(p11;p13) (*MOZ/CBP*)

AML with t(8;16) is associated with coagulopathy, extramedullary disease, monocytic differentiation, and erythrophagocytosis by blasts (18–20). The translocation involves *MOZ* at 8p11 and *CBP* at 16p13. Genetic variants and masked translocations have been reported, all involving *MOZ*. Translocations involving *MOZ* should not be confused with those involving *FGFR1*, also at 8p11, which is involved in the 8p11 myeloproliferative syndrome. The prognosis is generally poor.

Acute Myeloid Leukemia with t(8;21)(q22;q22) (*AML1/ETO*)

AML with t(8;21) is associated with young age at onset, extramedullary disease, Auer rods, and marrow eosinophilia (21–27). Approximately 90% of cases show neutrophilic differentiation (FAB M2); the remainder shows predominantly monocytic or minimal differentiation. Bone marrow aspirate smears reveal numerous dysplastic neutrophils and precursors. A peculiar type of homogeneous, salmon-pink cytoplasm has been reported in the neoplastic cells (28). Cases with less than 10% marrow blasts may be diagnosed as MDS rather than AML; this may not be a biologically meaningful distinction (29–31).

Flow cytometry shows expression of CD15, CD19, CD56, HLA-DR, and MPO. CD13 and CD34 expression are variable. CD14 and CD33 are typically not expressed. The finding of MPO expression is particularly helpful in cases lacking expression of both CD13 and CD33 (32–34).

Genetic studies demonstrate translocations of *ETO* at 8q22 and *AML1* at 21q22. Many genetic variants and masked translocations have been reported, all involving *ETO* and *AML1* (35–39). The prognosis is relatively good.

Acute Myeloid Leukemia with t(9;22)(q34;q11) (*BCR/ABL*)

AML with t(9;22) often has stem cell characteristics: little or no morphologic differentiation; expression of CD7, CD34, TdT, and lymphoid-associated antigens; and nonspecific rearrangements of *IgH* and *TCR* (40–46). The translocation involves *ABL* at 9q34 and *BCR* at 22q11. Many genetic variants and masked translocations have been reported, all involving *ABL* and *BCR*. The BCR/ABL fusion protein may be p190 (190 kd), p210, both p190 and p210, or, rarely, p230. Other karyotypic anomalies are often present. The prognosis is poor.

Acute Myeloid Leukemia with Anomalies of Chromosome 11q23 and/or *MLL*

AML of this type has variable characteristics, depending on the precise karyotypic anomaly and the involvement of *MLL*, located at 11q23 (47–56).

AML with t(11)(q23) is associated with young age, extramedullary disease, leukocytosis, myelomonocytic or monocytic differentiation, and expression of lymphoid-associated antigens. It accounts for 35% to 50% of AML cases in infants, 90% of which show myelomonocytic or monocytic differentiation.

AML with del(11)(q23) is also associated with leukocytosis but has a lower incidence of monocytic differentiation and less expression of lymphoid-associated antigens.

AML with *MLL* rearrangement is associated with monocytic differentiation. It accounts for 66% of AML cases in infants, 90% of which show myelomonocytic or monocytic differentiation. In adults, it represents 20% of AML with little morphologic differentiation (FAB M1) and 60% of acute monocytic leukemia cases.

Flow cytometry in these cases is similar, showing expression of CD4 (dim), CD11b, CD13, CD15, CD33, and/or HLA-DR. Other lymphoid-associated and stem cell antigens may be expressed, including CD2, CD3, CD7, CD34, and CD56.

Genetic studies show a surprising discrepancy between karyotypic 11q23 anomalies and *MLL* gene rearrangement. Of cases with 11q23 anomalies, only 60% show *MLL* gene rearrangement; conversely, of cases with *MLL* gene rearrangement, only 30% to 50% show 11q23 anomalies. *MLL* translocates with many different partner genes. The most common translocation is t(4;11). The prognosis in adults is poor, with the exception of cases showing t(9;11) and *MLL* translocation.

Acute Myeloid Leukemia with t(15;17)(q22;q12) (*PML/RAR*α)

Although AML with t(15;17) shows promyelocytic morphology in more than 98% of cases, it is not synonymous with APL (57–61). Occasional cases show neutrophilic (nonpromyelocytic), monocytic, megakaryocytic, eosinophilic, or only minimal differentiation.

Flow cytometry tends to demonstrate antigen expression in keeping with the stage of morphologic differentiation (62–65). Hypergranular cells usually express CD13 and/or CD33, but not CD14, CD15, CD34, CD117, or HLA-DR. Microgranular cells often express CD2, CD13, CD19, CD33, CD34, CD56, and HLA-DR. Atypical or undifferentiated cells may express of CD117 and TdT.

Genetic studies show involvement of *PML* at 15q24 and *RAR*α at 17q21. Masked translocations are associated with promyelocytic morphology and a therapeutic response to all-*trans*-retinoic acid (ATRA). Variant translocations involving *RAR*α tend to show atypical morphology and may or may not respond to ATRA (66–70). Three isoforms of the PML protein have been described, corresponding to different breakpoints in *PML* (64,71). The bcr1 isoform is the most common. The bcr3 isoform is associated with childhood onset, microgranular morphology, and worse prognosis. The prognosis is relatively good in ATRA–responsive cases.

Acute Myeloid Leukemia with inv(16)(p13q22) or t(16;16) (*CBF*β/*MYH11*)

AML with inversion or translocation involving chromosome bands 16p13 and 16q22 accounts for 3% to 5% of all AML cases (72–77). This type of AML shows increased and abnormal eosinophils in 85% of cases and is classifiable as AMML with eosinophilia (FAB M4Eo) in approximately 50% of cases. The remainder shows granulocytic (noneosinophilic), myelomonocytic, monocytic, megakaryocytic, or only minimal differentiation. Some cases show a low blast percentage and thus may be diagnosed as MDS rather than AML (78,79).

Flow cytometry shows expression of CD13, CD33, CD34, and CD117. CD2 expression is variable.

Genetic studies show inversion or translocation involving *MYH11* at 16p13 and *CBF*β (also called *PEBP2*β) at 16q22. Numerous variants and masked translocations have

been reported, all involving *MYH11* and *CBF*β (80–87). Trisomy 22 is present in some cases and may be a marker for masked translocation (88). AML with del(16q), although genetically similar, does not show the eosinophilia or good prognosis of AML with inv(16). AML with inv(16) not involving *MYH11* and *CBF*β probably represents a different disease (89).

The prognosis of AML with inv(16) or t(16;16) is relatively good, independent of morphologic differentiation.

Acute Myeloid Leukemia with t(16;21)(p11;q22) (*TLS/ERG*)

This type of AML is associated with young age, hemophagocytosis by blasts, and very poor prognosis (90–94). The blasts may show granulocytic, myelomonocytic, monocytic, megakaryocytic, or only minimal differentiation. Eosinophils may be increased and abnormal. Flow cytometry shows expression of CD11b, CD13, CD33, CD34, CD56, CD117, and HLA-DR (variable). Genetic studies show translocation of *TLS* (also known as *FUS*) at 16p11 and *ERG* at 21q22. AML with t(16;21) involving *TLS* and *ERG* should not be confused with AML with t(16;21) involving *AML1*, which is a variant of AML with t(8;21) (35,36).

Acute Myeloid Leukemia with Loss of Chromosome 17p

Loss of 17p is a characteristic finding in myelodysplastic syndromes, treated myeloproliferative disorders, and AML. It is associated with neutrophil dysplasia, including small size, hypogranularity, vacuolization, and nuclear hyposegmentation (Pelger-Huët anomaly) (95–98). The tumor suppressor gene *p53* is located in the centromeric portion of chromosome 17 and is lost in 17p deletions. Loss of 17p often occurs in myelodysplastic syndromes and treated myeloproliferative disorders and is associated with rapid progression to AML. Several genetic lesions result in loss of 17p: monosomy 17, del(17)(p), unbalanced t(17)(p), and i(17)(q). In many cases, the remaining *p53* allele shows an inactivating mutation. The prognosis is poor.

Acute Myeloid Leukemia with Constitutional Trisomy 21

AML with constitutional trisomy 21 (c21+) accounts for approximately 10% of childhood AML cases (99–114). Patients born at term with complete trisomy have the morphologic characteristics of Down syndrome; however, patients born prematurely, those with trisomy 21 mosaicism, and those with partial duplication of chromosome 21 may lack Down syndrome features. In the fetus, AML with c21+

is associated with cardiac hydrops, hepatic and pancreatic fibrosis, and a fatal outcome. In infants, it is associated with hematologic abnormalities, with approximately 50% of AML cases preceded by MDS.

Peripheral blood and bone marrow aspirate smears show abundant blasts and megakaryocytic, erythroid, and myeloid precursors. These cells have overlapping morphologic and immunophenotypic features and are thus difficult to classify precisely. More than 50% of cases show megakaryocytic differentiation. The remainder may show erythroid, myelomonocytic, eosinophilic, or only minimal differentiation. Histologic sections of the bone marrow show a heterogeneous population of early and abnormal cells and, in cases with megakaryocytic differentiation, fibrosis.

Flow cytometry usually shows expression of erythroid, megakaryocytic, and myeloid antigens, including CD1a, CD2, CD7 (variable), CD13, CD36, CD41, CD42, CD61, and glycophorin A.

Genetic studies show constitutional complete or partial trisomy of chromosome 21, in particular duplication of band 21q11 (115). In cases of trisomy 21 mosaicism, AML may arise in either a constitutionally abnormal cell or a normal cell (116,117). The neoplastic cells may show genetic evidence of clonal evolution or, rarely, multiclonal disease (118–122). AML with c21+ should be distinguished from AML with acquired chromosome 21 anomalies, although the two may be clinically and pathologically identical (123,124).

The prognosis may be relatively favorable, at least initially. Spontaneous remission occurs during fetal life or infancy in 10% of cases. This phenomenon has been reported in the literature as transient myeloproliferative disorder and leukemoid reaction. These are misnomers because the disease is clonal and relapses within 4 years in 25% of cases. The disease is better viewed as AML with spontaneous, but often transient, remission.

REFERENCES

General Features

1. Jaffe ES, Harris NL, Stein H, et al., eds. *Pathology and genetics of haematopoietic and lymphoid tissues.* Lyon: IARC Press, 2001.
2. Bennett JM. World Health Organization classification of the acute leukemias and myelodysplastic syndrome. *Int J Hematol* 2000;72:131–133.
3. Bennett JM, Catovsky D, Daniel MT, et al. Proposals for the classification of the acute leukaemias. French-American-British (FAB) co-operative group. *Br J Haematol* 1976;33:451–458.
4. Bennett JM, Catovsky D, Daniel MT, et al. Proposals for the classification of the myelodysplastic syndromes. *Br J Haematol* 1982;51:189–199.
5. Bennett JM, Catovsky D, Daniel MT, et al. Criteria for the diagnosis of acute leukemia of megakaryocyte lineage (M7). A report of the French-American-British Cooperative Group. *Ann Intern Med* 1985;103:460–462.
6. Bennett JM, Catovsky D, Daniel MT, et al. Proposal for the recognition of minimally differentiated acute myeloid leukaemia (AML-M0). *Br J Haematol* 1991;78:325–329.
7. Monpoux F, Lacour JP, Hatchuel Y, et al. Congenital leukemia cutis preceding monoblastic leukemia by 3 months. *Pediatr Dermatol* 1996;13:472–476.
8. Miyamoto T, Weissman IL, Akashi K. AML1/ETO-expressing nonleukemic stem cells in acute myelogenous leukemia with 8;21 chromosomal translocation. *Proc Natl Acad Sci U S A* 2000;97:7521–7526.
9. Dinulos JG, Hawkins DS, Clark BS, et al. Spontaneous remission of congenital leukemia. *J Pediatr* 1997;131:300–303.
10. Grundy RG, Martinez A, Kempski H, et al. Spontaneous remission of congenital leukemia: a case for conservative treatment. *J Pediatr Hematol Oncol* 2000;22:252–255.
11. Mora J, Dobrenis AM, Bussel JB, et al. Spontaneous remission of congenital acute nonlymphoblastic leukemia with normal karyotype in twins. *Med Pediatr Oncol* 2000;35:110–113.
12. Weintraub M, Kaplinsky C, Amariglio N, et al. Spontaneous regression of congenital leukaemia with an 8;16 translocation. *Br J Haematol* 2000;111:641–643.
13. Tzankov A, Ludescher C, Duba HC, et al. Spontaneous remission in a secondary acute myelogenous leukaemia following invasive pulmonary aspergillosis. *Ann Hematol* 2001;80:423–425.
14. Mitterbauer M, Fritzer-Szekeres M, Mitterbauer G, et al. Spontaneous remission of acute myeloid leukemia after infection and blood transfusion associated with hypergammaglobulinaemia. *Ann Hematol* 1996;73:189–193.
15. Martelli MP, Latagliata R, Spadea A, et al. Molecular and cytogenetic remission in a case of subtype M4E acute myelogenous leukemia with minimal monochemotherapy: high sensitivity or spontaneous remission? *Eur J Haematol* 2000;65:203–206.
16. Shimohakamada Y, Shinohara K, Fukuda N. Remission of acute myeloblastic leukemia after severe pneumonia treated with high-dose methylprednisolone. *Int J Hematol* 2001;74:173–177.
17. Surico G, Muggeo P, Muggeo V, et al. Polyclonal hypergammaglobulinemia at the onset of acute myeloid leukemia in children. *Ann Hematol* 1999;78:445–448.
18. Ferrara F, Di Noto R, Viola A, et al. Complete remission in acute myeloid leukaemia with t(8;21) following treatment with G-CSF: flow cytometric analysis of *in vivo* and *in vitro* effects on cell maturation. *Br J Haematol* 1999;106:520–523.
19. Katayama Y, Deguchi S, Shinagawa K, et al. Bone marrow necrosis in a patient with acute myeloblastic leukemia during administration of G-CSF and rapid hematologic recovery after allotransplantation of peripheral blood stem cells. *Am J Hematol* 1998;57:238–240.
20. Jeha S, Chan KW, Aprikyan AG, et al. Spontaneous remission of granulocyte colony-stimulating factor-associated leukemia in a child with severe congenital neutropenia. *Blood* 2000;96:3647–3649.
21. Weinkauff R, Estey EH, Starostik P, et al. Use of peripheral blood blasts vs bone marrow blasts for diagnosis of acute leukemia. *Am J Clin Pathol* 1999;111:733–740.
22. Tamura H, Ogata K, Yokose N, et al. Autoimmune hemolytic anemia in patients with de novo acute myelocytic leukemia. *Ann Hematol* 1996;72:45–47.
23. Nagai K, Kohno T, Chen YX, et al. Diagnostic criteria for hypocellular acute leukemia: a clinical entity distinct from overt acute leukemia and myelodysplastic syndrome. *Leuk Res* 1996;20:563–574.
24. Tuzuner N, Cox C, Rowe JM, et al. Hypocellular acute myeloid leukemia: the Rochester (New York) experience. *Hematol Pathol* 1995;9:195–203.
25. Richard G, Brody J, Sun T. A case of acute megakaryocytic leukemia with hematogones. *Leukemia* 1993;7:1900–1903.

26. Alliot C, Barrios M, Franck F. Malignancy case report: systemic sarcoidosis preceding acute myeloid leukemia. *Hematology* 2000;5:127–128.

27. Pagano L, Visani G, Ferrara F, et al. Contemporaneous acute myeloid leukaemia and sarcoidosis. Report of three cases. *Sarcoidosis Vasc Diffuse Lung Dis* 1998;15:67–70.

28. Egeler RM, Neglia JP, Puccetti DM, et al. Association of Langerhans cell histiocytosis with malignant neoplasms. *Cancer* 1993;71:865–873.

29. Lai R, Arber DA, Brynes RK, et al. Untreated chronic lymphocytic leukemia concurrent with or followed by acute myelogenous leukemia or myelodysplastic syndrome. A report of five cases and review of the literature. *Am J Clin Pathol* 1999;111:373–378.

30. Xie XY, Filie AC, Jasper GA, et al. Diagnosis of unexpected acute myeloid leukemia and chronic lymphocytic leukemia: a case report demonstrating the perils of restricted panels in flow cytometric immunophenotyping. *Cytometry* 2000;42:114–117.

31. Yenerel MN, Hatemi I, Keskin H. Concomitant chronic lymphocytic leukemia and acute myeloid leukemia diagnosed by two color flow cytometric analysis. *Haematologica* 1999;84:766–767.

32. Suh YK, Shin SS, Koo CH. Synchronous Hodgkin's disease and granulocytic sarcoma with no prior therapy. *Hum Pathol* 1996;27:1103–1106.

33. Nagata T, Mugishima H, Yoden A, et al. A case of monoclonal gammopathy associated with acute myelomonocytic leukemia with eosinophilia suggested to be the result of lineage infidelity. *Am J Hematol* 2000;65:66–71.

34. Anderson CM, Bueso-Ramos CE, Wallner SA, et al. Primary myeloid leukemia presenting concomitantly with primary multiple myeloma: two cases and an update of the literature. *Leuk Lymphoma* 1999;32:385–390.

35. Tsukasaki K, Koba T, Iwanaga M, et al. Possible association between adult T-cell leukemia/lymphoma and acute myeloid leukemia. *Cancer* 1998;82:488–494.

36. Jain NC, Cox C, Bennett JM. Auer rods in the acute myeloid leukemias: frequency and methods of demonstration. *Hematol Oncol* 1987;5:197–202.

37. Luno E, Payer AR, Luengo JR, et al. Trisomy 10 in acute myeloid leukemia: report of a new case. *Cancer Genet Cytogenet* 1998;100:84–87.

38. Ma SK, Yip SF, Wan TS, et al. Acute myeloid leukaemia with giant granules: association with t(10;11)(p13;q14) and disseminated intravascular coagulation. *Clin Lab Haematol* 2000;22:303–305.

39. Mehta AB, Bain BJ, Fitchett M, et al. Trisomy 13 and myeloid malignancy—characteristic blast cell morphology: a United Kingdom Cancer Cytogenetics Group survey. *Br J Haematol* 1998;101:749–752.

40. Au WY, Ma SK, Chan AC, et al. Near tetraploidy in three cases of acute myeloid leukemia associated with mediastinal granulocytic sarcoma. *Cancer Genet Cytogenet* 1998;102:50–53.

41. Kaplan SS, Rybka WB, Blom J, et al. Tetraploidy in acute myeloid leukemia secondary to large cell lymphoma. *Leuk Lymphoma* 1998;31:617–623.

42. Kwong YL, Wong KF. Hyperdiploid acute myeloid leukemia. Relationship between blast size and karyotype demonstrated by fluorescence *in situ* hybridization. *Cancer Genet Cytogenet* 1995;83:1–4.

43. Lemez P, Michalova K, Zemanova Z, et al. Three cases of near-tetraploid acute myeloid leukemias originating in pluripotent myeloid progenitors. *Leuk Res* 1998;22:581–588.

44. Xue Y, He J, Wang Y, et al. Secondary near-pentaploidy and/or near-tetraploidy characterized by the duplication of 8;21 translocation in the M2 subtype of acute myeloid leukemia. *Int J Hematol* 2000;71:359–365.

45. Yeh SP, Wang Y, Su J, et al. Near-tetraploid minimally differentiated acute myeloid leukemia with extensive erythrophagocytosis by leukemic blasts. *Ann Hematol* 2000;79:36–39.

46. Domingo-Claros A, Alonso E, Aventin A, et al. Oligoblastic leukaemia with (8;21) translocation and haemophagocytic syndrome and granulocytic cannibalism. *Leuk Res* 1996;20:517–521.

47. Mori H, Tawara M, Yoshida Y, et al. Minimally differentiated acute myeloid leukemia (AML-M0) with extensive erythrophagocytosis and del(20)(q11) chromosome abnormality. *Leuk Res* 2000;24:87–90.

48. Rosenthal NS, Farhi DC. Special stains in the diagnosis of acute leukemia. *Clin Lab Med* 2000;20:29–38.

49. Kheiri SA, MacKerrell T, Bonagura VR, et al. Flow cytometry with or without cytochemistry for the diagnosis of acute leukemias? *Cytometry* 1998;34:82–86.

50. Bahia DM, Yamamoto M, Chauffaille MD, et al. Acute myeloid leukemia: a high frequency of aberrant phenotypes and its clinical significance. *Haematologica* 2001;86:801–806.

51. Bene MC, Bernier M, Casasnovas RO, et al. The reliability and specificity of c-kit for the diagnosis of acute myeloid leukemias and undifferentiated leukemias. The European Group for the Immunological Classification of Leukemias (EGIL). *Blood* 1998;92:596–599.

52. Casasnovas RO, Campos L, Mugneret F, et al. Immunophenotypic patterns and cytogenetic anomalies in acute non-lymphoblastic leukemia subtypes: a prospective study of 432 patients. *Leukemia* 1998;12:34–43.

53. Cascavilla N, Musto P, D'Arena G, et al. CD117 (c-kit) is a restricted antigen of acute myeloid leukemia and characterizes early differentiative levels of M5 FAB subtype. *Haematologica* 1998;83:392–397.

54. Hans CP, Finn WG, Singleton TP, et al. Usefulness of anti-CD117 in the flow cytometric analysis of acute leukemia. *Am J Clin Pathol* 2002;117:301–305.

55. Huh YO, Smith TL, Collins P, et al. Terminal deoxynucleotidyl transferase expression in acute myelogenous leukemia and myelodysplasia as determined by flow cytometry. *Leuk Lymphoma* 2000;37:319–331.

56. Kaleem Z, Crawford E, Pathan MH, et al. Flow cytometric analysis of acute leukemias. Diagnostic utility and critical analysis of data. *Arch Pathol Lab Med* 2003;127:42–48.

57. Khalidi HS, Medeiros LJ, Chang KL, et al. The immunophenotype of adult acute myeloid leukemia: high frequency of lymphoid antigen expression and comparison of immunophenotype, French-American-British classification, and karyotypic abnormalities. *Am J Clin Pathol* 1998;109:211–220.

58. Nakase K, Sartor M, Bradstock K. Detection of myeloperoxidase by flow cytometry in acute leukemia. *Cytometry* 1998;34:198–202.

59. Paredes-Aguilera R, Romero-Guzman L, Lopez-Santiago N, et al. Flow cytometric analysis of cell-surface and intracellular antigens in the diagnosis of acute leukemia. *Am J Hematol* 2001;68:69–74.

60. Thalhammer-Scherrer R, Mitterbauer G, Simonitsch I, et al. The immunophenotype of 325 adult acute leukemias: relationship to morphologic and molecular classification and proposal for a minimal screening program highly predictive for lineage discrimination. *Am J Clin Pathol* 2002;117:380–389.

61. Venditti A, Del Poeta G, Buccisano F, et al. Prognostic relevance of the expression of Tdt and CD7 in 335 cases of acute myeloid leukemia. *Leukemia* 1998;12:1056–1063.

62. Raspadori D, Damiani D, Lenoci M, et al. CD56 antigenic expression in acute myeloid leukemia identifies patients with poor clinical prognosis. *Leukemia* 2001;15:1161–1164.

63. Baer MR, Stewart CC, Dodge RK, et al. High frequency of immunophenotype changes in acute myeloid leukemia at relapse: implications for residual disease detection (Cancer and Leukemia Group B Study 8361). *Blood* 2001;97:3574–3580.

64. Hur M, Chang YH, Lee DS, et al. Immunophenotypic and cytogenetic changes in acute leukaemia at relapse. *Clin Lab Haematol* 2001;23:173–179.

65. McIlwain L, Sokol L, Moscinski LC, et al. Acute myeloid leukemia mimicking primary testicular neoplasm. Presentation of a case with review of literature. *Eur J Haematol* 2003;70: 242–245.

66. Dunphy CH, Polski JM, Evans HL, et al. Evaluation of bone marrow specimens with acute myelogenous leukemia for CD34, CD15, CD117, and myeloperoxidase. *Arch Pathol Lab Med* 2001;125:1063–1069.

67. Dastugue N, Payen C, Lafage-Pochitaloff M, et al. Prognostic significance of karyotype in de novo adult acute myeloid leukemia. The BGMT group. *Leukemia* 1995;9:1491–1498.

68. Farhi DC. Fluorescence DNA hybridization in the evaluation of clonal myeloid disease. *J Clin Ligand Assay* 2002;24:192–200.

69. Fleischman EW, Reshmi S, Sokova OI, et al. Increased karyotype precision using fluorescence in situ hybridization and spectral karyotyping in patients with myeloid malignancies. *Cancer Genet Cytogenet* 1999;108:166–170.

70. Grimwade D, Walker H, Oliver F, et al. The importance of diagnostic cytogenetics on outcome in AML: analysis of 1,612 patients entered into the MRC AML 10 trial. The Medical Research Council Adult and Children's Leukaemia Working Parties. *Blood* 1998;92:2322–2333.

71. Raimondi SC, Chang MN, Ravindranath Y, et al. Chromosomal abnormalities in 478 children with acute myeloid leukemia: clinical characteristics and treatment outcome in a cooperative pediatric oncology group study POG 8821. *Blood* 1999;94:3707–3716.

72. Martinez-Climent JA, Garcia-Conde J. Chromosomal rearrangements in childhood acute myeloid leukemia and myelodysplastic syndromes. *J Pediatr Hematol Oncol* 1999;21:91–102.

73. Perkins D, Brennan S, Carstairs K, et al. Regional cancer cytogenetics: a report on 1,143 diagnostic cases. *Cancer Genet Cytogenet* 1997;96:64–80.

74. Tanaka K, Arif M, Eguchi M, et al. Interphase fluorescence in situ hybridization overcomes pitfalls of G-banding analysis with special reference to underestimation of chromosomal aberration rates. *Cancer Genet Cytogenet* 1999;115:32–38.

75. Wong KF, Kwong YL, Tang KC. Biclonal acute monoblastic leukemia showing del(7q) and trisomies 9 and 22. *Cancer Genet Cytogenet* 1995;82:70–72.

76. Launder TM, Bray RA, Stempora L, et al. Lymphoid-associated antigen expression by acute myeloid leukemia. *Am J Clin Pathol* 1996;106:185–191.

77. Schmidt CA, Przybylski G, Seeger K, et al. TCR delta gene rearrangements in acute myeloid leukemia with T-lymphoid antigen expression. *Leuk Lymphoma* 1995;20:45–49.

78. Tien HF, Wang CH, Lin MT, et al. Correlation of cytogenetic results with immunophenotype, genotype, clinical features, and ras mutation in acute myeloid leukemia. A study of 235 Chinese patients in Taiwan. *Cancer Genet Cytogenet* 1995;84:60–68.

79. Lillington DM, Jaju RJ, Shankar AG, et al. Cytogenetic and molecular evidence of marrow involvement in extramedullary acute myeloid leukaemia. *Br J Haematol* 2000;110: 547–551.

80. Kuwabara H, Nagai M, Yamaoka G, et al. Specific skin manifestations in CD56 positive acute myeloid leukemia. *J Cutan Pathol* 1999;26:1–5.

81. Byrd JC, Weiss RB, Arthur DC, et al. Extramedullary leukemia adversely affects hematologic complete remission rate and overall survival in patients with t(8;21)(q22;q22): results from Cancer and Leukemia Group B 8461. *J Clin Oncol* 1997;15:466–475.

82. Jenkin RD, Al-Shabanah M, Al-Nasser A, et al. Extramedullary myeloid tumors in children: the limited value of local treatment. *J Pediatr Hematol Oncol* 2000;22:34–40.

83. Schwyzer R, Sherman GG, Cohn RJ, et al. Granulocytic sarcoma in children with acute myeloblastic leukemia and t(8;21). *Med Pediatr Oncol* 1998;31:144–149.

84. Johansson B, Fioretos T, Kullendorff CM, et al. Granulocytic sarcomas in body cavities in childhood acute myeloid leukemias with 11q23/MLL rearrangements. *Genes Chromosomes Cancer* 2000;27:136–142.

85. Lestringant GG, Masouye I, El-Hayek M, et al. Diffuse calcinosis cutis in a patient with congenital leukemia and leukemia cutis. *Dermatology* 2000;200:147–150.

86. Linn YC, Goh YT, Tan HC. Relapse of leukemia and lymphoma after marrow transplant: a review of cases with extramedullary relapse. *Leuk Lymphoma* 2000;38:137–146.

87. Menasce LP, Banerjee SS, Beckett E, et al. Extra-medullary myeloid tumour (granulocytic sarcoma) is often misdiagnosed: a study of 26 cases. *Histopathology* 1999;34:391–398.

88. Sadahira Y, Sugihara T, Yawata Y, et al. Cutaneous granulocytic sarcoma mimicking immunoblastic large cell lymphoma. *Pathol Int* 1999;49:347–353.

89. Ashfaq R, Weinberg AG, Argyle CA. Acute megakaryoblastic leukemia simulating carcinoma. *Am J Clin Pathol* 1992;98: 55–60.

90. Karayalcin G, Khanijou A, Kim KY, et al. Monocytosis in congenital syphilis. *Am J Dis Child* 1977;131:782–783.

91. Moraes M, Wilkes J, Lowder JN. Monocytic leukemoid reaction, glucocorticoid therapy, and myelodysplastic syndrome. *Cleve Clin J Med* 1990;57:571–574.

92. Weitberg AB. A monocytic leukemoid reaction in a patient with myelodysplasia. *CA Cancer J Clin* 1985;35:308–310.

93. Ahmed MA. Promyelocytic leukaemoid reaction: an atypical presentation of mycobacterial infection. *Acta Haematol* 1991;85:143–145.

94. Bottom KS, Adams DM, Mann KP, et al. Trilineage hematopoietic toxicity associated with valproic acid therapy. *J Pediatr Hematol Oncol* 1997;19:73–76.

95. Gilbert-Barness E, Barness LA. Isovaleric acidemia with promyelocytic myeloproliferative syndrome. *Pediatr Dev Pathol* 1999;2:286–291.

96. Rizzatti EG, Garcia AB, Portieres FL, et al. Expression of CD117 and CD11b in bone marrow can differentiate acute promyelocytic leukemia from recovering benign myeloid proliferation. *Am J Clin Pathol* 2002;118:31–37.

97. Singh ZN, Kotwal J, Choudhry VP, et al. Leukemoid reaction simulating acute promyelocytic leukemia. *J Assoc Physicians India* 1999;47:1031–1032.

98. Dreskin SC, Iberti TJ, Watson-Williams EJ. Pseudoleukemia due to infection. A case report. *J Med* 1983;14:147–155.

99. Friedman HD, Landaw SA. Recent-onset myelodysplastic syndrome mimicking acute leukemia during infection. *Ann Hematol* 1996;72:85–88.

100. Ko WS, Chen LM, Chao TY, et al. Myeloblastic leukemoid reaction in paroxysmal nocturnal hemoglobinuria associated with myelodysplasia. *Acta Haematol* 1992;87:75–77.

101. Levine PH, Weintraub LW. Pseudoleukemia during recovery from dapsone-induced agranulocytosis. *Ann Intern Med* 1968;68:1060–1065.

102. Lin SJ, Jaing TH. Thrombocytopenia in systemic-onset juvenile chronic arthritis: report of two cases with unusual bone marrow features. *Clin Rheumatol* 1999;18:241–243.

103. Tamayose K, Sugimoto K, Ando M, et al. Mononucleosis syndrome and acute monocytic leukemia. *Eur J Haematol* 2002; 68:236–238.

104. Baer MR, Bernstein SH, Brunetto VL, et al. Biological effects of recombinant human granulocyte colony-stimulating factor in patients with untreated acute myeloid leukemia. *Blood* 1996;87:1484–1494.

105. Inukai T, Sugita K, Iijima K, et al. Leukemic cells with 11q23 translocations express granulocyte colony-stimulating factor (G-CSF) receptor and their proliferation is stimulated with G-CSF. *Leukemia* 1998;12:382–389.

106. Meyerson HJ, Farhi DC, Rosenthal NS. Transient increase in blasts mimicking acute leukemia and progressing myelodysplasia in patients receiving growth factor. *Am J Clin Pathol* 1998;109:675–681.

107. Ranaghan L, Drake M, Humphreys MW, et al. Leukaemoid monocytosis in M4 AML following chemotherapy and G-CSF. *Clin Lab Haematol* 1998;20:49–51.

108. Bunworasate U, Arnouk H, Minderman H, et al. Erythropoietin-dependent transformation of myelodysplastic syndrome to acute monoblastic leukemia. *Blood* 2001;98:3492–3494.

109. Dokal IS, Cox TM, Galton DA. Vitamin B-12 and folate deficiency presenting as leukaemia. *BMJ* 1990;300:1263–1264.

110. Boyd JE, Parmley RT, Langevin AM, et al. Neuroblastoma presenting as acute monoblastic leukemia. *J Pediatr Hematol Oncol* 1996;18:206–212.

111. Santos-Machado TM, Zerbini MC, Cristofani LM, et al. Simultaneous occurrence of advanced neuroblastoma and acute myeloid leukemia. *Pediatr Hematol Oncol* 2001;18:129–135.

Morphologic and Immunophenotypic Subtypes

1. Astall E, Yarranton H, Arno J, et al. Granulocytic sarcoma preceding AML M0 and the diagnostic value of CD34. *J Clin Pathol* 1999;52:705–707.

2. Cohen PL, Hoyer JD, Kurtin PJ, et al. Acute myeloid leukemia with minimal differentiation. A multiple parameter study. *Am J Clin Pathol* 1998;109:32–38.

3. Costello R, Mallet F, Chambost H, et al. The immunophenotype of minimally differentiated acute myeloid leukemia (AML-M0): reduced immunogenicity and high frequency of CD34+/CD38- leukemic progenitors. *Leukemia* 1999;13:1513–1518.

4. Huang SY, Tang JL, Jou ST, et al. Minimally differentiated acute myeloid leukemia in Taiwan: predominantly occurs in children less than 3 years and adults between 51 and 70 years. *Leukemia* 1999;13:1506–1512.

5. Kotylo PK, Seo IS, Smith FO, et al. Flow cytometric immunophenotypic characterization of pediatric and adult minimally differentiated acute myeloid leukemia (AML-M0). *Am J Clin Pathol* 2000;113:193–200.

6. Traweek ST, Liu J, Braziel RM, et al. Detection of myeloperoxidase gene expression in minimally differentiated acute myelogenous leukemia (AML-M0) using in situ hybridization. *Diagn Mol Pathol* 1995;4:212–219.

7. Venditti A, Del Poeta G, Buccisano F, et al. Minimally differentiated acute myeloid leukemia (AML-M0): comparison of 25 cases with other French-American-British subtypes. *Blood* 1997;89:621–629.

8. Ysebaert L, Carli PM, Casasnovas RO, et al. Minimally differentiated acute myeloid leukemia (AML-MO) with lymphoid presentation at relapse: a case report. *Leukemia* 2001;15:1673–1674.

9. Poirel H, Rack K, Delabesse E, et al. Incidence and characterization of MLL gene (11q23) rearrangements in acute myeloid leukemia M1 and M5. *Blood* 1996;87:2496–2505.

10. Stass SA, Lanham GR, Butler D, et al. Auer rods in mature granulocytes: a unique morphologic feature of acute myelogenous leukemia with maturation. *Am J Clin Pathol* 1984;81: 662–665.

11. del Mar Bellido M, Nomdedeu JF. Adult de novo acute myeloid leukemias with MLL rearrangements. *Leuk Res* 1999;23: 585–588.

12. Allford S, Grimwade D, Langabeer S, et al. Identification of the t(15;17) in AML FAB types other than M3: evaluation of the role of molecular screening for the PML/RARalpha rearrangement in newly diagnosed AML. The Medical Research Council (MRC) Adult Leukaemia Working Party. *Br J Haematol* 1999;105: 198–207.

13. Avvisati G, Lo Coco F, Mandelli F. Acute promyelocytic leukemia: clinical and morphologic features and prognostic factors. *Semin Hematol* 2001;38:4–12.

14. Castoldi GL, Liso V, Specchia G, et al. Acute promyelocytic leukemia: morphological aspects. *Leukemia* 1994;8:1441–1446.

15. Exner M, Thalhammer R, Kapiotis S, et al. The "typical" immunophenotype of acute promyelocytic leukemia (APL-M3): does it prove true for the M3-variant? *Cytometry* 2000;42: 106–109.

16. Foley R, Soamboonsrup P, Carter RF, et al. CD34-positive acute promyelocytic leukemia is associated with leukocytosis, microgranular/hypogranular morphology, expression of CD2 and bcr3 isoform. *Am J Hematol* 2001;67:34–41.

17. Girodon F, Carli PM, Favre B, et al. Acute myeloid leukemia with hypergranular cytoplasm: a differential diagnosis of acute promyelocytic leukemia. *Leuk Res* 2000;24:979–982.

18. Guglielmi C, Martelli MP, Diverio D, et al. Immunophenotype of adult and childhood acute promyelocytic leukaemia: correlation with morphology, type of PML gene breakpoint and clinical outcome. A cooperative Italian study on 196 cases. *Br J Haematol* 1998;102:1035–1041.

19. Kaleem Z, Watson MS, Zutter MM, et al. Acute promyelocytic leukemia with additional chromosomal abnormalities and absence of Auer rods. *Am J Clin Pathol* 1999;112:113–118.

20. Neame PB, Soamboonsrup P, Leber B, et al. Morphology of acute promyelocytic leukemia with cytogenetic or molecular evidence for the diagnosis: characterization of additional microgranular variants. *Am J Hematol* 1997;56:131–142.

21. Oren H, Duzovali O, Yuksel E, et al. Development of acute promyelocytic leukemia with isochromosome 17q after BCR/ABL positive chronic myeloid leukemia. *Cancer Genet Cytogenet* 1999;109:141–143.

22. Spell DW, Velagaleti GV, Jones DV, et al. Translocation (15;17) and trisomy 21 in the microgranular variant of acute promyelocytic leukemia. *Cancer Genet Cytogenet* 2002;132:74–76.

23. Orfao A, Chillon MC, Bortoluci AM, et al. The flow cytometric pattern of CD34, CD15 and CD13 expression in acute myeloblastic leukemia is highly characteristic of the presence of PML-RARalpha gene rearrangements. *Haematologica* 1999;84: 405–412.

24. Tallman MS, Hakimian D, Snower D, et al. Basophilic differentiation in acute promyelocytic leukemia. *Leukemia* 1993;7: 521–526.

25. Invernizzi R, Iannone AM, Bernuzzi S, et al. Acute promyelocytic leukemia toluidine blue subtype. *Leuk Lymphoma* 1995;18: 57–60.

26. Nagendra S, Meyerson H, Skallerud G, et al. Leukemias resembling acute promyelocytic leukemia, microgranular variant. *Am J Clin Pathol* 2002;117:651–657.

27. Symes PH, Williams ME, Flessa HC, et al. Acute promyelocytic leukemia with the pseudo-Chediak-Higashi anomaly and molecular documentation of t(15;17) chromosomal translocation. *Am J Clin Pathol* 1993;99:622–627.

28. Mori A, Wada H, Okada M, et al. Acute promyelocytic leukemia with marrow fibrosis at initial presentation: possible involvement of transforming growth factor-beta(1). *Acta Haematol* 2000; 103:220–223.

29. Stasi R, Bruno A, Venditti A, et al. A microgranular variant of acute promyelocytic leukemia with atypical morphocytochemical features and an early myeloid immunophenotype. *Leuk Res* 1997;21:575–580.

30. Nagendra S, Meyerson H, Skallerud G, et al. Leukemias resembling acute promyelocytic leukemia, microgranular variant. *Am J Clin Pathol* 2002;117:651–657.

31. Rizzatti EG, Garcia AB, Portieres FL, et al. Expression of CD117 and CD11b in bone marrow can differentiate acute promyelocytic leukemia from recovering benign myeloid proliferation. *Am J Clin Pathol* 2002;118:31–37.

32. Canioni D, Fraitag S, Thomas C, et al. Skin lesions revealing neonatal acute leukemias with monocytic differentiation. A report of 3 cases. *J Cutan Pathol* 1996;23:254–258.

33. Cimino G, Rapanotti MC, Elia L, et al. ALL-1 gene rearrangements in acute myeloid leukemia: association with M4-M5 French-American-British classification subtypes and young age. *Cancer Res* 1995;55:1625–1628.

34. Hernandez JM, Gonzalez MB, Granada I, et al. Detection of inv(16) and t(16;16) by fluorescence in situ hybridization in acute myeloid leukemia M4Eo. *Haematologica* 2000;85:481–485.

35. Cazzaniga G, Tosi S, Aloisi A, et al. The tyrosine kinase abl-related gene ARG is fused to ETV6 in an AML-M4Eo patient with a t(1;12)(q25;p13): molecular cloning of both reciprocal transcripts. *Blood* 1999;94:4370–4373.

36. Dengler R, Walther JU, Emmerich B. Trisomy 21 as the sole clonal aberration in a patient with acute myelomonocytic leukemia with abnormal bone marrow eosinophils and extramedullary involvement. *Ann Hematol* 1994;68:93–95.

37. Fung H, Shepherd JD, Naiman SC, et al. Acute monocytic leukemia: a single institution experience. *Leuk Lymphoma* 1995; 19:259–265.

38. Esteve J, Rozman M, Campo E, et al. Leukemia after true histiocytic lymphoma: another type of acute monocytic leukemia with histiocytic differentiation (AML-M5c)? *Leukemia* 1995; 9:1389–1391.

39. Lima M, Orfao A, Coutinho J, et al. An unusual acute myeloid leukemia associated with hyper IgE: another case of AML-M5c? *Haematologica* 2001;86:216–217.

40. Davey FR, Abraham N Jr, Brunetto VL, et al. Morphologic characteristics of erythroleukemia (acute myeloid leukemia; FAB-M6): a CALGB study. *Am J Hematol* 1995;49:29–38.

41. Day DS, Gay JN, Kraus JS, et al. Erythroleukemia of childhood and infancy: a report of two cases. *Ann Clin Lab Sci* 1997;27:142–150.

42. Domingo-Claros A, Larriba I, Rozman M, et al. Acute erythroid neoplastic proliferations. A biological study based on 62 patients. *Haematologica* 2002;87:148–153.

43. Garand R, Duchayne E, Blanchard D, et al. Minimally differentiated erythroleukaemia (AML M6 'variant'): a rare subset of AML distinct from AML M6. Groupe Francais d'Hematologie Cellulaire. *Br J Haematol* 1995;90:868–875.

44. Goldberg SL, Noel P, Klumpp TR, et al. The erythroid leukemias: a comparative study of erythroleukemia (FAB M6) and Di Guglielmo disease. *Am J Clin Oncol* 1998;21:42–47.

45. Hadjiyannakis A, Fletcher WA, Lebrun DP, et al. Congenital erythroleukemia in a neonate with severe hypoxic ischemic encephalopathy. *Am J Perinatol* 1998;15:689–694.

46. Hasserjian RP, Howard J, Wood A, et al. Acute erythremic myelosis (true erythroleukaemia): a variant of AML FAB-M6. *J Clin Pathol* 2001;54:205–209.

47. Kwong YL. Translocation (3;5)(q21;q34) in erythroleukemia: a molecular and *in situ* hybridization study. *Cancer Genet Cytogenet* 1998;103:15–19.

48. Linari S, Vannucchi AM, Ciolli S, et al. Coexpression of erythroid and megakaryocytic genes in acute erythroblastic (FAB M6) and megakaryoblastic (FAB M7) leukaemias. *Br J Haematol* 1998;102:1335–1337.

49. Mazzella FM, Alvares C, Kowal-Vern A, et al. The acute erythroleukemias. *Clin Lab Med* 2000;20:119–137.

50. Mazzella FM, Kowal-Vern A, Shrit MA, et al. Acute erythroleukemia: evaluation of 48 cases with reference to classification, cell proliferation, cytogenetics, and prognosis. *Am J Clin Pathol* 1998;110:590–598.

51. Michiels JJ, van der Meulen J, Brederoo P. The natural history of trilinear myelodysplastic syndrome and erythroleukemia. *Haematologica* 1997;82:452–454.

52. Tsuji M, Tamai M, Terada N, et al. Anerythremic form of acute erythremic myelosis (Di Guglielmo's syndrome) causing hepatosplenomegaly due to the infiltration of hemoglobin-bearing blast cells: an autopsy case. *Pathol Int* 1995;45:310–314.

53. Lorsbach RB, Folkerth RD, Pinkus GS. Relapse of acute myelogenous leukemia as a cerebellar myeloblastoma showing megakaryoblastic differentiation. *Mod Pathol* 1999;12:1186–1191.

54. Abrahamsson J, Swolin B, Mellander L. Bone marrow fibrosis and radiological changes of the long bones in children with acute megakaryocytic leukaemia. *Acta Paediatr* 1998;87:1093–1096.

55. Fisher D, Ruchlemer R, Hiller N, et al. Aggressive bone destruction in acute megakaryocytic leukaemia: a rare presentation. *Pediatr Radiol* 1997;27:20–22.

56. Gassmann W, Loffler H. Acute megakaryoblastic leukaemia. *Leuk Lymphoma* 1995;18:69–73.

57. Helleberg C, Knudsen H, Hansen PB, et al. CD34+ megakaryoblastic leukaemic cells are CD38-, but CD61+ and glycophorin A+: improved criteria for diagnosis of AML-M7? *Leukemia* 1997;11:830–834.

58. Ito E, Kasai M, Toki T, et al. Expression of erythroid specific genes in megakaryoblastic disorders. *Leuk Lymphoma* 1996;23:545–550.

59. Kozlowski K, Halimun E. Generalised bone disease with abundant periosteal reaction in megakaryocytic leukaemia. *Eur J Pediatr* 1997;156:845–847.

60. Paulien S, Busson-Le Coniat M, Berger R. Acute megakaryocytic leukaemia with acquired polysomy 21 and translocation t(1;21). *Ann Genet* 2000;43:99–104.

61. Pelloso LA, Baiocchi OC, Chauffaille ML, et al. Megakaryocytic blast crisis as a first presentation of chronic myeloid leukemia. *Eur J Haematol* 2002;69:58–61.

62. Polski JM, Galambos C, Gale GB, et al. Acute megakaryoblastic leukemia after transient myeloproliferative disorder with clonal karyotype evolution in a phenotypically normal neonate. *J Pediatr Hematol Oncol* 2002;24:50–54.

63. Tallman MS, Neuberg D, Bennett JM, et al. Acute megakaryocytic leukemia: the Eastern Cooperative Oncology Group experience. *Blood* 2000;96:2405–2411.

64. Xue Y, Lu D, Lu D, et al. A case of acute megakaryocytic leukemia presenting as peripheral acute leukemia with complex karyotypic abnormalities. *Cancer Genet Cytogenet* 1998;105:83–85.

65. Abe A, Emi N, Tanimoto M, et al. Fusion of the platelet-derived growth factor receptor beta to a novel gene CEV14 in acute myelogenous leukemia after clonal evolution. *Blood* 1997;90:4271–4277.

66. La Starza R, Trubia M, Testoni N, et al. Clonal eosinophils are a morphologic hallmark of ETV6/ABL1 positive acute myeloid leukemia. *Haematologica* 2002;87:789–794.

67. Lepretre S, Jardin F, Buchonnet G, et al. Eosinophilic leukemia associated with t(2;5)(p23;q31). *Cancer Genet Cytogenet* 2002; 133:164–167.

68. Loffler H, Gassmann W, Haferlach T. AML M1 and M2 with eosinophilia and AML M4Eo: diagnostic and clinical aspects. *Leuk Lymphoma* 1995;18:61–63.

69. Menssen HD, Renkl HJ, Rieder H, et al. Distinction of eosinophilic leukaemia from idiopathic hypereosinophilic syndrome by analysis of Wilms' tumour gene expression. *Br J Haematol* 1998;101:325–334.

70. Salmon-Nguyen F, Busson M, Daniel M, et al. CALM-AF10 fusion gene in leukemias: simple and inversion-associated translocation (10;11). *Cancer Genet Cytogenet* 2000;122:137–140.

71. Yagasaki F, Jinnai I, Yoshida S, et al. Fusion of TEL/ETV6 to a novel ACS2 in myelodysplastic syndrome and acute myelogenous leukemia with t(5;12)(q31;p13). *Genes Chromosomes Cancer* 1999;26:192–202.

72. Yahata N, Ohyashiki K, Ohyashiki JH, et al. Late appearance of t(5;12)(q31;p12) in acute myeloid leukemia associated with eosinophilia. *Cancer Genet Cytogenet* 1998;107:147–150.

73. Yu RQ, Huang W, Chen SJ, et al. A case of acute eosinophilic granulocytic leukemia with PML-RAR alpha fusion gene expression and response to all-trans retinoic acid. *Leukemia* 1997;11:609–611.

74. Bernini JC, Timmons CF, Sandler ES. Acute basophilic leukemia in a child. Anaphylactoid reaction and coagulopathy secondary to vincristine-mediated degranulation. *Cancer* 1995;75: 110–114.

75. Dastugue N, Duchayne E, Kuhlein E, et al. Acute basophilic leukaemia and translocation t(X;6)(p11;q23). *Br J Haematol* 1997;98:170–176.

76. Duchayne E, Demur C, Rubie H, et al. Diagnosis of acute basophilic leukemia. *Leuk Lymphoma* 1999;32:269–278.

77. Giagounidis AA, Hildebrandt B, Heinsch M, et al. Acute basophilic leukemia. *Eur J Haematol* 2001;67:72–76.

78. Lertprasertsuke N, Tsutsumi Y. An unusual form of chronic myeloproliferative disorder. Aleukemic basophilic leukemia. *Acta Pathol Jpn* 1991;41:73–81.

79. Mitev L, Apostolov P, Manolova Y. Case of acute monocytic leukemia with 47,XY,+X,t(2;10)(q21.1;q26.1) and basophilia. *Cancer Genet Cytogenet* 1996;86:80–82.

80. Peterson LC, Parkin JL, Arthur DC, et al. Acute basophilic leukemia. A clinical, morphologic, and cytogenetic study of eight cases. *Am J Clin Pathol* 1991;96:160–170.

81. Scolyer RA, Brun M, D'Rozario J, et al. Acute basophilic leukemia presenting with abnormal liver function tests and the absence of blast cells in the peripheral blood. *Pathology* 2000; 32:52–55.

82. Shekhter-Levin S, Penchansky L, Wollman MR, et al. An abnormal clone with monosomy 7 and trisomy 21 in the bone marrow of a child with congenital agranulocytosis (Kostmann disease) treated with granulocyte colony-stimulating factor. Evolution towards myelodysplastic syndrome and acute basophilic leukemia. *Cancer Genet Cytogenet* 1995;84:99–104.

83. Shvidel L, Shaft D, Stark B, et al. Acute basophilic leukaemia: eight unsuspected new cases diagnosed by electron microscopy. *Br J Haematol* 2003;120:774–781.

84. Yamagata T, Miwa A, Eguchi M, et al. Transformation into acute basophilic leukaemia in a patient with myelodysplastic syndrome. *Br J Haematol* 1995;89:650–652.

85. Yokohama A, Tsukamoto N, Hatsumi N, et al. Acute basophilic leukemia lacking basophil-specific antigens: the importance of cytokine receptor expression in differential diagnosis. *Int J Hematol* 2002;75:309–313.

86. Kahl C, Florschutz A, Muller G, et al. Prognostic significance of dysplastic features of hematopoiesis in patients with de novo acute myelogenous leukemia. *Ann Hematol* 1997;75:91–94.

87. Lemez P, Galikova J, Haas T. Erythroblastic and/or megakaryocytic dysplasia in de novo acute myeloid leukemias M0-M5 show relation to myelodysplastic syndromes and delimit two main categories. *Leuk Res* 2000;24:207–215.

88. Lima CS, Vassalo J, Lorand-Metze I, et al. The significance of trilineage myelodysplasia in de novo acute myeloblastic leukemia: clinical and laboratory features. *Haematologia* 1997;28:85–95.

89. Meckenstock G, Aul C, Hildebrandt B, et al. Dyshematopoiesis in de novo acute myeloid leukemia: cell biological features and prognostic significance. *Leuk Lymphoma* 1998;29:523–531.

90. Taguchi J, Miyazaki Y, Yoshida S, et al. Allogeneic bone marrow transplantation improves the outcome of de novo AML with trilineage dysplasia (AML-TLD). *Leukemia* 2000;14:1861–1866.

91. Hudson MM, Poquette CA, Lee J, et al. Increased mortality after successful treatment for Hodgkin's disease. *J Clin Oncol* 1998;16:3592–3600.

92. Kollmannsberger C, Beyer J, Droz JP, et al. Secondary leukemia following high cumulative doses of etoposide in patients treated for advanced germ cell tumors. *J Clin Oncol* 1998;16:3386–3391.

93. Kushner BH, Heller G, Cheung NK, et al. High risk of leukemia after short-term dose-intensive chemotherapy in young patients with solid tumors. *J Clin Oncol* 1998;16:3016–3020.

94. Loning L, Zimmermann M, Reiter A, et al. Secondary neoplasms subsequent to Berlin-Frankfurt-Munster therapy of acute lymphoblastic leukemia in childhood: significantly lower risk without cranial radiotherapy. *Blood* 2000;95:2770–2775.

95. Kolte B, Baer AN, Sait SN, et al. Acute myeloid leukemia in the setting of low dose weekly methotrexate therapy for rheumatoid arthritis. *Leuk Lymphoma* 2001;42:371–378.

96. McCarthy CJ, Sheldon S, Ross CW, et al. Cytogenetic abnormalities and therapy-related myelodysplastic syndromes in rheumatic disease. *Arthritis Rheum* 1998;41:1493–1496.

97. Orchard JA, Bolam S, Oscier DG. Association of myelodysplastic changes with purine analogues. *Br J Haematol* 1998;100: 677–679.

98. Pagano L, Annino L, Ferrari A, et al. Secondary haematological neoplasm after treatment of adult acute lymphoblastic leukemia: analysis of 1170 adult ALL patients enrolled in the GIMEMA trials. Gruppo Italiano Malattie Ematologiche Maligne dell'Adulto. *Br J Haematol* 1998;100:669–676.

99. Psiachou-Leonard E, Bain BJ. Persistent bone marrow failure with dysplastic features following pentostatin therapy for hairy cell leukaemia. *Clin Lab Haematol* 1998;20:195–197.

100. Rigolin GM, Cuneo A, Roberti MG, et al. Exposure to myelotoxic agents and myelodysplasia: case-control study and correlation with clinicobiological findings. *Br J Haematol* 1998; 103:189–197.

101. Schneider DT, Hilgenfeld E, Schwabe D, et al. Acute myelogenous leukemia after treatment for malignant germ cell tumors in children. *J Clin Oncol* 1999;17:3226–3233.

102. Seymour JF, Juneja SK, Campbell LJ, et al. Secondary acute myeloid leukemia with inv(16): report of two cases following paclitaxel-containing chemotherapy and review of the role of intensified ara-C therapy. *Leukemia* 1999;13:1735–1740.

103. Smith MA, Rubinstein L, Anderson JR, et al. Secondary leukemia or myelodysplastic syndrome after treatment with epipodophyllotoxins. *J Clin Oncol* 1999;17:569–577.

104. Turker A, Guler N. Therapy related acute myeloid leukemia after exposure to 5-fluorouracil: a case report. *Hematol Cell Ther* 1999;41:195–196.

105. Zompi S, Legrand O, Bouscary D, et al. Therapy related acute

myeloid leukaemia after successful therapy for acute promyelocytic leukaemia with t(15;17): a report of two cases and a review of the literature. *Br J Haematol* 2000;110:610–613.

106. Andersen MK, Johansson B, Larsen SO, et al. Chromosomal abnormalities in secondary MDS and AML. Relationship to drugs and radiation with specific emphasis on the balanced rearrangements. *Haematologica* 1998;83:483–488.

107. Dann EJ, Rowe JM. Biology and therapy of secondary leukaemias. *Best Pract Res Clin Haematol* 2001;14:119–137.

108. Olney HJ, Mitelman F, Johansson B, et al. Unique balanced chromosome abnormalities in treatment-related myelodysplastic syndromes and acute myeloid leukemia: report from an international workshop. *Genes Chromosomes Cancer* 2002;33:413–423.

109. Dissing M, Le Beau MM, Pedersen-Bjergaard J. Inversion of chromosome 16 and uncommon rearrangements of the CBFB and MYH11 genes in therapy-related acute myeloid leukemia: rare events related to DNA-topoisomerase II inhibitors? *J Clin Oncol* 1998;16:1890–1896.

110. Takeyama K, Seto M, Uike N, et al. Therapy-related leukemia and myelodysplastic syndrome: a large-scale Japanese study of clinical and cytogenetic features as well as prognostic factors. *Int J Hematol* 2000;71:144–152.

111. Andersen MK, Christiansen DH, Jensen BA, et al. Therapy-related acute lymphoblastic leukaemia with MLL rearrangements following DNA topoisomerase II inhibitors, an increasing problem: report on two new cases and review of the literature since 1992. *Br J Haematol* 2001;114:539–543.

112. Nasr F, Macintyre E, Venuat AM, et al. Translocation t(4;11)(q21;q23) and MLL gene rearrangement in acute lymphoblastic leukemia secondary to anti topoisomerase II anticancer agents. *Leuk Lymphoma* 1997;25:399–401.

113. Ohsaka A, Kato K, Hikiji K. Phenotypic conversion from t(8;21) acute myeloid leukemia to MLL gene rearrangement-positive acute lymphoblastic leukemia. *Hematopathol Mol Hematol* 1998;11:185–192.

114. Abe T. Infantile leukemia and soybeans—a hypothesis. *Leukemia* 1999;13:317–320.

115. Ishii E, Eguchi M, Eguchi-Ishimac M, et al. *In vitro* cleavage of the MLL gene by topoisomerase II inhibitor (etoposide) in normal cord and peripheral blood mononuclear cells. *Int J Hematol* 2002;76:74–79.

116. Severson RK, Ross JA. The causes of acute leukemia. *Curr Opin Oncol* 1999;11:20–24.

117. Strick R, Strissel PL, Borgers S, et al. Dietary bioflavonoids induce cleavage in the MLL gene and may contribute to infant leukemia. *Proc Natl Acad Sci U S A* 2000;97:4790–4795.

118. Cuneo A, Ferrant A, Michaux JL, et al. Cytogenetic and clinico-biological features of acute leukemia with stem cell phenotype: study of nine cases. *Cancer Genet Cytogenet* 1996;92:31–36.

119. Nagata T, Higashigawa M, Nagai M, et al. A child case of CD34+, CD33-, HLA-DR-, CD7+, CD56+ stem cell leukemia with thymic involvement. *Leuk Res* 1996;20:983–985.

120. Tien HF, Wang CH. CD7 positive hematopoietic progenitors and acute myeloid leukemia and other minimally differentiated leukemia. *Leuk Lymphoma* 1998;31:93–98.

121. Yoshida T, Kimura N, Sawada H, et al. CD56+CD7+ stem cell leukemia/lymphoma with D2-Jdelta1 rearrangement. *Intern Med* 1999;38:547–555.

122. Fleming DR, Doukas MA, Jennings DC, et al. Diagnostic and clinical implications of lineage fidelity in acute leukemia patients undergoing allogeneic stem cell transplantation. *Leuk Lymphoma* 2000;36:309–313.

123. Inoue T, Fujiyama Y, Kitamura S, et al. Trisomy 10 as the sole abnormality in biphenotypic leukemia. *Leuk Lymphoma* 2000;39:405–409.

124. Legrand O, Perrot JY, Simonin G, et al. Adult biphenotypic acute leukaemia: an entity with poor prognosis which is related to unfavourable cytogenetics and P-glycoprotein over-expression. *Br J Haematol* 1998;100:147–155.

125. Manabe A, Mori T, Ebihara Y, et al. Characterization of leukemic cells in CD2/CD19 double positive acute lymphoblastic leukemia. *Int J Hematol* 1998;67:45–52.

126. Uckun FM, Gaynon P, Sather H, et al. Clinical features and treatment outcome of children with biphenotypic CD2+ CD19+ acute lymphoblastic leukemia: a Children's Cancer Group study. *Blood* 1997;89:2488–2493.

127. Gloeckner-Hofmann K, Ottesen K, Schmidt S, et al. T-cell/natural killer cell lymphoblastic lymphoma with an unusual co-expression of B-cell antigens. *Ann Hematol* 2000;79:635–639.

128. Ino T, Tsuzuki M, Okamoto M, et al. Acute leukemia with the phenotype of a natural killer/T cell bipotential precursor. *Ann Hematol* 1999;78:43–47.

129. Paietta E, Neuberg D, Richards S, et al. Rare adult acute lymphocytic leukemia with CD56 expression in the ECOG experience shows unexpected phenotypic and genotypic heterogeneity. *Am J Hematol* 2001;66:189–196.

130. Ravandi F, Cortes J, Estrov Z, et al. CD56 expression predicts occurrence of CNS disease in acute lymphoblastic leukemia. *Leuk Res* 2002;26:643–649.

131. Handa H, Motohashi S, Isozumi K, et al. CD7+ and CD56+ myeloid/natural killer cell precursor acute leukemia treated with idarubicin and cytosine arabinoside. *Acta Haematol* 2002;108:47–52.

132. Inaba T, Shimazaki C, Sumikuma T, et al. Clinicopathological features of myeloid/natural killer (NK) cell precursor acute leukemia. *Leuk Res* 2001;25:109–113.

133. Kahl C, Pelz AF, Bartsch R, et al. Myeloid/natural killer cell precursor blast crisis of chronic myelogenous leukemia with two Philadelphia (Ph-1) chromosomes. *Ann Hematol* 2001;80:58–61.

134. Lee JJ, Kim HJ, Chung IJ, et al. Secondary myeloid/natural killer cell acute leukemia following T-cell lymphoma. *Leuk Lymphoma* 2001;41:457–460.

135. Lee PS, Lin CN, Liu C, et al. Acute leukemia with myeloid, B-, and natural killer cell differentiation. *Arch Pathol Lab Med* 2003;127:E93–E95.

136. Matsuo Y, Drexler HG, Kaneda K, et al. Megakaryoblastic leukemia cell line MOLM-16 derived from minimally differentiated acute leukemia with myeloid/NK precursor phenotype. *Leuk Res* 2003;27:165–171.

137. Nagai M, Bandoh S, Tasaka T, et al. Secondary myeloid/natural killer cell precursor acute leukemia following essential thrombocythemia. *Hum Pathol* 1999;30:868–871.

138. Suzuki R, Nakamura S. Malignancies of natural killer (NK) cell precursor: myeloid/NK cell precursor acute leukemia and blastic NK cell lymphoma/leukemia. *Leuk Res* 1999;23:615–624.

139. Suzuki R, Yamamoto K, Seto M, et al. CD7+ and CD56+ myeloid/natural killer cell precursor acute leukemia: a distinct hematolymphoid disease entity. *Blood* 1997;90:2417–2428.

140. Tezuka K, Nakayama H, Honda K, et al. Treatment of a child with myeloid/NK cell precursor acute leukemia with L-asparaginase and unrelated cord blood transplantation. *Int J Hematol* 2002;75:201–206.

141. Nakase K, Kita K, Miwa H, et al. Expression pattern of hybrid phenotype in adult acute lymphoblastic leukemia. *Cancer Detect Prev* 2001;25:394–405.

142. Bellido M, Martino R, Aventin A, et al. Leukemic relapse as T-acute lymphoblastic leukemia in a patient with acute myeloid leukemia and a minor T-cell clone at diagnosis. *Haematologica* 2000;85:1083–1086.

143. Lounici A, Cony-Makhoul P, Dubus P, et al. Lineage switch from acute myeloid leukemia to acute lymphoblastic leukemia: report of an adult case and review of the literature. *Am J Hematol* 2000;65:319–321.

144. Ysebaert L, Carli PM, Casasnovas RO, et al. Minimally differentiated acute myeloid leukemia (AML-MO) with lymphoid presentation at relapse: a case report. *Leukemia* 2001;15:1673–1674.

145. Bouabdallah R, Abena P, Chetaille B, et al. True histiocytic lymphoma following B-acute lymphoblastic leukaemia: case report with evidence for a common clonal origin in both neoplasms. *Br J Haematol* 2001;113:1047–1050.

146. Dunphy CH, Gardner LJ, Evans HL, et al. CD15(+) acute lymphoblastic leukemia and subsequent monoblastic leukemia: persistence of t(4;11) abnormality and B-cell gene rearrangement. *Arch Pathol Lab Med* 2001;125:1227–1230.

147. Fujisaki H, Hara J, Takai K, et al. Lineage switch in childhood leukemia with monosomy 7 and reverse of lineage switch in severe combined immunodeficient mice. *Exp Hematol* 1999;27:826–833.

148. Hashimoto S, Toba K, Aoki S, et al. Acute T-lymphoblastic leukemia relapsed with the character of myeloid/natural killer cell precursor phenotype: a case report. *Leuk Res* 2002;26:215–219.

149. Kawakami K, Miyanishi S, Amakawa R, et al. A case of T-lineage lymphoblastic lymphoma/leukemia with t(4;11)(q21;p15) that switched to myelomonocytic leukemia at relapse. *Int J Hematol* 1999;69:196–199.

150. Tsuboi K, Yazaki M, Miwa H, et al. Lineage conversion from acute lymphoblastic leukemia to acute myeloid leukemia on re-arrangement of the IgH gene in a patient with Down syndrome. *Int J Hematol* 2002;76:69–73.

151. Bierings M, Szczepanski T, van Wering ER, et al. Two consecutive immunophenotypic switches in a child with immunogenotypically stable acute leukaemia. *Br J Haematol* 2001;113:757–762.

Genotypic Subtypes

1. Bernstein J, Dastugue N, Haas OA, et al. Nineteen cases of the t(1;22)(p13;q13) acute megakaryblastic leukaemia of infants/children and a review of 39 cases: report from a t(1;22) study group. *Leukemia* 2000;14:216–218.

2. Dickstein JI, Davis EM, Roulston D. Localization of the chromosome 22 breakpoints in two cases of acute megakaryoblastic leukemia with t(1;22)(p13;q13). *Cancer Genet Cytogenet* 2001;129:150–154.

3. Ma Z, Morris SW, Valentine V, et al. Fusion of two novel genes, RBM15 and MKL1, in the t(1;22)(p13;q13) of acute megakaryoblastic leukemia. *Nat Genet* 2001;28:220–221.

4. Mercher T, Busson-Le Coniat M, Khac FN, et al. Recurrence of OTT-MAL fusion in t(1;22) of infant AML-M7. *Genes Chromosomes Cancer* 2002;33:22–28.

5. Ng KC, Tan AM, Chong YY, et al. Congenital acute megakaryoblastic leukemia (M7) with chromosomal t(1;22)(p13;q13) translocation in a set of identical twins. *J Pediatr Hematol Oncol* 1999;21:428–430.

6. Rieder H, Kolbus U, Koop U, et al. Translocation t(1;22) mimicking t(1;19) in a child with acute lymphoblastic leukemia as revealed by chromosome painting. *Leukemia* 1993;7:1663–1666.

7. Wong KF, So CC, Lau G. Precursor T-lymphoblastic leukemia with a novel t(1;22)(p34;q13). *Cancer Genet Cytogenet* 2002;136:146–148.

8. Chang VT, Aviv H, Howard LM, et al. Acute myelogenous leukemia associated with extreme symptomatic thrombocytosis and chromosome 3q translocation: case report and review of literature. *Am J Hematol* 2003;72:20–26.

9. Johansson B, Fioretos T, Mitelman F. Cytogenetic and molecular genetic evolution of chronic myeloid leukemia. *Acta Haematol* 2002;107:76–94.

10. Lindquist R, Forsblom AM, Ost A, et al. Mutagen exposures and chromosome 3 aberrations in acute myelocytic leukemia. *Leukemia* 2000;14:112–118.

11. Testoni N, Borsaru G, Martinelli G, et al. 3q21 and 3q26 cytogenetic abnormalities in acute myeloblastic leukemia: biological and clinical features. *Haematologica* 1999;84:690–694.

12. Adachi Y, Pavlakis GN, Copeland TD. Identification and characterization of SET, a nuclear phosphoprotein encoded by the translocation break point in acute undifferentiated leukemia. *J Biol Chem* 1994;269:2258–2262.

13. Alsabeh R, Brynes RK, Slovak ML, et al. Acute myeloid leukemia with t(6;9) (p23;q34): association with myelodysplasia, basophilia, and initial CD34 negative immunophenotype. *Am J Clin Pathol* 1997;107:430–437.

14. Fornerod M, Boer J, van Baal S, et al. Interaction of cellular proteins with the leukemia specific fusion proteins DEK-CAN and SET-CAN and their normal counterpart, the nucleoporin CAN. *Oncogene* 1996;13:1801–1808.

15. Makita M, Azuma T, Hamaguchi H, et al. Leukemia-associated fusion proteins, dek-can and bcr-abl, represent immunogenic HLA-DR-restricted epitopes recognized by fusion peptide-specific CD4+ T lymphocytes. *Leukemia* 2002;16:2400–2407.

16. Soekarman D, von Lindern M, Daenen S, et al. The translocation (6;9) (p23;q34) shows consistent rearrangement of two genes and defines a myeloproliferative disorder with specific clinical features. *Blood* 1992;79:2990–2997.

17. von Lindern M, Breems D, van Baal S, et al. Characterization of the translocation breakpoint sequences of two DEK-CAN fusion genes present in t(6;9) acute myeloid leukemia and a SET-CAN fusion gene found in a case of acute undifferentiated leukemia. *Genes Chromosomes Cancer* 1992;5:227–234.

18. Kitabayashi I, Aikawa Y, Yokoyama A, et al. Fusion of MOZ and p300 histone acetyltransferases in acute monocytic leukemia with a t(8;22)(p11;q13) chromosome translocation. *Leukemia* 2001;15:89–94.

19. Panagopoulos I, Isaksson M, Lindvall C, et al. Genomic characterization of MOZ/CBP and CBP/MOZ chimeras in acute myeloid leukemia suggests the involvement of a damage-repair mechanism in the origin of the t(8;16)(p11;p13). *Genes Chromosomes Cancer* 2003;36:90–98.

20. Sun T, Wu E. Acute monoblastic leukemia with t(8;16): a distinct clinicopathologic entity; report of a case and review of the literature. *Am J Hematol* 2001;66:207–212.

21. Andrieu V, Radford-Weiss I, Troussard X, et al. Molecular detection of t(8;21)/AML1-ETO in AML M1/M2: correlation with cytogenetics, morphology and immunophenotype. *Br J Haematol* 1996;92:855–865.

22. Haferlach T, Bennett JM, Loffler H, et al. Acute myeloid leukemia with translocation (8;21). Cytomorphology, dysplasia and prognostic factors in 41 cases. AML Cooperative Group and ECOG. *Leuk Lymphoma* 1996;23:227–234.

23. Khalidi HS, Medeiros LJ, Chang KL, et al. The immunophenotype of adult acute myeloid leukemia: high frequency of lymphoid antigen expression and comparison of immunophenotype, French-American-British classification, and karyotypic abnormalities. *Am J Clin Pathol* 1998;109:211–220.

24. Ma SK, Au WY, Kwong YL, et al. Hematological features and treatment outcome in acute myeloid leukemia with t(8;21). *Hematol Oncol* 1997;15:93–103.

25. Schwyzer R, Sherman GG, Cohn RJ, et al. Granulocytic sarcoma in children with acute myeloblastic leukemia and t(8;21). *Med Pediatr Oncol* 1998;31:144–149.

26. Molero MT, Gomez Casares MT, Valencia JM, et al. Detection of

a t(8;21)(q22;q22) in a case of M5 acute monoblastic leukemia. *Cancer Genet Cytogenet* 1998;100:176–178.

27. Ferrara F, Di Noto R, Annunziata M, et al. Immunophenotypic analysis enables the correct prediction of t(8;21) in acute myeloid leukaemia. *Br J Haematol* 1998;102:444–448.

28. Nakamura H, Kuriyama K, Sadamori N, et al. Morphological subtyping of acute myeloid leukemia with maturation (AML-M2): homogeneous pink-colored cytoplasm of mature neutrophils is most characteristic of AML-M2 with t(8;21). *Leukemia* 1997;11:651–655.

29. Bernheim A, Duverger A, Fouquet F, et al. FISH diagnosis of t(8;21) in a myelodysplasia secondary to Hodgkin lymphoma. *Leukemia* 1995;9:107–108.

30. Kojima K, Omoto E, Hara M, et al. Myelodysplastic syndrome with translocation (8;21): a distinct myelodysplastic syndrome entity or M2-acute myeloid leukemia with extensive myeloid maturation? *Ann Hematol* 1998;76:279–282.

31. Taj AS, Ross FM, Vickers M, et al. t(8;21) myelodysplasia, an early presentation of M2 AML. *Br J Haematol* 1995;89:890–892.

32. Arber DA, Glackin C, Lowe G, et al. Presence of t(8;21)(q22;q22) in myeloperoxidase-positive, myeloid surface antigen-negative acute myeloid leukemia. *Am J Clin Pathol* 1997;107:68–73.

33. Garcia Vela JA, Martin M, Delgado I, et al. Acute myeloid leukemia M2 and t(8;21)(q22;q22) with an unusual phenotype: myeloperoxidase(+), CD13(−), CD14(−), and CD33(−). *Ann Hematol* 1999;78:237–240.

34. Hirai K, Torimoto Y, Moriichi K, et al. Discordant expression of myeloid antigens and myeloperoxidase in a case of t(8;21) positive AML expressing CD7. *Int J Hematol* 1999;70:30–35.

35. Berger R, Le Coniat M, Romana SP, et al. Secondary acute myeloblastic leukemia with t(16;21) (q24;q22) involving the AML1 gene. *Hematol Cell Ther* 1996;38:183–186.

36. Gamou T, Kitamura E, Hosoda F, et al. The partner gene of AML1 in t(16;21) myeloid malignancies is a novel member of the MTG8(ETO) family. *Blood* 1998;91:4028–4037.

37. Harrison CJ, Radford-Weiss I, Ross F, et al. Fluorescence *in situ* hybridization analysis of masked (8;21)(q22;q22) translocations. *Cancer Genet Cytogenet* 1999;112:15–20.

38. Mitterbauer M, Kusec R, Schwarzinger I, et al. Comparison of karyotype analysis and RT-PCR for AML1/ETO in 204 unselected patients with AML. *Ann Hematol* 1998;76:139–143.

39. Taviaux S, Brunel V, Dupont M, et al. Simple variant t(8;21) acute myeloid leukemias harbor insertions of the AML1 or ETO genes. *Genes Chromosomes Cancer* 1999;24:165–171.

40. Chen Z, Morgan R, Notohamiprodjo M, et al. The Philadelphia chromosome as a secondary change in leukemia: three case reports and an overview of the literature. *Cancer Genet Cytogenet* 1998;101:148–151.

41. Cuneo A, Ferrant A, Michaux JL, et al. Philadelphia chromosome-positive acute myeloid leukemia: cytoimmunologic and cytogenetic features. *Haematologica* 1996;81:423–427.

42. Lim LC, Heng KK, Vellupillai M, et al. Molecular and phenotypic spectrum of de novo Philadelphia positive acute leukemia. *Int J Mol Med* 1999;4:665–667.

43. Paietta E, Racevskis J, Bennett JM, et al. Biologic heterogeneity in Philadelphia chromosome-positive acute leukemia with myeloid morphology: the Eastern Cooperative Oncology Group experience. *Leukemia* 1998;12:1881–1885.

44. Haskovec C, Ponzetto C, Polak J, et al. P230 BCR/ABL protein may be associated with an acute leukaemia phenotype. *Br J Haematol* 1998;103:1104–1108.

45. Veelken H, Licht T, Lais A, et al. Drug resistance of secondary acute myeloid leukemia with megakaryoblastic features and p190 BCR-ABL rearrangement. *Leuk Res* 1998;22:1021–1027.

46. Yamashita S, Umemura T, Sadamura S, et al. Acute leukemias expressing p210- and p190-type bcr/abl mRNAs: report of two cases and review of the literature. *Acta Haematol* 1996;96:99–104.

47. Baer MR, Stewart CC, Lawrence D, et al. Acute myeloid leukemia with 11q23 translocations: myelomonocytic immunophenotype by multiparameter flow cytometry. *Leukemia* 1998;12:317–325.

48. Chessells JM, Harrison CJ, Kempski H, et al. Clinical features, cytogenetics and outcome in acute lymphoblastic and myeloid leukaemia of infancy: report from the MRC Childhood Leukaemia working party. *Leukemia* 2002;16:776–784.

49. Harbott J, Mancini M, Verellen-Dumoulin C, et al. Hematological malignancies with a deletion of 11q23: cytogenetic and clinical aspects. European 11q23 Workshop participants. *Leukemia* 1998;12:823–827.

50. Hilden JM, Smith FO, Frestedt JL, et al. MLL gene rearrangement, cytogenetic 11q23 abnormalities, and expression of the NG2 molecule in infant acute myeloid leukemia. *Blood* 1997;89:3801–3805.

51. Ibrahim S, Estey EH, Pierce S, et al. 11q23 abnormalities in patients with acute myelogenous leukemia and myelodysplastic syndrome as detected by molecular and cytogenetic analyses. *Am J Clin Pathol* 2000;114:793–797.

52. Mrozek K, Heinonen K, Lawrence D, et al. Adult patients with de novo acute myeloid leukemia and t(9;11)(p22;q23) have a superior outcome to patients with other translocations involving band 11q23: a cancer and leukemia group B study. *Blood* 1997;90:4532–4538.

53. Poirel H, Rack K, Delabesse E, et al. Incidence and characterization of MLL gene (11q23) rearrangements in acute myeloid leukemia M1 and M5. *Blood* 1996;87:2496–2505.

54. Satake N, Maseki N, Nishiyama M, et al. Chromosome abnormalities and MLL rearrangements in acute myeloid leukemia of infants. *Leukemia* 1999;13:1013–1017.

55. Secker-Walker LM. General Report on the European Union Concerted Action Workshop on 11q23, London, UK, May 1997. *Leukemia* 1998;2:776–778.

56. Tien HF, Hsiao CH, Tang JL, et al. Characterization of acute myeloid leukemia with MLL rearrangements—no increase in the incidence of coexpression of lymphoid-associated antigens on leukemic blasts. *Leukemia* 2000;14:1025–1030.

57. Allford S, Grimwade D, Langabeer S, et al. Identification of the t(15;17) in AML FAB types other than M3: evaluation of the role of molecular screening for the PML/RARalpha rearrangement in newly diagnosed AML. The Medical Research Council (MRC) Adult Leukaemia Working Party. *Br J Haematol* 1999;105:198–207.

58. Morgan DL, Dunn DM, Cobos E, et al. Translocation t(15;17) in acute myelogenous leukemia with atypical megakaryoblastic features: diagnostic, clinical, and therapeutic implications. *Cancer Genet Cytogenet* 1996;92:50–53.

59. Neame PB, Soamboonsrup P, Leber B, et al. Morphology of acute promyelocytic leukemia with cytogenetic or molecular evidence for the diagnosis: characterization of additional microgranular variants. *Am J Hematol* 1997;56:131–142.

60. Varella-Garcia M, Brizard F, Roche J, et al. Aml1/ETO and Pml/RARA rearrangements in a case of AML-M2 acute myeloblastic leukemia with t(15;17). *Leuk Lymphoma* 1999;33:403–406.

61. Yu RQ, Huang W, Chen SJ, et al. A case of acute eosinophilic granulocytic leukemia with PML-RAR alpha fusion gene expression and response to all-trans retinoic acid. *Leukemia* 1997;11:609–611.

62. Exner M, Thalhammer R, Kapiotis S, et al. The "typical" immunophenotype of acute promyelocytic leukemia (APL-M3):

does it prove true for the M3-variant? *Cytometry* 2000;42: 106–109.

63. Foley R, Soamboonsrup P, Carter RF, et al. CD34-positive acute promyelocytic leukemia is associated with leukocytosis, micro-granular/hypogranular morphology, expression of CD2 and bcr3 isoform. *Am J Hematol* 2001;67:34–41.

64. Guglielmi C, Martelli MP, Diverio D, et al. Immunophenotype of adult and childhood acute promyelocytic leukaemia: correlation with morphology, type of PML gene breakpoint and clinical outcome. A cooperative Italian study on 196 cases. *Br J Haematol* 1998;102:1035–1041.

65. Stasi R, Bruno A, Venditti A, et al. A microgranular variant of acute promyelocytic leukemia with atypical morpho-cytochemical features and an early myeloid immunophenotype. *Leuk Res* 1997;21:575–580.

66. Grimwade D, Gorman P, Duprez E, et al. Characterization of cryptic rearrangements and variant translocations in acute promyelocytic leukemia. *Blood* 1997;90:4876–4885.

67. Jansen JH, de Ridder MC, Geertsma WM, et al. Complete remission of t(11;17) positive acute promyelocytic leukemia induced by all-trans retinoic acid and granulocyte colony-stimulating factor. *Blood* 1999;94:39–45.

68. Wan TS, Chim CS, So CK, et al. Complex variant 15;17 translocations in acute promyelocytic leukemia. A case report and review of three-way translocations. *Cancer Genet Cytogenet* 1999; 111:139–143.

69. Yamamoto K, Hamaguchi H, Kobayashi M, et al. Terminal deletion of the long arm of chromosome 9 in acute promyelocytic leukemia with a cryptic PML/RAR alpha rearrangement. *Cancer Genet Cytogenet* 1999;113:120–125.

70. Yamamoto K, Hamaguchi H, Nagata K, et al. A new complex translocation (15;20;17)(q22;p13;q21) in acute promyelocytic leukemia. *Cancer Genet Cytogenet* 1998;101:89–94.

71. Lim LC, Vellupillai M, Ghafar AA. Clinico-biological features of 30 patients with acute promyelocytic leukemia and response to combination induction chemotherapy with all-trans retinoic acid and anthracycline. *Med Oncol* 2000;17:301–306.

72. Asou N, Osato M, Okubo T, et al. Acute myelomonoblastic leukemia carrying the PEBP2beta/MYH11 fusion gene. *Leuk Lymphoma* 1998;31:81–91.

73. Costello R, Sainty D, Lecine P, et al. Detection of CBFbeta/MYH11 fusion transcripts in acute myeloid leukemia: heterogeneity of cytological and molecular characteristics. *Leukemia* 1997;11:644–650.

74. Marlton P, Keating M, Kantarjian H, et al. Cytogenetic and clinical correlates in AML patients with abnormalities of chromosome 16. *Leukemia* 1995;9:965–971.

75. Mitterbauer M, Laczika K, Novak M, et al. High concordance of karyotype analysis and RT-PCR for CBF beta/MYH11 in unselected patients with acute myeloid leukemia. A single center study. *Am J Clin Pathol* 2000;113:406–410.

76. Monahan BP, Rector JT, Liu PP, et al. Clinical aspects of expression of inversion 16 chromosomal fusion transcript CBFB/MYH11 in acute myelogenous leukemia subtype M1 with abnormal bone marrow eosinophilia. *Leukemia* 1996;10: 1653–1654.

77. Tobal K, Johnson PR, Saunders MJ, et al. Detection of CBFB/MYH11 transcripts in patients with inversion and other abnormalities of chromosome 16 at presentation and remission. *Br J Haematol* 1995;91:104–108.

78. Inaba T, Shimazaki C, Inaba E, et al. Inversion of chromosome 16 and eosinophilia in refractory anemia with ring sideroblasts: report of a case. *Am J Hematol* 1993;44:134–138.

79. Miyamoto T, Akashi K, Hayashi S, et al. Pericentric inversion of chromosome 16 and eosinophilia in chronic myelomonocytic leukemia. *Cancer Genet Cytogenet* 1997;94:99–102.

80. Dierlamm J, Stul M, Vranckx H, et al. FISH identifies inv(16)(p13q22) masked by translocations in three cases of acute myeloid leukemia. *Genes Chromosomes Cancer* 1998;22:87–94.

81. Maarek O, Salabelle A, Le Coniat MB, et al. Chromosome 16 inversion-associated translocation: two new cases. *Cancer Genet Cytogenet* 1999;114:126–129.

82. Martinez-Climent JA, Comes AM, Vizcarra E, et al. Variant three-way translocation of inversion 16 in AML-M4Eo confirmed by fluorescence in situ hybridization analysis. *Cancer Genet Cytogenet* 1999;110:111–114.

83. O'Reilly J, Chipper L, Springall F, et al. A unique structural abnormality of chromosome 16 resulting in a CBF beta-MYH11 fusion transcript in a patient with acute myeloid leukemia, FAB M4. *Cancer Genet Cytogenet* 2000;121:52–55.

84. Pirc-Danoewinata H, Dauwerse HG, Konig M, et al. CBFB/MYH11 fusion in a patient with AML-M4Eo and cytogenetically normal chromosomes 16. *Genes Chromosomes Cancer* 2000;29:186–191.

85. Reddy KS, Wang S, Montgomery P, et al. Fluorescence in situ hybridization identifies inversion 16 masked by t(10;16)(q24;q22), t(7;16)(q21;q22), and t(2;16)(q37;q22) in three cases of AML-M4Eo. *Cancer Genet Cytogenet* 2000;116:148–152.

86. Ritter M, Thiede C, Schakel U, et al. Underestimation of inversion (16) in acute myeloid leukaemia using standard cytogenetics as compared with polymerase chain reaction: results of a prospective investigation. *Br J Haematol* 1997;98:969–972.

87. Viswanatha DS, Chen I, Liu PP, et al. Characterization and use of an antibody detecting the CBFbeta-SMMHC fusion protein in inv(16)/t(16;16)-associated acute myeloid leukemias. *Blood* 1998;91:1882–1890.

88. Wong KF, Kwong YL. Trisomy 22 in acute myeloid leukemia: a marker for myeloid leukemia with monocytic features and cytogenetically cryptic inversion 16. *Cancer Genet Cytogenet* 1999;109:131–133.

89. Sotomatsu M, Ogawa C, Shimoda M, et al. Molecular analysis of minimally differentiated acute myeloid leukemia with chromosome 16 inversion. *Leuk Lymphoma* 1997;24:319–325.

90. Imashuku S, Hibi S, Sako M, et al. Hemophagocytosis by leukemic blasts in 7 acute myeloid leukemia cases with t(16;21)(p11;q22): common morphologic characteristics for this type of leukemia. *Cancer* 2000;88:1970–1975.

91. Kong XT, Ida K, Ichikawa H, et al. Consistent detection of TLS/FUS-ERG chimeric transcripts in acute myeloid leukemia with t(16;21)(p11;q22) and identification of a novel transcript. *Blood* 1997;90:1192–1199.

92. Sharma P, Watson N, Robson L, et al. Novel chromosome 16 abnormality—der(16)del(16)(q13)t(16;21)(p11.2;q22)—associated with acute myeloid leukemia. *Cancer Genet Cytogenet* 1999;113:25–28.

93. Shikami M, Miwa H, Nishii K, et al. Myeloid differentiation antigen and cytokine receptor expression on acute myelocytic leukaemia cells with t(16;21)(p11;q22): frequent expression of CD56 and interleukin-2 receptor alpha chain. *Br J Haematol* 1999;105:711–719.

94. Sadamori N, Yao E, Tagawa M, et al. 16;21 translocation in acute nonlymphocytic leukemia with abnormal eosinophils: a unique subtype. *Acta Haematol* 1990;84:212–216.

95. McClure RF, Dewald GW, Hoyer JD, et al. Isolated isochromosome 17q: a distinct type of mixed myeloproliferative disorder/myelodysplastic syndrome with an aggressive clinical course. *Br J Haematol* 1999;106:445–454.

96. Merlat A, Lai JL, Sterkers Y, et al. Therapy-related myelodysplastic syndrome and acute myeloid leukemia with 17p deletion. A report on 25 cases. *Leukemia* 1999;13:250–257.

97. Soenen V, Preudhomme C, Roumier C, et al. 17p deletion in acute myeloid leukemia and myelodysplastic syndrome. Analysis

of breakpoints and deleted segments by fluorescence *in situ. Blood* 1998;91:1008–1015.

98. Watson N, Dunlop L, Robson L, et al. 17p- syndrome arising from a novel dicentric translocation in a patient with acute myeloid leukemia. *Cancer Genet Cytogenet* 2000;118:159–162.

99. Baschat AA, Wagner T, Malisius R, et al. Prenatal diagnosis of a transient myeloproliferative disorder in trisomy 21. *Prenat Diagn* 1998;18:731–736.

100. Bozner P. Transient myeloproliferative disorder with erythroid differentiation in Down syndrome. *Arch Pathol Lab Med* 2002;126:474–477.

101. Girodon F, Favre B, Couillaud G, et al. Immunophenotype of a transient myeloproliferative disorder in a newborn with trisomy 21. *Cytometry* 2000;42:118–122.

102. Hartung J, Chaoui R, Wauer R, et al. Fetal hepatosplenomegaly: an isolated sonographic sign of trisomy 21 in a case of myeloproliferative disorder. *Ultrasound Obstet Gynecol* 1998;11:453–455.

103. Holt SE, Brown EJ, Zipursky A. Telomerase and the benign and malignant megakaryoblastic leukemias of Down syndrome. *J Pediatr Hematol Oncol* 2002;24:14–17.

104. Karandikar NJ, Aquino DB, McKenna RW, et al. Transient myeloproliferative disorder and acute myeloid leukemia in Down syndrome. An immunophenotypic analysis. *Am J Clin Pathol* 2001;116:204–210.

105. Kempski HM, Craze JL, Chessels JM, et al. Cryptic deletions and inversions of chromosome 21 in a phenotypically normal infant with transient abnormal myelopoiesis: a molecular cytogenetic study. *Br J Haematol* 1998;103:473–479.

106. Kusanagi Y, Ochi H, Matsubara K, et al. Hypereosinophilic syndrome in a trisomy 21 fetus. *Obstet Gynecol* 1998;92:701–702.

107. Lange BJ, Kobrinsky N, Barnard DR, et al. Distinctive demography, biology, and outcome of acute myeloid leukemia and myelodysplastic syndrome in children with Down syndrome: Children's Cancer Group Studies 2861 and 2891. *Blood* 1998;91: 608–615.

108. Liang DC, Ma SW, Lu TH, et al. Transient myeloproliferative disorder and acute myeloid leukemia: study of six neonatal cases with long-term follow-up. *Leukemia* 1993;7:1521–1524.

109. Ohnishi H, Taki T, Tabuchi K, et al. Down's syndrome with myelodysplastic syndrome showing t(7;11)(p13;p14). *Am J Hematol* 2000;65:62–65.

110. Ohta T, Nakano M, Tsujita T, et al. Isolation of a cosmid clone corresponding to an inv(21) breakpoint of a patient with transient abnormal myelopoiesis. *Am J Hum Genet* 1996;58: 544–550.

111. Ridgway D, Benda GI, Magenis E, et al. Transient myeloproliferative disorder of the Down type in the normal newborn. *Am J Dis Child* 1990;144:1117–1119.

112. Schwab M, Niemeyer C, Schwarzer U. Down syndrome, transient myeloproliferative disorder, and infantile liver fibrosis. *Med Pediatr Oncol* 1998;31:159–165.

113. Zipursky A, Brown EJ, Christensen H, et al. Transient myeloproliferative disorder (transient leukemia) and hematologic manifestations of Down syndrome. *Clin Lab Med* 1999;19: 157–167.

114. Zubizarreta P, Felice MS, Alfaro E, et al. Acute myelogenous leukemia in Down's syndrome: report of a single pediatric institution using a BFM treatment strategy. *Leuk Res* 1998;22: 465–472.

115. Cavani S, Perfumo C, Argusti A, et al. Cytogenetic and molecular study of 32 Down syndrome families: potential leukaemia predisposing role of the most proximal segment of chromosome 21q. *Br J Haematol* 1998;103:213–216.

116. Kempski HM, Chessells JM, Reeves BR. Deletions of chromosome 21 restricted to the leukemic cells of children with Down syndrome and leukemia. *Leukemia* 1997;11:1973–1977.

117. Sato A, Imaizumi M, Koizumi Y, et al. Acute myelogenous leukaemia with t(8;21) translocation of normal cell origin in mosaic Down's syndrome with isochromosome 21q. *Br J Haematol* 1997;96:614–616.

118. Duflos-Delaplace D, Lai JL, Nelken B, et al. Transient leukemoid disorder in a newborn with Down syndrome followed 19 months later by an acute myeloid leukemia: demonstration of the same structural change in both instances with clonal evolution. *Cancer Genet Cytogenet* 1999;113:166–171.

119. Granzen B, Bernhard B, Reinisch I, et al. Transient myeloproliferative disorder with 11q23 aberration in two neonates with Down syndrome. *Ann Hematol* 1998;77:51–54.

120. Kounami S, Aoyagi N, Tsuno H, et al. Additional chromosome abnormalities in transient abnormal myelopoiesis in Down's syndrome patients. *Acta Haematol* 1997;98:109–112.

121. Kounami S, Aoyagi N, Tsuno H, et al. Myelodysplastic syndrome after regression of transient abnormal myelopoiesis in a Down syndrome infant: different clonal origin? *Cancer Genet Cytogenet* 1998;104:115–118.

122. Malkin D, Brown EJ, Zipursky A. The role of p53 in megakaryocyte differentiation and the megakaryocytic leukemias of Down syndrome. *Cancer Genet Cytogenet* 2000;116:1–5.

123. Paulien S, Busson-Le Coniat M, Berger R. Acute megakaryocytic leukaemia with acquired polysomy 21 and translocation t(1;21). *Ann Genet* 2000;43:99–104.

124. Worth LL, Zipursky A, Christensen H, et al. Transient leukemia with extreme basophilia in a phenotypically normal infant with blast cells containing a pseudodiploid clone, 46,XY i(21)(q10). *J Pediatr Hematol Oncol* 1999;21:63–66.

20

ACUTE LYMPHOID LEUKEMIA

GENERAL FEATURES

Classification

Acute lymphoid (lymphocytic, lymphoblastic) leukemia (ALL) is classified primarily according to immunophenotypic and genetic characteristics. The most recent classification of ALL is that adopted by the World Health Organization, which groups ALL with solid tumors of lymphoblasts or lymphoblastic lymphoma (Table 20-1) (1). This classification is based primarily on immunophenotype. The earlier French-American-British (FAB) classification is based primarily on morphologic characteristics and is no longer used extensively, although the blast descriptions are still very useful in recognizing the spectrum of neoplastic lymphoblasts (2,3). The classification in this chapter is based primarily on immunophenotypic and genetic characteristics (Table 20-2).

ALL is currently diagnosed at a peripheral blood or bone marrow blast percentage of at least 20%. This definition may be expected to change because methods of blast enumeration and quantitative criteria continue to evolve.

Clinical Course

ALL occurs predominantly in children 2 to 10 years old and then shows a small but steadily rising incidence with age (4). Patients present with evidence of marrow replacement, lymphadenopathy, hepatosplenomegaly, and/or coagulopathy. A distinctive subset of patients presents with prominent bone pain, skeletal lesions, low white blood cell count, and few circulating blasts; the prognosis in this type of ALL is relatively good (5,6). Another distinctive subset presents with an aplastic anemia-like prodrome, initiated by viral infection in some cases (7–12).

ALL has a generally downhill course, complicated by the sequelae of bone marrow failure. Combination chemother-

TABLE 20-1. CLASSIFICATION OF ACUTE LYMPHOID LEUKEMIA ACCORDING TO THE WORLD HEALTH ORGANIZATION

Precursor B lymphoblastic leukemia/lymphoma
Precursor T lymphoblastic leukemia/lymphoma

TABLE 20-2. ORGANIZATION OF ACUTE LYMPHOID LEUKEMIA IN THIS CHAPTER

Immunophenotypic subtypes
  Precursor B-cell ALL
  Mature B-cell ALL
  T-cell ALL
  Natural killer cell ALL

Genotypic subtypes
  ALL with hypodiploidy
  ALL with high hyperdiploidy
  ALL with t(1;19)(q23;p13) (PBX1/E2A)
  ALL with t(9;22)(q34;q11) (BCR/ABL)
  ALL with anomalies of chromosome 11q23 and/or MLL
  ALL with t(12;21)(p13;q22) (ETV6/AML1)
  ALL with t(14;18) (IgH/BCL2)
  ALL with constitutional trisomy 21

ALL, acute lymphoid leukemia.

apy induces remission in 80% to 90% of patients, but relapses occur in most adult patients (13). Stem cell transplantation offers the best chance for lasting remission in adults.

Spontaneous (or nearly spontaneous) remission has rarely been reported in ALL in association with severe infection, blood transfusion, and granulocyte colony-stimulating factor therapy (14–17).

Peripheral Blood

The peripheral blood usually shows anemia and thrombocytopenia. Red blood cell and platelet morphology is usually unremarkable. The white blood cell count and peripheral blast percentage are highly variable. In cases with prominent skeletal involvement, both may be very low. In cases of pancytopenia, the peripheral blood smear should be carefully searched for blasts. The peripheral blood may show other abnormalities, including eosinophilia, basophilia cyclic neutropenia, and thrombocytosis (18–24). ALL presenting with thrombocytosis should be distinguished from chronic myeloid leukemia presenting in lymphoid blast crisis (25).

Bone Marrow

Bone marrow aspirate smears show 20% or more (usually >70%) blasts. The myeloid:erythroid ratio is typically

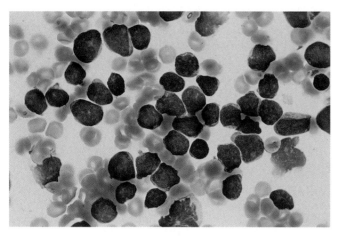

FIGURE 20-1. Bone marrow aspirate smear, acute lymphoblastic leukemia (FAB L1). This is the most common type of childhood acute lymphoid leukemia, with numerous small, lymphocyte-like blasts admixed with larger blasts. The chromatin is fine and smooth, and the cytoplasm is nearly imperceptible.

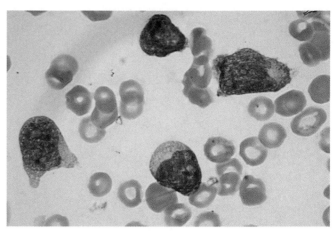

FIGURE 20-3. Bone marrow aspirate, acute lymphoblastic leukemia (FAB L2). In this specimen, the blasts are large and show coarse chromatin. This morphology may suggest an erroneous diagnosis of B-cell or T-cell malignant lymphoma.

unevaluable because of the preponderance of blasts. Normal hematopoietic cells often persist but do not show myelodysplastic changes. Histologic sections show hypercellularity for site and age. Some cases present with hypocellularity and an aplastic anemia-like prodrome.

Other bone marrow findings in ALL include necrosis, fibrosis, and pseudo-Gaucher cells (26–28). Persistence of blasts in the bone marrow after initiation of chemotherapy is a poor prognostic sign (29–31). Langerhans cell histiocytosis has been reported to follow remission of ALL (32,33).

Blast Morphology

Blast morphology is variable in ALL, a fact reflected in the FAB classification of ALL (2,3) (Figs. 20-1 through 20-6).

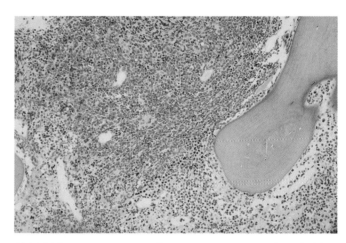

FIGURE 20-4. Bone marrow biopsy specimen, acute lymphoblastic leukemia. The bone marrow is replaced by a diffuse infiltrate of small blasts.

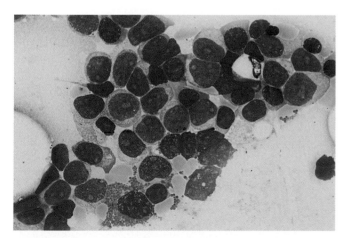

FIGURE 20-2. Bone marrow aspirate smear, acute lymphoblastic leukemia (FAB L2). This type of acute lymphoid leukemia is characterized by large blasts with variable chromatin, prominent nucleoli, and scant to moderate amounts of agranular cytoplasm.

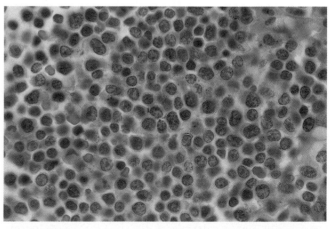

FIGURE 20-5. Bone marrow biopsy specimen, acute lymphoblastic leukemia (FAB L1). The infiltrate is composed of small, monotonous blasts without distinguishing characteristics.

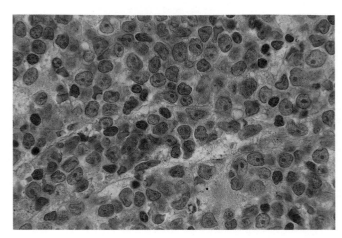

FIGURE 20-6. Bone marrow biopsy specimen, acute lymphoblastic leukemia (FAB L2). The infiltrate is composed of larger blasts with prominent nucleoli.

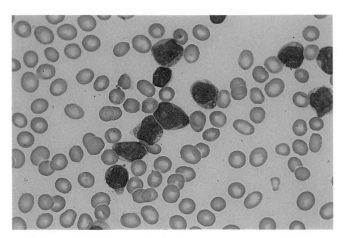

FIGURE 20-7. Bone marrow aspirate, granular acute lymphoblastic leukemia (FAB L2). The blast cytoplasm contains irregular reddish granules.

The most common blast type predominates in childhood ALL (FAB L1). These small to moderate-sized blasts are relatively monomorphous. The nucleus is generally round, with moderately condensed to dispersed chromatin, inconspicuous or absent nucleoli, and scant agranular cytoplasm. These blasts may be difficult to differentiate from normal lymphocytes and chronic lymphocytic leukemia.

The next most common blast type is seen in most cases of adult ALL (FAB L2). The blasts are larger and more heterogeneous than those in FAB L1. The nucleus is larger and more irregular, with moderately dispersed chromatin, one or more nucleoli, and scant to moderately abundant agranular cytoplasm. The prognosis may be less favorable than the usual type of ALL (34). The differential diagnosis includes acute myeloid leukemia (AML) with minimal differentiation (FAB M0), which is morphologically indistinguishable from this type of ALL.

Rarely, blasts show Burkitt-type morphology (FAB L3). The blasts are round, with deeply basophilic cytoplasm containing numerous vacuoles. Such cases may present with features of leukemia and/or lymphoma (see Chapter 24, Burkitt lymphoma/leukemia).

Other morphologic variants have been described. Granular ALL is characterized by blasts containing reddish cytoplasmic granules or inclusions (Fig. 20-7). These are lysosomes, which may stain positive for periodic acid–Schiff but negative for Sudan black B, myeloperoxidase, nonspecific esterase, and chloroacetate esterase (35–37). Some cases of ALL show convoluted blast nuclei; this finding occurs in both precursor B-cell and precursor T-cell ALL.

Cytochemistry

Cytochemical stains have been largely supplanted by immunophenotyping by flow cytometry for the diagnosis of ALL (38). Stains for granulocytic differentiation and mono-

cytic differentiation are typically negative in ALL blasts, with the exception of nonspecific esterase positivity, partially inhibitable with sodium fluoride, seen in the blasts of precursor T-cell ALL (39). In addition, rare cases of ALL have been described showing weak positivity for Sudan black B and chloroacetate esterase (39).

Flow Cytometry

Immunophenotyping by flow cytometry is the most important method of diagnosis and prognosis in ALL (40,41). Precursor B-cell immunophenotype is found in approximately 80% of both childhood and adult ALL, and precursor T-cell immunophenotype in most of the remainder (32). These immunophenotypic subtypes are further discussed below.

Other immunophenotypic findings may have a bearing on clinicopathologic features, including prognosis. CD34 expression is found in approximately 50% of adult ALL and is associated with older age, hepatomegaly, myeloid antigen expression, and poor prognosis (42). CD45 expression is found in approximately 90% of childhood ALL; CD45-negative cases are more likely to show precursor B-cell than the precursor T-cell phenotype (43). CD56 expression, found in approximately 3% to 8% of ALL, is associated with FAB L2 morphology and the central nervous system disease (44,45). Terminal deoxynucleotidyl transferase (TdT) expression is found in more than 95% of ALL cases; the rare TdT-negative cases may show either precursor B-cell or precursor T-cell phenotype (46,47).

Myeloid-associated antigen expression is found in approximately 30% to 35% of ALL cases and is directly correlated with precursor B-cell phenotype, t(9;22), and rearrangements of *MLL* and *ETV6/TEL* (48–50). CD13 and CD33 are each expressed in approximately 15% of childhood ALL cases, CD15 in 7%, and CD14 in 1% (51). Myeloperoxidase expression and myeloperoxidase mRNA may be found in precursor B-cell ALL, especially in cases with t(4;11) or t(9;22), but is not necessarily accompanied by myeloid antigen expression (52–55). CD117 is not expressed (56). No prognostic significance is attached to the expression of myeloid antigens in ALL.

Immunophenotype is not necessarily stable in ALL. At presentation, a single clone may show multiple immunophenotypes (57). At relapse, approximately 50% of cases show immunophenotypic changes (58). Common changes include gain or loss of the myeloid antigens CD13 and CD33. Immunophenotype switching from lymphoid to myeloid immunophenotype has been reported, especially in cases with t(4;11) (59–66).

Immunohistochemistry

Immunophenotyping by immunohistochemistry may be helpful in the diagnosis and classification of ALL, especially in combination with molecular methods when material for flow cytometry is not available (67).

Genetic Analysis

Genetic analysis is used to assess clonality and to detect prognostically important lesions and minimal residual disease in ALL. Clonal karyotypic abnormalities are found in approximately 75% of cases; the figure is higher when more sensitive molecular methods are used (50,68–76). Among the most common anomalies are gains of chromosomes X, 4, 6, 10, 14, 17, 18, and 21 and rearrangements of 6q, 8q24, 9p, 11q23, 12p, and the immunoglobulin and T-cell receptor (TCR) genes. Oligoclonality has been reported in 20% to 30% of ALL cases (77).

Immunoglobulin heavy chain (*IgH*) and/or *TCR* gene rearrangements are found in the vast majority of ALL cases but are not necessarily lineage-specific (78–85). Precursor B-cell ALL shows *IgH* gene rearrangement in more than 90% of cases as well as *TCR* δ-chain gene rearrangement in more than 70% of childhood and 45% of adult cases. Precursor T-cell ALL shows *TCR* gene rearrangements in more than 95% of cases, and *IgH* gene rearrangement in approximately 20% of cases. In cases with *TCR* gene rearrangement, the β-chain gene is rearranged in 30%, the γ-chain gene in 25%, and the δ-chain gene in 90% to 95% of cases. Immunoglobulin and *TCR* gene rearrangements change over time in approximately 30% of cases, most commonly in the κ-light chain gene, followed by the *TCR* γ-chain gene, the *IgH* gene, and the *TCR* δ-chain gene (86,87).

Precursor B-cell ALL arises at several genetically defined developmental stages (88). From the earliest to latest stage of B-cell development, these are (a) the stage before *IgH* gene rearrangement; (b) the stage at which recombinations of IgH variable, joining, and diversity segments occur; and (c) the stage at which *IgH* gene rearrangement is completed.

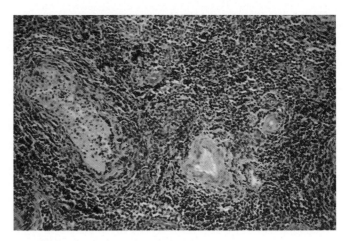

FIGURE 20-8. Testis, acute lymphoblastic leukemia. The seminiferous tubules are separated by a diffuse, monomorphous infiltrate of lymphoblasts.

Extramedullary Disease

Extramedullary disease may occur at initial presentation or at relapse, especially after stem cell transplantation (89–91) (Fig. 20-8). ALL classically recurs in the central nervous system and gonads but also in the breast, body cavities, skin, joints, and other sites (92–97). Concomitant bone marrow disease may be present.

Differential Diagnosis

The differential diagnosis of ALL includes conditions producing increased lymphoblasts or lymphocytes in the peripheral blood or bone marrow (Table 20-3).

Nonneoplastic conditions resembling ALL include precursor B-cell hyperplasia, reactive lymphocytosis of the peripheral blood and bone marrow, acute infectious lymphocytosis, and infectious mononucleosis. It should be kept in mind that these conditions may coexist with ALL.

Neoplastic conditions resembling ALL include malignant lymphoma with leukemic phase, especially the blastic

TABLE 20-3. DIFFERENTIAL DIAGNOSIS OF ACUTE LYMPHOID LEUKEMIA

Nonneoplastic conditions
  Precursor B-cell hyperplasia
  Reactive lymphocytosis
  Acute infectious lymphocytosis
  Infectious mononucleosis

Neoplastic conditions
  Acute myeloid leukemia
  Chronic lymphocytic leukemia
  Malignant lymphoma with leukemic phase
  Embryonal rhabdomyosarcoma
  Ewing sarcoma
  Medulloblastoma
  Neuroblastoma
  Neuroendocrine carcinoma

variant of mantle cell lymphoma, and aggressive natural killer (NK) cell leukemia/lymphoma. Chronic lymphocytic leukemia can be surprisingly difficult to distinguish from cases of ALL in which the blasts show somewhat condensed nuclear chromatin. Nonhematolymphoid tumors mimicking ALL include embryonal rhabdomyosarcoma, Ewing sarcoma, medulloblastoma, neuroblastoma, and neuroendocrine carcinoma. Immunophenotyping by flow cytometry is invaluable in making the correct diagnosis.

IMMUNOPHENOTYPIC SUBTYPES

ALL typically shows differentiation along B-cell, T-cell, or NK cell lineage. ALL with differentiation along multiple lymphoid and/or myeloid lineage is discussed with acute biphenotypic leukemia (see Chapter 19).

Precursor B-Cell Acute Lymphoid Leukemia

Precursor B-cell ALL accounts for 20% of ALL in infants but more than 95% of ALL in children aged 2 to 9 years old (1–9) (Fig. 20-9). The blasts are relatively small and monomorphous in approximately 80% (FAB L1) and larger and more pleomorphic in the remainder (FAB L2).

Flow cytometry shows expression of CD13 and/or CD33 in 11%, CD34 in 70%, CD45 in 87%, and TdT in 97% of cases. CD2 expression is rare, and most CD2-positive cases are reported as acute biphenotypic leukemia. Immunophenotyping permits classification of precursor B-cell ALL into three developmental stages. The earliest stage is represented by pro–B-cell ALL, which shows expression of CD19 and CD34 but typically lacks expression of CD10, CD20, and both surface and cytoplasmic immunoglobulin. This phenotype is associated with adult onset, CD15 expression, t(4;11), t(9;22), and a very poor prognosis. The second stage

is pre–B-cell ALL, which expresses CD10, CD19, CD20 (in approximately 25% of cases), CD34, and cytoplasmic immunoglobulin but typically lacks expression of surface immunoglobulin. This phenotype is found in more than 80% of childhood ALL and is associated with a relatively good prognosis. The third, and rarest, stage is mature B-cell ALL (see below).

Genetic analysis shows *IgH* gene rearrangements in almost 90% of cases and *TCR* gene rearrangements in 60%. *TCR* gene rearrangement is directly correlated with the presence of t(9;22), t(12;21), and, to a lesser extent, t(4;11).

Mature B-Cell Acute Lymphoid Leukemia

Mature B cell ALL is rare and occurs predominantly in adults (10–18) (Fig. 20-10). The morphology may be monomorphous or pleomorphic (FAB L1 or FAB L2) or, less often, Burkitt-like (FAB L3). Flow cytometry shows expression of CD19, CD20, CD34, TdT, and both surface and cytoplasmic immunoglobulin. Genetic studies show an association with t(1;19) and with translocations involving the *BCL-2, c-myc,* and immunoglobulin genes, e.g., t(2;8), t(8;14), t(8;22), t(14;18). A rare case with t(9;22) has been reported. The prognosis is poor.

T-Cell Acute Lymphoid Leukemia

T-cell ALL accounts for 10% to 15% of ALL cases among both children and adults (3,6,7,19–29) (Fig. 20-11). In younger patients, it is associated with male gender, mediastinal mass, lymphadenopathy, hepatosplenomegaly, and marked leukocytosis. Patients older than 60 years of age tend to lack evidence of bulky disease, and the blasts express myeloid antigens more commonly than those in younger patients.

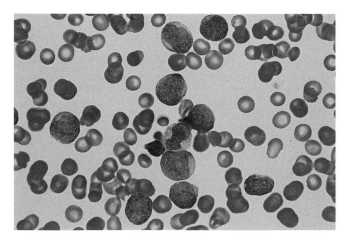

FIGURE 20-9. Peripheral blood smear, acute lymphoblastic leukemia with pre–B-cell phenotype. The blasts are a mixture of L1 and L2 type cells.

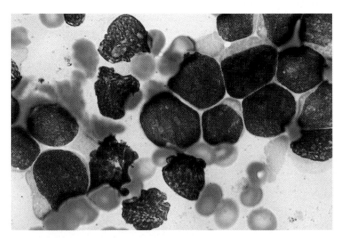

FIGURE 20-10. Bone marrow aspirate, acute lymphoid leukemia with a mature B-cell phenotype. The blasts in this specimen are large and somewhat pleomorphic.

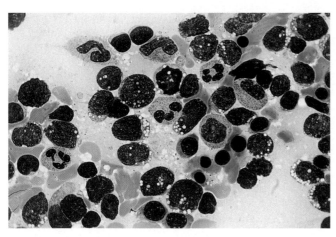

FIGURE 20-11. Bone marrow aspirate, acute lymphoblastic leukemia with pre–T-cell phenotype. The blasts show variable, predominantly L2 morphology and prominent cytoplasmic vacuolation, which may suggest an erroneous diagnosis of Burkitt lymphoma/leukemia.

Flow cytometry shows expression of CD10 in 18%, CD13 and/or CD33 in 10% to 20%, CD45 in 96%, and CD79a in approximately 35% to 40% of cases. Immunophenotyping permits classification of precursor T-cell ALL into three developmental stages. The earliest stage is represented by pro–T-cell ALL, which shows a stem cell–like phenotype with expression of CD7 and TdT but not CD2, CD3, or CD5. The prognosis is very poor. The second stage is pre–T-cell ALL, which usually expresses CD4, CD7, and TCR γ/δ, and variably expresses CD2, CD3, CD5, and CD8. The third and rarest stage is mature T-cell ALL, which shows expression of CD2, CD3, CD5, CD7, and TCR α/β.

Genetic studies may show cryptic t(5;14) and various other karyotypic abnormalities involving 11q23, 14q11, and 14q32. Molecular analysis shows various *TCR* and *IgH* gene rearrangements, depending on the developmental stage of disease. Pro–T-cell ALL shows (in decreasing order) *TCR* δ-chain, *TCR* γ-chain, and *IgH* and *TCR* β-chain gene rearrangements. Pre–T-cell ALL usually shows *TCR* γ- and δ-chain gene rearrangements. Mature T-cell ALL may show *TCR* β-chain gene rearrangements.

Natural Killer Cell Acute Lymphoid Leukemia

Acute NK cell leukemia is essentially indistinguishable from NK cell lymphoma/leukemia (also reported as blastic NK cell lymphoma) and is discussed with NK cell neoplasms (see Chapter 28). Flow cytometry shows expression of CD2, CD7, and CD56. CD3, CD19, and CD20 are not expressed. Occasional cases have been reported with coexpression of B-cell, T-cell, and/or myeloid antigens (see Chapter 19, Acute Biphenotypic Leukemia).

GENOTYPIC SUBTYPES

Acute Lymphoid Leukemia with Hypodiploidy

ALL with hypodiploidy (less than 46 chromosomes) is relatively uncommon and carries a notably poor prognosis (1–5).

Acute Lymphoid Leukemia with High Hyperdiploidy

ALL with high hyperdiploidy (51 to 65 chromosomes) accounts for approximately 10% of ALL cases and is associated with young age, pre–B-cell phenotype, and good prognosis (3–7). Genetic studies typically show gains of chromosomes 4, 6, 10, 14, 17, 18, 21, and X.

Acute Lymphoid Leukemia with t(1;19)(q23;p13) (*PBX1/E2A*)

ALL with t(1;19) accounts for 5% to 10% of childhood and 3% of adult ALL cases (2,8–11). In childhood ALL, this karyotypic anomaly is found predominantly in patients older than 10 years of age. Flow cytometry usually shows a pre–B-cell phenotype, rarely a mature B-cell phenotype. Genetic studies show translocation of *PBX1* at 1q23 and *E2A* at 19p13. A subset of cases also shows t(14;18) (see below). The prognosis is poor.

Acute Lymphoid Leukemia with t(9;22)(q34;q11) (*BCR/ABL*)

ALL with t(9;22) is associated with older age, leukocytosis, pre–B-cell phenotype, and poor prognosis (2,4,12–29). The (9;22) translocation is found in less than 5% of childhood cases but in 25% to 50% of cases in adults older than age 60. Flow cytometry shows expression of CD10, CD13, CD19, and CD34, with a pre–B-cell phenotype in more than 90% of cases, a pre–T-cell phenotype in most of the remainder, and rarely a mature B-cell phenotype. CD20 and CD38 are variably expressed.

Genetic studies show translocation of *ABL* at 9q34 and *BCR* at 22q21, which may be karyotypically inapparent or masked. The *BCR* breakpoint site is variable, yielding a 190-kd BCR/ABL fusion protein (p190) in approximately 77% of cases, p210 in 20%, and both p190 and p210 in 3%. The breakpoint site and lineage appear to be related because p190 is associated with lymphoid differentiation and p210 with both lymphoid and myeloid differentiation. However, even cases with only p190 production may show neoplastic granulocytes, suggesting that apparent ALL with t(9;22) is often biphenotypic. Additional genetic lesions are present in more than 50% of cases.

The differential diagnosis includes chronic myeloid leukemia presenting in lymphoid blast crisis. After successful induction therapy, ALL with t(9;22), p210 production, and evidence of multilineage differentiation converts to chronic phase chronic myeloid leukemia in 15% to 20% of cases.

Acute Lymphoid Leukemia with Anomalies of Chromosome 11q23 and/or *MLL*

ALL with anomalies of chromosome 11q23 and/or *MLL* occurs predominantly in infants and older adults and is associated with male gender and hyperleukocytosis (2–4,30–37). Flow cytometry typically shows a pro–B-cell phenotype, often with expression of the myeloid antigens CD13, CD15, and/or CD33. Genetic studies may show a normal karyotype with masked *MLL* translocation or a clonal 11q23 anomaly with translocation of *MLL* and one or more partner genes. The most common karyotypic anomaly of infant ALL, and the most common translocation affecting *MLL,* is t(4;11)(q21;q23), involving *AF4* at 4q21. The prognosis is very poor.

Acute Lymphoid Leukemia with t(12;21)(p13;q22) (*ETV6/AML1*)

ALL with t(12;21) is the most common type of childhood ALL, accounting for 20% to 40% of cases (37–46). At least 50% of cases arise *in utero*. It is rare in adults and occurs rarely, if at all, in patients with constitutional trisomy 21. The white blood cell count is relatively low, and the blasts are monomorphous (FAB L1). Flow cytometry shows a characteristic pre–B-cell phenotype, with relatively intense CD10 and HLA-DR expression and relatively low CD20, CD34, and CD45 expression. CD13 is often expressed. Genetic studies usually show no karyotypic anomaly, but molecular analysis shows a cryptic translocation involving *ETV6/TEL* at 12p13 and *AML1* at 21q22 and deletion of the second *ETV6/TEL* allele. The prognosis is relatively good.

Acute Lymphoid Leukemia with t(14;18) (*IgH/BCL2*)

ALL with t(14;18) is a rare but distinctive disease of adults, not associated with a history of malignant lymphoma (47–55). Patients tend to be adults rather than children and present with prominent nodal, extranodal, and bone marrow involvement. Morphologically, the malignant cells are usually monomorphous or pleomorphic lymphoblasts (FAB L1 and L2), occasionally Burkitt-type cells (FAB L3). Flow cytometry shows a mature B-cell, rarely pre-B cell, phenotype. Genetic studies show abnormalities involving *IgH* at 14q32 and *BCL-2* at 18q21. Other findings include frequent *c-MYC* anomalies and, in some cases, coexistent t(1;19). The prognosis is very poor.

Acute Lymphoid Leukemia with Constitutional Trisomy 21

ALL with constitutional trisomy 21 (c21+) accounts for approximately 1% to 2% of childhood ALL (56–61). It occurs in a slightly older age group than other childhood ALL. Patients may present with the clinical features of Down syndrome, if complete trisomy 21 is present and the patient is not a premature neonate. Flow cytometry usually shows a pre-B, rarely pro-B, phenotype; conversion to myeloid phenotype has been reported. Genetic studies may show t(8;14). Hyperdiploidy and t(12;21), both common anomalies in childhood ALL, are not found. Spontaneously remitting disease, similar to that observed in acute myeloid leukemia with c21+, has rarely been reported. The prognosis is poor. The differential diagnosis includes ALL with acquired trisomy 21 (62).

REFERENCES

General Features

 1. Jaffe ES, Harris NL, Stein H, et al., eds. *Pathology and genetics of haematopoietic and lymphoid tissues.* Lyon: IARC Press, 2001.
 2. Bennett JM, Catovsky D, Daniel MT, et al. The morphological classification of acute lymphoblastic leukaemia: concordance among observers and clinical correlations. *Br J Haematol* 1981;47:553–561.
 3. Childs CC, Stass SA, Bennett JM. The morphologic classification of acute lymphoblastic leukemia in childhood. Observations on concordance using a simple scoring system. *Am J Clin Pathol* 1986;86:503–506.
 4. Farhi DC, Rosenthal NS. Acute lymphoblastic leukemia. *Clin Lab Med* 2000;17–28.
 5. Kayser R, Mahlfeld K, Nebelung W, et al. Vertebral collapse and normal peripheral blood cell count at the onset of acute lymphatic leukemia in childhood. *J Pediatr Orthop B* 2000;9:55–57.
 6. Muller HL, Horwitz AE, Kuhl J. Acute lymphoblastic leukemia with severe skeletal involvement: a subset of childhood leukemia with a good prognosis. *Pediatr Hematol Oncol* 1998;15:121–133.
 7. Atra A, Abboudi Z, Farahat N, et al. Quantitative flow cytometry can predict childhood acute lymphoblastic leukaemia presenting with aplasia. *Leuk Lymphoma* 1997;27:173–177.
 8. Heegaard ED, Madsen HO, Schmiegelow K. Transient pancytopenia preceding acute lymphoblastic leukaemia (pre-ALL) precipitated by Parvovirus B19. *Br J Haematol* 2001;114:810–813.
 9. Hirose Y, Masaki Y, Ebata K, et al. T-cell type acute lymphoblastic leukemia following cyclosporin A therapy for aplastic anemia. *Int J Hematol* 2001;73:226–229.
10. Kikuchi M, Ohsaka A, Chiba Y, et al. Bone marrow aplasia with prominent atypical plasmacytic proliferation preceding acute lymphoblastic leukemia. *Leuk Lymphoma* 1999;35:213–217.
11. Rafel M, Cobo F, Cervantes F, et al. Transient pancytopenia after non-A non-B non-C acute hepatitis preceding acute lymphoblastic leukemia. *Haematologica* 1998;83:564–566.
12. Suzan F, Terre C, Garcia I, et al. Three cases of typical aplastic anaemia associated with a Philadelphia chromosome. *Br J Haematol* 2001;112:385–387.
13. Litzow MR. Acute lymphoblastic leukemia in adults. *Curr Treat Options Oncol* 2000;1:19–29.
14. Charak BS, Parikh PM, Giri N, et al. Spontaneous complete remission in acute lymphoblastic leukaemia. *Indian J Cancer* 1989;26:10–13.

15. Hatta Y, Iwata T, Takeuchi J, et al. Complete remission in a patient with hypoplastic acute lymphoblastic leukemia induced by granulocyte-colony-stimulating factor. *Acta Haematol* 1995;94:39–43.

16. Lefrere F, Hermine O, Radford-Weiss I, et al. A spontaneous remission of lymphoid blast crisis in chronic myelogenous leukaemia following blood transfusion and infection. *Br J Haematol* 1994;88:621–622.

17. Yetgin S, Tuncer AM, Guler E, et al. Spontaneous complete remission in a child with acute lymphoblastic leukemia. *Turk J Pediatr* 1996;38:227–229.

18. Bjerregaard LL, Rosthooj S. Vertebral compression and eosinophilia in a child with acute lymphatic leukemia. *J Pediatr Hematol Oncol* 2002;24:313–315.

19. Ghosh K, Hiwase D, Muirhead D. Intense eosinophilia with abnormal ultrastructure as presenting manifestation of acute lymphoblastic leukemia. *Haematologia* 2000;30:137–141.

20. Jain P, Kumar R, Gujral S, et al. Granular acute lymphoblastic leukemia with hypereosinophilic syndrome. *Ann Hematol* 2000;79:272–274.

21. Narayanan G, Hussain BM, Chandralekha B, et al. Hypereosinophilic syndrome in acute lymphoblastic leukaemia–case report and literature review. *Acta Oncol* 2000;39:241–243.

22. Parker D, Graham-Pole J, Malpas JS, Paxton A. Acute lymphoblastic leukemia with eosinophilia and basophilia. *Am J Pediatr Hematol Oncol* 1979;1:195–199.

23. Goraya JS, Virdi VS, Marwaha N, et al. Acute lymphoblastic leukemia presenting as cyclic neutropenia. *Pediatr Hematol Oncol* 2002;19:279–282.

24. Blatt J, Penchansky L, Horn M. Thrombocytosis as a presenting feature of acute lymphoblastic leukemia in childhood. *Am J Hematol* 1989;31:46–49.

25. Hajjar KA. Philadelphia chromosome-positive chronic myelogenous leukemia following apparent acute lymphoblastic leukemia. *Clin Pediatr (Phila)* 1985;24:402–405.

26. Knox-Macaulay H, Bhusnurmath S, Alwaily A. Pseudo-Gaucher's cells in association with common acute lymphoblastic leukemia. *South Med J* 1997;90:69–71.

27. Thomas X, Le QH, Danaila C, et al. Bone marrow biopsy in adult acute lymphoblastic leukemia: morphological characteristics and contribution to the study of prognostic factors. *Leuk Res* 2002;26:909–918.

28. Yetgin S, Olcay L, Yel L, et al. T-ALL with monoclonal gammopathy and hairy cell features. *Am J Hematol* 2000;65:166–170.

29. Coustan-Smith E, Sancho J, Behm FG, et al. Prognostic importance of measuring early clearance of leukemic cells by flow cytometry in childhood acute lymphoblastic leukemia. *Blood* 2002;100:52–58.

30. Dworzak MN, Froschl G, Printz D, et al. Prognostic significance and modalities of flow cytometric minimal residual disease detection in childhood acute lymphoblastic leukemia. *Blood* 2002;99:1952–1958.

31. Sandlund JT, Harrison PL, Rivera G, et al. Persistence of lymphoblasts in bone marrow on day 15 and days 22 to 25 of remission induction predicts a dismal treatment outcome in children with acute lymphoblastic leukemia. *Blood* 2002;100:43–47.

32. Chiles LR, Christian MM, McCoy DK, et al. Langerhans cell histiocytosis in a child while in remission for acute lymphocytic leukemia. *J Am Acad Dermatol* 2001;45[Suppl 6]:S233–S234.

33. Raj A, Bendon R, Moriarty T, et al. Langerhans cell histiocytosis following childhood acute lymphoblastic leukemia. *Am J Hematol* 2001;68:284–286.

34. Kanerva J, Saarinen-Pihkala UM, Riikonen P, et al. Reemphasis on lymphoblast L2 morphology as a poor prognostic factor in childhood acute lymphoblastic leukemia. *Med Pediatr Oncol* 1999;33:388–394.

35. Cap J, Babusikova O, Kaiserova E, et al. Granular acute lymphoblastic leukemia in a 15-year-old boy. *Med Oncol* 2000;17:144–146.

36. Jain P, Kumar R, Gujral S, et al. Granular acute lymphoblastic leukemia with hypereosinophilic syndrome. *Ann Hematol* 2000;79:272–274.

37. Sharma S, Narayan S, Kaur M. Acute lymphoblastic leukaemia with giant intracytoplasmic inclusions—a case report. *Indian J Pathol Microbiol* 2000;43:485–487.

38. Kheiri SA, MacKerrell T, Bonagura VR, et al. Flow cytometry with or without cytochemistry for the diagnosis of acute leukemias? *Cytometry* 1998;34:82–86.

39. Rosenthal NS, Farhi DC. Special stains in the diagnosis of acute leukemia. *Clin Lab Med* 2000;20:29–38.

40. Czuczman MS, Dodge RK, Stewart CC, et al. Value of immunophenotype in intensively treated adult acute lymphoblastic leukemia: cancer and leukemia group B study 8364. *Blood* 1999;93:3931–3939.

41. Riley RS, Massey D, Jackson-Cook C, et al. Immunophenotypic analysis of acute lymphocytic leukemia. *Hematol Oncol Clin North Am* 2002;16:245–299.

42. Cacciola E, Guglielmo P, Cacciola E, et al. CD34 expression in adult acute lymphoblastic leukemia. *Leuk Lymphoma* 1995;18 [Suppl 1]:31–36.

43. Ratei R, Sperling C, Karawajew L, et al. Immunophenotype and clinical characteristics of CD45-negative and CD45-positive childhood acute lymphoblastic leukemia. *Ann Hematol* 1998;77:107–114.

44. Paietta E, Neuberg D, Richards S, et al. Rare adult acute lymphocytic leukemia with CD56 expression in the ECOG experience shows unexpected phenotypic and genotypic heterogeneity. *Am J Hematol* 2001;66:189–196.

45. Ravandi F, Cortes J, Estrov Z, et al. CD56 expression predicts occurrence of CNS disease in acute lymphoblastic leukemia. *Leuk Res* 2002;26:643–649.

46. Faber J, Kantarjian H, Roberts MW, et al. Terminal deoxynucleotidyl transferase-negative acute lymphoblastic leukemia. *Arch Pathol Lab Med* 2000;124:92–97.

47. Kaleem Z, Crawford E, Pathan MH, et al. Flow cytometric analysis of acute leukemias. Diagnostic utility and critical analysis of data. *Arch Pathol Lab Med* 2003;127:42–48.

48. Faderl S, Kantarjian HM, Thomas DA, et al. Outcome of Philadelphia chromosome-positive adult acute lymphoblastic leukemia. *Leuk Lymphoma* 2000;36:263–273.

49. Firat H, Favier R, Adam M, et al. Determination of myeloid antigen expression on childhood acute lymphoblastic leukaemia cells: discrepancies using different monoclonal antibody clones. *Leuk Lymphoma* 2001;42:75–82.

50. Khalidi HS, Chang KL, Medeiros LJ, et al. Acute lymphoblastic leukemia. Survey of immunophenotype, French-American-British classification, frequency of myeloid antigen expression, and karyotypic abnormalities in 210 pediatric and adult cases. *Am J Clin Pathol* 1999;111:467–476.

51. Pui CH, Rubnitz JE, Hancock ML, et al. Reappraisal of the clinical and biologic significance of myeloid-associated antigen expression in childhood acute lymphoblastic leukemia. *J Clin Oncol* 1998;16:3768–3773.

52. Arber DA, Snyder DS, Fine M, et al. Myeloperoxidase immunoreactivity in adult acute lymphoblastic leukemia. *Am J Clin Pathol* 2001;116:25–33.

53. Austin GE, Alvarado CS, Austin ED, et al. Prevalence of myeloperoxidase gene expression in infant acute lymphocytic leukemia. *Am J Clin Pathol* 1998;110:575–581.

54. Nakase K, Sartor M, Bradstock K. Detection of myeloperoxidase by flow cytometry in acute leukemia. *Cytometry* 1998;34:198–202.

55. Serrano J, Lo Coco F, Sprovieri T, et al. Myeloperoxidase gene expression in non-infant pro-B acute lymphoblastic leukaemia with or without ALL1/AF4 transcript. *Br J Haematol* 2000;111:1065–1070.

56. Hans CP, Finn WG, Singleton TP, et al. Usefulness of anti-CD117 in the flow cytometric analysis of acute leukemia. *Am J Clin Pathol* 2002;117:301–305.

57. Miura T, Ouhira M, Koseki N, et al. Childhood T-cell acute lymphoblastic leukemia with four distinct immunophenotypes representing different stages of T-cell development. *Pediatr Hematol Oncol* 2001;18:267–272.

58. Guglielmi C, Cordone I, Boecklin F, et al. Immunophenotype of adult and childhood acute lymphoblastic leukemia: changes at first relapse and clinico-prognostic implications. *Leukemia* 1997;11:1501–1507.

59. Bierings M, Szczepanski T, van Wering ER, et al. Two consecutive immunophenotypic switches in a child with immunogenotypically stable acute leukaemia. *Br J Haematol* 2001;113:757–762.

60. Bouabdallah R, Abena P, Chetaille B, et al. True histiocytic lymphoma following B-acute lymphoblastic leukaemia: case report with evidence for a common clonal origin in both neoplasms. *Br J Haematol* 2001;113:1047–1050.

61. Dunphy CH, Gardner LJ, Evans HL, et al. CD15(+) acute lymphoblastic leukemia and subsequent monoblastic leukemia: persistence of t(4;11) abnormality and B-cell gene rearrangement. *Arch Pathol Lab Med* 2001;125:1227–1230.

62. Fujisaki H, Hara J, Takai K, et al. Lineage switch in childhood leukemia with monosomy 7 and reverse of lineage switch in severe combined immunodeficient mice. *Exp Hematol* 1999;27:826–833.

63. Hashimoto S, Toba K, Aoki S, et al. Acute T-lymphoblastic leukemia relapsed with the character of myeloid/natural killer cell precursor phenotype: a case report. *Leuk Res* 2002;26:215–219.

64. Kawakami K, Miyanishi S, Amakawa R, et al. A case of T-lineage lymphoblastic lymphoma/leukemia with t(4;11)(q21;p15) that switched to myelomonocytic leukemia at relapse. *Int J Hematol* 1999;69:196–199.

65. Matsumoto Y, Kawano C, Kametaka M, et al. Phenotypic conversion of T-lineage lymphoblasts in the lymph node to myeloblasts in the bone marrow during relapse after allogeneic bone marrow transplantation. *Int J Hematol* 2000;72:253–254.

66. Tsuboi K, Yazaki M, Miwa H, et al. Lineage conversion from acute lymphoblastic leukemia to acute myeloid leukemia on rearrangement of the IgH gene in a patient with Down syndrome. *Int J Hematol* 2002;76:69–73.

67. Krober SM, Greschniok A, Kaiserling E, et al. Acute lymphoblastic leukaemia: correlation between morphological/immunohistochemical and molecular biological findings in bone marrow biopsy specimens. *Mol Pathol* 2000;53:83–87.

68. Elghezal H, Le Guyader G, Radford-Weiss I, et al. Reassessment of childhood B-lineage lymphoblastic leukemia karyotypes using spectral analysis. *Genes Chromosomes Cancer* 2001;30:383–392.

69. Jalal SM, Law ME, Stamberg J, et al. Detection of diagnostically critical, often hidden, anomalies in complex karyotypes of haematological disorders using multicolour fluorescence in situ hybridization. *Br J Haematol* 2001;112:975–980.

70. Kerndrup GB, Kjeldsen E. Acute leukemia cytogenetics: an evaluation of combining G-band karyotyping with multi-color spectral karyotyping. *Cancer Genet Cytogenet* 2001;124:7–11.

71. Mathew S, Rao PH, Dalton J, et al. Multicolor spectral karyotyping identifies novel translocations in childhood acute lymphoblastic leukemia. *Leukemia* 2001;15:468–472.

72. Nordgren A, Heyman M, Sahlen S, et al. Spectral karyotyping and interphase FISH reveal abnormalities not detected by conventional G-banding. Implications for treatment stratification of childhood acute lymphoblastic leukaemia: detailed analysis of 70 cases. *Eur J Haematol* 2002;68:31–41.

73. Ribera JM, Ortega JJ, Oriol A, et al. Prognostic value of karyotypic analysis in children and adults with high-risk acute lymphoblastic leukemia included in the PETHEMA ALL-93 trial. *Haematologica* 2002;87:154–166.

74. Schneider NR, Carroll AJ, Shuster JJ, et al. New recurring cytogenetic abnormalities and association of blast cell karyotypes with prognosis in childhood T-cell acute lymphoblastic leukemia: a pediatric oncology group report of 343 cases. *Blood* 2000;96:2543–2549.

75. Scholz I, Popp S, Granzow M, et al. Comparative genomic hybridization in childhood acute lymphoblastic leukemia: correlation with interphase cytogenetics and loss of heterozygosity analysis. *Cancer Genet Cytogenet* 2001;124:89–97.

76. Verdorfer I, Brecevic L, Saul W, et al. Comparative genomic hybridization-aided unraveling of complex karyotypes in human hematopoietic neoplasias. *Cancer Genet Cytogenet* 2001;124:1–6.

77. Moreira I, Papaioannou M, Mortuza FY, et al. Heterogeneity of VH-JH gene rearrangement patterns: an insight into the biology of B cell precursor ALL. *Leukemia* 2001;15:1527–1536.

78. Brumpt C, Delabesse E, Beldjord K, et al. The incidence of clonal T-cell receptor rearrangements in B-cell precursor acute lymphoblastic leukemia varies with age and genotype. *Blood* 2000;96:2254–2261.

79. Kimura N, Akiyoshi T, Uchida T, et al. High prevalence of T cell receptor D delta 2(D delta)J delta rearrangement in CD7-positive early T cell acute lymphoblastic leukemia. *Leukemia* 1996;10:650–657.

80. Li AH, Rosenquist R, Forestier E, et al. Clonal rearrangements in childhood and adult precursor B acute lymphoblastic leukemia: a comparative polymerase chain reaction study using multiple sets of primers. *Eur J Haematol* 1999;63:211–218.

81. Scrideli CA, Simoes AL, Defavery R, et al. Childhood B lineage acute lymphoblastic leukemia clonality study by the polymerase chain reaction. *J Pediatr Hematol Oncol* 1997;19:516–522.

82. Szczepanski T, Beishuizen A, Pongers-Willemse MJ, et al. Cross-lineage T cell receptor gene rearrangements occur in more than ninety percent of childhood precursor-B acute lymphoblastic leukemias: alternative PCR targets for detection of minimal residual disease. *Leukemia* 1999;13:196–205.

83. Szczepanski T, Langerak AW, Wolvers-Tettero IL, et al. Immunoglobulin and T cell receptor gene rearrangement patterns in acute lymphoblastic leukemia are less mature in adults than in children: implications for selection of PCR targets for detection of minimal residual disease. *Leukemia* 1998;12:1081–1088.

84. Szczepanski T, Pongers-Willemse MJ, Langerak AW, et al. Unusual immunoglobulin and T-cell receptor gene rearrangement patterns in acute lymphoblastic leukemias. *Curr Top Microbiol Immunol* 1999;246:205–213.

85. van der Burg M, Barendregt BH, Szczepanski T, et al. Immunoglobulin light chain gene rearrangements display hierarchy in absence of selection for functionality in precursor-B-ALL. *Leukemia* 2002;16:1448–1453.

86. Szczepanski T, Willemse MJ, Kamps WA, et al. Molecular discrimination between relapsed and secondary acute lymphoblastic leukemia: proposal for an easy strategy. *Med Pediatr Oncol* 2001;36:352–358.

87. Szczepanski T, Willemse MJ, Brinkhof B, et al. Comparative analysis of Ig and TCR gene rearrangements at diagnosis and at relapse of childhood precursor-B-ALL provides improved strategies for selection of stable PCR targets for monitoring of minimal residual disease. *Blood* 2002;99:2315–2323.

88. Weston VJ, McConville CM, Mann JR, et al. Molecular analysis of single colonies reveals a diverse origin of initial clonal proliferation

in B-precursor acute lymphoblastic leukemia that can precede the t(12;21) translocation. *Cancer Res* 2001;61:8547–8553.

89. Li CK, Shing MM, Chik KW, et al. Isolated testicular relapse after bone marrow transplant with total body irradiation and testicular boost in acute lymphoblastic leukemia. *Bone Marrow Transplant* 1998;22:397–399.

90. Savasan S, Abella E, Karanes C, et al. Recurrent breast relapses in a patient with acute lymphoblastic leukaemia following allogeneic bone marrow transplantation. *Acta Haematol* 1998;99:95–97.

91. Ueda S, Kanamori H, Sasaki S, et al. Isolated extramedullary relapse in knee joint after allogeneic bone marrow transplantation for Ph ALL. *Bone Marrow Transplant* 1998;21:319–321.

92. Chim CS, Shek TW, Liang R. Isolated relapse of acute lymphoblastic leukemia in the breast masquerading as gynecomastia. *Am J Med* 2000;108:677–679.

93. Dix DB, Anderson RA, McFadden DE, et al. Pleural relapse during hematopoietic remission in childhood acute lymphoblastic leukemia. *J Pediatr Hematol Oncol* 1997;19:470–472.

94. Franck P, Duffner U, Schulze-Seemann W, et al. Testicular relapse after 13 years of complete remission of acute lymphoblastic leukemia. *Urol Int* 1998;60:239–241.

95. Lyman MD, Neuhauser TS. Precursor T-cell acute lymphoblastic leukemia/lymphoma involving the uterine cervix, myometrium, endometrium, and appendix. *Ann Diagn Pathol* 2002;6:125–128.

96. Millot F, Robert A, Bertrand Y, et al. Cutaneous involvement in children with acute lymphoblastic leukemia or lymphoblastic lymphoma. The Children's Leukemia Cooperative Group of the European Organization of Research and Treatment of Cancer (EORTC). *Pediatrics* 1997;100:60–64.

97. van den Berg H, Odink AE, Behrendt H. Delayed craniospinal irradiation for a first isolated central nervous relapse of acute lymphoblastic leukemia: report on 14 cases. *Med Pediatr Oncol* 2000;34:402–406.

Immunophenotypic Subtypes

1. Brumpt C, Delabesse E, Beldjord K, et al. The incidence of clonal T-cell receptor rearrangements in B-cell precursor acute lymphoblastic leukemia varies with age and genotype. *Blood* 2000;96:2254–2261.

2. Consolini R, Legitimo A, Rondelli R, et al. Clinical relevance of CD10 expression in childhood ALL. The Italian Association for Pediatric Hematology and Oncology (AIEOP). *Haematologica* 1998;83:967–973.

3. Kaleem Z, Crawford E, Pathan MH, et al. Flow cytometric analysis of acute leukemias. Diagnostic utility and critical analysis of data. *Arch Pathol Lab Med* 2003;127:42–48.

4. Lenormand B, Bene MC, Lesesve JF, et al. PreB1 (CD10-) acute lymphoblastic leukemia: immunophenotypic and genomic characteristics, clinical features and outcome in 38 adults and 26 children. *Leuk Lymphoma* 1998;28:329–342.

5. Ludwig WD, Rieder H, Bartram CR, et al. Immunophenotypic and genotypic features, clinical characteristics, and treatment outcome of adult pro-B acute lymphoblastic leukemia: results of the German multicenter trials GMALL 03/87 and 04/89. *Blood* 1998;92:1898–1909.

6. Pui CH, Rubnitz JE, Hancock ML, et al. Reappraisal of the clinical and biologic significance of myeloid-associated antigen expression in childhood acute lymphoblastic leukemia. *J Clin Oncol* 1998;16:3768–3773.

7. Ratei R, Sperling C, Karawajew L, et al. Immunophenotype and clinical characteristics of CD45-negative and CD45-positive childhood acute lymphoblastic leukemia. *Ann Hematol* 1998;77:107–114.

8. Secker-Walker LM, Prentice HG, Durrant J, et al. Cytogenetics adds independent prognostic information in adults with acute lymphoblastic leukaemia on MRC trial UKALL XA. MRC Adult Leukaemia Working Party. *Br J Haematol* 1997;96:601–610.

9. Uckun FM, Sather H, Gaynon P, et al. Prognostic significance of the CD10+CD19+CD34+ B-progenitor immunophenotype in children with acute lymphoblastic leukemia: a report from the Children's Cancer Group. *Leuk Lymphoma* 1997;27:445–457.

10. Chan NP, Ma ES, Wan TS, et al. The spectrum of acute lymphoblastic leukemia with mature B-cell phenotype. *Leuk Res* 2003;27:231–234.

11. Dunphy CH, van Deventer HW, Carder KJ, et al. Mature B-cell acute lymphoblastic leukemia with associated translocations (14;18)(q32;q21) and (8;9)(q24;p13)—a Burkitt variant? *Arch Pathol Lab Med* 2003;127:610–613.

12. Gunduz C, Cogulu O, Cetingul N, et al. New chromosome rearrangement in acute lymphoblastic leukemia. *Cancer Genet Cytogenet* 2002;137:150–152.

13. Kouides PA, Phatak PD, Wang N, et al. B-cell acute lymphoblastic leukemia with L1 morphology and coexistence of t(1;19) and t(14;18) chromosome translocations. *Cancer Genet Cytogenet* 1994;78:23–27.

14. Mann G, Trebo MM, Haas OA, et al. Philadelphia chromosome-positive mature B-cell (Burkitt cell) leukaemia. *Br J Haematol* 2002;118:559–562.

15. Ohtsuki T, Ogawa Y, Izumi T, et al. Two cases of mature B-cell acute lymphocytic leukemia with normal karyotype in adults. *Acta Haematol* 1996;96:258–261.

16. Rowe D, Devaraj PE, Irving JA, et al. A case of mature B-cell ALL with coexistence of t(1;19) and t(14;18) and expression of the E2A/PBX1 fusion gene. *Br J Haematol* 1996;94:133–135.

17. Stamatoullas A, Buchonnet G, Lepretre S, et al. De novo acute B cell leukemia/lymphoma with t(14;18). *Leukemia* 2000;14:1960–1966.

18. Vasef MA, Brynes RK, Murata-Collins JL, et al. Surface immunoglobulin light chain-positive acute lymphoblastic leukemia of FAB L1 or L2 type: a report of 6 cases in adults. *Am J Clin Pathol* 1998;110:143–149.

19. Attarbaschi A, Mann G, Dworzak M, et al. Mediastinal mass in childhood T-cell acute lymphoblastic leukemia: significance and therapy response. *Med Pediatr Oncol* 2002;39:558–565.

20. Conde-Sterling DA, Aguilera NS, Nandedkar MA, et al. Immunoperoxidase detection of CD10 in Precursor T-lymphoblastic lymphoma/leukemia: a clinicopathologic study of 24 cases. *Arch Pathol Lab Med* 2000;124:704–708.

21. Consolini R, Legitimo A, Rondelli R, et al. Clinical relevance of CD10 expression in childhood ALL. The Italian Association for Pediatric Hematology and Oncology (AIEOP). *Haematologica* 1998;83:967–973.

22. Heerema NA, Sather HN, Sensel MG, et al. Frequency and clinical significance of cytogenetic abnormalities in pediatric T-lineage acute lymphoblastic leukemia: a report from the Children's Cancer Group. *J Clin Oncol* 1998;16:1270–1278.

23. Helias C, Leymarie V, Entz-Werle N, et al. Translocation t(5;14)(q35;q32) in three cases of childhood T cell acute lymphoblastic leukemia: a new recurring and cryptic abnormality. *Leukemia* 2002;16:7–12.

24. Kimura N, Akiyoshi T, Uchida T, et al. High prevalence of T cell receptor D delta 2(D delta)J delta rearrangement in CD7-positive early T cell acute lymphoblastic leukemia. *Leukemia* 1996;10:650–657.

25. Lai R, Juco J, Lee SF, et al. Flow cytometric detection of CD79a expression in T-cell acute lymphoblastic leukemias. *Am J Clin Pathol* 2000;113:823–830.

26. Langerak AW, Wolvers-Tettero IL, van den Beemd MW, et al.

Immunophenotypic and immunogenotypic characteristics of TCRgammadelta+ T cell acute lymphoblastic leukemia. *Leukemia* 1999;13:206–214.

27. Onciu M, Lai R, Vega F, et al. Precursor T-cell acute lymphoblastic leukemia in adults: age-related immunophenotypic, cytogenetic, and molecular subsets. *Am J Clin Pathol* 2002;117:252–258.

28. Szczepanski T, Langerak AW, Willemse MJ, et al. T cell receptor gamma (TCRG) gene rearrangements in T cell acute lymphoblastic leukemia reflect 'end-stage' recombinations: implications for minimal residual disease monitoring. *Leukemia* 2000;14:1208–1214.

29. Uckun FM, Gaynon PS, Sensel MG, et al. Clinical features and treatment outcome of childhood T-lineage acute lymphoblastic leukemia according to the apparent maturational stage of T-lineage leukemic blasts: a Children's Cancer Group study. *J Clin Oncol* 1997;15:2214–2221.

Genotypic Subtypes

1. Heerema NA, Nachman JB, Sather HN, et al. Hypodiploidy with less than 45 chromosomes confers adverse risk in childhood acute lymphoblastic leukemia: a report from the Children's Cancer Group. *Blood* 1999;94:4036–4045.

2. Raimondi SC, Zhou Y, Mathew S, et al. Reassessment of the prognostic significance of hypodiploidy in pediatric patients with acute lymphoblastic leukemia. *Cancer* 2003;98:2715–2722.

3. Chessels JM, Swansbury GJ, Reeves B, et al. Cytogenetics and prognosis in childhood lymphoblastic leukaemia: results of MRC UKALL X. Medical Research Council Working Party in Childhood Leukaemia. *Br J Haematol* 1997;99:93–100.

4. Forestier E, Johansson B, Gustafsson G, et al. Prognostic impact of karyotypic findings in childhood acute lymphoblastic leukaemia: a Nordic series comparing two treatment periods. For the Nordic Society of Paediatric Haematology and Oncology (NOPHO) Leukaemia Cytogenetic Study Group. *Br J Haematol* 2000;110:147–153.

5. Secker-Walker LM, Prentice HG, Durrant J, et al. Cytogenetics adds independent prognostic information in adults with acute lymphoblastic leukaemia on MRC trial UKALL XA. MRC Adult Leukaemia Working Party. *Br J Haematol* 1997;96:601–610.

6. Heerema NA, Sather HN, Sensel MG, et al. Prognostic impact of trisomies of chromosomes 10, 17, and 5 among children with acute lymphoblastic leukemia and high hyperdiploidy (>50 chromosomes). *J Clin Oncol* 2000;18:1876–1887.

7. Nordgren A, Farnebo F, Johansson B, et al. Identification of numerical and structural chromosome aberrations in 15 high hyperdiploid childhood acute lymphoblastic leukemias using spectral karyotyping. *Eur J Haematol* 2001;66:297–304.

8. Foa R, Vitale A, Mancini M, et al. E2A-PBX1 fusion in adult acute lymphoblastic leukaemia: biological and clinical features. *Br J Haematol* 2003;120:484–487.

9. Khalidi HS, O'Donnell MR, Slovak ML, et al. Adult precursor-B acute lymphoblastic leukemia with translocations involving chromosome band 19p13 is associated with poor prognosis. *Cancer Genet Cytogenet* 1999;109:58–65.

10. Sharma P, Watson N, Sartor M, et al. Fifteen cases of t(1;19)(q23;p13.3) identified in an Australian series of 122 children and 80 adults with acute lymphoblastic leukemia. *Cancer Genet Cytogenet* 2001;124:132–136.

11. Uckun FM, Sensel MG, Sather HN, et al. Clinical significance of translocation t(1;19) in childhood acute lymphoblastic leukemia in the context of contemporary therapies: a report from the Children's Cancer Group. *J Clin Oncol* 1998;16:527–535.

12. Arico M, Valsecchi MG, Camitta B, et al. Outcome of treatment in children with Philadelphia chromosome-positive acute lymphoblastic leukemia. *N Engl J Med* 2000;342:998–1006.

13. Fabbiano F, Santoro A, Felice R, et al. Bcr-abl rearrangement in adult T-lineage acute lymphoblastic leukemia. *Haematologica* 1998;856–857.

14. Faderl S, Kantarjian HM, Thomas DA, et al. Outcome of Philadelphia chromosome-positive adult acute lymphoblastic leukemia. *Leuk Lymphoma* 2000;36:263–273.

15. Gleissner B, Gokbuget N, Bartram CR, et al. Leading prognostic relevance of the BCR-ABL translocation in adult acute B-lineage lymphoblastic leukemia: a prospective study of the German Multicenter Trial Group and confirmed polymerase chain reaction analysis. *Blood* 2002;99:1536–1543.

16. Kasprzyk A, Harrison CJ, Secker-Walker LM. Investigation of clonal involvement of myeloid cells in Philadelphia-positive and high hyperdiploid acute lymphoblastic leukemia. *Leukemia* 1999;13:2000–2006.

17. Ko BS, Tang JL, Tsai W, et al. Philadelphia chromosome-positive acute lymphoblastic leukemia in Taiwan. *Ann Hematol* 2001;80:510–515.

18. Lim LC, Heng KK, Vellupillai M, et al. Molecular and phenotypic spectrum of *de novo* Philadelphia positive acute leukemia. *Int J Mol Med* 1999;4:665–667.

19. Mann G, Trebo MM, Haas OA, et al. Philadelphia chromosome-positive mature B-cell (Burkitt cell) leukaemia. *Br J Haematol* 2002;118:559–562.

20. Onciu M, Bueso-Ramos C, Medeiros LJ, et al. Acute lymphoblastic leukemia in elderly patients the Philadelphia chromosome may not be a significant adverse prognostic factor. *Am J Clin Pathol* 2002;117:716–720.

21. Pajor L, Vass JA, Kereskai L, et al. The existence of lymphoid lineage restricted Philadelphia chromosome-positive acute lymphoblastic leukemia with heterogeneous bcr-abl rearrangement. *Leukemia* 2000;14:1122–1126.

22. Radich JP. Philadelphia chromosome-positive acute lymphocytic leukemia. *Hematol Oncol Clin North Am* 2001;15:21–36.

23. Ribera JM, Ortega JJ, Oriol A, et al. Prognostic value of karyotypic analysis in children and adults with high-risk acute lymphoblastic leukemia included in the PETHEMA ALL-93 trial. *Haematologica* 2002;87:154–166.

24. Rieder H, Bonwetsch C, Janssen LA, et al. High rate of chromosome abnormalities detected by fluorescence in situ hybridization using BCR and ABL probes in adult acute lymphoblastic leukemia. *Leukemia* 1998;12:1473–1481.

25. Schenk TM, Keyhani A, Bottcher S, et al. Multilineage involvement of Philadelphia chromosome positive acute lymphoblastic leukemia. *Leukemia* 1998;12:666–674.

26. Tabernero MD, Bortoluci AM, Alaejos I, et al. Adult precursor B-ALL with BCR/ABL gene rearrangements displays a unique immunophenotype based on the pattern of CD10, CD34, CD13 and CD38 expression. *Leukemia* 2001;15:406–414.

27. Thalhammer-Scherrer R, Mitterbauer G, Simonitsch I, et al. The immunophenotype of 325 adult acute leukemias: relationship to morphologic and molecular classification and proposal for a minimal screening program highly predictive for lineage discrimination. *Am J Clin Pathol* 2002;117:380–389.

28. Thomas X, Thiebaut A, Olteanu N, et al. Philadelphia chromosome positive adult acute lymphoblastic leukemia: characteristics, prognostic factors and treatment outcome. *Hematol Cell Ther* 1998;40:119–128.

29. Uckun FM, Nachman JB, Sather HN, et al. Clinical significance of Philadelphia chromosome positive pediatric acute lymphoblastic leukemia in the context of contemporary intensive therapies: a report from the Children's Cancer Group. *Cancer* 1998;83:2030–2039.

30. Armstrong SA, Staunton JE, Silverman LB, et al. MLL translocations specify a distinct gene expression profile that distinguishes a unique leukemia. *Nat Genet* 2002;30:41–47.

31. Bertrand FE, Vogtenhuber C, Shah N, et al. Pro-B-cell to pre-B-cell development in B-lineage acute lymphoblastic leukemia expressing the MLL/AF4 fusion protein. *Blood* 2001;98:3398–3405.

32. Borkhardt A, Wuchter C, Viehmann S, et al. Infant acute lymphoblastic leukemia—combined cytogenetic, immunophenotypical and molecular analysis of 77 cases. *Leukemia* 2002;16:1685–1690.

33. Chessells JM, Harrison CJ, Kempski H, et al. Clinical features, cytogenetics and outcome in acute lymphoblastic and myeloid leukaemia of infancy: report from the MRC Childhood Leukaemia working party. *Leukemia* 2002;16:776–784.

34. Harbott J, Mancini M, Verellen-Dumoulin C, et al. Hematological malignancies with a deletion of 11q23: cytogenetic and clinical aspects. European 11q23 Workshop participants. *Leukemia* 1998;12:823–827.

35. Sharma P, Jarvis A, Jauch A, et al. Complex variant t(4;11) characterized by fluorescence in situ hybridization in infant acute lymphoblastic leukemia. *Cancer Genet Cytogenet* 2001;127:177–180.

36. von Bergh A, Gargallo P, De Prijck B, et al. Cryptic t(4;11) encoding MLL-AF4 due to insertion of 5′ MLL sequences in chromosome 4. *Leukemia* 2001;15:595–600.

37. Pui CH, Rubnitz JE, Hancock ML, et al. Reappraisal of the clinical and biologic significance of myeloid-associated antigen expression in childhood acute lymphoblastic leukemia. *J Clin Oncol* 1998;16:3768–3773.

38. Codrington R, O'Connor HE, Jalali GR, et al. Analysis of ETV6/AML1 abnormalities in acute lymphoblastic leukaemia: incidence, alternative spliced forms and minimal residual disease value. *Br J Haematol* 2000;111:1071–1079.

39. De Zen L, Orfao A, Cazzaniga G, et al. Quantitative multiparametric immunophenotyping in acute lymphoblastic leukemia: correlation with specific genotype. I. ETV6/AML1 ALLs identification. *Leukemia* 2000;14:1225–1231.

40. Ford AM, Fasching K, Panzer-Grumayer ER, et al. Origins of "late" relapse in childhood acute lymphoblastic leukemia with TEL-AML1 fusion genes. *Blood* 2001;98:558–564.

41. Jabber Al-Obaidi MS, Martineau M, Bennett CF, et al. ETV6/AML1 fusion by FISH in adult acute lymphoblastic leukemia. *Leukemia* 2002;16:669–674.

42. Jamil A, Theil KS, Kahwash S, et al. TEL/AML-1 fusion gene. its frequency and prognostic significance in childhood acute lymphoblastic leukemia. *Cancer Genet Cytogenet* 2000;122:73–78.

43. McHale CM, Wiemels JL, Zhang L, et al. Prenatal origin of TEL-AML1-positive acute lymphoblastic leukemia in children born in California. *Genes Chromosomes Cancer* 2003;37:36–43.

44. Seyfarth J, Madsen HO, Nyvold C, et al. Post-induction residual disease in translocation t(12;21)-positive childhood ALL. *Med Pediatr Oncol* 2003;40:82–87.

45. Tsang KS, Li CK, Chik KW, et al. TEL/AML1 rearrangement and the prognostic significance in childhood acute lymphoblastic leukemia in Hong Kong. *Am J Hematol* 2001;68:91–98.

46. Weston VJ, McConville CM, Mann JR, et al. Molecular analysis of single colonies reveals a diverse origin of initial clonal proliferation

47. Berger R, Flexor M, Le Coniat M, et al. Presence of three recurrent chromosomal rearrangements, t(2;3)(p12;q37), del(8)(q24), and t(14;18), in an acute lymphoblastic leukemia. *Cancer Genet Cytogenet* 1996;86:76–79.

48. Collett JM, Begley CG, Sammann ME, et al. Two cases of de novo precursor B-cell acute lymphoblastic leukemia with t(14;18), but without cytogenetic evidence of an associated Burkitt's or Burkitt's variant translocation. *Am J Clin Pathol* 1994;101:587–589.

49. Dunphy CH, van Deventez HW, Carder KJ, et al. Mature B-cell acute lymphoblastic leukemia with associated translocations (14;18)(q32;q21) and (8;9)(q24;p13)—a Burkitt variant? *Arch Pathol Lab Med* 2003;127:610–613.

50. Kouides PA, Phatak PD, Wang N, et al. B-cell acute lymphoblastic leukemia with L1 morphology and coexistence of t(1;19) and t(14;18) chromosome translocations. *Cancer Genet Cytogenet* 1994;78:23–27.

51. Nakamura F, Tatsumi E, Tani K, et al. Coexpression of cell-surface immunoglobulin (sIg), terminal deoxynucleotidyl transferase (TdT) and recombination activating gene 1 (RAG-1): two cases and derived cell lines. *Leukemia* 1996;10:1159–1163.

52. Rowe D, Devaraj PE, Irving JA, et al. A case of mature B-cell ALL with coexistence of t(1;19) and t(14;18) and expression of the E2A/PBX1 fusion gene. *Br J Haematol* 1996;94:133–135.

53. Stamatoullas A, Buchonnet G, Lepretre S, et al. De novo acute B-cell leukemia/lymphoma with t(14;18). *Leukemia* 2000;14:1960–1966.

54. Velangi MR, Reid MM, Bown N, et al. Acute lymphoblastic leukaemia of the L3 subtype in adults in the Northern health region of England 1983-99. *J Clin Pathol* 2002;55:591–595.

55. Wlodarska I, Stul M, De Wolf-Peeters C, et al. t(1;19) without detectable E2A rearrangements in two t(14;18)-positive lymphoma/leukemia cases. *Genes Chromosomes Cancer* 1994;10:171–176.

56. Chessells JM, Harrison G, Richards SM, et al. Down's syndrome and acute lymphoblastic leukaemia: clinical features and response to treatment. *Arch Dis Child* 2001;85:321–325.

57. Dordelmann M, Schrappe M, Reiter A, et al. Down's syndrome in childhood acute lymphoblastic leukemia: clinical characteristics and treatment outcome in four consecutive BFM trials Berlin-Frankfurt-Munster Group. *Leukemia* 1998;12:645–651.

58. Fernandez de Castro M, Salas S, Martinez A, et al. Transitory T-lymphoblastic leukemoid reaction in a neonate with Down syndrome. *Am J Pediatr Hematol Oncol* 1990;12:71–73.

59. Kaleem Z, Shuster JJ, Carroll AJ, et al. Acute lymphoblastic leukemia with an unusual t(8;14)(q11.2;q32): a Pediatric Oncology Group Study. *Leukemia* 2000;14:238–240.

60. Reynolds P, Von Behren J, Elkin EP. Birth characteristics and leukemia in young children. *Am J Epidemiol* 2002;155:603–613.

61. Tsuboi K, Yazaki M, Miwa H, et al. Lineage conversion from acute lymphoblastic leukemia to acute myeloid leukemia on rearrangement of the IgH gene in a patient with Down syndrome. *Int J Hematol* 2002;76:69–73.

62. Loncarevic IF, Roitzheim B, Ritterbach J, et al. Trisomy 21 is a recurrent secondary aberration in childhood acute lymphoblastic leukemia with TEL/AML1 gene fusion. *Genes Chromosomes Cancer* 1999;24:272–277.

in B-precursor acute lymphoblastic leukemia that can precede the t(12;21) translocation. *Cancer Res* 2001;61:8547–8553.

MYELODYSPLASTIC SYNDROMES

ANDREW S. EDELMAN
DIANE C. FARHI

GENERAL CONSIDERATIONS

Definition

The myelodysplastic syndromes (MDS) is a group of clonal disorders of hematopoietic stem cells and thus may involve all lineages of hematopoietic origin: granulocytes, monocytes, erythroid cells, megakaryocytes, mast cells, dendritic cells, and lymphocytes. MDS usually presents with decreased cell counts and may be asymptomatic or present with symptoms referable to cytopenias (1–6). The hematopoietic stem cells show increased proliferative activity, but differentiation persists. Classically, there is dysplasia and ineffective hematopoiesis of one or more cell lines as well as an increased apoptotic rate, leading to a discrepancy between hypercellular bone marrow and peripheral cytopenias. In some cases, proliferation outstrips apoptosis, and increased marrow cellularity coexists with increased peripheral cell counts. Such cases are easily mistaken for myeloproliferative disorders or are termed mixed myeloproliferative/myelodysplastic syndromes.

MDS occurs predominantly in adults (median age, 70 years) with an incidence of approximately three in 100,000. Although MDS can also occur in children, the frequency of various forms of MDS is different. In children, the majority of cases show cytopenias, with a minority showing increased peripheral cell counts. Risk factors in both children and adults include a wide variety of constitutional disorders, environmental exposures, medical therapy, and other conditions (see Chapter 18).

Clinical Course

MDS occurs *de novo* and as a transformation of aplastic anemia, pure red cell aplasia, paroxysmal nocturnal hemoglobinuria, or myeloproliferative disorders (MPD). MDS may also occur as a secondary disease either therapy-related or owing to environmental exposure to toxins (7,8). The clinical and cytogenetic aspects differ in *de novo* MDS and secondary MDS (7,8). MDS as secondary disease usually has a worse prognosis and a higher rate of cytogenetic abnor-

malities compared with *de novo* MDS. The presence of cytogenetic abnormalities, such as balanced translocations, is much more common in MDS as a secondary disease process (7,8). MDS in children has distinct features with regard to cytogenetics, morphology, and other disease associations.

MDS and acute leukemia represent different points on a continuum and are thus not clearly separable. In general, MDS shows more differentiation with correspondingly fewer blasts. Transformation of MDS to acute leukemia is well-known. The phenotype is usually myeloid but may be lymphoid (9–14). Although progression to overt leukemia occurs in approximately 30% of all patients with MDS, the risk of leukemic transformation depends on age, the number and severity of cytopenias, the extent and degree of dysplasia, the percentage of blasts, drug resistance, genetic anomalies, and many other factors (15–24). Acute leukemia is recognized, by current convention, when peripheral blood or marrow blasts reach 20% of total cells; however, it should be kept in mind that the biologic behavior of high-grade MDS may be indistinguishable from that of acute leukemia.

Other outcomes include aplastic anemia (25), spontaneous remission (25–31), and remission after colony-stimulating factor and/or immunosuppressive therapy (32,33).

Classification and Prognosis

Classification of MDS is in flux because of the large amount of data available and the great number of prognostically relevant variables (3,6,34–37) (Tables 21-1 through 21-3). The first well-delineated classification of MDS was developed by the French-American-British (FAB) Working Group (38). This classification has been recently modified by the World Health Organization (WHO) (37). A morphologic outline has been used in this chapter to help the diagnostician determine the best classification for a given case (Table 21-3).

The original FAB classification is primarily based on morphologic features and the percentage of blasts. The absolute monocyte count and the presence and percentage of ringed

TABLE 21-1. CLASSIFICATION OF MYELODYSPLASTIC SYNDROMES ACCORDING TO THE FRENCH-AMERICAN-BRITISH WORKING GROUP

Disease	Blood Findings	Bone Marrow Findings
Refractory anemia	Anemia[a] <1% Blasts	<5% Blasts <15% Ringed sideroblasts
Refractory anemia with ringed sideroblasts	Anemia <1% Blasts	<5% Blasts >15% Ringed sideroblasts
Refractory anemia with excess blasts	Anemia (cytopenias) <5% Blasts	5%–20% Blasts
Refractory anemia with excess blasts in transformation	Cytopenias <5% Blasts[b] Auer rods[b]	21%–30% Blasts[b] Auer rods[b]
Chronic myelomonocytic leukemia	<5% Blasts >1000 monocytes/mL ($>1 \times 10^9$/L)[c]	<20% Blasts

[a]Other single lineage cytopenias included in this category.
[b]Only one of these findings required for the classification of refractory anemia with excess blasts in transformation.
[c]Other causes of monocytosis need to be excluded. Neutrophilia with anemia and thrombocytopenia are often present.
Adapted from Bennett JM, Catovsky D, Daniel MT, et al. Proposals for the classification of the myelodysplastic syndromes. *Br J Haematol* 1982;51;189–199.

TABLE 21-2. CLASSIFICATION OF MYELODYSPLASTIC SYNDROMES ACCORDING TO THE WORLD HEALTH ORGANIZATION

Disease	Blood Findings	Bone Marrow Findings
Refractory anemia	Anemia, rare blasts	Erythroid dysplasia only, <5% blasts, <15% ringed sideroblasts
Refractory anemia with ringed sideroblasts	Anemia, no blasts	Erythroid dysplasia only, <5% blasts, $\geq$15% ringed sideroblasts
Refractory cytopenia with multilineage dysplasia	Cytopenias (bi-/pancytopenia), rare blasts, no Auer rods, $<1 \times 10^9$ monocytes	Dysplasia[a] in two or more cell lines, <5% blasts, <15% ringed sideroblasts, no Auer rods
Refractory cytopenia with multilineage dysplasia and ringed sideroblasts	Cytopenias (bi-/pancytopenia), rare blasts, no Auer rods, $<1 \times 10^9$ monocytes	Dysplasia[a] in two or more cell lines, <5% blasts, $\geq$15% ringed sideroblasts, no Auer rods
Refractory anemia with excess blasts-I	Cytopenias, <5% blasts, no Auer rods, $<1 \times 10^9$ monocytes	Uni-/multilineage dysplasia, 5%–9% blasts, no Auer rods
Refractory anemia with excess blasts-II	Cytopenias, 5%–19% blasts[b], $\pm$Auer rods[b], $<1 \times 10^9$ monocytes	Uni-/multilineage dysplasia, 10%–19% blasts[b], $\pm$Auer rods[b]
Myelodysplastic syndrome, unclassified	Cytopenias, rare blasts, no Auer rods	Unilineage dysplasia, <5% blasts, no Auer rods
Myelodysplastic syndromes associated with isolated del(5q)	Anemia, <5% blasts, platelets normal or increased	<5% blasts, isolated del(5q) cytogenetic abnormality, no Auer rods, normal to increased megakaryocytes with hypolobated nuclei

[a]Dysplasia is defined as the presence of dysplastic features in 10% or more of the cells in a given lineage.
[b]Patients with 5% to 19% blasts in the blood or with Auer rods are classified as refractory anemia with excess blasts-II even if bone marrow blast counts are less than 10%.
Adapted from Vardiman JW, Harris NL, Brunning RD. The World Health Organization (WHO) classification of the myeloid neoplasms. *Blood* 2002;100:2292–2302 and Brunning RD, Bennett JM, Flandrin G, et al. Myelodysplastic syndromes. In: Jaffe ES, Harris NL, Stein H, et al., eds. *World Health Organization classification of tumors: pathology and genetics of tumours of haematopoietic and lymphoid tissues.* Lyon: IARC Press, 2001:61–74.

TABLE 21-3. ORGANIZATION OF MYELODYSPLASTIC SYNDROMES IN THIS CHAPTER

Myelodysplastic Syndromes with Cytopenias
  Refractory Anemia
  Refractory Anemia with Ringed Sideroblasts
  Refractory Cytopenia with Multilineage Dysplasia
  Refractory Anemia with Excess Blasts
  Refractory Anemia with Excess Blasts in Transformation
  5q- Syndrome
  Myelodysplastic Syndrome, Unclassified
  Acute Myelodysplastic Syndrome with Fibrosis

Myelodysplastic Syndromes with Increased Peripheral Cell
    Counts and Myelodysplastic Syndromes/Myeloproliferative
    Disorders
  Myelodysplastic Syndrome with Neutrophilia
  Myelodysplastic Syndrome with Monocytosis
  Myelodysplastic Syndrome with Eosinophilia
  Myelodysplastic Syndrome with Basophilia
  Myelodysplastic Syndrome with Mastocytosis
  Myelodysplastic Syndrome with Thrombocytosis

Special Types of Myelodysplastic Syndrome
  Secondary Myelodysplastic Syndrome
  Myelodysplastic Syndrome in Childhood
  Paroxysmal Nocturnal Hemoglobinuria

Disorders Associated with Myelodysplastic Syndromes

---

sideroblasts are used to subclassify some of the disorders. Although five morphologic subtypes are used, the FAB classification divides MDS into only two prognostic categories: low-grade MDS consisting of refractory anemia (RA), RA with ringed sideroblasts (RARS) and high-grade MDS, consisting of RA with excess blasts (RAEB), RAEB in transformation (RAEB-T), and chronic myelomonocytic leukemia (CMML) (Table 21-1).

The WHO classification modifies the FAB classification by the addition of multilineage dysplasia (either bi- or trilineage) and the separation of CMML into a category of diseases that have combined features of MDS and MPD (MDS/MPD category). The WHO categories further separate pure RA, either without or with ringed sideroblasts (RARS), from refractory cytopenias with multilineage dysplasia (RCMD), also without or with ringed sideroblasts. Subclassification based on the percentage of blasts divides RAEB into two groups: RAEB-I (5% to 9% blasts) and RAEB-II (10% to 19% blasts). Finally, the WHO reduces the percentage of blasts necessary for the diagnosis of acute myeloid leukemia (AML) from 30% to 20%, thus eliminating the category of RAEB-T. The WHO clearly notes, however, that this reclassification of patients does not imply the need to change treatment options for the patients with 20% to 30% blasts but allows their inclusion in clinical trials or treatment with AML protocols, if deemed appropriate for a given patient. Some special situations are separately classified and include MDS-U (unclassified) and the 5q— syndrome [MDS with isolated del(5q)] Table 21-2.

Although both the FAB and WHO systems are useful for classification, better separation of risk groups can be obtained by the addition of cytogenetic data (39). The International Prognostic Scoring System (IPSS) for MDS incorporates the percentage of blasts, the karyotype, and the number of cytopenias to determine the IPSS score. Four risk groups have been identified based on this score: low, intermediate 1, intermediate 2, and high (Table 21-4). Further patient stratification based on bone marrow dysplasia has also been proposed (40).

An outline of MDS as discussed in this chapter is given to assist the reader in locating information according to clinical and morphologic findings (Table 21-3).

Genetic and Phenotypic Findings

Genetic studies show clonal karyotypic anomalies in more than 50% of cases, and more anomalies in cases studied by fluorescent methods (41–43). Multiclonality may occur (41,44). The anomalies are often multiple and/or complex, especially in therapy-related MDS. A wide variety of

---

TABLE 21-4. INTERNATIONAL PROGNOSTIC SCORING SYSTEM FOR MYELODYSPLASTIC SYNDROMES

Prognostic Variable	Score Value[a]				
	0	0.5	1.0	1.5	2.0
Bone marrow blasts (%)	<5	5–10		11–20	21–30
Karyotype[b]	Good	Intermediate	Poor		
Cytopenias[c]	0–1	2–3			

[a]Total scores for risk groups are as follows: low, 0; intermediate-1, 0.5–1.0; intermediate-2, 1.5–2.0; high, ≥2.5.
[b]Good, normal, -Y, del(5q), del(20q); poor, complex (three or more abnormalities) or chromosome 7 abnormalities; intermediate, other abnormalities.
[c]Cytopenias defined as hemoglobin less than 10g/dL, absolute neutrophil count less than 1,500/μL, platelets less than 100,000/μL.
Adapted from Greenberg P, Cox C, LeBeau MM, et al. International scoring system for evaluating prognosis in myelodysplastic syndromes. *Blood* 1997;89:2079–2088.

anomalies has been reported, and additional anomalies frequently appear over time (clonal evolution) (45–51). Common findings include trisomy 1q, del(5q), monosomy 7 (especially in children), del(7q), trisomy 8, monosomy 17, and del(17p) (5,41,52–57). Rarely, t(9;22)(q34;q11) and/or *BCR/ABL* gene rearrangement may be present, but the other features of chronic myeloid leukemia are lacking (58,59). The isolated finding of a del(5q), listed previously, defines a special form of MDS, 5q- syndrome, which has distinct clinical and prognostic features.

Although not promoted in the past, many recent studies have advocated the use of flow cytometry data to aid in the diagnosis and classification of MDS (60–65). Some studies have shown subtle abnormalities, including an increased percentage of immature myeloid cells expressing CD13, CD33, CD34, and HLA-DR and reduced CD11b expression (65). Others have identified reduced expression of CD10 on mature granulocytes (60). Phenotypic abnormalities of the blast populations in MDS (61) as well as the composite phenotypes of the myeloid and monocytic populations (64) have been shown to be of prognostic significance. One common factor is the expression of CD7 on myeloid or monocytic cells. A flow cytometry scoring system has been proposed, which correlates well with clinical outcome and IPSS score (64).

Immunostains and cytochemical stains aid in the identification of cellular elements. They may show expression of myeloid antigens, including α_1-antitrypsin, α_1-antichymotrypsin, lysozyme, and myeloperoxidase; and markers of immaturity, such as CD34 and p53 protein (66–69). Cytochemical stains may show abnormal results for myeloperoxidase, chloroacetate esterase, and nonspecific esterase (70,71). Aberrant periodic acid–Schiff staining of erythroid precursors is found in some cases of MDS.

Morphologic Findings

General Aspects

The hallmarks of MDS are the morphologic dysplastic features that accompany these disorders. The erythroid lineage is affected in virtually all these diseases, with variable involvement of the myeloid and megakaryocytic elements. In rare cases, the dysplasia does not involve the red cell elements, and there is selective cytopenia of either granulocytes or platelets.

A major challenge in the diagnosis of MDS is to determine whether the presence of morphologic dysplasia is truly owing to a clonal disorder or other factors. Numerous disorders can cause the same or similar changes in hematopoietic cells, including vitamin deficiencies (B$_{12}$, folate), toxic factors (accidental or therapeutic), and infections (e.g., Parvovirus) (see Chapter 18). The differential diagnosis of nonsideroblastic MDS includes nonclonal constitutional and acquired myelodysplasia (1–11), blast proliferation owing

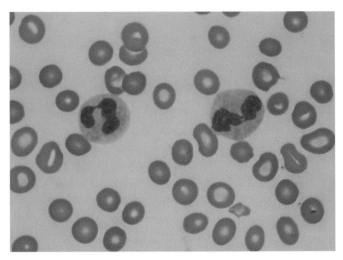

FIGURE 21-1. Peripheral blood with aniso- and poikilocytosis, hypogranular neutrophils, and no of platelets (Wright stain).

to endogenous (12) and exogenous (13,14) hematopoietic colony-stimulating factors, aplastic anemia (15–21), MPD and acute leukemia. The differential diagnosis of RARS consists of nonclonal constitutional and acquired sideroblastic anemias (22–38). A trial of pyridoxine may be helpful in putative cases of RARS because pyridoxine responsiveness is more characteristic of nonclonal than clonal sideroblastic anemia. Rarely, nonclonal sideroblastic anemia may evolve to clonal MDS (32).

Peripheral Blood

The peripheral blood shows one or more cytopenias, which may be cyclic (39–41). All three cell lines may show morphologic abnormalities (Figs. 21-1 through 21-5).

Anemia may be accompanied by red blood cell (RBC) morphologic abnormalities. The RBCs are typically macrocytic and may include schistocytes and elliptocytes (42–44). Delayed maturation of immature RBCs may cause pseudoreticulocytosis (45–47) with coarse basophilic stippling and Howell-Jolly bodies. Nucleated RBCs may be present, showing megaloblastoid change and/or abnormal nuclear shape.

Granulocytes and precursors show abnormal nuclear morphology, including hypolobation (pseudo–Pelger-Huët anomaly), hyperlobation, and/or abnormal nuclear contours, including ring forms. Cytoplasmic abnormalities commonly include profound hypogranularity, but hypergranularity and/or abnormal granule size and shape may also be seen. Monocytes and precursors may show abnormal nuclear morphology and phagocytic activity (48). Blasts may be present but constitute less than 20% of cells seen.

Dysplasia within the megakaryocyte/platelet lineage is primarily demonstrated by abnormal platelets within the blood. Platelets are of abnormal size, often pleomorphic,

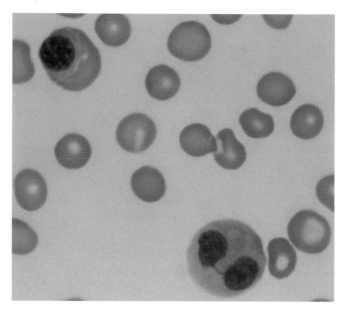

FIGURE 21-2. This blood smear also demonstrated some degree of erythroid dysmorphia. A nucleated red blood cell and a hypogranular pseudo–Pelger-Huët neutrophil are present. There is an absence of platelets in this smear (Wright stain).

and most frequently large and hypogranular. Megakaryocytic fragments and micromegakaryocytes can also be found in some patients.

Bone Marrow Aspirate

Analysis of a properly prepared bone marrow aspirate allows careful morphologic evaluation of hematopoietic precursors (Figs. 21-6 through 21-13). Bone marrow aspirate smears are variably cellular, depending on marrow cellularity and fibrosis. The myeloid:erythroid ratio is variable and often decreased.

The RBC dysplastic changes described previously are present throughout all maturational stages. In addition, erythroid precursors may show nuclear abnormalities, including multilobation, nuclear budding, and internuclear bridging. Cytoplasmic changes include basophilia, vacuolization,

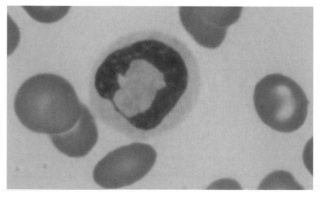

FIGURE 21-3. A dysplastic neutrophil with a ring nucleus is shown (Wright stain).

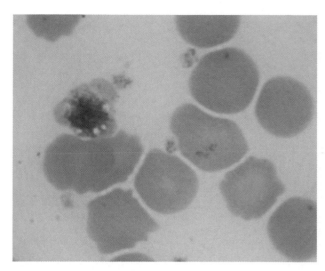

FIGURE 21-4. Platelet dysplasia as indicated by the large/giant platelet. Basophilic stippling within many of the erythrocytes were also seen in this case (Wright stain).

identification of perinuclear rings of iron-containing mitochondria (ringed sideroblasts) by iron staining, and coarse or fine periodic acid–Schiff-positive granules.

Dysplastic features of peripheral granulocytes are also present in the marrow. Blasts constitute as many as 20% of cells, at which point the diagnosis changes to acute leukemia. Phagocytic activity by blasts has been reported (49). Megakaryocytes may be of abnormal size (usually small) and show nuclear hypolobation and separation of nuclear lobes. Megakaryocytic abnormalities may be better appreciated in the biopsy specimen.

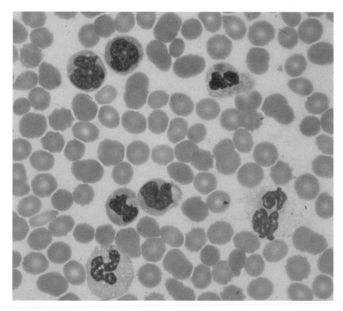

FIGURE 21-5. Dysplastic monocytes and neutrophils are seen in this smear from a patient with chronic myelomonocytic leukemia (Wright stain).

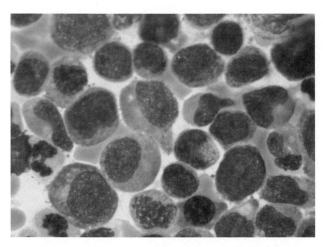

FIGURE 21-6. High cellularity of this bone marrow aspirate is accompanied by multilineage dysplasia and a lack of maturation in this patient with a refractory anemia with excess blasts (Wright stain).

Bone Marrow Biopsy

Histologic sections are most useful for evaluating cellularity, architectural disorder (i.e., precursor localization and fibrosis), and megakaryocytic abnormalities (Figs. 21-14 through 21-20). The bone marrow usually shows increased cellularity for the site and age. Hypocellularity has been reported; however, many studies fail to correct cellularity for age (15–21). Cellularity is rarely low once age is taken into account, and hypocellularity has not been shown to affect prognosis (21).

Dyserythropoietic changes are less obvious in the biopsy specimen compared with the smears but are shown by the presence of erythroid hyperplasia and disorganized erythroid colony formation. Dysplasia in the myeloid lineage is noted by intratrabecular clusters of myeloid precursors, monocytes, and/or blasts (50–52), which has been termed "abnormal localization of immature precursors (ALIP)."

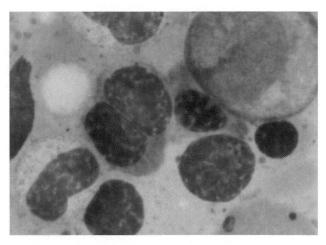

FIGURE 21-8. Dyserythropoiesis in this marrow aspirate as evidenced by a binucleated erythroblast (Wright stain).

Findings within the megakaryocyte lineage are often quite striking. Megakaryocytic hyperplasia is accompanied with morphologic abnormalities in many cases. The megakaryocytes are often smaller than normal, with micromegakaryocytes, and are usually mononuclear. Megakaryocyte clusters are also common. Occasionally, enlarged, hyperlobated forms can be seen.

Other bone marrow findings include mastocytosis (53), lymphocytosis (54), lymphoid aggregates (55), fibrosis (54,56–62), increased histiocytes (63,64), pseudo-Gaucher histiocytes (65), and frank hemophagocytic syndrome (66).

MYELODYSPLASTIC SYNDROMES WITH CYTOPENIAS

Refractory Anemia

RA, defined by the FAB classification as showing less than 1% peripheral blasts and less than 5% marrow blasts, is one of the

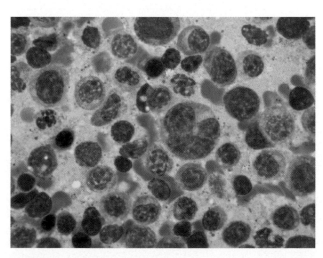

FIGURE 21-7. Erythroid hyperplasia and multilineage dysplasia is noted in this marrow aspirate (Wright stain).

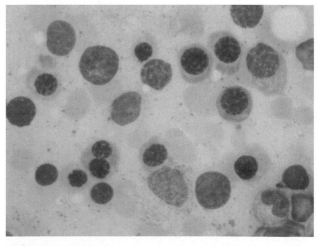

FIGURE 21-9. This smear shows considerable erythroid hyperplasia with dysplastic maturation and binucleation of a maturing cell (Wright stain).

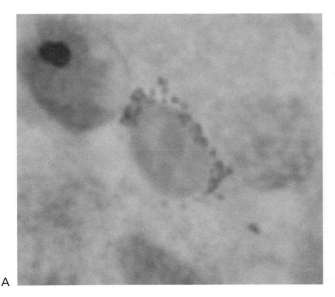
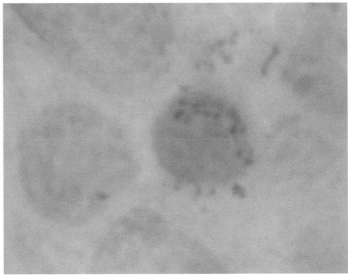

A
B

FIGURE 21-10. A, B: Two bone marrow aspirate smears demonstrate the presence of ringed sidero-blasts in refractory anemia (Prussian blue stain).

most common FAB categories of MDS (1,2). Although cases of isolated refractory thrombocytopenia and neutropenia are meant to be included in RA (by the FAB classification), they tend to be overlooked and are thus discussed separately. RA shows a highly variable extent and degree of dysplasia, ranging from subtle unilineal involvement to marked trilineal changes. The clinical course is likewise variable.

For this reason, the WHO reserves the classification of RA for cases with pure RBC dysplasia and anemia (3). Blast counts are the same as defined previously. Multiple or other isolated cytopenias are placed in separate categories (discussed later). This restriction causes RA to be relatively uncommon and often becomes a diagnosis of exclusion, given

the minimal morphologic changes. Genetic abnormalities are seen in a minority of cases (25%), and there is a protracted clinical course with a low progression to acute leukemia (approximately 6%).

Refractory Anemia with Ringed Sideroblasts

RARS is defined in both the FAB and WHO classifications by superimposing the presence of ringed sideroblasts in cases of RA. Thus, RARS shows less than 1% peripheral blasts, less than 5% marrow blasts, and numerous (>15% of erythroid precursors) marrow ringed sideroblasts (1). The ring is formed by perinuclear, iron-laden mitochondria, the

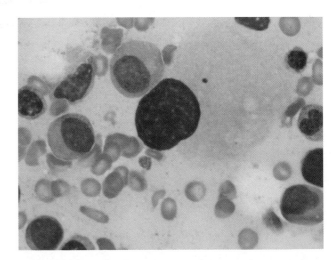

FIGURE 21-11. As seen in the peripheral blood, hypogranular pseudo–Pelger-Huët neutrophils can be identified in this bone marrow aspirate smear (Wright stain).

FIGURE 21-12. A dysplastic mononuclear megakaryocyte is centrally located in this smear. Dysmorphic erythrocytes are also noted (Wright stain).

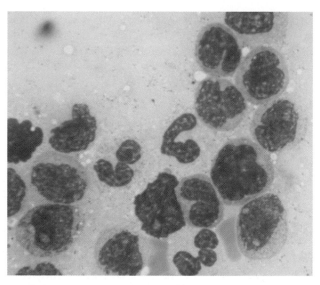

FIGURE 21-13. Dysplastic monocytes and neutrophils are seen in this aspirate from a patient with chronic myelomonocytic leukemia. These findings are similar to those seen in the peripheral blood in Figure 21-5) (Wright stain).

result of mutations in mitochondrial genes encoding oxidative enzymes (4–6). The clinical course is usually indolent, although transformation to more aggressive disease has been reported (7–9). With unilineage dysplasia (WHO classification), progression to acute leukemia occurs in approximately 1% to 2% of cases (3).

Refractory Cytopenia with Multilineage Dysplasia

RCMD, as defined by the WHO, has a low blast count like RA, but there is the presence of multiple cytopenias in the

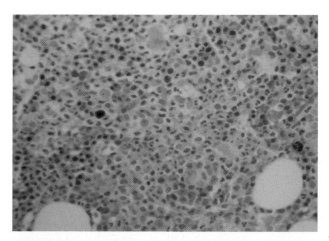

FIGURE 21-14. A classic bone marrow section from a patient with myelodysplasia. Even at this relatively low power, erythroid hyperplasia and dysplasia can be appreciated. Numerous dysplastic, small and mononuclear megakaryocytes can be seen. Abnormal localization of myeloid precursors is also present at approximately the 6-o'clock position (hematoxylin and eosin stain). (A higher power view of this is shown in Figure 21-17.)

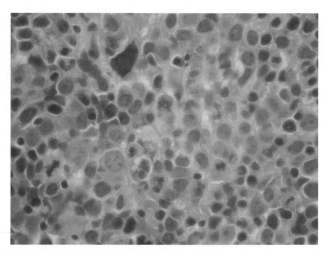

FIGURE 21-15. A higher power view of Bone marrow shown in Figure 21-14 reveals trilineage dysplasia and a lack of maturation in this patient with refractory anemia with excess blasts (hematoxylin and eosin stain).

blood, and dysplasia of two or all three cell lines within the bone marrow. This removes some of the more aggressive RA cases under the FAB classification and gives an intermediate prognosis to these patients. The presence of 15% ringed sideroblasts leads to the diagnosis of RCMD with ringed sideroblasts but is of little or no clinical significance.

In this group, approximately 50% of cases have cytogenetic abnormalities, and the overall frequency of progression to acute leukemia is approximately 11%. Marked dysplasia is associated with a prognosis between that of less dysplastic RA and RAEB (10), but patients with complex karyotypes have a survival rate similar to that of RAEB.

Refractory Anemia with Excess Blasts

RAEB, defined by both the FAB and WHO classifications as showing less than 5% peripheral blasts (most cases) and

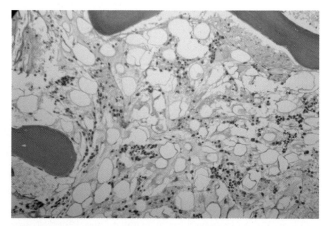

FIGURE 21-16. Hypocellular myelodysplastic syndrome is shown in this section at relatively low power. The main cellular elements are dysplastic erythroid cells and immature dysplastic myeloid cells (hematoxylin and eosin stain).

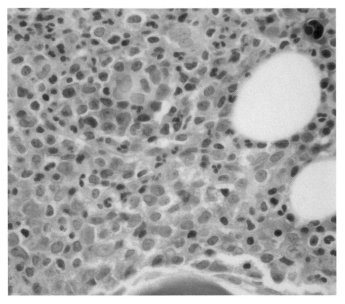

FIGURE 21-17. Abnormal localization of immature (myeloid) precursors is present in Figure (hematoxylin and eosin stain).

between 5% and 20% marrow blasts (1), accounts for many cases in adults and approximately 33% in children (11). RAEB is further subdivided by the WHO into RAEB-I and RAEB-II based on bone marrow blast counts (5% to 9% and 10% to 19%, respectively). Patients with 5% to 19% blasts in the peripheral blood or the presence of Auer rods are classified as having RAEB-II regardless of bone marrow blast count (<20%). Virtually all RAEB cases show multilineage dysplasia in both peripheral blood and bone marrow.

RAEB is not a distinct clinicopathologic syndrome but forms a seamless continuum with acute leukemia; many cases are clinically indistinguishable from overt acute leukemia (12–15). RAEB often progresses to a state showing 20% or

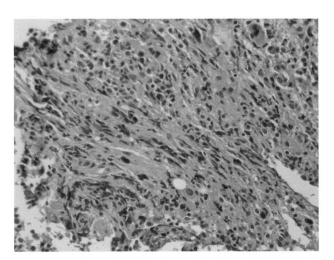

FIGURE 21-18. Early marrow fibrosis can be appreciated in this section by the cellular streaming effect. Dysplastic megakaryocytes can be identified even at this low power (hematoxylin and eosin stain).

more blasts, at which point it is diagnosed as acute leukemia by the WHO classification. Clonal cytogenetic abnormalities are found in approximately 40% of cases, and the progression to acute leukemia is 25% to 33%.

Refractory Anemia with Excess Blasts in Transformation

RAEB-T was defined by the FAB classification as showing more than 5% peripheral blasts, 20% to 30% marrow blasts, and/or Auer rods in granulocytic precursors in either the peripheral blood or marrow (1,16). The WHO criteria for acute leukemia place the cases with more than 20% blasts into the category of AML with multilineage dysplasia (17). There is no significant clinical difference between patients with 20% to 30% blasts and those with more than 30% of blasts within this subgroup of AML. Those cases of RAEB-T with less than 20% blasts but with Auer rods are placed into the RAEB-II category of the WHO classification.

5q- Syndrome

5q- syndrome refers to MDS with del(5)(q) as the sole karyotypic anomaly, a disorder that appears to represent a distinct clinicopathologic entity (3,18–23). It usually occurs in older women and often presents with severe anemia and thrombocytosis; neutropenia and thrombocytopenia are uncommon. The typical marrow findings are megaloblastic erythropoiesis, megakaryocytic hyperplasia, and monolobation of megakaryocyte nuclei. Most cases fulfill criteria for RA, but some show criteria consistent with RARS, RAEB, or RAEB-T. The differential diagnosis includes other clonal myeloid disorders with del(5q), especially those harboring cryptic t(5;11) (24) and essential thrombocythemia (19,25,26). This syndrome is associated with long-term survival and a low progression rate to acute leukemia.

Myelodysplastic Syndrome, Unclassified

MDS, unclassified, is the final category that is recognized by the WHO. It includes all other MDS that do not fall into the previous categories. Often there is unilineage dysplasia (other than anemia). Entities include refractory thrombocytopenia and refractory neutropenia. Refractory thrombocytopenia is an MDS with thrombocytopenia as the sole cytopenia (27–31). Marrow dysplasia is variable in degree and extent. Progression to acute leukemia may occur. The differential diagnosis includes immune-mediated thrombocytopenia; confusion between the two is compounded by the fact that refractory thrombocytopenia may show a transient and/or partial response to corticosteroid therapy and may occur as a complication of immune-mediated thrombocytopenia (30). Refractory neutropenia is an MDS with neutropenia as the dominant finding, a relatively rare event (32).

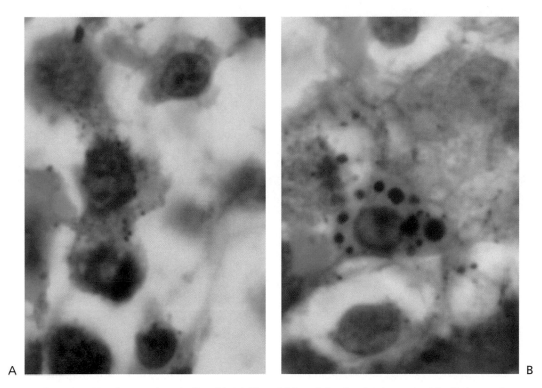

A

B

FIGURE 21-19. Abnormal periodic acid–Schiff positivity of the dysplastic erythroid cells is seen in these two biopsy specimens. A fine granular stain is seen in (**A**) compared with the course staining seen in (**B**).

Acute Myelodysplastic Syndrome with Fibrosis

Acute MDS with fibrosis, deserves a separate discussion (Fig. 21-21). It has often been reported as acute or malignant myelofibrosis or myelosclerosis; the term used here is similar to one formerly proposed (33), which duly emphasizes the primary nature of the disease as acute MDS with secondary marrow fibrosis. Acute MDS with fibrosis may arise *de novo* or as a transformation of a preexisting MDS (7,8).

It usually occurs in males and is accompanied by little or no splenomegaly (33–40). The peripheral blood shows marked cytopenias and evidence of trilineal dysplasia. The marrow is hypercellular and shows marked trilineal dysplasia, a prominent increase in atypical megakaryocytes, increased blasts (but less than 20% of cells), marked fibrosis, and variable osteosclerosis. The stromal changes are likely the result of cytokine secretion by abnormal megakaryocytes. Genetic

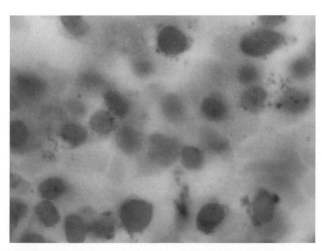

FIGURE 21-20. This bone marrow clot section shows numerous ringed sideroblasts (Prussian blue stain).

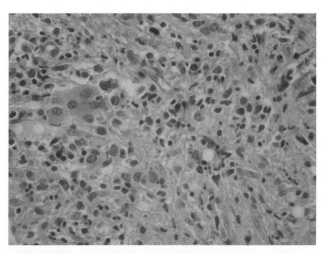

FIGURE 21-21. A bone marrow section in a case of acute myelofibrosis. Most of the cells present are dysplastic megakaryocytes and immature, dysplastic myeloid blasts.

studies usually show multiple, complex clonal anomalies. The clinical course is rapidly progressive and usually fatal, with or without eventual transformation to overt acute leukemia. The differential diagnosis includes RA with trilineage dysplasia, MPD, and acute megakaryoblastic leukemia (38,41). The WHO classification for this disorder is acute panmyelosis with myelofibrosis and is considered a rare form of AML (17).

MYELODYSPLASTIC SYNDROMES WITH INCREASED PERIPHERAL CELL COUNTS AND MYELODYSPLASTIC SYNDROMES/MYELOPROLIFERATIVE DISORDERS

MDS with increased cell counts are relatively less well-recognized than those with cytopenias. They are treated separately here to emphasize their occurrence and facilitate their distinction from MPD. The WHO classification also places some of these disorders into a separate MDS/MPD category of diseases (1) (Table 21-5).

The white blood cell (WBC) and platelet counts depend on a balance of proliferation, differentiation, and apoptosis. Cases initially showing normal (2) or low (3–6) counts may develop leukocytosis and/or thrombocytosis and vice versa. Some cases of MDS show WBC and platelet counts within the normal range (2). The actual WBC and platelet counts in a given case should not impair recognition of a disorder as MDS, and MDS cases with increased peripheral cell counts may not differ significantly from other cases of MDS in biology, morphology, or outcome.

The terminology for MDS with leukocytosis and/or thrombocytosis has been confusing and includes atypical chronic myeloid leukemia, mixed myeloproliferative-myelodysplastic syndrome (MPS/MPD), and overlap syndrome (3,4,6–9). Special terms like these are probably unnecessary for true MDS. Use of these terms as part of the WHO classification should be clearly stated as such, with strict adherence to the WHO classification criteria to avoid confusion with common MPD or other MDS.

Variants of MDS with increased peripheral cell counts are briefly discussed according to the lineage most affected.

MDS with Neutrophilia

MDS with neutrophilia has usually been reported as chronic neutrophilic leukemia, a term used in the literature for neutrophilic leukemoid reaction, a specific MPD, and MDS

TABLE 21-5. CLASSIFICATION OF MDS/MPD DISEASES ACCORDING TO THE WHO

Disease	Diagnostic Criteria
Chronic myelomonocytic leukemia	1. Persistent monocytosis >1 × 10^9/L 2. No Philadelphia chromosome or *BCR/ABL* fusion gene 3. <20% blasts (including promonocytes) in blood and bone marrow 4. Dysplasia in one or more lineages or clonal cytogenetic abnormality or monocytosis for ≥3 mo with other causes excluded
Atypical chronic myeloid leukemia	1. Leukocytosis owing to increased neutrophils 2. Prominent dysgranulopoiesis 3. No Philadelphia chromosome or *BCR/ABL* fusion gene 4. Neutrophilic precursors ≥10% of WBCs 5. Minimal basophilia (<2% of WBCs) 6. Minimal monocytosis (<10% of WBCs) 7. Hypercellular marrow with granulocytic proliferation and dysplasia 8. <20% blasts in blood and bone marrow
Juvenile myelomonocytic leukemia	1. Persistent monocytosis >1 × 10^9/L 2. No Philadelphia chromosome or *BCR/ABL* fusion gene 3. <20% blasts (including promonocytes) in blood and bone marrow 4. Two or more of the following: Hemoglobin F increased for age Immature granulocytes in the peripheral blood WBCs >10 × 10^9/L Clonal cytogenetic abnormality (including monosomy 7) Granulocyte-monocyte colony-stimulating factor hypersensitivity of myeloid progenitors *in vitro*)
Myelodysplastic/myeloproliferative disease, unclassifiable	1. Features of MDS with <20% blasts and features of MPD (i.e., increased cell counts), and no history of MDS; MPD; cytotoxic treatment; Philadelphia chromosome or *BCR/ABL* fusion gene; del(5q), t(3;3)(q21;q26) or inv(3)(q21q26) or 2. Mixed MDS/MPD features and cannot be assigned to other category of MDS, MPD or MDS/MPD

WBCs, white blood cells; MDS, myelodysplastic syndrome; MPD, myeloproliferative disease.
Adapted from Vardiman JW. Myelodysplastic/myeloproliferative diseases. In: Jaffe ES, Harris NL, Stein H, et al., eds. *World Health Organization classification of tumors: pathology and genetics of tumours of haematopoietic and lymphoid tissues.* Lyon: IARC Press, 2001:45–59.

with neutrophilia. The term MDS with neutrophilia is used here to identify clearly those cases with MDS characteristics (10–15). MDS with neutrophilia may arise *de novo* or in the course of other MDS (5). Individual cases may be classifiable according to the FAB criteria (8) as RAEB or other MDS. The WHO system classifies most of these cases as atypical chronic myeloid leukemia (1).

The peripheral blood shows neutrophilia, anemia, and thrombocytopenia. The neutrophils are clearly dysplastic, displaying many of the features previously described. RBCs may be macrocytic and show aniso- and poikilocytosis. Platelets may be morphologically abnormal. The marrow is hypercellular with increased neutrophils and precursors. Dysplastic changes may involve only the neutrophil lineage or multiple lineages. Genetic studies show clonal karyotypic anomalies characteristic of MDS; *BCR/ABL* gene rearrangement is absent. Transformation to acute leukemia is relatively common, as in other forms of MDS.

Myelodysplastic Syndrome with Monocytosis

MDS with monocytosis, with or without neutrophilia (CMML), occurs in children and adults (16–32). Other terms used for CMML include juvenile myelomonocytic leukemia (JMML) in the pediatric population, which often has monosomy 7 (monosomy 7 syndrome). The WHO system classifies these two entities separately, although there are many common features (1).

CMML is heterogeneous and forms a continuum with regard to both neutrophil and blast counts. Cases of CMML showing monocytosis without leukocytosis may be classified according to FAB criteria as RA, RA with monocytosis (2,33,34), or RAEB (2). Individual cases may progress from normal or low to increased WBC counts (2,32,33,35). By modified FAB criteria, cases with WBC counts of less than 13×10^9/L have been termed dysplastic as opposed to proliferative CMML (24); however, this division does not define separate clinicopathologic entities.

The WHO classification separates CMML into two subcategories, CMML-1 and CMML-2, based on blast counts (1). CMML-1 has less than 5% peripheral blood blasts and less than 10% bone marrow blasts (RA-type CMML). For CMML-2, the blasts count criteria are the same as for RAEB; 5% to 19% in blood and 10% to 19% in bone marrow or the presence of Auer rods with less than 20% blasts in the blood.

The peripheral blood shows monocytosis, leukocytosis (50% of cases), anemia, and thrombocytopenia. Eosinophilia may be present and is a separate subset of the WHO classification because of specific cytogenetic and clinical features (1). The granulocytes, monocytes, and myeloid precursors are dysplastic. The neutrophil (leukocyte) alkaline phosphatase score is variable and may be as low as that seen in chronic myeloid leukemia (21). RBCs are frequently macrocytic, with aniso- and poikilocytosis; nucleated

RBCs may show dysplastic nuclei. Platelets may be dysplastic. The marrow is hypercellular and shows dysplasia of granulocytes, monocytes, erythroid cells, and megakaryocytes. Clusters of monocytes may be found (29). Blasts constitute less than 20% of cells; at 20%, acute leukemia is diagnosed. Fibrosis may be present (27).

Immunologic studies show expression of granulocytic and monocytic markers. p53 Protein may be expressed (26). Genetic studies show clonal karyotypic anomalies characteristic of MDS. Isolated monosomy 7 is especially common in childhood cases (19,25,30). Rarely, t(9;22)(q34;q11) and/or *BCR/ABL* gene rearrangement may be present (must be absent according to WHO classification criteria), but other features of chronic myeloid leukemia are lacking (16,20, 23,32).

Extramedullary disease has frequently been reported in CMML. The skin is often affected, but virtually any site, including body cavities, may be involved (17,36–43). Transformation of CMML to acute leukemia occurs. The phenotype is usually myeloid but may be lymphoid (20,44,45). Other outcomes include spontaneous remission (46). The differential diagnosis includes reactive conditions (30,47–49), osteopetrosis (50), MPD (especially essential thrombocythemia and chronic myeloid leukemia) (9,51–53), and acute leukemia.

JMML is a term used for CMML (see previously) in infancy and childhood, which is strongly associated with underlying neurofibromatosis type 1 and xanthomas (54–60). Although the WHO separates this entity from CMML, there are many similarities (1). Specific diagnostic criteria are given (Table 21-4). No subclassification of JMML is recommended by the WHO as it does for CMML.

Myelodysplastic Syndrome with Eosinophilia

MDS with eosinophilia is characterized by peripheral and/or marrow eosinophilia with dysplastic eosinophils (44,51,61–77). Individual cases may be classifiable according to FAB or WHO criteria as RA (75,76), RARS (65), RAEB (72,74), or CMML (69,70,77). MDS with eosinophilia may not be distinguishable from chronic eosinophilic leukemia. The peripheral blood shows variable eosinophilia and anemia, with either thrombocytopenia or thrombocytosis. Monocytosis and/or basophilia may also be present. The marrow is hypercellular and shows increased and dysplastic eosinophils and precursors. Blasts constitute less than 20% of cells; at 20%, acute leukemia is diagnosed. Genetic studies may show t(1;5) (63), t(1;7) (64,68,51), t(2;18;2) (75), t(5;12) or variant (62,71,77), other chromosome 5 and/or 7 anomalies (61,75,76), trisomy 8 (74), inv(16) (65,69), del(16)(q22) (73), monosomy 17 (66), iso(17)(q) (74), and/or t(12;21) (76). Additional anomalies have been described in cases reported as chronic eosinophilic leukemia.

Myelodysplastic Syndrome with Basophilia

MDS with basophilia is characterized by peripheral and/or marrow basophilia with dysplastic basophils (72,78–82). Individual cases may be classifiable according to FAB or WHO criteria as RARS (78), RAEB (72,80,82), or other MDS. The peripheral blood shows basophilia, anemia, and thrombocytopenia. Eosinophilia may also be present. The marrow is hypercellular and shows increased and dysplastic basophils and precursors. Blasts constitute less than 20% of cells; at 20%, acute leukemia is diagnosed. Genetic studies show various clonal karyotypic anomalies, including t(5;12) (82).

Myelodysplastic Syndrome with Mastocytosis

MDS with mastocytosis may occur *de novo* (83) or in the course of other MDS (84). Such cases may be classifiable according to FAB or WHO criteria as RAEB (83) or other MDS. MDS with mastocytosis may not be distinguishable from chronic and/or systemic mast cell disease with MPD or MDS.

Myelodysplastic Syndrome with Thrombocytosis

MDS with thrombocytosis shows an increased platelet count rather than the usual thrombocytopenia (52,85–90). Individual cases may be classifiable according to FAB or WHO criteria as RARSs (85,87), 5q–syndrome, RAEB (72), CMML (85), or other MDS. The peripheral blood shows anemia and either leukopenia or leukocytosis. Eosinophilia may be present. The marrow is hypercellular and shows hematopoietic dysplasia, sometimes including ringed sideroblasts. Genetic studies may show 1p34 anomalies (86) or del(5q) (72,88). Differentiation of MDS with thrombocytosis from essential thrombocythemia may be difficult in some cases (51,52).

SPECIAL TYPES OF MYELODYSPLASTIC SYNDROME

Secondary Myelodysplastic Syndrome

As mentioned previously, MDS occurs both *de novo* and secondary to a known exposure to cytotoxic agents. The most common form of secondary MDS is that related to therapy for other malignant disease with cytotoxic agents or radiation (t-MDS). T-MDS is closely related and sometimes inseparable from therapy-related AML and is often included in a single diagnostic category of t-MDS/AML (1).

Patients with therapy-related disease have a high incidence of clonal cytogenetic abnormalities and fairly short overall survival. In large studies, more than 90% of patients with t-MDS/AML will show clonal cytogenetic abnormal-

ities. The vast majority involves chromosomes 5 and/or 7. Balanced translocations are also commonly identified and are usually seen in the more aggressive (AML) cases. Balanced translocations are uncommon in *de novo* MDS. Occupational and environmental exposure to toxins and radiation leads to similar cytogenetic abnormalities (2).

Myelodysplastic Syndromes in Childhood

Terminology for MDS in childhood has a complicated history. Terms used for childhood cases include JMML, juvenile chronic myeloid leukemia, and monosomy 7 syndrome, named for an isolated genetic anomaly seen in both childhood and adult MDS, which does not describe a specific clinicopathologic entity in either age category.

Current thinking divides the pediatric MDS and MPD into three main groups: MDS/MPD disorders, Down syndrome–associated disorders, and pure MDS. A recent proposal, based on international study group analysis, is patterned after the WHO classification of these disorders (Table 21-6) (3).

The MDS/MPD category uses the JMML designation for the pediatric equivalent of adult CMML. It is the most common of the MDS/MPD disorders in children and has very specific diagnostic criteria. Many of these cases are characterized by isolated monosomy 7, previously classified as a distinct syndrome. CMML classification is reserved for secondary cases only, and *BCR/ABL*-negative CML is extremely rare and may represent JMML cases.

The Down syndrome disorders are primarily leukemic in nature, although there may be MDS features (3,4). Transient abnormal myelopoiesis, also referred to as transient MPD, is increasingly recognized as a form of AML and is discussed in Chapter 19.

Pure MDS in children is similar to the adult counterparts but often lacks anemia. For this reason, the term refractory cytopenia may be more appropriate (3). Furthermore, ringed sideroblasts are extremely rare in children. The classification of RAEB is the same as in adult MDS, but subclassification based on blast count is of uncertain usefulness in the pediatric population. Similarly, the removal of RAEB-T is not recommended for pediatric MDS at this time. The presence of cytogenetic abnormalities associated with AML [e.g., t(15:17), t(8:21), inv(16), t(9:11)], however, warrant the diagnosis of AML regardless of blast count (even <20%).

Secondary MDS may also occur in childhood and is often associated with a constitutional condition (3). Conditions associated with JMML include neurofibromatosis type 1, Noonan syndrome, and trisomy 8 mosaicism. Those associated with other childhood MDS include Fanconi anemia, Kostmann syndrome, Shwachman-Diamond syndrome, and Blackfan-Diamond syndrome. Familial MDS (at least one first-degree relative with MDS/AML) is also associated with MDS in children. With the exception of Down syndrome and Fanconi anemia, MDS with constitutional

TABLE 21-6. DIAGNOSTIC CATEGORIES OF MYELODYSPLASTIC AND MYELOPROLIFERATIVE DISEASES IN CHILDREN

Category	Diseases
Myelodysplastic/myeloproliferative diseases	Juvenile myelomonocytic leukemia Chronic myelomonocytic leukemia (secondary only) *BCR/ABL*-negative chronic myeloid leukemia
Down syndrome–associated diseases	Transient abnormal myelopoiesis Myeloid leukemia of Down syndrome
Myelodysplastic syndromes	Refractory cytopenia (PB blasts, <2%; BM blasts, <5%) Refractory anemia with excess blasts (PB blasts, 2%–19% or BM blasts, 5%–19%) Refractory anemia with excess blasts in transformation (PB or BM blasts, 20%–29%)

PB, peripheral blood; BM, bone marrow.
Adapted from Hasle H, Niemeyer CM, Chessells JM, et al. A pediatric approach to the WHO classification of myelodysplastic and myeloproliferative diseases. *Leukemia* 2003;17:277—282.

abnormalities appears to behave no differently than MDS without an abnormality.

Prognostic factors and scoring systems have been proposed for pediatric MDS (5,6). The finding of increased hemoglobin F (>10%) has been repeatedly identified as a significant negative prognostic indicator. The significance of the other factors of the proposed FPC scoring system (6), platelet count, and cytogenetic abnormalities require further investigation.

Paroxysmal Nocturnal Hemoglobinuria

Paroxysmal nocturnal hemoglobinuria (PNH) is a clonal hematopoietic stem cell disorder caused by acquired mutation of *PIG-A* (7–10). The mutation occurs in a hematopoietic stem cell and is carried by all clonally derived lineages: erythroid cells, granulocytes, monocytes, megakaryocytes, and lymphocytes (11,12). *PIG-A* encodes the glycosyl phosphatidyl inositol anchor for many surface molecules. PNH is characterized by hemolysis, a consequence of glycosyl phosphatidyl inositol–anchored protein deficiencies, and thromboembolism of obscure origin. PNH occurs *de novo* and as a complication of aplastic anemia (13,14) and MDS (15–17). Conversely, transformation of PNH to aplastic anemia, MDS, and acute leukemia has often been reported (18–25). *PIG-A* mutation is present in approximately 20% of patients with aplastic anemia and MDS (14,15).

The peripheral blood cell counts may be normal but are more often decreased (26,27). Functional tests for hypersensitivity to complement-mediated lysis (Ham test, sugar-water test) are positive in full-blown PNH but may be negative in early cases (26). Bone marrow aspirate smears and sections may show megaloblastic change, erythroid hyperplasia or hypoplasia, or MDS (15,28). Reactive mastocytosis may be present (29).

Flow cytometry is much more sensitive than functional tests for complement lysis and is the preferred method of making the diagnosis of PNH (15,26,27,30,31). Immunophenotyping shows decreased expression of glycosyl phosphatidyl inositol–anchored molecules, including CD14, CD16, CD24, CD48, CD55, CD57, CD58, CD59, and CD66b. Deficiencies of these antigens vary in severity and in the lineages affected. Defective expression of the complement inhibitors CD55 and CD59 (the most commonly analyzed antigens for diagnosis) lead to the complement hypersensitivity and hemolysis for which PNH is named.

Genetic studies usually show no karyotypic anomalies unless overt MDS or acute leukemia is present (16,18–20,32). Multiple *PIG-A* mutations may occur (33,34). PNH, like MDS, may be accompanied by immune-mediated disorders (35,36) and clonal lymphoplasmacytic disease (21,37). The differential diagnosis includes a rare constitutional PNH-like disorder (38) and non-PNH hemolytic anemias.

DISORDERS ASSOCIATED WITH MYELODYSPLASTIC SYNDROMES

MDS, with either decreased or increased cell counts, is accompanied by autoimmune disorders in more than 10% of patients, owing, at least in part, to lymphoid differentiation and the production of self-reactive CD5/19-positive B cells (1–4). These disorders include arthritides, autoimmune cytopenias, connective tissue diseases (especially relapsing polychondritis), glomerulopathy, hyper- and hypogammaglobulinemia, inflammatory bowel disease, neuropathy, panniculitis, plasmacytosis, thyroiditis, and vasculitides (1–13). Other disorders accompanying MDS include acquired hemoglobinopathies (14,15), coagulopathies (16–18), nephrotic syndrome (19), sarcoidosis (20), increased hemoglobin F (especially in pediatric cases) (5,6), PNH (21), and Kaposi sarcoma (22).

Clonal B-cell, T-cell, and plasma cell disorders reported in MDS include chronic lymphocytic leukemia (23–30), Hodgkin lymphoma (31), other malignant lymphomas (23,28–32), mono- and biclonal gammopathy (30–33), multiple myeloma (23,34–36), systemic amyloidosis (33,37), T lymphoblastic lymphoma, and other T-cell lymphomas. The lymphoid and plasma cell populations in MDS may be either clonally related (2–4,36–40) or unrelated (24–26).

Histiocytic differentiation is possible in MDS (41), and Langerhans cell abnormalities have been reported (42). Histiocytic disorders reported with CMML include xanthomas (33,43–45), Langerhans cell tumor (46), and nodal histiocytic proliferation (47). As CMML involves monocytes and their derivatives, clonal identity of CMML and accompanying histiocytic lesions is possible but remains unproven.

Extramedullary disease occurs in MDS, as in other clonal hematopoietic disorders, producing solid tumors and body cavity effusions in virtually every site, but especially the skin (48–53).

REFERENCES

General Considerations

1. Aul C, Bowen DT, Yoshida Y. Pathogenesis, etiology and epidemiology of myelodysplastic syndromes. *Haematologica* 1998;83: 71–86.
2. Dansey R. Myelodysplasia. *Curr Opin Oncol* 2000;12:13–21.
3. Heaney ML, Golde DW, WHO. Critical evaluation of the World Health Organization classification of myelodysplasia and acute myeloid leukemia. *Curr Oncol Rep* 2000;2:140–143.
4. Lowenthal RM, Marsden KA. Myelodysplastic syndromes. *Int J Hematol* 1997;65:319–338.
5. Luna-Fineman S, Shannon KM, Atwater SK, et al. Myelodysplastic and myeloproliferative disorders of childhood: a study of 167 patients. *Blood* 1999;93:459–466.
6. Mielot F, Buisine J, Duchayne E, et al. Myelodysplastic syndromes in childhood: is the FAB classification relevant? Report of 81 children from a French multicentre study. French Group of Cellular Hematology. *Leuk Lymphoma* 1998;28:531–540.
7. Smith SM, Le Beau MM, Huo D, et al. Clinical-cytogenetic associations in 306 patients with therapy-related myelodysplasia and myeloid leukemia: The University of Chicago series. *Blood* 2003;102:43–52.
8. West RR, Stafford DA, White AD, et al. Cytogenetic abnormalities in the myelodysplastic syndromes and occupational or environmental exposure. *Blood* 2002;95:2093–2097.
9. Tien HF, Wang CH, Chuang SM, et al. Acute leukemic transformation of myelodysplastic syndrome—immunophenotypic, genotypic, and cytogenetic studies. *Leuk Res* 1995;19:595–603.
10. Abruzzese E, Buss D, Rainer R, et al. Progression of a myelodysplastic syndrome to pre-B acute lymphoblastic leukemia: a case report and cell lineage study. *Ann Hematol* 1996;73:35–38.
11. Dunphy CH, Kitchen S, Saravia O, et al. Acute myelofibrosis terminating in acute lymphoblastic leukemia: case report and review of the literature. *Am J Hematol* 1996;51:85–89.
12. Escudier SM, Albitar M, Robertson LE, et al. Acute lymphoblastic leukemia following preleukemic syndromes in adults. *Leukemia* 1996;10:473–477.
13. Pajor L, Matolcsy A, Vass JA, et al. Phenotypic and genotypic analyses of blastic cell population suggest that pure B-lymphoblastic leukemia may arise from myelodysplastic syndrome. *Leuk Res* 1998;22:13–17.
14. Rossbach HC, Sutcliffe MJ, Chamizo W, et al. Pre-B acute lymphoblastic leukemia in a 3-year-old boy with pre-acute myelogenous leukemia myelodysplastic syndrome: cytogenetic evidence of common early progenitor cell ontogeny. *J Pediatr Hematol Oncol* 1998;20:347–352.
15. Balduini CL, Guarnone R, Pecci A, et al. The myelodysplastic syndromes: predictive value of eight prognostic systems in 143 cases from a single institution. *Haematologica* 1999;84:12–16.
16. Greenberg PL. Risk factors and their relationship to prognosis in myelodysplastic syndromes. *Leuk Res* 1998;22[Suppl 1]:S3–S6.
17. Gupta P, Niehans GA, LeRoy SC, et al. Fas ligand expression in the bone marrow in myelodysplastic syndromes correlates with FAB subtype and anemia, and predicts survival. *Leukemia* 1999;13: 44–53.
18. Hiddemann W, Jahns-Streubel G, Verbeek W, et al. Intensive therapy for high-risk myelodysplastic syndromes and the biological significance of karyotype abnormalities. *Leuk Res* 1998;22[Suppl 1]: S23–S26.
19. Lee JJ, Kim HJ, Chung IJ, et al. Comparisons of prognostic scoring systems for myelodysplastic syndromes: a Korean multicenter study. *Leuk Res* 1999;23:425–432.
20. Lepelley P, Poulain S, Grardel N, et al. Expression of lung resistance protein and correlation with other drug resistance proteins and outcome in myelodysplastic syndromes. *Leuk Lymphoma* 1998;29:547–551.
21. Maes B, Meeus P, Michaux L, et al. Application of the International Prognostic Scoring System for myelodysplastic syndromes. *Ann Oncol* 1999;10:825–829.
22. Matsuda A, Jinnai I, Yagasaki F, et al. New system for assessing the prognosis of refractory anemia patients. *Leukemia* 1999;13:1727–1734.
23. Pfeilstocker M, Reisner R, Nosslinger T, et al. Cross-validation of prognostic scores in myelodysplastic syndromes on 386 patients from a single institution confirms importance of cytogenetics. *Br J Haematol* 1999;106:455–463.
24. Shimazaki K, Ohshima K, Suzumiya J, et al. Evaluation of apoptosis as a prognostic factor in myelodysplastic syndromes. *Br J Haematol* 2000;110:584–590.
25. Bader-Meunier B, Mielot F, Tchernia G, et al. Myelodysplastic syndromes in childhood: report of 49 patients from a French multicentre study. French Society of Paediatric Haematology and Immunology. *Br J Haematol* 1996;92:344–350.
26. Benaim E, Hvizdala EV, Papenhausen P, et al. Spontaneous remission in monosomy 7 myelodysplastic syndrome. *Br J Haematol* 1995;89:947–948.
27. Chu JY, Batanian JR, Gale GB, et al. Spontaneous resolution of myelodysplastic cytogenetic abnormality developed during the treatment of leukemia. *J Pediatr Hematol Oncol* 1998;20: 88–90.
28. Dervenoulas JG, Tsirigotis P, Bollas G, et al. Spontaneous remission in myelodysplastic syndrome. *Ann Hematol* 1999;78: 89–90.
29. Mantadakis E, Shannon KM, Singer DA, et al. Transient monosomy 7: a case series in children and review of the literature. *Cancer* 1999;85:2655–26561.
30. Renneboog B, Hansen V, Heimann P, et al. Spontaneous remission in a patient with therapy-related myelodysplastic syndrome (t-MDS) with monosomy 7. *Br J Haematol* 1996;92:696–698.

31. Scheurlen W, Borkhardt A, Ritterbach J, et al. Spontaneous hematological remission in a boy with myelodysplastic syndrome and monosomy 7. *Leukemia* 1994;8:1435–1438.

32. Tamayose K, Sugimoto K, Ando M, et al. Disappearance of chromosomal abnormalities and recovery of hematopoiesis after immunosuppressive therapy for hypoplastic refractory anemia with excess of blasts. *Blood* 2001;97:2524.

33. Samuelsson J, Larfars G. Unusual clinical presentation in a patient with myelodysplastic syndrome, with subsequent hematological remission and suppression of the malignant clone following treatment with cyclosporine A, erythropoietin and granulocyte colony-stimulating factor. *Leuk Res* 1999;23:513–517.

34. Mijovic A, Mufti GJ. The myelodysplastic syndromes: towards a functional classification. *Blood Rev* 1998;12:73–83.

35. Ramos F, Fernandez-Ferrero S, Suarez D, et al. Myelodysplastic syndrome: a search for minimal diagnostic criteria. *Leuk Res* 1999;23:283–290.

36. Vallespi T, Imbert M, Mecucci C, et al. Diagnosis, classification, and cytogenetics of myelodysplastic syndromes. *Haematologica* 1998;83:258–275.

37. Vardiman JW, Harris NL, Brunning RD. The World Health Organization (WHO) classification of the myeloid neoplasms. *Blood* 2002;100:2292–2302.

38. Bennett JM, Catovsky D, Daniel MT, et al. Proposals for the classification of the myelodysplastic syndromes. *Br J Haematol* 1982;51;189–199.

39. Greenberg P, Cox C, LeBeau MM, et al. International scoring system for evaluating prognosis in myelodysplastic syndromes. *Blood* 1997;89:2079–2088.

40. Tassin F, Dewe W, Schaaf N, et al. A four-parameter index of marrow dysplasia has predictive value for the survival in myelodysplastic syndromes. *Leuk Lymphoma* 200;36:485–496.

41. Haase D, Fonatsch C, Freund M, et al. Cytogenetic findings in 179 patients with myelodysplastic syndromes. *Ann Hematol* 1995;70:171–187.

42. Jotterand M, Parlier V. Diagnostic and prognostic significance of cytogenetics in adult primary myelodysplastic syndromes. *Leuk Lymphoma* 1996;23:253–266.

43. Mohr B, Bornhauser M, Thiede C, et al. Comparison of spectral karyotyping and conventional cytogenetics in 39 patients with acute myeloid leukemia and myelodysplastic syndrome. *Leukemia* 2000;14:1031–1038.

44. Schmetzer HM, Poleck B, Duell T, et al. Cytogenetic and Southern blot analysis to demonstrate clonality and to estimate prognosis in patients with myelodysplastic syndromes. *Ann Hematol* 2000;79:20–29.

45. Chen Z, Richkind K, Roherty S, et al. A group of previously not recognized cytogenetic abnormalities in myeloid hematological malignancies. *Cancer Genet Cytogenet* 1999;113:162–165.

46. Gancberg D, Kentos A, Dargent JL, et al. Trisomy 21 as the sole abnormality in a refractory anemia with ring sideroblasts. *Cancer Genet Cytogenet* 1999;113:180–182.

47. Hatano Y, Miura I, Nakamura T, et al. Molecular heterogeneity of the NUP98/HOXA9 fusion transcription myelodysplastic syndromes associated with t(7;11)(p15;p15). *Br J Haematol* 1999;107:600–604.

48. Keung YK, Cobos E, Tonk V, et al. Translocation (1;22) in refractory anemia and the prognostic significance of karyotypic abnormalities in refractory anemia. *Cancer Genet Cytogenet* 1998;106:72–75.

49. Martinez-Climent JA, Garcia-Conde J. Chromosomal rearrangements in childhood acute myeloid leukemia and myelodysplastic syndromes. *J Pediatr Hematol Oncol* 1999;21:91–102.

50. Mohamed AN, Varterasian ML, Dobin SM, et al. Trisomy 6 as a primary karyotypic aberration in hematologic disorders. *Cancer Genet Cytogenet* 1998;106:152–155.

51. Vasef MA, Murata-Collins JL, Alsabeh R, et al. Trisomy 14 in myelodysplastic syndromes: report of two cases and review of the literature. *Arch Pathol Lab Med* 1998;122:77–83.

52. Kikukawa M, Aoki N, Sakamoto Y, et al. Study of p53 in elderly patients with myelodysplastic syndromes by immunohistochemistry and DNA analysis. *Am J Pathol* 1999;155:717–721.

53. Acar H, Caliskan U, Cora T. Paediatric myelodysplastic syndrome (MDS) and juvenile chronic myelogenous leukaemia (JCML) detected by cytogenetic and FISH techniques. *Clin Lab Haematol* 1999;21:403–406.

54. Arif M, Tanaka K, Damodaran C, et al. Hidden monosomy 7 in acute myeloid leukemia and myelodysplastic syndrome detected by interphase fluorescence *in situ* hybridization. *Leuk Res* 1996;20:709–716.

55. Hasle H, Arico M, Basso G, et al. Myelodysplastic syndrome, juvenile myelomonocytic leukemia, and acute myeloid leukemia associated with complete or partial monosomy 7. European Working Group on MDS in Childhood (EWOG-MDS). *Leukemia* 1999;13:376–385.

56. Lessard M, Herry A, Berthou C, et al. FISH investigation of 5q and 7q deletions in MDS/AML reveals hidden translocations, insertions and fragmentations of the same chromosomes. *Leuk Res* 1998;22:303–312.

57. Pedersen B. MDS and AML with trisomy 8 as the sole chromosome aberration show different sex ratios and prognostic profiles: a study of 115 published cases. *Am J Hematol* 1997;56:224–229.

58. Villegas A, Anguita E, Gonzalez FA, et al. Occurrence of BCR-ABL rearrangement in a Philadelphia chromosome-negative patient with 5q and 13q deletions and myeloproliferative syndrome. *Cancer Genet Cytogenet* 1998;100:1–4.

59. Xue Y, Zhang R, Guo Y, et al. Acquired amegakaryocytic thrombocytopenic purpura with a Philadelphia chromosome. *Cancer Genet Cytogenet* 1993;69:51–56.

60. Chang CC, Cleveland RP. Decreased CD10-positive mature granulocytes in bone marrow from patients with myelodysplastic syndrome. *Arch Pathol Lab Med* 2000;124:1152–1156.

61. Ogata K, Nakamura K, Yokose N, et al. Clinical significance of phenotypic features of blasts in patients with myelodysplastic syndrome. *Blood* 2002;100:3887–3896.

62. Stetler-Stevenson M, Arthur DC, Jabbour N, et al. Diagnostic utility of flow cytometric immunophenotyping in myelodysplastic syndrome. *Blood* 2001;98:979–987.

63. Todd WM. Acute myeloid leukemia and related conditions. *Hematol Oncol Clin North Am* 2002;16:301–319.

64. Wells DA, Benesch M, Loken MR, et al. Myeloid and monocytic dyspoiesis as determined by flow cytometric scoring in myelodysplastic syndrome correlates with the IPSS and with outcome after hematopoietic stem cell transplantation. *Blood* 2003;102:394–403.

65. Elghetany MT. Surface marker abnormalities in myelodysplastic syndromes. *Haematologica* 1998;83:1104–1115.

66. Lambertenghi Deliliers G, Annaloro C, Soligo D, et al. The diagnostic and prognostic value of bone marrow immunostaining in myelodysplastic syndromes. *Leuk Lymphoma* 1998;28:231–239.

67. Elghetany MT, Vyas S, Yuoh G. Significance of p53 overexpression in bone marrow biopsies from patients with bone marrow failure: aplastic anemia, hypocellular refractory anemia, and hypercellular refractory anemia. *Ann Hematol* 1998;77:261–264.

68. Kikukawa M, Aoki N, Sakamoto Y, et al. Study of p53 in elderly patients with myelodysplastic syndromes by immunohistochemistry and DNA analysis. *Am J Pathol* 1999;155:717–721.

69. Baur AS, Meuge-Moraw C, Schmidt PM, et al. CD34/QBEND 10 immunostaining in bone marrow biopsies: an additional parameter for the diagnosis and classification of myelodysplastic syndromes. *Eur J Haematol* 2000;64:71–79.
70. Elghetany MT, Peterson B, MacCallum J, et al. Double esterase staining and other neutrophilic granule abnormalities in 237 patients with the myelodysplastic syndrome studied by the Cancer and Leukemia Group B. *Acta Haematol* 1998;100:13–16.
71. Elghetany MT, Peterson B, MacCallum J, et al. Deficiency of neutrophilic granule membrane glycoproteins in the myelodysplastic syndromes: a common deficiency in 216 patients studied by the Cancer and Leukemia Group B. *Leuk Res* 1997;21:801–806.

Morphologic Findings

1. Bader-Meunier B, Mielot F, Tchernia G, et al. Myelodysplastic syndromes in childhood: report of 49 patients from a French multicentre study. French Society of Paediatric Haematology and Immunology. *Br J Haematol* 1996;92:344–350.
2. Bader-Meunier B, Rieux-Laucat F, Croisille L, et al. Dyserythropoiesis associated with a Fas-deficient condition in childhood. *Br J Haematol* 2000;108:300–304.
3. Banerjee R, Halil O, Bain BJ, et al. Neutrophil dysplasia caused by mycophenolate mofetil. *Transplantation* 2000;70:1608–1610.
4. Baurmann H, Schwarz TF, Oertel J, et al. Acute Parvovirus B19 infection mimicking myelodysplastic syndrome of the bone marrow. *Ann Hematol* 1992;64:43–45.
5. Hasle H, Kerndrup G, Jacobsen BB, et al. Chronic Parvovirus infection mimicking myelodysplastic syndrome in a child with subclinical immunodeficiency. *Am J Pediatr Hematol Oncol* 1994;16:329–333.
6. Hirose M, Taguchi Y, Makimoto A, et al. New variant of congenital dyserythropoietic anemia with trilineage myelodysplasia. *Acta Haematol* 1995;94:102–104.
7. Katsarou O, Terpos E, Patsouris E, et al. Myelodysplastic features in patients with long-term HIV infection and haemophilia. *Haemophilia* 2001;7:47–52.
8. Miyahara M, Shimamoto Y, Yamada H, et al. Cytomegalovirus-associated myelodysplasia and thrombocytopenia in an immunocompetent adult. *Ann Hematol* 1997;74:99–101.
9. Rinn R, Chow WS, Pinkerton PH. Transient acquired myelodysplasia associated with Parvovirus B19 infection in a patient with congenital spherocytosis. *Am J Hematol* 1995;50:71–72.
10. Tchernia G, Bader-Meunier B, Lavergne JM, et al. Myelodysplasia in childhood may be a polyclonal disease. *Hematol Cell Ther* 1996;38:325–330.
11. Wollman MR, Penchansky L, Shekhter-Levin S. Transient 7q- in association with megaloblastic anemia due to dietary folate and vitamin B12 deficiency. *J Pediatr Hematol Oncol* 1996;18:162–165.
12. Ko WS, Chen LM, Chao TY, et al. Myeloblastic leukemoid reaction in paroxysmal nocturnal hemoglobinuria associated with myelodysplasia. *Acta Haematol* 1992;87:75–77.
13. Meyerson HJ, Farhi DC, Rosenthal NS. Transient increase in blasts mimicking acute leukemia and progressing myelodysplasia in patients receiving growth factor. *Am J Clin Pathol* 1998;109:675–681.
14. Scagni P, Saracco P, Timeus F, et al. Use of recombinant granulocyte colony-stimulating factor in Fanconi's anemia. *Haematologica* 1998;83:432–437.
15. Goyal R, Qawi H, Ali I, et al. Biologic characteristics of patients with hypocellular myelodysplastic syndromes. *Leuk Res* 1999;23:357–364.
16. Jameel T, Anwar M, Abdi SI, et al. Aplastic anemia or aplastic preleukemic syndrome? *Ann Hematol* 1997;75:189–193.
17. Jonasova A, Neuwirtova R, Cermak J, et al. Cyclosporin A therapy in hypoplastic MDS patients and certain refractory anaemias without hypoplastic bone marrow. *Br J Haematol* 1998;100:304–309.
18. Maschek H, Kaloutsi V, Rodriguez-Kaiser M, et al. Hypoplastic myelodysplastic syndrome: incidence, morphology, cytogenetics, and prognosis. *Ann Hematol* 1993;66:117–122.
19. Orazi A, Albitar M, Heerema NA, et al. Hypoplastic myelodysplastic syndromes can be distinguished from acquired aplastic anemia by CD34 and PCNA immunostaining of bone marrow biopsy specimens. *Am J Clin Pathol* 1997;107:268–274.
20. Otawa M, Kawanishi Y, Iwase O, et al. Comparative multi-color flow cytometric analysis of cell surface antigens in bone marrow hematopoietic progenitors between refractory anemia and aplastic anemia. *Leuk Res* 2000;24:359–366.
21. Tuzuner N, Cox C, Rowe JM, et al. Hypocellular myelodysplastic syndromes (MDS): new proposals. *Br J Haematol* 1995;91:612–617.
22. Bader-Meunier B, Mielot F, Breton-Gorius J, et al. Hematologic involvement in mitochondrial cytopathies in childhood: a retrospective study of bone marrow smears. *Pediatr Res* 1999;46:158–162.
23. Bazarbachi A, Muakkit S, Ayas M, et al. Thiamine-responsive myelodysplasia. *Br J Haematol* 1998;102:1098–1100.
24. Chan GC, Head DR, Wang WC. Refractory anemia with ringed sideroblasts in children: two diseases with a similar phenotype? *J Pediatr Hematol Oncol* 1999;21:418–423.
25. Cotter PD, May A, Fitzsimons EJ, et al. Late-onset X-linked sideroblastic anemia. Missense mutations in the erythroid delta-aminolevulinate synthase (ALAS2) gene in two pyridoxine-responsive patients initially diagnosed with acquired refractory anemia and ringed sideroblasts. *J Clin Invest* 1995;96:2090–2096.
26. Cotter PD, May A, Li L, et al. Four new mutations in the erythroid-specific 5-aminolevulinate synthase (ALAS2) gene causing X-linked sideroblastic anemia: increased pyridoxine responsiveness after removal of iron overload by phlebotomy and coinheritance of hereditary hemochromatosis. *Blood* 1999;93:1757–1769.
27. Demiroglu H, Dundar S. Vitamin B6 responsive sideroblastic anaemia in a patient with tuberculosis. *Br J Clin Pract* 1997;51:51–52.
28. Fiske DN, McCoy HE 3rd, Kitchens CS. Zinc-induced sideroblastic anemia: report of a case, review of the literature, and description of the hematologic syndrome. *Am J Hematol* 1994;46:147–150.
29. Harigae H, Furuyama K, Kudo K, et al. A novel mutation of the erythroid-specific gamma-aminolevulinate synthase gene in a patient with non-inherited pyridoxine-responsive sideroblastic anemia. *Am J Hematol* 1999;62:112–114.
30. Inbal A, Avissar N, Shaklai M, et al. Myopathy, lactic acidosis, and sideroblastic anemia: a new syndrome. *Am J Med Genet* 1995;55:372–378.
31. Jackson N, Hamizah I. Sideroblastic anemia recurring during two pregnancies. *Int J Hematol* 1996;65:85–88.
32. Kardos G, Veerman AJ, de Waal FC, et al. Familial sideroblastic anemia with emergence of monosomy 5 and myelodysplastic syndrome. *Med Pediatr Oncol* 1996;26:54–56.
33. Lynch SA, de Berker D, Lehmann AR, et al. Trichothiodystrophy with sideroblastic anaemia and developmental delay. *Arch Dis Child* 1995;73:249–251.
34. May A, Bishop DF. The molecular biology and pyridoxine responsiveness of X-linked sideroblastic anaemia. *Haematologica* 1998;83:56–70.

35. Perry AR, Pagliuca A, Fitzsimons EJ, et al. Acquired sideroblastic anaemia induced by a copper-chelating agent. *Int J Hematol* 1996;64:69–72.

36. Smith OP, Hann IM, Woodward CE, et al. Pearson's marrow/pancreas syndrome: haematological features associated with deletion and duplication of mitochondrial DNA. *Br J Haematol* 1995;90:469–472.

37. Soliman AT, Bappal B, Darwish A, et al. Growth hormone deficiency and empty sella in DIDMOAD syndrome: an endocrine study. *Arch Dis Child* 1995;73:251–253.

38. Tuckfield A, Ratnaike S, Hussein S, et al. A novel form of hereditary sideroblastic anaemia with macrocytosis. *Br J Haematol* 1997;97:279–285.

39. Abe Y, Hirase N, Muta K, et al. Adult onset cyclic hematopoiesis in a patient with myelodysplastic syndrome. *Int J Hematol* 2000;71:40–45.

40. Crown JP, Jhanwar S, Haimi J, et al. Acquired cyclic haematopoiesis associated with a radiation-induced chromosomal abnormality with clonal, morphologically normal circulating leucocytes. *Acta Haematol* 1991;86:103–106.

41. Pavord S, Sivakumaran M, Furber P, et al. Cyclical thrombocytopenia as a rare manifestation of myelodysplastic syndrome. *Clin Lab Haematol* 1996;18:221–223.

42. Hartz JW, Buss DH, White DR, et al. Marked elliptocytosis and schistocytosis in hematopoietic dysplasia. *Am J Clin Pathol* 1984;82:354–359.

43. Ideguchi H, Yamada Y, Kondo S, et al. Abnormal erythrocyte band 4.1 protein in myelodysplastic syndrome with elliptocytosis. *Br J Haematol* 1993;85:387–392.

44. Ishida F, Shimodaira S, Kobayashi H, et al. Elliptocytosis in myelodysplastic syndrome associated with translocation (1;5) (p10;q10) and deletion of 20q. *Cancer Genet Cytogenet* 1999;108:162–165.

45. Carulli G, Marini A, Azzara A, et al. Pseudoreticulocytosis in a case of myelodysplastic syndrome. *Acta Haematol* 1998;100:156–158.

46. de Pree C, Cabrol C, Frossard JL, et al. Pseudoreticulocytosis in a case of myelodysplastic syndrome with translocation t(1;14) (q42;q32). *Semin Hematol* 1995;32:232–236.

47. Sher GD, Pinkerton PH, Ali MA, et al. Myelodysplastic syndrome with prolonged reticulocyte survival mimicking hemolytic disease. *Am J Clin Pathol* 1994;101:149–153.

48. Cohen AM, Alexandrova S, Bessler H, et al. Ultrastructural observations on bone marrow cells of 26 patients with myelodysplastic syndromes. *Leuk Lymphoma* 1997;27:165–172.

49. Kuyama J, Fushino M, Take H, et al. Myelodysplastic syndrome associated with erythrophagocytosis by blasts and myeloid cells. *Int J Hematol* 1995;62:243–246.

50. De Wolf-Peeters C, Stessens R, Desmet V, et al. The histological characterization of ALIP in the myelodysplastic syndromes. *Pathol Res Pract* 1986;181:402–407.

51. Lambertenghi Deliliers G, Annaloro C, Soligo D, et al. The diagnostic and prognostic value of bone marrow immunostaining in myelodysplastic syndromes. *Leuk Lymphoma* 1998;28:231–239.

52. Mongkonsritragoon W, Letendre L, Qian J, et al. Nodular lesions of monocytic component in myelodysplastic syndrome. *Am J Clin Pathol* 1998;110:154–162.

53. Prokocimer M, Polliack A. Increased bone marrow mast cells in preleukemic syndromes, acute leukemia, and lymphoproliferative disorders. *Am J Clin Pathol* 1981;75:34–38.

54. Gottlieb CA, Maeda K, Hawley RC, et al. Myelodysplasia with bone marrow lymphocytosis and fibrosis mimicking recurrent Hodgkin's disease. *Am J Clin Pathol* 1989;91:6–11.

55. Mongkonsritragoon W, Letendre L, Li CY. Multiple lymphoid nodules in bone marrow have the same clonality as underlying myelodysplastic syndrome recognized with fluorescent *in situ* hybridization technique. *Am J Hematol* 1998;59:252–257.

56. Guenova M, Taskov H, Zechev J. CD4+ acute undifferentiated leukaemia, probably early monoblastic type, developing in a patient with myelodysplastic syndrome and bone marrow fibrosis. *Leuk Lymphoma* 1997;26:399–403.

57. Imbert M, Nguyen D, Sultan C. Myelodysplastic syndromes (MDS) and acute myeloid leukemias (AML) with myelofibrosis. *Leuk Res* 1992;16:51–54.

58. Kamei S, Shinohara K, Oeda E. Myelodysplastic syndrome associated with myelofibrosis, a report of 3 cases. *Intern Med* 1993;32:668–671.

59. Maschek H, Georgii A, Kaloutsi V, et al. Myelofibrosis in primary myelodysplastic syndromes: a retrospective study of 352 patients. *Eur J Haematol* 1992;48:208–214.

60. Sahu S, Shah SS, Srivastava A, et al. Pediatric hyperfibrotic myelodysplasia: an unusual clinicopathologic entity. *Pediatric Hematol Oncol* 1997;14:133–139.

61. Suvajdzic N, Marisavljevic D, Jovanovic V, et al. Pure red cell aplasia evolving through the hyperfibrotic myelodysplastic syndrome to the acute myeloid leukemia: some pathogenetic aspects. *Hematol Cell Ther* 1999;41:27–29.

62. Verhoef GE, De Wolf-Peeters C, Ferrant A, et al. Myelodysplastic syndromes with bone marrow fibrosis: a myelodysplastic disorder with proliferative features. *Ann Hematol* 1991;63:235–241.

63. Kitagawa M, Kamiyama R, Kasuga T. Increase in number of bone marrow macrophages in patients with myelodysplastic syndromes. *Eur J Haematol* 1993;51:56–58.

64. Reza S, Dar S, Andric T, et al. Biologic characteristics of 164 patients with myelodysplastic syndromes. *Leuk Lymphoma* 1999;33:281–287.

65. Stewart AJ, Jones RD. Pseudo-Gaucher cells in myelodysplasia. *J Clin Pathol* 1999;52:917–918.

66. Karasuno T, Teshima H, Hiraoka A, et al. Successful bone marrow transplantation in an adult patient with reactive hemophagocytic syndrome associated with myelodysplastic syndrome. *Int J Hematol* 2000;71:180–183.

Myelodysplastic Syndromes with Cytopenias

1. Bennett JM, Catovsky D, Daniel MT, et al. Proposals for the classification of the myelodysplastic syndromes. *Br J Haematol* 1982;51:189–199.

2. Bauduer F, Ducout L, Dastugue N, et al. Epidemiology of myelodysplastic syndromes in a French general hospital of the Basque country. *Leuk Res* 1998;22:205–208.

3. Brunning RD, Bennett JM, Flandrin G, et al. Myelodysplastic syndromes. In: Jaffe ES, Harris NL, Stein H, et al., eds. *World Health Organization classification of tumors: pathology and genetics of tumours of haematopoietic and lymphoid tissues.* Lyon: IARC Press, 2001:61–74.

4. Broker S, Meunier B, Rich P, et al. MtDNA mutations associated with sideroblastic anaemia cause a defect of mitochondrial cytochrome c oxidase. *Eur J Biochem* 1998;258:132–138.

5. Gattermann N. From sideroblastic anemia to the role of mitochondrial DNA mutations in myelodysplastic syndromes. *Leuk Res* 2000;24:141–151.

6. Wang YL, Choi HK, Aul C, et al. The MERRF mutation of mitochondrial DNA in the bone marrow of a patient with acquired idiopathic sideroblastic anemia. *Am J Hematol* 1999;60:83–84.

7. Bested AC, Cheng G, Pinkerton PH, et al. Idiopathic acquired

sideroblastic anaemia transforming to acute myelosclerosis. *J Clin Pathol* 1984;37:1032–1034.

8. Butler WM, Taylor HG, Viswanathan U. Idiopathic acquired sideroblastic anemia terminating in acute myelosclerosis. *Cancer* 1982;49:2497–2499.

9. Hattori M, Tanaka M, Yamazaki Y, et al. Detection of major and minor bcr/abl fusion gene transcripts in a patient with acute undifferentiated leukemia secondary to treatment with an alkylating agent. *Leuk Res* 1995;19:389–396.

10. Matsuda A, Jinnai I, Yagasaki F, et al. Refractory anemia with severe dysplasia: clinical significance of morphological features in refractory anemia. *Leukemia* 1998;12:482–485.

11. Hasle H, Kerndrup G, Jacobsen BB. Childhood myelodysplastic syndrome in Denmark: incidence and predisposing conditions. *Leukemia* 1995;9:1569–1572.

12. Bernstein SH, Brunetto VL, Davey FR, et al. Acute myeloid leukemia-type chemotherapy for newly diagnosed patients without antecedent cytopenias having myelodysplastic syndrome as defined by French-American-British criteria: a Cancer and Leukemia Group B Study. *J Clin Oncol* 1996;14:2486–2494.

13. Chan GC, Wang WC, Raimondi SC, et al. Myelodysplastic syndrome in children: differentiation from acute myeloid leukemia with a low blast count. *Leukemia* 1997;11:206–211.

14. Estey E, Thall P, Beran M, et al. Effect of diagnosis (refractory anemia with excess blasts, refractory anemia with excess blasts in transformation, or acute myeloid leukemia [AML]) on outcome of AML-type chemotherapy. *Blood* 1997;90:2969–2977.

15. Guerci AP, Feldmann L, Humbert JC, et al. Refractory anemia with excess of blasts: a multivariate analysis of prognostic factors in 91 patients and a simplified scoring system for predicting survival. *Eur J Haematol* 1995;54:241–244.

16. Weisdorf DJ, Oken MM, Johnson GJ, et al. Auer rod positive dysmyelopoietic syndrome. *Am J Hematol* 1981;11:397–402.

17. Brunning RD, Matutes E, Harris NL, et al. Acute myeloid leukaemias. In: Jaffe ES, Harris NL, Stein H, et al., eds. *World Health Organization classification of tumors: pathology and genetics of tumours of haematopoietic and lymphoid tissues.* Lyon: IARC Press, 2001:75–107.

18. Jaju RJ, Boultwood J, Oliver FJ, et al. Molecular cytogenetic delineation of the critical deleted region in the 5q- syndrome. *Genes Chromosomes Cancer* 1998;22:251–256.

19. Koike T, Uesugi Y, Toba K, et al. 5q- Syndrome presenting as essential thrombocythemia: myelodysplastic syndrome or chronic myeloproliferative disorders? *Leukemia* 1995;9:517–518.

20. Lewis S, Oscier D, Boultwood J, et al. Hematological features of patients with myelodysplastic syndromes associated with a chromosome 5q deletion. *Am J Hematol* 1995;49:194–200.

21. Mathew P, Tefferi A, Dewald GW, et al. The 5q- syndrome: a single-institution study of 43 consecutive patients. *Blood* 1993;81:1040–1045.

22. Nilsson L, Astrand-Grundstrom I, Arvidsson I, et al. Isolation and characterization of hematopoietic progenitor/stem cells in 5q-deleted myelodysplastic syndromes: evidence for involvement at the hematopoietic stem cell level. *Blood* 2000;96:2012–2021.

23. Pedersen B. Anatomy of the 5q- deletion: different sex ratios and deleted 5q bands in MDS and AML. *Leukemia* 1996;10:1883–1890.

24. Jaju RJ, Haas OA, Neat M, et al. A new recurrent translocation, t(5;11)(q35;p15.5), associated with del(5q) in childhood acute myeloid leukemia. The UK Cancer Cytogenetics Group. *Blood* 1999;94:773–780.

25. Reis MD, Sher GD, Lakhani A, et al. Deletion of the long arm of chromosome 5 in essential thrombocythemia. *Cancer Genet Cytogenet* 1992;61:93–95.

26. Takahashi H, Furukawa T, Hashimoto S, et al. 5q- Syndrome pre-

senting chronic myeloproliferative disorders-like manifestation: a case report. *Am J Hematol* 2000;64:120–123.

27. Menke DM, Colon-Otero G, Cockerill KJ, et al. Refractory thrombocytopenia. A myelodysplastic syndrome that may mimic immune thrombocytopenic purpura. *Am J Clin Pathol* 1992;98:502–510.

28. Najean Y, Lecompte T. Chronic pure thrombocytopenia in elderly patients: an aspect of the myelodysplastic syndrome. *Cancer* 1989;64:2506–2510.

29. Ridell B, Kutti J, Swolin B, et al. Dysplastic megakaryopoiesis with thrombocytopenia and chromosomal aberration. *Am J Clin Pathol* 1992;98:227–230.

30. Samuelsson J, Larfars G. Unusual clinical presentation in a patient with myelodysplastic syndrome, with subsequent hematological remission and suppression of the malignant clone following treatment with cyclosporine A, erythropoietin and granulocyte colony-stimulating factor. *Leuk Res* 1999;23:513–517.

31. Tricot G, Criel A, Verwilghen RL. Thrombocytopenia as presenting symptom of preleukaemia in 3 patients. *Scand J Haematol* 1982;28:243–250.

32. Auner HW, Klintschar M, Crevenna R, et al. Two case studies of chronic idiopathic neutropenia preceding acute myeloid leukaemia. *Br J Haematol* 1999;105:431–433.

33. Sultan C, Sigaux F, Imbert M, et al. Acute myelodysplasia with myelofibrosis: a report of eight cases. *Br J Haematol* 1981;49:11–16.

34. Allen EF, Lunde JH, McNally R, et al. A case of acute myelofibrosis with complex karyotypic changes: a type of myelodysplastic syndrome. *Cancer Genet Cytogenet* 1996;90:24–28.

35. Bearman RM, Pangalis GA, Rappaport H. Acute ("malignant") myelosclerosis. *Cancer* 1979;43:279–293.

36. Clare N, Elson D, Manhoff L. Cytogenetic studies of peripheral myeloblasts and bone marrow fibroblasts in acute myelofibrosis. *Am J Clin Pathol* 1982;77:762–766.

37. Das S, Prabhakar BR. Acute myelofibrosis. *Ind J Pathol Microbiol* 1997;40:527–530.

38. Hruban RH, Kuhajda FP, Mann RB. Acute myelofibrosis: immunohistochemical study of four cases and comparison with acute megakaryocytic leukemia. *Am J Clin Pathol* 1987;88:578–588.

39. Oyen WJ, Raemaekers JM, Corstens FH. Acute myelofibrosis mimicking multiple bone metastases on Tc-99m MDP bone imaging. *Clin Nucl Med* 1998;23:1–2.

40. Truong LD, Saleem A, Schwartz MR. Acute myelofibrosis: a report of four cases and review of the literature. *Medicine* 1984;63:182–187.

41. Bain BJ, Catovsky D, O'Brien M, et al. Megakaryoblastic leukemia presenting as acute myelofibrosis—a study of four cases with the platelet-peroxidase reaction. *Blood* 1981;58:206–213.

Myelodysplastic Syndromes with Increased Peripheral Cell Counts and Myelodysplastic Syndromes/Myeloproliferative Disorders

1. Vardiman JW. Myelodysplastic/myeloproliferative diseases. In: Jaffe ES, Harris NL, Stein H, et al., eds. *World Health Organization classification of tumors: pathology and genetics of tumours of haematopoietic and lymphoid tissues.* Lyon: IARC Press, 2001:45–59.

2. Rigolin GM, Cuneo A, Roberti MG, et al. Myelodysplastic syndromes with monocytic component: hematologic and cytogenetic characterization. *Haematologica* 1997;82:25–30.

3. Neuwirtova R, Mocikova K, Musilova J, et al. Mixed myelodysplastic and myeloproliferative syndromes. *Leuk Res* 1996;20: 717–726.

4. Oscier DG. Atypical chronic myeloid leukaemia, a distinct clinical entity related to the myelodysplastic syndrome? *Br J Haematol* 1996;92:582–586.

5. Pascucci M, Dorion P, Makary A, et al. Chronic neutrophilic leukemia evolving from a myelodysplastic syndrome. *Acta Haematol* 1997;98:163–166.

6. Tefferi A, Inwards DJ, Hoyer JD. Spontaneous remission of anemia associated with a myelodysplastic syndrome with disease evolution into a myeloproliferative state. *Acta Haematol* 1999;101:50–52.

7. Bain BJ. The relationship between the myelodysplastic syndromes and the myeloproliferative disorders. *Leuk Lymphoma* 1999;34:443–449.

8. Bennett JM, Catovsky D, Daniel MT, et al. Proposals for the classification of the myelodysplastic syndromes. *Br J Haematol* 1992;51:189–199.

9. Bennett JM, Catovsky D, Daniel MT, et al. The chronic myeloid leukaemias: guidelines for distinguishing chronic granulocytic, atypical chronic myeloid, and chronic myelomonocytic leukaemia: proposals by the French-American-British Cooperative Leukaemia Group. *Br J Haematol* 1994;87:746–754.

10. Kojima K, Yasukawa M, Hara M, et al. Familial occurrence of chronic neutrophilic leukaemia. *Br J Haematol* 1999;105: 428–430.

11. Matano S, Nakamura S, Kobayashi K, et al. Deletion of the long arm of chromosome 20 in a patient with chronic neutrophilic leukemia: cytogenetic findings in chronic neutrophilic leukemia. *Am J Hematol* 1997;54:72–75.

12. Ota S, Tanaka J, Kobayashi S, et al. Evolution to acute myeloblastic leukemia from chronic neutrophilic leukemia with dysplastic features in granulocytic lineage. *Acta Haematol* 2000;104: 207–211.

13. Takamatsu Y, Kondo S, Inoue M, et al. Chronic neutrophilic leukemia with dysplastic features mimicking myelodysplastic syndromes. *Int J Hematol* 1996;63:65–69.

14. Terre C, Garcia I, Bastie JN, et al. A case of chronic neutrophilic leukemia with deletion (11)(q23). *Cancer Genet Cytogenet* 1999;110:70–71.

15. Tohda S, Koyama N, Tanaka M, et al. A case of atypical chronic myeloid leukemia regarded as MDS with myeloproliferative features. *Acta Haematol* 1998;100:191–194.

16. Acar H, Caliskan U, Cora T. Paediatric myelodysplastic syndrome (MDS) and juvenile chronic myelogenous leukaemia (JCML) detected by cytogenetic and FISH techniques. *Clin Lab Haematol* 1999;21:403–406.

17. Aul C, Gattermann N, Germing U, et al. Fatal hyperleukocytic syndrome in a patient with chronic myelomonocytic leukemia. *Leuk Res* 1997;21:249–253.

18. Cambier N, Baruchel A, Schlageter MH, et al. Chronic myelomonocytic leukemia: from biology to therapy. *Hematol Cell Ther* 1997;39:41–48.

19. Cotter FE. Childhood myeloproliferative disorders. *Baillieres Clin Haematol* 1998;11:875–898.

20. Dautel MM, Francois S, Bertheas MF, et al. Successive transformation of chronic myelomonocytic leukaemia into acute myeloblastic then lymphoblastic leukaemia, both with minor-bcr rearrangement. *Br J Haematol* 1997;98:210–212.

21. Farhi DC, Luckey CN, Siddiqui AM. Breakpoint cluster region, immunoglobulin, and T-cell receptor gene rearrangement analysis in juvenile chronic myelogenous leukemia. *Mod Pathol* 1995;8:389–393.

22. Fugazza G, Bruzzone R, Dejana AM, et al. Cytogenetic clonality in chronic myelomonocytic leukemia studied with fluorescence in situ hybridization. *Leukemia* 1995;9:109–114.

23. Garay CA, Al-Saleem T, Testa JR, et al. Coexisting myelodysplasia and myeloproliferative features in a single clone containing 5q-, Ph and i(17q). *Leuk Res* 1999;23:965–967.

24. Germing U, Gattermann N, Minning H, et al. Problems in the classification of CMML—dysplastic versus proliferative type. *Leuk Res* 1998;22:871–878.

25. Hasle H, Arico M, Basso G, et al. Myelodysplastic syndrome, juvenile myelomonocytic leukemia, and acute myeloid leukemia associated with complete or partial monosomy 7. European Working Group on MDS in Childhood (EWOG-MDS). *Leukemia* 1999;13:376–385.

26. Kikukawa M, Aoki N, Sakamoto Y, et al. Study of p53 in elderly patients with myelodysplastic syndromes by immunohistochemistry and DNA analysis. *Am J Pathol* 1999;155:717–721.

27. Krishnan K, Sheldon S. A new translocation, t(3;6)(q12;24) associated with chronic myelomonocytic leukaemia and marrow fibrosis. *Clin Lab Haematol* 1996;18:47–49.

28. Misialek MJ, Pechet L. A diagnostic dilemma: chronic myelomonocytic leukemia versus atypical chronic myeloid leukemia. A case report and review of the literature. *Acta Haematol* 1997; 98:221–227.

29. Mongkonsritragoon W, Letendre L, Qian J, et al. Nodular lesions of monocytic component in myelodysplastic syndrome. *Am J Clin Pathol* 1998;110:154–162.

30. Niemeyer CM, Arico M, Basso G, et al. Chronic myelomonocytic leukemia in childhood: a retrospective analysis of 110 cases. European Working Group on Myelodysplastic Syndromes in Childhood (EWOG-MDS). *Blood* 1997;89:3534–3543.

31. Novitzky N. Myelodysplastic syndromes in children. A critical review of the clinical manifestations and management. *Am J Hematol* 2000;63:212–222.

32. Roumier C, Daudignon A, Soenen V, et al. p190 bcr-abl rearrangement: a secondary cytogenetic event in some chronic myeloid disorders? *Haematologica* 1999;84:1075–1080.

33. Yavorkovsky LL, Zain J, Wu CD, et al. Monocytic leukemia cutis diagnosed simultaneously with refractory anemia with monocytosis: a case report. *Am J Hematol* 2001;66:120–122.

34. Horton YM, Johnson PR. Trisomy 14 in myeloid malignancies: report of two cases and review of the literature. *Cancer Genet Cytogenet* 2001;124:172–174.

35. Shirota T, Hayashi O, Uchida H, et al. Myelodysplastic syndrome associated with relapsing polychondritis: unusual transformation from refractory anemia to chronic myelomonocytic leukemia. *Ann Hematol* 1993;67:45–47.

36. Vadillo M, Jucgla A, Podzamczer D, et al. Pyoderma gangrenosum with liver, spleen and bone involvement in a patient with chronic myelomonocytic leukaemia. *Br J Dermatol* 1999;141: 541–543.

37. Bourantas KL, Tsiara S, Panteli A, et al. Pleural effusion in chronic myelomonocytic leukaemia. *Acta Haematol* 1998;99:34–37.

38. Braga D, Manganoni AM, Boccaletti V, et al. Specific skin infiltration as first sign of chronic myelomonocytic leukemia with an unusual phenotype. *J Am Acad Dermatol* 1996;35:804–807.

39. Hancock JC, Prchal JT, Bennett JM, et al. Trilineage extramedullary myeloid cell tumor in myelodysplastic syndrome. *Arch Pathol Lab Med* 1997;121:520–523.

40. Horiuchi Y, Masuzawa M, Nozaki O, et al. Unusual cutaneous lesions associated with chronic myelomonocytic leukaemia. *Clin Exp Dermatol* 1992;17:121–124.

41. Lieutaud T, Mejean A, Prayssac P, et al. Renal and adrenal gland localization of chronic myelomonocytic leukemia presenting as a kidney tumor. *Leuk Lymphoma* 1999;34:405–408.

42. Saxena A, Saidman B, Greenwald D, et al. Testicular

extramedullary myeloid cell tumor in a patient with myelodysplastic syndrome. *Arch Pathol Lab Med* 1996;120:389–392.

43. Sires UI, Mallory SB, Hess JL, et al. Cutaneous presentation of juvenile chronic myelogenous leukemia: a diagnostic and therapeutic dilemma. *Pediatr Dermatol* 1995;12:364–368.

44. Follows GA, Owen RG, Ashcroft AJ, et al. Eosinophilic myelodysplasia transforming to acute lymphoblastic leukaemia. *J Clin Pathol* 1999;52:388–389.

45. Kouides PA, Bennett JM. Transformation of chronic myelomonocytic leukemia to acute lymphoblastic leukemia: case report and review of the literature of lymphoblastic transformation of myelodysplastic syndrome. *Am J Hematol* 1995;49:157–162.

46. Fukuda M, Horibe K, Miyajima Y, et al. Spontaneous remission of juvenile chronic myelomonocytic leukemia in an infant with Noonan syndrome. *J Pediatr Hematol Oncol* 1997;19:177–179.

47. Arico M, Biondi A, Pui C-H. Differentiating juvenile myelomonocytic leukemia from infectious disease: response. *Blood* 1998;91:365.

48. Herrod HG, Dow LW, Sullivan JL. Persistent Epstein-Barr virus infection mimicking juvenile chronic myelogenous leukemia: immunologic and hematologic studies. *Blood* 1983;61:1098–1104.

49. Niemeyer CM, Fenu S, Hasle H, et al. Differentiating juvenile myelomonocytic leukemia from infectious disease: response. *Blood* 1998;91:365–367.

50. Toren A, Neumann Y, Meyer JJ, et al. Malignant osteopetrosis manifested as juvenile chronic myeloid leukemia. *Pediatr Hematol Oncol* 1993;10:187–189.

51. Yamada T, Tsurumi H, Murakami N, et al. Werner's syndrome developing acute megakaryoblastic leukemia with der(1;7). *Rinsho Ketsueki* 1997;38:28–32.

52. Takahashi H, Furukawa T, Hashimoto S, et al. 5q− syndrome presenting chronic myeloproliferative disorders-like manifestation: a case report. *Am J Hematol* 2000;64:120–123.

53. Mahon FX, Labouyrie E, Aurich-Costa J, et al. Philadelphia negative BCR-ABL positive chronic myeloid leukemia mimicking juvenile chronic myeloid leukemia in a 2-year-old child. *Leuk Lymphoma* 1997;26:615–619.

54. Arico M, Biondi A, Pui C-H. Juvenile myelomonocytic leukemia. *Blood* 1997;90:479–488.

55. Cooper LJ, Shannon KM, Loken MR, et al. Evidence that juvenile myelomonocytic leukemia can arise from a pluripotent stem cell. *Blood* 2000;96:2310–2313.

56. Jang KA, Choi JH, Sung KJ, et al. Juvenile chronic myelogenous leukemia, neurofibromatosis 1, and xanthoma. *J Dermatol* 1999;26:33–35.

57. Kai S, Sumita H, Fujioka K, et al. Loss of heterozygosity of NF1 gene in juvenile chronic myelogenous leukemia with neurofibromatosis type 1. *Int J Hematol* 1998;68:53–60.

58. Luna-Fineman S, Shannon KM, Atwater SK, et al. Myelodysplastic and myeloproliferative disorders of childhood: a study of 167 patients. *Blood* 1999;93:459–466.

59. Side LE, Emanuel PD, Taylor B, et al. Mutations of the *NF1* gene in children with juvenile myelomonocytic leukemia without clinical evidence of neurofibromatosis, type 1. *Blood* 1998;92:267–272.

60. Zvulunov A, Barak Y, Metzker A. Juvenile xanthogranuloma, neurofibromatosis, and juvenile chronic myelogenous leukemia. World statistical analysis. *Arch Dermatol* 1995;131:904–908.

61. Bakotic BW, Poniecka AW, Dominguez CJ, et al. Myelodysplastic syndrome with atypical eosinophilia in association with ring chromosome 7. A case report. *Cancer Genet Cytogenet* 1999;115:19–22.

62. Baranger L, Szapiro N, Gardais J, et al. Translocation t(5;12)(q31-q33;p12-p13): a non-random translocation associated with a myeloid disorder with eosinophilia. *Br J Haematol* 1994;88:343–347.

63. Darbyshire PJ, Shortland D, Swansbury GJ, et al. A myeloproliferative disease in two infants associated with eosinophilia and chromosome t(1;5) translocation. *Br J Haematol* 1987;66:483–486.

64. Forrest DL, Horsman DE, Jensen CL, et al. Myelodysplastic syndrome with hypereosinophilia and a nonrandom chromosomal abnormality dic(1;7): confirmation of eosinophil clonal involvement by fluorescence *in situ* hybridization. *Cancer Genet Cytogenet* 1998;107:65–68.

65. Inaba T, Shimazaki C, Inaba E, et al. Inversion of chromosome 16 and eosinophilia in refractory anemia with ring sideroblasts: report of a case. *Am J Hematol* 1993;44:134–138.

66. Kobayashi H, Kitano K, Shimodaira S, et al. Eosinophilia in myelodysplastic syndrome with a (12;21)(q23;q22) translocation. *Cancer Genet Cytogenet* 1993;68:95–98.

67. Koike M, Ishiyama T, Yokoyama A, et al. Increased proliferation of eosinophil clusters in myelodysplastic syndromes. *Leuk Res* 1995;19:915–920.

68. Ma SK, Wong KF, Chan JK, et al. Refractory cytopenia with t(1;7),+8 abnormality and dysplastic eosinophils showing intranuclear Charcot-Leyden crystals: a fluorescence *in situ* hybridization study. *Br J Haematol* 1995;90:216–218.

69. Miyamoto T, Akashi K, Hayashi S, et al. Pericentric inversion of chromosome 16 and eosinophilia in chronic myelomonocytic leukemia. *Cancer Genet Cytogenet* 1997;94:99–102.

70. Muroi K, Miyata T, Saito M, et al. Therapy-related chronic myelomonocytic leukaemia with bone marrow eosinophilia associated with der(11)t(1;11)(q21;q14). *Acta Haematol* 1996;96:251–254.

71. Pellier I, Le Moine PJ, Rialland X, et al. Myelodysplastic syndrome with t(5;12)(q31;p12-13) and eosinophilia: a pediatric case with review of literature. *J Pediatr Hematol Oncol* 1996;18:285–288.

72. Saigo K, Sugimoto T, Ryo R, et al. Hematologic improvement by alpha-interferon in a case of the 5q− syndrome with basophilia and eosinophilia. *Rinsho Ketsueki* 1995;36:18–22.

73. Takimoto Y, Imanaka F, Hayashi Y, et al. A patient with basophilic-eosinophilic myeloproliferative disorder showing monosomy 7 and hyperhistaminemia. *Acta Haematol* 1997;98:37–41.

74. Tanabe J, Sasaki S, Tamura T, et al. Myelodysplastic syndrome associated with marked eosinophilia and basophilia. *Rinsho Ketsueki* 1992;33:189–193.

75. Viniou N, Abazis D, Yataganas X, et al. A novel chromosomal abnormality involving chromosomes 2 and 18 in a patient with myelodysplastic syndrome. *Cancer Genet Cytogenet* 1997;96:7–12.

76. Viniou N, Yataganas X, Abazis D, et al. Hypereosinophilia associated with monosomy 7. *Cancer Genet Cytogenet* 1995;80:68–71.

77. Wlodarska I, Mecucci C, Marynen P, et al. TEL gene is involved in myelodysplastic syndromes with either the typical t(5;12)(q33;p13) translocation or its variant t(10;12)(q24;p13). *Blood* 1995;85:2848–2852.

78. el-Rifai W, Pettersson T, Larramendy ML, et al. Lineage involvement and karyotype in a patient with myelodysplasia and blood basophilia. *Eur J Haematol* 1994;53:288–292.

79. Ma SK, Chan JC, Wan TS, et al. Myelodysplastic syndrome with myelofibrosis and basophilia: detection of trisomy 8 in basophils by fluorescence *in-situ* hybridization. *Leuk Lymphoma* 1998;31:429–432.

80. Shirakawa C, Ohno M, Sugishima H, et al. Overt leukemia from MDS associated with marked basophilia. *Rinsho Ketsueki* 1992;33:1031–1035.

81. Tinegate H, Chetty M. Basophilia as a feature of the myelodysplastic syndrome. *Clin Lab Haematol* 1986;8:269–271.

82. Yagasaki F, Jinnai I, Yoshida S, et al. Fusion of TEL/ETV6 to a novel ACS2 in myelodysplastic syndrome and acute myelogenous leukemia with t(5;12)(q31;p13). *Genes Chromosomes Cancer* 1999;26:192–202.

83. Wimazal F, Sperr WR, Horny HP, et al. Hyperfibrinolysis in a case of myelodysplastic syndrome with leukemic spread of mast cells. *Am J Hematol* 1999;61:66–77.

84. Dror Y, Leaker M, Caruana G, et al. Mastocytosis cells bearing a c-kit activating point mutation are characterized by hypersensitivity to stem cell factor and increased apoptosis. *Br J Haematol* 2000;108:729–736.

85. Gupta R, Abdalla SH, Bain BJ. Thrombocytosis with sideroblastic erythropoiesis: a mixed myeloproliferative myelodysplastic syndrome. *Leuk Lymphoma* 1999;34:615–619.

86. Jondeau K, Bouscary D, Viguie F, et al. Thrombocytemia and abnormal megakaryopoiesis associated with abnormality of chromosome 1p34 in myelodysplastic syndromes. *Leukemia* 1996;10:1692–1695.

87. Patel K, Kelsey P. Primary acquired sideroblastic anemia, thrombocytosis, and trisomy 8. *Ann Hematol* 1997;74:199–201.

88. Reis MD, Sher GD, Lakhani A, et al. Deletion of the long arm of chromosome 5 in essential thrombocythemia. *Cancer Genet Cytogenet* 1992;61:93–95.

89. Tefferi A, Inwards DJ, Hoyer JD. Spontaneous remission of anemia associated with a myelodysplastic syndrome with disease evolution into a myeloproliferative state. *Acta Haematol* 1999;101:50–52.

90. Tison T, Vianello F, Radossi P, et al. Myelodysplastic syndrome and thrombocytosis: a random association? *Haematologica* 1994;79:534–535.

91. Aguiar RC, Chase A, Coulthard S, et al. Abnormalities of chromosome band 8p11 in leukemia: two clinical syndromes can be distinguished on the basis of MOZ involvement. *Blood* 1997;90:3130–3135.

92. Chaffanet M, Popovici C, Leroux D, et al. t(6;8), t(8;9) and t(8;13) translocations associated with stem cell myeloproliferative disorders have close or identical breakpoints in chromosome region 8p11-12. *Oncogene* 1998;16:945–949.

93. Martinez-Climent JA, Vizcarra E, Benet I, et al. Cytogenetic response induced by interferon alpha in the myeloproliferative disorder with eosinophilia, T cell lymphoma and the chromosomal translocation t(8;13). *Leukemia* 1998;12:999–1000.

94. Nakayama H, Inamitsu T, Ohga S, et al. Chronic myelomonocytic leukaemia with t(8;9)(p11;q34) in childhood: an example of the 8p11 myeloproliferative disorder? *Br J Haematol* 1996;92:692–695.

95. Popovici C, Zhang B, Gregoire MJ, et al. The t(6;8)(q27;p11) translocation in a stem cell myeloproliferative disorder fuses a novel gene, FOP, to fibroblast growth factor receptor 1. *Blood* 1999;93:1381–1389.

96. Reiter A, Sohal J, Kulkarni S, et al. Consistent fusion of ZNF198 to the fibroblast growth factor receptor-1 in the t(8;13)(p11;q12) myeloproliferative syndrome. *Blood* 1998;92:1735–1742.

97. Sano K, Goji J, Kosaka Y, et al. Translocation (10;12)(q24;q15) in a T-cell lymphoblastic lymphoma with myeloid hyperplasia. *Cancer Genet Cytogenet* 1998;105:168–171.

Special Types of Myelodysplastic Syndromes

1. Latagliata R, Petti MC, Fenu S, et al. Therapy-related myelodysplastic syndrome-acute myelogenous leukemia in patients treated for acute promyelocytic leukemia: an emerging problem. *Blood* 2002;99:822–224.

2. West RR, Stafford DA, White AD, et al. Cytogenic abnormalities in the myelodysplastic syndromes and occupational or environmental exposure. *Blood* 2000;95:2093–2097.

3. Hasle H, Niemeyer CM, Chessells JM, et al. A pediatric approach to the WHO classification of myelodysplastic and myeloproliferative diseases. *Leukemia* 2003;17:277–282.

4. Lange BJ, Kobrinsky N, Barnard DR, et al. Distinctive demography, biology, and outcome of acute myeloid leukemia and myelodysplastic syndrome in children with down syndrome: children's cancer group studies 2861 and 2891. *Blood* 1998;91:608–615.

5. Luna-Fineman S, Shannon KM, Atwater SK, et al. Myelodysplastic and myeloproliferative disorders of childhood: a study of 167 patients. *Blood* 1999;93:459–466.

6. Passmore SJ, Hann IM, Stiller CA, et al. Pediatric myelodysplasia: a study of 68 children and a new prognostic scoring system. *Blood* 1995;85:1742–1750.

7. Bessler M, Hillmen P. Somatic mutation and clonal selection in the pathogenesis and in the control of paroxysmal nocturnal hemoglobinuria. *Semin Hematol* 1998;35:149–167.

8. Boccuni P, Del Vecchio L, Di Noto R, et al. Glycosyl phosphatidylinositol (GPI)-anchored molecules and the pathogenesis of paroxysmal nocturnal hemoglobinuria. *Crit Rev Oncol Hematol* 2000;33:25–43.

9. Nishimura J, Murakami Y, Kinoshita T. Paroxysmal nocturnal hemoglobinuria: an acquired genetic disease. *Am J Hematol* 1999;62:175–182.

10. Rosti V. The molecular basis of paroxysmal nocturnal hemoglobinuria. *Haematologica* 2000;85:82–87.

11. Basara N, Antunovic P, Sefer D, et al. Megakaryocyte progenitors in paroxysmal nocturnal haemoglobinuria are sensitive to complement. *Eur J Haematol* 1996;57:227–229.

12. Richards SJ, Norfolk DR, Swirsky DM, et al. Lymphocyte subset analysis and glycosylphosphatidylinositol phenotype in patients with paroxysmal nocturnal hemoglobinuria. *Blood* 1998;92:1799–1806.

13. Azenishi Y, Ueda E, Machii T, et al. CD59-deficient blood cells and PIG-A gene abnormalities in Japanese patients with aplastic anaemia. *Br J Haematol* 1999;104:523–529.

14. Vu T, Griscelli-Bennaceur A, Gluckman E, et al. Aplastic anaemia and paroxysmal nocturnal haemoglobinuria: a study of the GPI-anchored proteins on human platelets. *Br J Haematol* 1996;93:586–589.

15. Dunn DE, Tanawattanacharoen P, Boccuni P, et al. Paroxysmal nocturnal hemoglobinuria cells in patients with bone marrow failure syndromes. *Ann Intern Med* 1999;131:401–408.

16. Iwanaga M, Furukawa K, Amenomori T, et al. Paroxysmal nocturnal haemoglobinuria clones in patients with myelodysplastic syndromes. *Br J Haematol* 1998;102:465–474.

17. Viniou N, Michali E, Meletis J, et al. Trisomy 8 in a patient who responded to therapy with all-trans-retinoic acid and developed paroxysmal nocturnal haemoglobinuria. *Br J Haematol* 1997;97:135–136.

18. Longo L, Bessler M, Beris P, et al. Myelodysplasia in a patient with pre-existing paroxysmal nocturnal haemoglobinuria: a clonal disease originating from within a clonal disease. *Br J Haematol* 1994;87:401–403.

19. Mortazavi Y, Tooze JA, Gordon-Smith EC, et al. N-RAS gene mutation in patients with aplastic anemia and aplastic anemia/paroxysmal nocturnal hemoglobinuria during evolution to clonal disease. *Blood* 2000;95:646–650.

20. Parlier V, Tiainen M, Beris P, et al. Trisomy 8 detection in granulomonocytic, erythrocytic and megakaryocytic lineages by chromosomal *in situ* suppression hybridization in a case of refractory anaemia with ringed sideroblasts complicating the course of paroxysmal nocturnal haemoglobinuria. *Br J Haematol* 1992;81:296–304.

21. Harris JW, Koscick R, Lazarus HM, et al. Leukemia arising out of paroxysmal nocturnal hemoglobinuria. *Leuk Lymphoma* 1999;32:401–426.

22. Cornelis F, Montfort L, Osselaer JC, et al. Acute leukaemia in paroxysmal nocturnal haemoglobinuria. Case report and review of the literature. *Hematol Cell Ther* 1996;38:285–288.

23. Socie G, Mary JY, de Gramont A, et al. Paroxysmal nocturnal haemoglobinuria: long-term follow-up and prognostic factors. French Society of Haematology. *Lancet* 1996;348:573–577.

24. Uchida T, Ohashi H, Kinoshita T, et al. Hypermethylation of p15(INK4B) gene in a patient with acute myelogenous leukemia evolved from paroxysmal nocturnal hemoglobinuria. *Blood* 1998;92:2981–2983.

25. van Kamp H, Smit JW, van den Berg E, et al. Myelodysplasia following paroxysmal nocturnal haemoglobinuria: evidence for the emergence of a separate clone. *Br J Haematol* 1994;87: 399–400.

26. Fores R, Bautista G, Steegmann JL, et al. De novo smoldering paroxysmal nocturnal hemoglobinuria: a flow cytometric diagnosis. *Haematologica* 1997;82:695–697.

27. Pramoonjago P, Pakdeesuwan K, Siripanyaphinyo U, et al. Genotypic, immunophenotypic and clinical features of Thai patients with paroxysmal nocturnal haemoglobinuria. *Br J Haematol* 1999;105:497–504.

28. Parab RB. Paroxysmal nocturnal hemoglobinuria: a study of 17 cases. *J Postgrad Med* 1990;36:23–26.

29. Prokocimer M, Polliack A. Increased bone marrow mast cells in preleukemic syndromes, acute leukemia, and lymphoproliferative disorders. *Am J Clin Pathol* 1981;75:34–38.

30. Alfinito F, Del Vecchio L, Rocco S, et al. Blood cell flow cytometry in paroxysmal nocturnal hemoglobinuria: a tool for measuring the extent of the PNH clone. *Leukemia* 1996;10:1326–1330.

31. Hall SE, Rosse WF. The use of monoclonal antibodies and flow cytometry in the diagnosis of paroxysmal nocturnal hemoglobinuria. *Blood* 1996;87:5332–5340.

32. Gongora-Biachi RA, Gonzalez-Martinez P, Pinto-Escalante D, et al. Chromosomic findings in patients with paroxysmal nocturnal hemoglobinuria. *Int J Hematol* 1993;58:163–167.

33. Nafa K, Bessler M, Deeg HJ, et al. New somatic mutation in the PIG-A gene emerges at relapse of paroxysmal nocturnal hemoglobinuria. *Blood* 1998;92:3422–3427.

34. Purow DB, Howard TA, Marcus SJ, et al. Genetic instability and the etiology of somatic PIG-A mutations in paroxysmal nocturnal hemoglobinuria. *Blood Cells Mol Dis* 1999;25:81–91.

35. Conti L, Iurlo A, Gandolfo GM, et al. Evans' syndrome in paroxysmal nocturnal hemoglobinuria. *Acta Haematol* 1985;73: 210–211.

36. Mak SK, Wong PN, Lee KF, et al. IgA nephropathy in a patient with paroxysmal nocturnal haemoglobinuria. *Nephrol Dial Transplant* 1995;10:2126–2129.

37. Christou T, Subramanian S, Fung C. Paroxysmal nocturnal hemoglobinuria preceding malignant lymphoma. *Arch Intern Med* 1987;147:377–378.

38. Shichishima T, Saitoh Y, Terasawa T, et al. Complement sensitivity of erythrocytes in a patient with inherited complete deficiency of CD59 or with the Inab phenotype. *Br J Haematol* 1999;104: 303–306.

Disorders Associated with Myelodysplastic Syndromes

1. Okamoto T, Okada M, Mori A, et al. Correlation between immunological abnormalities and prognosis in myelodysplastic syndrome patients. *Int J Hematol* 1997;66:345–351.

2. Billstrom R, Johansson B, Strombeck B, et al. Clonal CD5-positive B lymphocytes in myelodysplastic syndrome with systemic vasculitis and trisomy 8. *Ann Hematol* 1997;74:37–40.

3. Okada M, Okamoto T, Takemoto Y, et al. Function and X chromosome inactivation analysis of B lymphocytes in myelodysplastic syndromes with immunological abnormalities. *Acta Haematol* 2000;102:124–130.

4. Okamoto T, Okada M, Itoh T, et al. Myelodysplastic syndrome with B cell clonality in a patient five years after renal transplantation. *Int J Hematol* 1998;68:61–65.

5. Ehrenfeld M, Gur H, Shoenfeld Y. Rheumatologic features of hematologic disorders. *Curr Opin Rheumatol* 1999;11:62–67.

6. Katsuki K, Shinohara K, Kameda N, et al. Two cases of myelodysplastic syndrome with extramedullary polyclonal plasma cell proliferation and autoantibody production: possible role of soluble Fas antigen for production of excessive self-reactive B cells. *Intern Med* 1998;37:973–977.

7. Komatsuda A, Miura I, Ohtani H, et al. Crescentic glomerulonephritis accompanied by myeloperoxidase-antineutrophil cytoplasmic antibodies in a patient having myelodysplastic syndrome with trisomy 7. *Am J Kidney Dis* 1998;31:336–340.

8. Myers B, Gould J, Dolan G. Relapsing polychondritis and myelodysplasia: a report of two cases and review of the current literature. *Clin Lab Haematol* 2000;22:45–48.

9. Pirayesh A, Verbunt RJ, Kluin PM, et al. Myelodysplastic syndrome with vasculitic manifestations. *J Intern Med* 1997;242: 425–431.

10. Aslangul-Castier E, Papo T, Amoura Z, et al. Systemic vasculitis with bilateral perirenal haemorrhage in chronic myelomonocytic leukaemia. *Ann Rheum Dis* 2000;59:390–393.

11. Kitahara M, Koike K, Kurokawa Y, et al. Lupus nephritis in juvenile myelomonocytic leukemia. *Clin Nephrol* 1999;51: 314–318.

12. Shimamoto Y, Narisawa Y, Suga K, et al. Relationship between autoantibody and dermatosis in myelodysplastic syndrome. *Haematologia (Budap)* 1993;25:253–261.

13. Vadillo M, Jucgla A, Podzamczer D, et al. Pyoderma gangrenosum with liver, spleen and bone involvement in a patient with chronic myelomonocytic leukaemia. *Br J Dermatol* 1999;141: 541–543.

14. Hoyle C, Kaeda J, Leslie J, et al. Acquired beta thalassaemia trait in MDS. *Br J Haematol* 1991;79:116–117.

15. Honig GR, Suarez CR, Vida LN, et al. Juvenile myelomonocytic leukemia (JMML) with the hematologic phenotype of severe beta thalassemia. *Am J Hematol* 1998;58:67–71.

16. Lin CK, Liang R, Liu HW, et al. Myelodysplastic syndrome and acquired factor VIII inhibitor with severe subcutaneous haemorrhage. *Acta Haematol* 1991;85:206–208.

17. Mittelman M, Zeidman A. Platelet function in the myelodysplastic syndromes. *Int J Hematol* 2000;71:95–98.

18. Evans G, Pasi KJ, Mehta A, et al. Recurrent venous thromboembolic disease and factor XI concentrate in a patient with severe factor XI deficiency, chronic myelomonocytic leukaemia, factor V Leiden and heterozygous plasminogen deficiency. *Blood Coagul Fibrinolysis* 1997;8:437–440.

19. Saitoh T, Murakami H, Uchiumi H, et al. Myelodysplastic syndromes with nephrotic syndrome. *Am J Hematol* 1999;60: 200–204.

20. Tunkel AR, Sebastianelli KJ, Pandit N, et al. Development of 5q- myelodysplasia in a patient with sarcoidosis. *Am J Hematol* 1990;34:225–227.

21. Hisatake K, Wada S, Iyota K, et al. Chronic myelomonocytic leukemia (CMMoL) with systemic lymph node swelling and paroxysmal nocturnal hemoglobinuria (PNH)-like complication. *Rinsho Ketsueki* 1989;30:1963–1968.

22. Tombuloglu M, Keskin A, Tobu M, et al. Kaposi's sarcoma in the course of juvenile myelodysplastic syndrome. *Acta Oncol* 1995;34:263–264.

23. Florensa L, Vallespi T, Woessner S, et al. Incidence and characteristics of lymphoid malignancies in untreated myelodysplastic syndromes. *Leuk Lymphoma* 1996;23:609–612.

24. Mitterbauer G, Schwarzmeier J, Mitterbauer M, et al. Myelodysplastic syndrome/acute myeloid leukemia supervening previously untreated chronic B-lymphocytic leukemia: demonstration of the concomitant presence of two different malignant clones by immunologic and molecular analysis. *Ann Hematol* 1997;74: 193–197.

25. Mossafa H, Fourcade C, Pulic M, et al. Chronic lymphocytic leukemia associated with myelodysplastic syndrome and/or chronic myeloid leukemia: evidence for independent clonal chromosomal evolution. *Leuk Lymphoma* 2001;41:337–341.

26. Sylvester LS, Nowell PC, Bonner H, et al. Concurrent diagnosis of chronic lymphocytic leukemia and myelodysplastic syndrome. *Leuk Res* 1997;21:619–621.

27. Elghetany MT. Hodgkin's disease coexisting with myelodysplastic syndrome prior to therapy: a case report and a review of the association of Hodgkin's disease with stem cell disorders. *Ann Hematol* 1997;75:231–234.

28. Romero MJ, Acin P, Avellaneda C. Sideroblastic refractory anemia and acute leukemia in Waldenstrom's macroglobulinemia. *Sangre (Barc)* 1998;43:464–465.

29. Uematsu M, Ochi H, Ueda Y, et al. Coexistent myelodysplastic syndrome and non-Hodgkin lymphoma. Report of a case and review of the literature. *Int J Hematol* 1995;62:45–51.

30. Majumdar G, Slater NG. Waldenstrom's macroglobulinaemia terminating in acute myeloid leukaemia: report of a case and review of the literature. *Leuk Lymphoma* 1993;9: 513–516.

31. Ornellas EP, LeBeau MM, Venkataraman M, et al. Coexistent double gammapathy, myeloproliferative disorder, and malignant lymphoma. *Am J Clin Pathol* 1990;93:132–137.

32. Shvidel L, Sigler E. Chronic myelomonocytic leukemia preceding high-grade immunoblastic lymphoma. *Eur J Haematol* 1995;54:270.

33. Cohen AM, Mittelman M, Gal R, et al. Chronic myelomonocytic leukemia associated with primary amyloidosis. *Leuk Lymphoma* 1994;16:183–187.

34. Hall R, Hopkinson N, Hamblin T. Relapsing polychondritis, smouldering non-secretory myeloma and early myelodysplastic syndrome in the same patient: three difficult diagnoses produce a life threatening illness. *Leuk Res* 2000;24:91–93.

35. Rios R, Sole F, Gascon F. Simultaneous occurrence of the 5q- syndrome and multiple myeloma. *Clin Lab Haematol* 2000; 22:49–53.

36. Schmetzer HM, Mittermuller J, Duell T, et al. Development of myeloma and secondary myelodysplastic syndrome from a common clone. *Cancer Genet Cytogenet* 1998;100:31–35.

37. Okuda T, Yumoto Y, Kamakari K, et al. Primary amyloidosis complicated with chronic myelomonocytic leukemia. *Rinsho Ketsueki* 1996;37:858–862.

38. Jaju RJ, Jones M, Boultwood J, et al. Combined immunophenotyping and FISH identifies the involvement of B-cells in 5q- syndrome. *Genes Chromosomes Cancer* 2000;29:276–280.

39. van Lom K, Hagemeijer A, Smit E, et al. Cytogenetic clonality analysis in myelodysplastic syndrome: monosomy 7 can be demonstrated in the myeloid and in the lymphoid lineage. *Leukemia* 1995;9:1818–1821.

40. Nakazawa T, Koike K, Agematsu K, et al. Cytogenetic clonality analysis in monosomy 7 associated with juvenile myelomonocytic leukemia: clonality in B and NK cells, but not in T cells. *Leuk Res* 1998;22:887–892.

41. Matteo Rigolin G, Howard J, Buggins A, et al. Phenotypic and functional characteristics of monocyte-derived dendritic cells from patients with myelodysplastic syndromes. *Br J Haematol* 1999;107:844–850.

42. Sepp N, Zwierzina H, Smolle J, et al. Epidermal Langerhans cells in myelodysplastic syndromes are abnormal. *J Invest Dermatol* 1991;96:932–936.

43. Marcoval J, Moreno A, Bordas X, et al. Diffuse plane xanthoma: clinicopathologic study of 8 cases. *J Am Acad Dermatol* 1998;39:439–442.

44. Miralles ES, Escribano L, Bellas C, et al. Cutaneous xanthomatous tumours as an expression of chronic myelomonocytic leukaemia? *Clin Exp Dermatol* 1996;21:145–147.

45. Vail JT Jr, Adler KR, Rothenberg J. Cutaneous xanthomas associated with chronic myelomonocytic leukemia. *Arch Dermatol* 1985; 121:1318–1320.

46. Kaiserling E, Horny HP. Dermal Langerhans' cell tumor in chronic myelomonocytic leukemia. *Ultrastruct Pathol* 1988;12:209–219.

47. Harris NL, Demirjian Z. Plasmacytoid T-zone cell proliferation in a patient with chronic myelomonocytic leukemia. *Am J Surg Pathol* 1991;15:87–95.

48. Avivi I, Rosenbaum H, Levy Y, et al. Myelodysplastic syndrome and associated skin lesions: a review of the literature. *Leuk Res* 1999;23:323–330.

49. Dabbagh V, Browne G, Parapia LA, et al. Granulocytic sarcoma of the rectum: a rare complication of myelodysplasia. *J Clin Pathol* 1999;52:865–866.

50. Drent M, Peters FP, Jacobs JA, et al. Pulmonary infiltration associated with myelodysplasia. *Ann Oncol* 1997;8:905–909.

51. Hurford MT, Gujral S, Schuster SJ, et al. Extramedullary myeloid cell tumor of the urinary bladder in a patient with myelodysplastic syndrome. *Pathol Res Pract* 1999;195:699–703.

52. Namba Y, Koizumi H, Nakamura H, et al. Specific cutaneous lesions of the scalp in myelodysplastic syndrome with deletion of 20q. *J Dermatol* 1999;26:220–224.

53. Ravandi-Kashani F, Cortes J, Giles FJ. Myelodysplasia presenting as granulocytic sarcoma of mediastinum causing superior vena cava syndrome. *Leuk Lymphoma* 2000;36:631–637.

MYELOPROLIFERATIVE DISORDERS

GENERAL FEATURES

Classification

The myeloproliferative disorders (MPDs) are characterized by increased peripheral blood cell counts and increased bone marrow cellularity, with preservation of hematopoietic maturation and differentiation (Tables 22-1 and 22-2) (1–10). In general, the peripheral blood and bone marrow blast counts and myelodysplastic features are less marked than in the myelodysplastic syndromes (MDSs); however, no clear dividing line exists between MPDs and MDSs. Cases with features of both may be diagnosed as unclassified MPD or mixed MPD/myelodysplastic disorder (see Chapter 21).

Most of the MPDs have been recognized for decades and are relatively common. Polycythemia vera (PV), essential thrombocythemia (ET), myelofibrosis with myeloid metaplasia (MMM), and chronic myeloid leukemia (CML) fit into this category. The remainder are rare or only recently recognized as belonging to this group. The classification of an MPD in a single patient may change over time from one entity to another.

Clinical Course

MPD usually presents with the insidious onset of non-specific complaints, abdominal pain referable to hepatosplenomegaly, and/or coagulopathy. Many patients are initially asymptomatic, and the diagnosis is made after routine peripheral blood screening. The course is generally indolent in the initial chronic phase of disease followed by a period of decreasing peripheral blood cell counts and

increasing blast percentage (accelerated phase), with eventual transformation to an MDS or acute leukemia (blast crisis) in some cases. Progression to acute leukemia occurs at a variable rate, depending on the specific type of MPD.

Many types of MPD are associated with lymphoid, plasma cell, and histiocytic neoplasms, both clonally related and unrelated. The clonally related neoplasms occur as a consequence of lymphoid or histiocytic differentiation of the neoplastic clone.

Peripheral Blood

The peripheral blood counts are variable but usually include at least one cell line that is increased. Neutrophilia, eosinophilia, basophilia, and thrombocytosis are common. Platelets often appear enlarged, abnormally shaped, and/or hypogranular. The blast percentage is less than 3% in the chronic phase and higher in the accelerated phase and leukemic transformation.

Bone Marrow

The bone marrow is typically hypercellular and shows hematopoietic maturation. The blast percentage is 3% or less in the chronic phase, higher in the accelerated phase, and

TABLE 22-1. CLASSIFICATION OF CHRONIC MYELOPROLIFERATIVE DISEASES ACCORDING TO THE WORLD HEALTH ORGANIZATION

Chronic myelogenous leukemia
Chronic neutrophilic leukemia
Chronic eosinophilic leukemia/hypereosinophilic syndrome
Polycythemia vera
Essential thrombocythemia
Chronic myeloproliferative disease, unclassifiable

TABLE 22-2. ORGANIZATION OF MYELOPROLIFERATIVE DISORDERS IN THIS CHAPTER

Morphologic
  Polycythemia vera
  Essential thrombocythemia
  Myelofibrosis with myeloid metaplasia
  Chronic eosinophilic leukemia
  Chronic basophilic leukemia
  Systemic mastocytosis and related disorders

Genotypic subtypes
  Chronic myeloid leukemia with t(9;22) (*BCR/ABL* and p210 ± p190)
  Chronic myeloid leukemia with t(9;22) (*BCR/ABL* and p190 only)
  Chronic neutrophilic leukemia with t(9;22) (*BCR/ABL* and p230)
  Myeloproliferative disorder with t(8p11) (*FGFR1*)

Unclassified myeloproliferative disorders

20% or more in leukemic transformation. Megakaryocytic hyperplasia and dysmegakaryopoiesis are characteristic. Hypervascularity, reticulin fibrosis, and osteosclerosis are frequently found. For unknown reasons, stainable iron stores are often absent; this finding does not indicate iron deficiency. Bone marrow findings tend to change over time, with increasing dysmyelopoiesis, more blasts, and worsening fibrosis and osteosclerosis. Some cases eventually convert to MDS and either acute myeloid or lymphoid leukemia.

Flow Cytometry

Flow cytometry is of limited value until accelerated phase or blast crisis occurs, when blast enumeration and immunophenotyping may be helpful. The peripheral blood shows a nonspecific increase in CD34+ cells in the chronic phase.

Genetic Analysis

Few MPDs are characterized or defined by a cytogenetic anomaly, and even in these cases, the anomaly alone is probably not sufficient for the development of disease (11–29).

PV and ET are not defined by a specific genetic anomaly; on the contrary, it has been conclusively established that many cases show polyclonal hematopoiesis. *PRV-1* is overexpressed but not mutated in nearly all cases of PV and ET. The pathogenesis of PV and ET and the related disorder MMM remains a mystery. Although clonal anomalies may be present at diagnosis or appear with time, they appear to be the result of clonal evolution and not a specific pathogenetic event. *BCR/ABL* is not present in PV, ET, or MMM, except when rarely acquired in the course of clonal evolution.

Systemic mastocytosis (SM) is characterized by activating mutations of *c-KIT;* this anomaly may eventually be required for diagnosis.

CML and chronic neutrophilic leukemia (CNL) show *BCR/ABL* translocations involving different breakpoints, producing fusion proteins of different length. Evidence suggests that *BCR/ABL* may be a sign of clonal evolution rather than an initial pathogenetic event, as *BCR/ABL*-negative clonal populations have been identified in cases of CML (30,31). Furthermore, the presence of *BCR/ABL* is not sufficient to cause CML, as this translocation has been reported in hematopoietic cells of individuals without clinical evidence of disease (32–35).

Extramedullary Disease

MPD is frequently, if not always, accompanied by extramedullary disease. The liver, spleen, and lymph nodes are most often affected, but virtually any organ or body cavity may be involved. Extramedullary disease may occur at any stage of MPD. The histologic findings may reflect the chronic phase, accelerated phase, or leukemic transformation regardless of concurrent bone marrow histology.

Differential Diagnosis

The diagnosis of MPD is usually based on a combination of clinical judgment, laboratory findings, and bone marrow examination. MPD in the chronic phase may be difficult to distinguish from reactive hematopoietic proliferations. MPD in the accelerated phase resembles MDS. MPD in leukemic transformation should be distinguished from *de novo* acute leukemia and malignant lymphoma.

MORPHOLOGIC SUBTYPES

Polycythemia Vera

PV is characterized primarily by erythrocytosis (1–20) (Figs. 22-1 through 22-6). It occurs in middle-aged and older adults, more often in males and rarely in adolescents. Clinical signs and symptoms are referable to hyperviscosity, coagulopathy, and excessive hematopoiesis and include arterial and venous thromboembolism, vasculopathy, neurologic deficits, and mild hepatosplenomegaly. Many patients are asymptomatic. PV occurs as a *de novo* disorder, a therapy-related disease, and a transformation of (or in conjunction with) ET, MMM, SM, and CML.

The clinical course is usually indolent, with eventual transformation to fibrosis and osteosclerosis, another MPD, MDS, and/or acute leukemia in approximately 1% to 5% of patients. The risk of transformation is related to the type and duration of therapy. Secondary MPDs reported after a diagnosis of PV include ET, MMM (this transformation is also known as postpolycythemic myelofibrosis or spent phase PV), chronic eosinophilic leukemia (CEL), SM, and CML. MDS with neutrophilia, an unusual type of MDS often reported as CNL, has often been described after PV. Clonally related and unrelated B-cell, plasma cell, and T-cell neoplasms have also been reported in patients with PV. Spontaneous remission has been rarely reported.

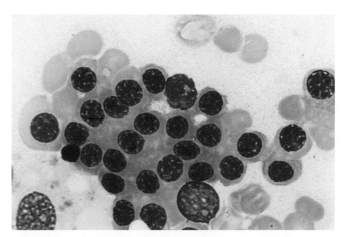

FIGURE 22-1. Bone marrow aspirate smear, polycythemia vera. Numerous erythroid precursors are present, showing no discernible morphologic abnormalities.

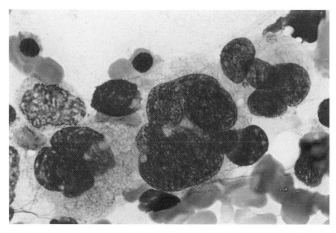

FIGURE 22-2. Bone marrow aspirate smear, polycythemia vera. Megakaryocytes are increased and show numerous nuclear lobations.

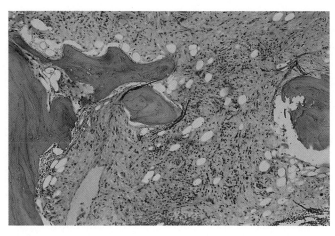

FIGURE 22-5. Bone marrow biopsy specimen, polycythemia vera with terminal fibrosis (spent phase). Osteosclerosis and marrow fibrosis are prominent.

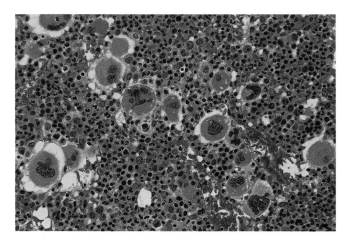

FIGURE 22-3. Bone marrow biopsy specimen, polycythemia vera. Megakaryocytes are increased and multilobated; erythroid precursors are also increased.

Laboratory studies reveal an increased packed red blood cell (RBC) volume or hematocrit (>60% in males, >56% in females), neutrophilia (>10 × 10^9/L in nonsmokers), and thrombocytosis (>400 × 10^9/L). The leukocyte (neutrophil) alkaline phosphatase (LAP) score is increased. Mild eosinophilia and basophilia are usually present. The RBC mass is increased but is difficult to measure and may be falsely low because of obesity. Serum erythropoietin is decreased. Circulating hematopoietic precursors capable of spontaneous erythroid colony formation are increased; however, in practice, this is a difficult test to perform reliably and is neither sensitive nor specific enough to use as a diagnostic criterion.

Cell counts in PV may be affected by concomitant hematopoietic disorders or other factors. The platelet count may be increased by iron deficiency and the hematocrit increased by hypoxia or renal disorders. Conversely, the hematocrit may be decreased by expanded plasma volume, megaloblastic anemia, iron deficiency, and/or renal failure.

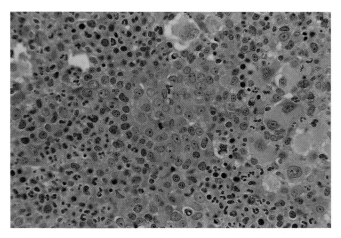

FIGURE 22-4. Bone marrow biopsy specimen, polycythemia vera with focal transformation to acute myeloid leukemia. An interstitial collection of blasts is present.

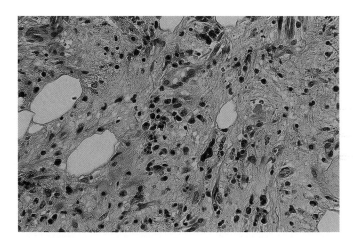

FIGURE 22-6. Bone marrow biopsy specimen, polycythemia vera with terminal fibrosis (spent phase). Fibrous tissue compresses the residual hematopoietic cells.

The peripheral blood smear shows normal RBC morphology in uncomplicated PV. Neutrophils may be morphologically normal or slightly dysplastic, with subtle abnormalities and increased nuclear lobation. Platelets are often normal in appearance but may include large and/or agranular forms.

Bone marrow aspirate smears show a myeloid:erythroid (M:E) ratio of 1:1 or less. Maturation is essentially unremarkable in the untreated patient. Megakaryocytes are plentiful and mature and include large forms with hyperlobated nuclei. Iron stores are decreased to absent, a finding that does not necessarily reflect true iron deficiency.

Histologic sections of the bone marrow show increased cellularity, most prominently affecting erythroid precursors and megakaryocytes. Megakaryocytes range from small to very large, with larger cells showing increased nuclear lobation and densely clumped chromatin. Reticulin fibrosis is often present. The trabeculae show irregular thickening to overt osteosclerosis. Other reported findings include benign lymphoid aggregates, reactive histiocytosis, and granulomas. Therapy reduces cellularity but does not necessarily reverse fibrosis.

Genetic studies show monoclonality in some, but not all, cases. Cases with monoclonality (as evidenced by chromosome X inactivation or other means) have overexpression of *PRV-1;* the significance of this finding is not yet known. The appearance of clonal karyotypic anomalies indicates clonal evolution and correlates with an increased risk of leukemic transformation. Commonly acquired anomalies include trisomies 8 and 9 and deletion of 20q and *p53. BCR/ABL* translocation is absent.

The differential diagnosis includes congenital, inherited, reactive, and idiopathic erythrocytosis; relative erythrocytosis owing to decreased plasma volume; and other MPDs, especially ET, MMM, and CML. Clinical history, laboratory values, and absence of *BCR/ABL* translocation are helpful in excluding other MPDs.

Essential Thrombocythemia

ET is characterized primarily by thrombocytosis (3,8,10,15, 21–53) (Figs. 22-7 through 22-10). It occurs in children and adults, more often in females. Clinical signs and symptoms are referable to coagulopathy and excessive hematopoiesis and include thromboembolism and mild hepatosplenomegaly. Many patients are asymptomatic. ET occurs as a *de novo* disorder, a therapy-related disease, and a transformation of PV.

The clinical course is usually indolent, with eventual transformation to fibrosis and osteosclerosis, another MPD or MDS, and/or acute leukemia in approximately 1% to 5% of patients. The risk of transformation is related to the type and duration of therapy. Secondary MPDs reported after a diagnosis of ET include PV, MMM, and SM. Clonally related and unrelated B-cell and plasma cell neoplasms have

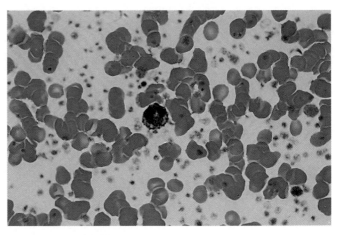

FIGURE 22-7. Peripheral blood smear, essential thrombocythemia. A basophil is surrounded by numerous platelets, some of which show abnormal shapes and hypogranularity.

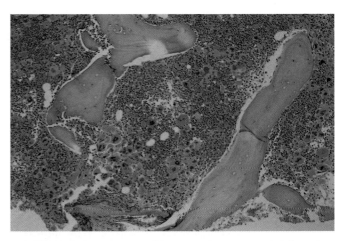

FIGURE 22-8. Bone marrow biopsy specimen, essential thrombocythemia. Osteosclerotic bone surrounds hypercellular bone marrow with increased and multilobated megakaryocytes.

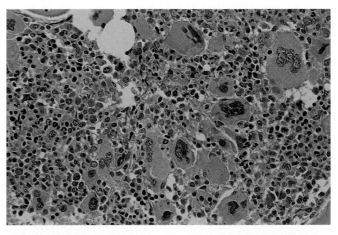

FIGURE 22-9. Bone marrow biopsy specimen, essential thrombocythemia. Megakaryocytes are increased, multilobated, and atypical; the intervening cells are a mixture of red and white blood cell precursors.

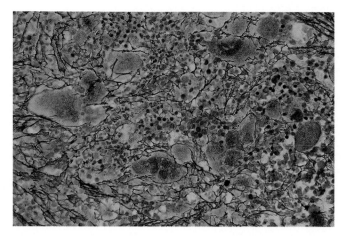

FIGURE 22-10. Bone marrow biopsy specimen, essential thrombocythemia. Reticulin fibers are increased and outline many of the abnormal megakaryocytes (silver stain for reticulin).

also been reported in patients with ET. Spontaneous remission has been reported during pregnancy.

Laboratory studies reveal thrombocytosis, neutrophilia, and a normal to decreased hematocrit. The LAP score is increased. Mild eosinophilia and basophilia are usually present. The platelet count is usually more than $500 \times 10^9/L$, but symptomatic ET has been reported with platelet counts as low as $300 \times 10^9/L$. Platelet function studies are often abnormal. Serum thrombopoietin is normal to increased. Circulating hematopoietic precursors capable of spontaneous erythroid colony formation are increased; however, in practice, this is a difficult test to perform reliably and is neither sensitive nor specific enough to use as a diagnostic criterion.

The peripheral blood smear shows normal RBC morphology in uncomplicated ET. Neutrophils may be morphologically normal or slightly dysplastic, with subtle abnormalities and increased nuclear lobation. Platelets are often normal in appearance but may include large and/or agranular forms.

Bone marrow aspirate smears show a variable M:E ratio. Maturation is essentially unremarkable in the untreated patient. Megakaryocytes are plentiful and mature and include large forms with hyperlobated nuclei. Iron stores are decreased to absent, a finding that does not necessarily reflect true iron deficiency.

Histologic sections of the bone marrow show increased cellularity, most prominently affecting megakaryocytes. Megakaryocytes range from small to very large, with larger cells showing increased nuclear lobation and densely clumped chromatin. Reticulin fibrosis may be present. The trabeculae show irregular thickening and thinning. Other reported findings include pure red cell aplasia, necrosis (possibly owing to antiphospholipid antibody syndrome), and reactive histiocytosis.

Genetic studies show monoclonality in some, but not all, cases. Cases with monoclonality (as evidenced by chromosome X inactivation or other means) show overexpression of *PRV-1*; the significance of this finding is not yet known. The appearance of clonal karyotypic anomalies indicates clonal evolution, and correlates with an increased risk of leukemic transformation. Commonly acquired anomalies include deletion of chromosome 17p and/or *p53* mutation. *BCR/ABL* translocation is absent.

The differential diagnosis includes reactive thrombocytosis; other MPDs, especially PV, the early (cellular) stage of MMM, and CML with thrombocytosis; and MDS with thrombocytosis. ET is distinguished from PV primarily by a higher platelet count and lower hematocrit, from MMM by thrombocytosis and relative lack of fibrosis, and from CML by the absence of *BCR/ABL* translocation. It may not always be possible to distinguish ET from PV or from MDS with thrombocytosis.

Myelofibrosis with Myeloid Metaplasia

MMM is characterized primarily by anemia and leukoerythroblastosis (15,35,51,54–77) (Figs. 22-11 through 22-14). It occurs predominantly in middle-aged to older adults. MMM has been diagnosed in children, but it is possible that in these rare cases, the disorder represents a congenital bone marrow failure syndrome, acute leukemia with fibrosis, or other disorder. Clinical signs and symptoms are referable to cytopenias, coagulopathy, and excessive extramedullary hematopoiesis. Palpable splenomegaly is found in approximately 75% and hepatomegaly in almost 50% of patients at diagnosis. Massive hepatosplenomegaly occurs late in the disease. MMM occurs as a *de novo* disorder and as a transformation of PV and ET.

The clinical course is relentlessly progressive, with worsening cytopenias and eventual transformation to PV, MDS, and/or acute leukemia. Survival is significantly worse than in PV or ET. The risk of transformation is related to the type and duration of therapy and is increased by splenectomy.

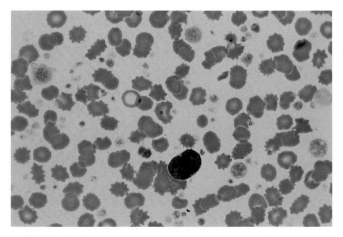

FIGURE 22-11. Peripheral blood smear, myelofibrosis with myeloid metaplasia. A micromegakaryocyte is present, surrounded by increased and abnormal platelets.

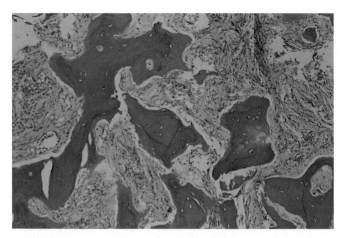

FIGURE 22-12. Bone marrow biopsy specimen, myelofibrosis with myeloid metaplasia. Osteosclerosis and marrow fibrosis are prominent.

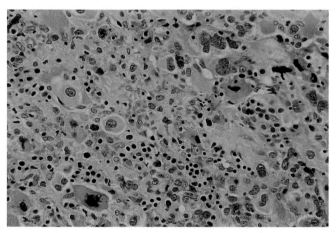

FIGURE 22-13. Bone marrow biopsy specimen, myelofibrosis with myeloid metaplasia. Cellularity is virtually 100% in the early, or cellular, phase of the disease. Abnormal megakaryocytes are prominent.

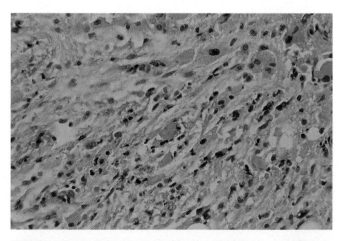

FIGURE 22-14. Bone marrow biopsy specimen, myelofibrosis with myeloid metaplasia. Fibrous tissue compresses atypical megakaryocytes and other residual hematopoietic cells. This appearance is indistinguishable from the terminal phase of polycythemia vera or essential thrombocythemia.

Clonal B-cell and plasma cell neoplasms have been reported with in patients with MMM. Spontaneous hematologic remission rarely occurs, followed in most cases by leukemic transformation.

The peripheral blood usually shows anemia, neutrophilia with immature cells, basophilia, and thrombocytosis with large, irregular, hypogranular platelets; naked megakaryocytic nuclei; and fragments of megakaryocytic cytoplasm. Over time, neutropenia, thrombocytopenia, and circulating blasts appear. RBCs characteristically show teardrop forms as well as more generalized aniso- and poikilocytosis. Granulocytes and precursors may show mild dysplastic changes.

Bone marrow aspirate smears may be hypercellular in the early stages of MMM (see later) and hypocellular in patients with advanced fibrosis. Megakaryocytes are increased and atypical, varying in size, maturation, nuclear shape, and nuclear lobation. Stainable iron may be absent, a finding that does not necessarily indicate iron deficiency.

Histologic sections show variable cellularity, depending on the stage of disease. Most cases are advanced at diagnosis and show hematopoietic hypocellularity. The M:E ratio is variable. Megakaryocytes are increased, distributed singly and in clusters, and atypical, with varying size and shape, bizarre forms, enlarged and hyperchromatic nuclei, and abnormal nuclear lobation. Stromal changes are usually marked. Reticulin fibrosis is present because of local cytokine secretion and proliferation of polyclonal fibroblast proliferation. In far advanced cases, collagen fibrosis may be found. Changes in trabecular bone parallel the degree of fibrosis. The trabeculae are thickened and irregular, sometimes to the point of overt osteosclerosis. Other findings include benign lymphoid aggregates, sea-blue histiocytosis, gelatinous transformation, and granulomas. Therapy may reduce the degree of fibrosis.

Early or cellular stage MMM may be difficult to recognize. Patients present with minimal to modest splenomegaly. The peripheral blood shows mild leukocytosis, therapy-refractory anemia with occasional teardrop forms, thrombocytosis, and relatively few myeloid and erythroid precursors. The bone marrow is hypercellular with an increased M:E ratio, increased immature myeloid cells, increased and atypical megakaryocytes, and little or no fibrosis. Cases with these features may be diagnosed as unclassifiable MPD until findings more characteristic of MMM emerge.

Genetic studies show clonal karyotypic anomalies in approximately 50% of patients, primarily trisomies of chromosome 1q, 8, and 9, and deletions of chromosomes 12p, 13q14, and 20q. Acquisition of additional anomalies is evidence of clonal progression and presages leukemic transformation. *BCR/ABL* translocation is typically absent but has been rarely reported in the course of clonal evolution.

The differential diagnosis includes reactive marrow fibrosis, other MPDs, MDS, and acute leukemia with fibrosis, and lymphoid and plasma cell neoplasia with fibrosis. MMM is distinguished from PV by a lower hematocrit, more atypical megakaryocyte morphology, and more prominent fibrosis; from ET by more atypical megakaryocyte morphology and prominent fibrosis; and from CML by the absence of *BCR/ABL* translocation. It may be difficult to distinguish MMM from MDS with fibrosis; helpful clues include, in MMM, a more insidious clinical course, more prominent splenomegaly, less impressive dysplasia, and fewer cytogenetic anomalies.

Chronic Eosinophilic Leukemia

CEL is a rare disorder characterized by persistent eosinophilia (78–113). Patients may be asymptomatic or present with visceral damage caused by the effects of prolonged eosinophilia. The clinical course is indolent to slowly progressive. Leukemic transformation to overt acute myeloid leukemia may occur, sometimes after many years and often in an extramedullary site. The term idiopathic hypereosinophilic syndrome refers to sustained eosinophilia of unknown cause and undetermined clonality; further laboratory investigation and/or the passage of time helps to classify such cases more precisely as either CEL or nonclonal eosinophilia.

Laboratory studies show sustained eosinophilia. Criteria commonly used for the diagnosis of CEL are idiopathic absolute eosinophilia greater than $1,500 \times 10^9/L$ for more than 6 months and symptoms of visceral damage; however, these criteria do not always distinguish CEL from nonclonal causes of chronic eosinophilia.

The peripheral blood smear usually shows increased eosinophils, with morphology ranging from normal to slightly dysplastic. Signs of dysplasia include hypogranularity, large or atypical granules, and abnormal nuclear lobation. Rarely, peripheral eosinophilia is absent, and the diagnosis is made based on bone marrow eosinophilia.

Bone marrow aspirate smears show eosinophilia. Histologic sections of the bone marrow show eosinophilia and, in many cases, fibrosis.

Genetic studies show clonal chromosome X inactivation. Karyotypic anomalies may be present during the chronic phase and/or leukemic transformation and often resemble those found in MDS and acute myeloid leukemia. *BCR/ABL* translocation is absent.

The differential diagnosis includes other causes of sustained eosinophilia. Reactive eosinophilia may accompany acute lymphoid leukemia and other B-cell, plasma cell, and T-cell neoplasms. Neoplastic eosinophilia occurs in other MPDs (especially PV, SM, CML, and 8p11 MPD), MDS, and acute myeloid leukemia. It is often difficult to distinguish CEL from reactive eosinophilia on morphologic grounds; demonstration of clonality is the most reliable way to establish a diagnosis of CEL. Compared with MDS with eosinophilic differentiation, CEL shows relatively little dysplasia and a long indolent phase; however, these are imprecise criteria, and each case must be judged individually.

Chronic Basophilic Leukemia

Chronic basophilic leukemia (CBL) appears to exist, but is an extremely rare disorder (114,115). Patients present with hyperhistaminic symptoms, such as gastrointestinal ulcers, pruritis, and coagulopathy. The peripheral blood and bone marrow typically show sustained basophilia with little or no increase in blasts; one case has been described in which peripheral basophilia was absent. Associated peripheral eosinophilia and bone marrow mastocytosis are frequent in CBL, apparently due to close relationships among these lineages, and may lead to a diagnosis of concurrent systemic mastocytosis. The bone marrow may show fibrosis. Genetic studies do not show evidence of *BCR/ABL* translocation, the hallmark of chronic myeloid leukemia. CBL has been reported to transform to more aggressive disease and acute myeloid leukemia.

The differential diagnosis includes basophilia seen in association with other myeloproliferative and myelodysplastic syndromes, and acute basophilic leukemia. CBL shows more prominent involvement of the basophil lineage than other clonal myeloid neoplasms, and pursues a more chronic course than acute basophilic leukemia.

Systemic Mastocytosis and Related Disorders

SM is part of a spectrum of neoplastic mastocytosis, which has recently been classified according to clinical and pathologic criteria (114–161) (Figs. 22-15 through 22-20). In its most limited presentation, neoplastic mastocytosis presents as skin disease (urticaria pigmentosa); however, even urticaria pigmentosa is often accompanied by molecular evidence of bone marrow involvement. A more advanced form of the disease is SM, which may present with skin lesions, bony abnormalities, soft-tissue masses, hepatosplenomegaly, and/or lymphadenopathy. Symptoms of mast cell activation and

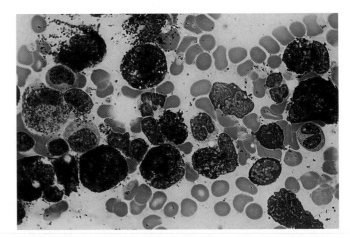

FIGURE 22-15. Bone marrow aspirate, systemic mastocytosis. Numerous enlarged and atypical mast cells are present.

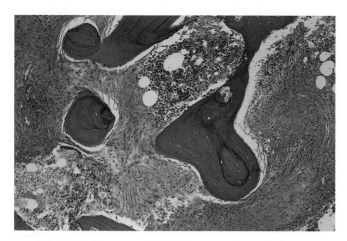

FIGURE 22-16. Bone marrow biopsy specimen, systemic mastocytosis. Osteosclerotic bone encloses hypercellular marrow with extensive replacement by spindled cells.

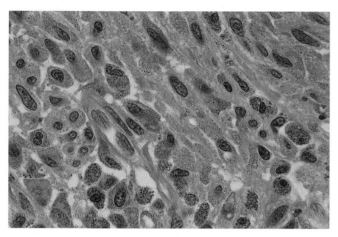

FIGURE 22-17. Bone marrow biopsy specimen, systemic mastocytosis. Densely packed mast cells are present, showing a range of forms from spindled to round. Scattered eosinophils are also present.

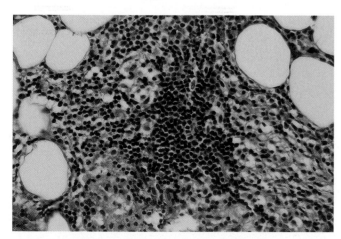

FIGURE 22-18. Bone marrow biopsy specimen, systemic mastocytosis. A lymphoid aggregate is present and composed of small round lymphocytes and surrounded by a rim of pale cells, likely histiocytes and mast cells. This type of targetoid lesion is typical of systemic mastocytosis.

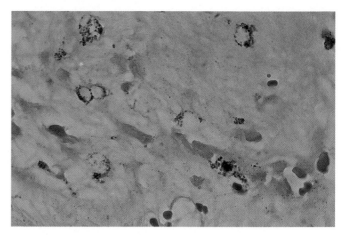

FIGURE 22-19. Bone marrow biopsy specimen, systemic mastocytosis. Dense fibrous tissue contains compressed mast cells, revealed by Giemsa staining.

degranulation may be present, including flushing, headache, diarrhea, hyperfibrinolysis, and vascular collapse. The most advanced forms of disease are aggressive SM and overt mast cell leukemia, which occur *de novo* and as a transformation of SM.

SM presents in both children and adults. The clinical course is variable, with progression and spontaneous regression. Cases with relatively slow progression have recently been labeled as smoldering mastocytosis. SM may be accompanied or followed by another clonally related MPD, MDS, histiocytic neoplasm, or acute myeloid or lymphoid leukemia. Many B-cell and plasma cell neoplasms have also been reported with SM; at least some are probably clonally related to coexistent SM. The prognosis is related to the extent and aggressiveness of disease.

The peripheral blood smear in SM and aggressive SM may show anemia, leukocytosis, thrombocytopenia, and/or eosinophilia. Recognizable mast cells are usually not identifiable, although they are detectable by molecular methods. In mast cell leukemia, circulating mast cells are found.

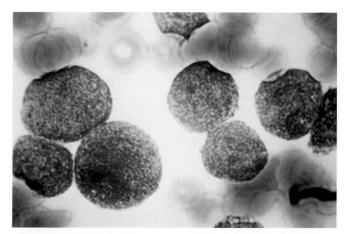

FIGURE 22-20. Bone marrow aspirate, mast cell leukemia. The mast cells stain metachromatically with toluidine blue.

Bone marrow involvement is present in more than 80% of neoplastic mastocytosis, regardless of age or clinical presentation, with mast cells usually constituting 5% or less of nucleated marrow cells. At a differential count of 20% or more, a diagnosis of mast cell leukemia is warranted. Mast cell morphology ranges from normal to atypical. Atypical features include large cell size, round or spindled contour, large and/or eccentric nucleus, bi- or multilobated nucleus, blastlike chromatin, and cytoplasmic hypogranularity. Cases with 5% or more of mast cells tend to show atypical features in at least 10% of mast cells.

Histologic sections of the bone marrow show increased cellularity and focal to diffuse mastocytosis. Focal disease may be perivascular, paratrabecular, or interatrabecular. The lesions are composed of dense clusters of spindled mast cells and lymphocytes, often ringed by eosinophils. The eosinophilic fibrohistiocytic lesion of bone marrow is now considered by some to represent a focal lesion of SM. Diffuse infiltration is characterized by spindled, hypogranular, and fibroblast-like mast cells enmeshed in reticulin fibers. In such cases, mast cells may be difficult to recognize, leading to an erroneous diagnosis of marrow fibrosis. Other findings include eosinophilia, other MPDs, MDS, and bony abnormalities ranging from osteoporosis to osteopetrosis.

Histochemical and cytochemical reactions of neoplastic mast cells include positivity for α_1-antichymotrypsin, α_1-antitrypsin, chloroacetate esterase, chymase, Giemsa, lysozyme, toluidine blue, tryptase, and vimentin but not myeloperoxidase. In aggressive SM and mast cell leukemia, staining reactions for lysozyme, toluidine blue, Giemsa, chloroacetate esterase, and chymase may be negative; however, tryptase and CD117 are usually positive.

Flow cytometry and immunostaining of SM show expression of CD2, CD11c, CD13, CD22, CD25, CD33, CD43, CD45, CD68, CD69, CD117, HLA-DR, and stem cell factor but not other B- or T-cell markers, CD34, or CD38. Coexpression of CD2 and CD25 is characteristic. In aggressive SM and mast cell leukemia, CD41 and/or CD61 may be expressed.

Genetic studies of SM show clonal X chromosome inactivation. Clonal karyotypic anomalies are uncommon and include loss of the Y chromosome and trisomies of chromosomes 8 and 9; additional changes are found in cases with clinical progression or MDS. The hallmark of SM is an activating mutation of *c-KIT,* which encodes the tyrosine kinase CD117. CD117 is the receptor for stem cell factor, a potent hematopoietic cytokine. The *c-KIT* mutation found in SM produces constitutive CD117 activation and thus hypersensitivity to stem cell factor. Rare cases of SM do not show an activating *c-KIT* mutation; it is possible that in such cases, hypersensitivity to stem cell factor occurs by another genetic route.

Genetic studies of aggressive SM and mast cell leukemia more often show clonal karyotypic anomalies, including tri-

somy 4 and t(8;21). Activating *c-KIT* mutations are typically absent, except in cases arising as a transformation of SM.

The differential diagnosis includes reactive mastocytosis, constitutional (familial) and childhood-onset mastocytosis, and MPD and MDS with mast cell differentiation. Reactive mastocytosis is usually found in association with stromal disease or low-grade lymphoma; the mast cells are few in number and morphologically normal. Therapy with stem cell factor may cause bone marrow mast cell hyperplasia mimicking SM. Constitutional (familial) and most, but not all, cases of childhood-onset mastocytosis are nonneoplastic. The lesions are typically limited to the skin and do not show activating *c-KIT* mutations or associated hematolymphoid disease. MPD and MDS with mast cell differentiation are said to have a more indolent course than SM and show individual mast cells scattered throughout the bone marrow, which lack CD2 and CD25 expression; however, in many instances such cases may not be biologically or pathologically distinguishable from SM with associated MPD or MDS.

GENOTYPIC SUBTYPES

Chronic Myeloid Leukemia with t(9;22) (*BCR/ABL* with p210 $\pm$ p190)

CML is a common neoplasm characterized by marked granulocytic proliferation at all stages of development (1,2) (Figs. 22-21 through 22-27). It occurs in children and adults from 2 years to old age, peaking at 45 to 60 years of age, and is more common in males. Patients may be asymptomatic or present with signs and symptoms referable to increased metabolism, coagulopathy, and extramedullary hematopoiesis. Splenomegaly is found in approximately 75% and hepatomegaly in approximately 35% of patients at diagnosis. CML occurs as a *de novo* disease, a therapy-related malignancy, and a transformation of other MPDs (3,4).

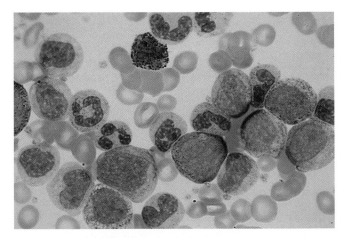

FIGURE 22-21. Peripheral blood smear, chronic myeloid leukemia. Numerous neutrophils, neutrophil precursors, and basophils are present.

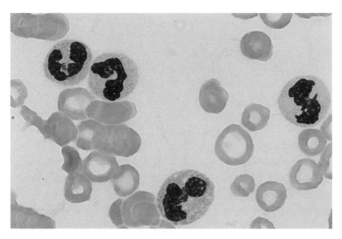

FIGURE 22-22. Peripheral blood smear, chronic myeloid leukemia. The segmented neutrophils show subtle abnormalities in nuclear lobation.

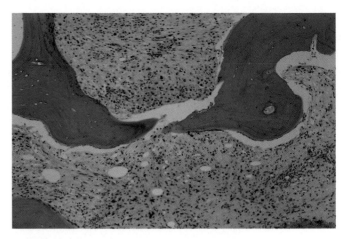

FIGURE 22-25. Bone marrow biopsy specimen, chronic myeloid leukemia. Osteosclerotic bone encloses fibrotic marrow almost devoid of fat cells.

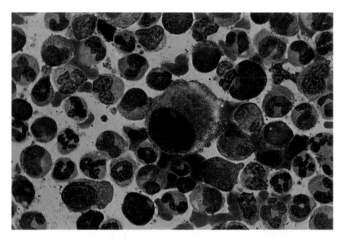

FIGURE 22-23. Bone marrow aspirate smear, chronic myeloid leukemia. Abundant neutrophils and neutrophil precursors are present as well as a characteristically small, hypolobated megakaryocyte.

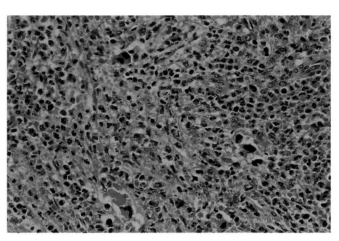

FIGURE 22-26. Bone marrow biopsy specimen, chronic myeloid leukemia. The marrow is packed with granulocytic precursors and small megakaryocytes. The compression of hematopoietic cells into a single-file arrangement is typical of reticulin fibrosis.

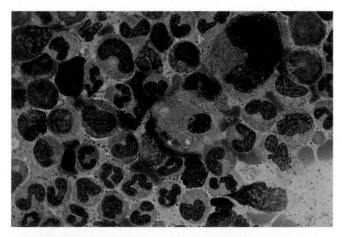

FIGURE 22-24. Bone marrow aspirate smear, chronic myeloid leukemia. A storage (pseudo-Gaucher) histiocyte is present as well as a typical megakaryocyte.

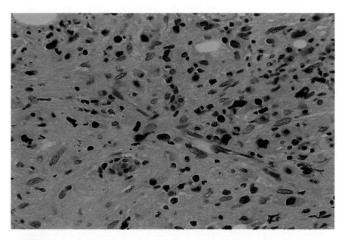

FIGURE 22-27. Bone marrow biopsy specimen, chronic myeloid leukemia. In later stage disease, dense marrow fibrosis encompasses residual hematopoietic precursors and small, atypical megakaryocytes.

The clinical course is progressive. The initial chronic phase is characterized by relatively stable peripheral blood cell counts and clinical status, with less than 5% peripheral blood and bone marrow blasts. An accelerated phase follows, characterized by worsening clinical status and approximately 5% to 10% blasts. CML terminates in an acute phase characterized by the onset of overt acute leukemia (leukemic transformation or blast crisis). CML rarely shows erythrocytosis or converts to PV (5–7). Another rare outcome is spontaneous remission from acute leukemia to the chronic phase or from the chronic phase to normal hematopoiesis (8–10). Other clonal diseases reported with CML include B-cell, plasma cell, and T-cell neoplasms (11–20). In some cases, these neoplasms are clonally related to CML.

CML in leukemic transformation usually shows a myeloid phenotype (21–32). Virtually all types of differentiation are represented, including promyelocytic, eosinophilic, basophilic, myelomonocytic, erythroid, megakaryocytic, mastocytic, and histiocytic. CML in lymphoid blast transformation shows a B-cell phenotype in 90% of cases and a T-cell, natural killer cell, or myeloid/natural killer cell phenotype in the remainder. Blast crisis may be the first manifestation of CML. It presents in an extramedullary site in approximately 10% of cases; this presentation is particularly likely after stem cell transplantation.

Laboratory studies usually show anemia, neutrophilia, eosinophilia, basophilia, and thrombocytosis (33). The mean white blood cell count at diagnosis is approximately $135 \times 10^9/L$; however, the white blood cell count is less than $50 \times 10^9/L$ in 30% of cases. Absolute eosinophilia is found in 80% to 90%, absolute basophilia in 85% to 100%, and absolute lymphocytosis in 50% to 55% of cases. The mean platelet count is $400 \times 10^9/L$; thrombocytosis is found in approximately 50% and thrombocytopenia in approximately 10% of cases. Nucleated RBCs are found in approximately 40% of cases.

The LAP score is usually very low (34–40). This finding correlates with increased serum granulocyte colony-stimulating factor levels and decreased neutrophil granularity; however, it is neither entirely specific nor sensitive for CML. An increased LAP may be found in CML with acute inflammation, advanced disease, or therapy, and a decreased score may be found in reactive disorders and MDS.

The peripheral blood findings are remarkably consistent among patients with CML in the chronic phase. Abundant granulocytes at all stages of maturation are found. The majority are segmented neutrophils and neutrophilic myelocytes, with approximately 2% to 5% promyelocytes and 1% to 2% blasts. The neutrophils and precursors show mild dysplasia, including hyperlobated and abnormally lobated nuclei and hypogranularity. Eosinophils, basophils, hybrid eosinophil-basophil forms, and their precursors are prominent (41,42). Eosinophilia and basophilia may be lacking in patients undergoing corticosteroid therapy for other conditions, and basophils may be difficult to identify when degran-

ulated. Platelets are abnormally large with bizarre shapes and hypogranularity. Small (dwarf, micro-) megakaryocytes and naked megakaryocytic nuclei are often present. CML with extreme thrombocytosis (platelet counts of 1,000 to 4,000 $\times$ $10^9/L$) may be mistaken for ET (43–49). Such cases have clinicopathologic findings more compatible with CML than ET and are diagnosed as CML based on *BCR/ABL* translocation.

Bone marrow aspirate smears show a M:E ratio of 8:1 or more. Mature neutrophils and myelocytes predominate; blasts constitute 1% to 2% of cells. Mature megakaryocytes are increased but may be difficult to appreciate because of their small size and hypolobation (50). As in the peripheral blood, eosinophil and basophil precursors are increased, and hybrid forms are present. Storage (pseudo-Gaucher) histiocytes are present in many cases. Stainable intracellular iron is absent in chronic phase CML, a finding not indicative of iron deficiency (51,52).

Histologic sections of the bone marrow show hypercellularity, usually reaching 100% (53–59). The M:E ratio is increased, owing to both proliferation of granulocytes and reduction of erythroid precursors. Granulocytic and erythroid maturation is preserved. Megakaryocytes appear decreased in approximately 30% and increased in approximately 50% of cases; they are typically small and hypolobated and thus may be difficult to identify. Mild to marked reticulin fibrosis is present, apparently the result of cytokine secretion from megakaryocytes and other cells; the fibroblasts are polyclonal. In advanced cases, collagen fibrosis may be found; rarely, fibrosis dominates the morphologic findings. The trabeculae are consistently thickened and irregular; in advanced cases, overt osteosclerosis is present. Other reported findings include pure red cell aplasia and granulomas. Therapy causes decreased cellularity, normalization of megakaryocyte morphology, and variable changes in fibrosis and osteosclerosis.

Flow cytometry of the peripheral blood and bone marrow shows increased early myeloid precursors in the chronic phase. In the accelerated phase and leukemic transformation, blasts are more numerous and may show either a myeloid or lymphoid phenotype.

Genetic studies show clonal t(9;22)(q34;q11) in 90%, a variant translocation involving chromosomes 9 and 22 in approximately 5%, and no karyotypic anomaly (masked translocation) in approximately 5% of cases (60–65). The common t(9;22) produces a shortened chromosome 22, known as the Philadelphia chromosome. Whatever the karyotypic findings, molecular studies show a rearrangement involving *ABL* at chromosome 9q34 and *BCR* at chromosome 22q11. *ABL* encodes a tyrosine kinase; *BCR* encodes a protein of unknown function. The fusion gene is usually found on chromosome 22 but may be found on chromosome 9 or elsewhere. *BCR/ABL* rearrangement has been demonstrated in all hematopoietic and lymphoid lineages, including histiocytes and osteoclasts.

Additional clonal anomalies are found in 20% to 25% of cases in the chronic phase and 70% of cases in the accelerated phase or leukemic transformation. Clonal evolution tends to follow predictable pathways, marked by the appearance of del(1p36), trisomy 8, additional t(9;22), iso(17q) and *p53* inactivation, trisomy 19, trisomy 21, t(3;21), and t(8;21). Loss of chromosome 17p is associated with pseudo–Pelger-Huët change in CML neutrophils. After stem cell transplantation, clonal evolution does not follow the usual sequence but is characterized by more random anomalies.

The fusion protein BCR/ABL is a constitutively activated tyrosine kinase, which appears to cause the clinical manifestations of CML (66–72). In CML, *BCR* is usually split at the major breakpoint cluster region (M-BCR), which produces a 210-kd fusion protein (p210). A smaller fusion protein (p190) is produced by splitting of *BCR* at the minor breakpoint cluster region (m-BCR) and by posttranscriptional splicing of p210. A larger fusion protein, p230, is produced by splitting of *BCR* at the micro-breakpoint cluster region (μ-BCR). Most cases of CML show p210 or a combination of p210 and p190. CML with p190 only may represent a distinct clinicopathologic entity (see later). CML with p230 only is rare (73,74); most cases of MPD with this fusion protein are classified as CNL.

The differential diagnosis of CML in the chronic phase includes other MPDs and MDS (75–79) (Table 22-3). Other MPDs enter the differential diagnosis when CML shows erythrocytosis or marked thrombocytosis. In distinguishing CML from MDS, it should be kept in mind that CML may have myelodysplastic features, especially with disease progression and after cytotoxic therapy; and that t(9;22) may appear as an acquired anomaly in MDS and other hematolymphoid neoplasms.

The differential diagnosis of CML in leukemic transformation includes *de novo* and therapy-related acute leukemia and malignant lymphoma (80–85). Helpful criteria for distinguishing CML with lymphoid blast crisis from *de novo* acute lymphoid leukemia with t(9;22) include lack of CD20 and CD34 expression in blasts, p230 production, and, after remission induction, appearance of chronic phase CML morphology and persistence of *BCR/ABL*. It should be kept in mind that CML may occur simultaneously with clonally unrelated acute leukemia and malignant lymphoma.

Chronic Myeloid Leukemia with t(9;22) (*BCR/ABL* and p190 Only)

CML with t(9;22) involving the minor breakpoint of *BCR* (m-bcr) is characterized by production of a 190-kd BCR/ABL fusion protein (p190) (86–95). This type of *BCR/ABL* translocation occurs in less than 1% of cases diagnosed as CML. Compared with usual CML, this variant tends to show prominent monocytosis and a lower neutrophil:monocyte ratio. Splenomegaly and basophilia may be absent.

The peripheral blood shows circulating myeloid precursors and a low LAP score. This variant of CML may present in the chronic phase, accelerated phase, or blast crisis. The differential diagnosis of cases presenting in the chronic phase is primarily chronic myelomonocytic leukemia.

TABLE 22-3. DIFFERENTIAL FEATURES OF CHRONIC MYELOID LEUKEMIA, CHRONIC NEUTROPHILIC LEUKEMIA, AND MYELODYSPLASTIC SYNDROME WITH NEUTROPHILIA

	CML	CNL	MDS with Neutrophilia
Clinical findings			
Splenomegaly	+++	Absent	Absent
Extramedullary disease	++–+++	Absent	±
Leukemic transformation	100%	Rare	50%
Peripheral blood findings			
White blood cell count ($\times -10^9$/L)	80–300	15–60	40–70
Platelet count ($\times -10^9$/L) 400–>1,000	700–1,300	<500	
Myeloid precursors	+++	Absent	+–++
Absolute eosinophilia	+++	Absent	±
Absolute basophilia	+++	Absent	±
Blast (%)	1–2	<1	0–10
Bone marrow findings			
Dysplasia	+	Absent	++–+++
Monolobated megakaryocytes	+++	Absent	±
Fibrosis/osteosclerosis	++–+++	Absent	±
Blast (%)	1–2	<3	0–19
Genetic findings			
BCR/ABL gene	+++	+++	Absent
BCR/ABL protein	p210 ± p190	p230	Absent

CML, chronic myeloid leukemia; CNL, chronic neutrophilic leukemia; MDS, myelodysplastic syndrome; +, occasionally present; ++, often present; +++, always present; ±, may or may not be present.

The differential diagnosis of cases presenting in lymphoid blast crisis is primarily *BCR/ABL*-positive acute lymphoblastic leukemia. In such cases, underlying CML may become evident only after remission is induced.

Chronic Neutrophilic Leukemia with t(9;22) (*BCR/ABL* and p230)

CNL, also termed neutrophilic chronic myeloid leukemia, is a rare disorder characterized by neutrophilia composed of mature segmented neutrophils (96–100). It occurs as a *de novo* disorder in young to elderly adults, with a marked female predominance. Patients are typically asymptomatic; mild splenomegaly may be present. The clinical course is usually indolent, with survival exceeding 10 years, and only rare leukemic transformation.

Laboratory studies show neutrophilia ranging, with rare exception, from 16 to 58 × 10^9/L. The white blood cell differential count shows 85% or more neutrophils, without eosinophilia, basophilia, myeloid precursors, or blasts. Thrombocytosis is often present, with reported platelet counts ranging as high as 1,240 × 10^9/L. The LAP score is normal to increased.

The peripheral blood shows mature, normal-appearing neutrophils without Döhle bodies, toxic granulation, or dysplasia. RBCs and platelets are morphologically unremarkable.

Bone marrow aspirate smears and histologic sections show increased neutrophils without myelodysplasia or increased blasts. Histologic sections of the bone marrow show hypercellularity, usually reaching 100%. The M:E ratio is greater than 10:1, and megakaryocytes are increased. Dysplastic changes, fibrosis, and osteosclerosis are absent. Blasts are not increased.

Genetic studies show *BCR/ABL* gene rearrangement involving the micro-breakpoint cluster region (μ-BCR) of *BCR,* the same breakpoint predominating in acute lymphoid leukemia with t(9;22). The translocation may be karyotypically inapparent (masked). Breakage at μ-BCR results in fusion of nearly the entire *BCR* gene with *ABL*. The fusion protein p230 is a constitutively activated tyrosine kinase. Other karyotypic abnormalities are rare. One instance of coexistent i(17q) has been reported in a patient with a low absolute neutrophil count and unusually aggressive disease; this case may be an example of clonal evolution in CNL or an example of MDS with acquired t(9;22).

The differential diagnosis includes neutrophilic leukemoid reaction and MDS with neutrophilia. In fact, the great majority of cases reported as CNL fall into one of these categories. Neutrophilic leukemoid reactions occur in a variety of settings, often as a result of tumor production of granulocyte colony-stimulating factor. Leukemoid reactions reported as CNL are usually due to underlying clonal lymphoplasmacytoid disorders, sarcomas, or carcinomas (101–104). The cause of a neutrophilic leukemoid reaction may not be evi-

dent for years; thus, reactive neutrophilia may easily be misdiagnosed as CNL. Unlike the neutrophils of CNL, those found in leukemoid reactions may show Döhle bodies and toxic granulation.

MDS with neutrophilia is often reported as CNL (105–125). The clinical history may include factors suggestive of MDS, such as myelotoxic exposure or a history of preexisting PV. The clinical course is aggressive, with frequent leukemic transformation. The peripheral blood shows marked neutrophilia. The bone marrow shows increased neutrophilic precursors and myelodysplasia. Genetic studies fail to reveal *BCR/ABL* but usually show other clonal karyotypic anomalies characteristic of MDS; in some cases, no karyotypic anomalies are identified.

It should be kept in mind that the presence of μ-BCR and production of p230 are not found exclusively in CNL but have been reported in CML and acute myeloid leukemia (126–128).

Myeloproliferative Disorder with t(8p11) (*FGFR1*)

MPD with 8p11 (or 8p11 MPD) is characterized by clonal myeloid and lymphoid proliferation (129–144). The peripheral blood shows eosinophilia. The bone marrow shows a disorder resembling CML or chronic myelomonocytic leukemia, which progresses to acute myeloid or stem cell leukemia. A lymph node or other extramedullary site shows lymphoblastic lymphoma with eosinophilic infiltration, usually of the T-cell phenotype but occasionally of the B-cell phenotype. Rare cases have been reported presenting with systemic mastocytosis or acute lymphoid leukemia, and eventually progressing to acute myeloid leukemia.

Genetic studies show translocation involving *FGFR1* at chromosome 8p11. This gene encodes fibroblast growth factor 1, a tyrosine kinase receptor. The usual translocation partner is *ZNF198,* located at chromosome 13q12. Thus, the most common translocation is t(8;13)(p11;q12); however, several variants have been reported, including t(6;8)(q27; p11), t(8;9)(p11;q33), t(8;11)(p11;p15), t(8;12)(p11;q15), t(8;17)(p11;q25), ins(12;8)(p11;p11p21), and t(8;22) (p11;q11).

The differential diagnosis includes biphenotypic T-cell myeloid lymphoblastic lymphoma, T-cell lymphoblastic lymphoma with coincidental myeloid hyperplasia, and clonal hematolymphoid disease bearing a chromosome 8p11 translocation but involving a different gene.

UNCLASSIFIED MYELOPROLIFERATIVE DISORDERS

Some MPDs are not classifiable according to the previously discussed diseases because they show insufficient or overlapping criteria or because they represent new or rare

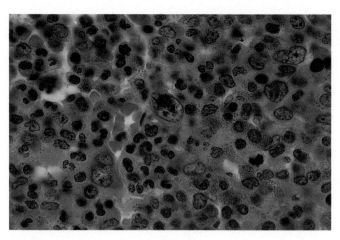

FIGURE 22-28. Bone marrow biopsy specimen, unclassified myeloproliferative disorder. The marrow is completely cellular, filled with maturing granulocytes, including numerous eosinophils, and occasional megakaryocytes. Karyotypic analysis disclosed a complex translocation involving chromosomes 7, 9, and 10.

clinicopathologic entities (1–6) (Fig. 22-28). In cases with insufficient or overlapping criteria, the passage of time may help to classify the disorder. In other cases, genetic criteria may eventually define new disorders.

REFERENCES

General Features

1. Andreasson B, Swolin B, Kutti J. Patients with idiopathic myelofibrosis show increased CD34+ cell concentrations in peripheral blood compared to patients with polycythaemia vera and essential thrombocythaemia. *Eur J Haematol* 2002;68:189–193.
2. Bench AJ, Cross NC, Huntly BJ, et al. Myeloproliferative disorders. *Best Pract Res Clin Haematol* 2001;14:531–551.
3. Lundberg LG, Lerner R, Sundelin P, et al. Bone marrow in polycythemia vera, chronic myelocytic leukemia, and myelofibrosis has an increased vascularity. *Am J Pathol* 2000;157:15–19.
4. Mesa RA. Clinical and scientific advances in the Philadelphia-chromosome negative chronic myeloproliferative disorders. *Int J Hematol* 2002;76[Suppl 2]:193–203.
5. Michiels JJ, Thiele J. Clinical and pathological criteria for the diagnosis of essential thrombocythemia, polycythemia vera, and idiopathic myelofibrosis (agnogenic myeloid metaplasia). *Int J Hematol* 2002;76:133–145.
6. Spivak JL. Diagnosis of the myeloproliferative disorders: resolving phenotypic mimicry. *Semin Hematol* 2003;40[1 Suppl 2]:1–5.
7. Tefferi A. Chronic myeloid disorders: classification and treatment overview. *Semin Hematol* 2001;38[1 Suppl 2]:1–4.
8. Tefferi A. The pathogenesis of chronic myeloproliferative diseases. *Int J Hematol* 2001;73:170–176.
9. Thiele J, Kvasnicka HM, Fischer R. Histochemistry and morphometry on bone marrow biopsies in chronic myeloproliferative disorders—aids to diagnosis and classification. *Ann Hematol* 1999;78:495–506.
10. Thiele J, Kvasnicka HM, Zankovich R, et al. Relevance of bone marrow features in the differential diagnosis between essential thrombocythemia and early stage idiopathic myelofibrosis. *Haematologica* 2000;85:1126–1134.
11. Chiusolo P, La Barbera EO, Laurenti L, et al. Clonal hemopoiesis and risk of thrombosis in young female patients with essential thrombocythemia. *Exp Hematol* 2001;29:670–676.
12. Crisan D, Mattson JC, O'Malley BA, et al. bcr gene rearrangement analysis in myeloproliferative disorders other than chronic myelogenous leukemia. *Cancer Detect Prev* 1996;20:263–269.
13. Damaj G, Delabesse E, Le Bihan C, et al. Typical essential thrombocythaemia does not express bcr-Abelson fusion transcript. *Br J Haematol* 2002;116:812–816.
14. El-Kassar N, Hetet G, Briere J, et al. Clonality analysis of hematopoiesis and thrombopoietin levels in patients with essential thrombocythemia. *Leuk Lymphoma* 1998;30:181–188.
15. Emilia E, Marasca R, Zucchini P, et al. BCR-ABL rearrangement is not detectable in essential thrombocythemia. *Blood* 2001;97:2187–2189.
16. Ferraris AM, Mangerini R, Racchi O, et al. Heterogeneity of clonal development in chronic myeloproliferative disorders. *Am J Hematol* 1999;60:158–160.
17. Gale RE. Basic sciences of the myeloproliferative diseases: pathogenic mechanisms of ET and PV. *Int J Hematol* 2002;76[Suppl 2]:305–310.
18. Hackwell S, Ross F, Cullis JO. Patients with essential thrombocythemia do not express bcr-abl transcripts. *Blood* 1999;93:2420.
19. Harrison CN, Gale RE, Machin SJ, et al. A large proportion of patients with a diagnosis of essential thrombocythemia do not have a clonal disorder and may be at lower risk of thrombotic complications. *Blood* 1999;93:417–424.
20. Herishanu Y, Lishner M, Bomstein Y, et al. Comparative genomic hybridization in polycythemia vera and essential thrombocytosis patients. *Cancer Genet Cytogenet* 2001;128:154–157.
21. Klippel S, Strunck E, Busse CE, et al. Biochemical characterization of PRV-1, a novel hematopoietic cell surface receptor, which is overexpressed in polycythemia rubra vera. *Blood* 2002;100:2441–2448.
22. Mesa RA. Clinical and scientific advances in the Philadelphia-chromosome negative chronic myeloproliferative disorders. *Int J Hematol* 2002;76[Suppl 2]:193–203.
23. Mitterbauer G, Winkler K, Gisslinger H, et al. Clonality analysis using X-chromosome inactivation at the human androgen receptor gene (Humara). Evaluation of large cohorts of patients with chronic myeloproliferative diseases, secondary neutrophilia, and reactive thrombocytosis. *Am J Clin Pathol* 1999;112:93–100.
24. Prchal JT. Pathogenetic mechanisms of polycythemia vera and congenital polycythemic disorders. *Semin Hematol* 2001;38[1 Suppl 2]:10–20.
25. Roumier C, Daudignon A, Soenen V, et al. p190 bcr-abl rearrangement: a secondary cytogenetic event in some chronic myeloid disorders? *Haematologica* 1999;84:1075–1080.
26. Shih LY, Lin TL, Dunn P, et al. Clonality analysis using X-chromosome inactivation patterns by HUMARA-PCR assay in female controls and patients with idiopathic thrombocytosis in Taiwan. *Exp Hematol* 2001;29:202–208.
27. Steensma DP, Tefferi A. Cytogenetic and molecular genetic aspects of essential thrombocythemia. *Acta Haematol* 2002;108:55–65.
28. Teofili L, Martini M, Luongo M, et al. Overexpression of the polycythemia rubra vera-1 gene in essential thrombocythemia. *J Clin Oncol* 2002;20:4249–4254.
29. Tiribelli M, Michelutti A, Damante G, et al. Screening of bcr-abl transcripts in Philadelphia negative essential thrombocythemia. *Leuk Lymphoma* 2000;39:339–341.
30. Luppi M, Morselli M, Emilia G, et al. Spontaneous loss of Ph chromosome with maintenance of clonal hemopoiesis in an untreated patient with myeloproliferative disease and a long survival. *Genes Chromosomes Cancer* 1995;12:237–240.

31. Raskind WH, Ferraris AM, Najfeld V, et al. Further evidence for the existence of a clonal Ph-negative stage in some cases of Ph-positive chronic myelocytic leukemia. *Leukemia* 1993;7: 1163–1167.

32. Basecke J, Griesinger F, Trumper L, et al. Leukemia- and lymphoma-associated genetic aberrations in healthy individuals. *Ann Hematol* 2002;81:64–75.

33. Biernaux C, Loos M, Sels A, et al. Detection of major bcr-abl gene expression at a very low level in blood cells of some healthy individuals. *Blood* 1995;86:3118–3122.

34. Bose S, Deininger M, Gora-Tybor J, et al. The presence of typical and atypical BCR-ABL fusion genes in leukocytes of normal individuals: biologic significance and implications for the assessment of minimal residual disease. *Blood* 1998;92:3362–3367.

35. Pajor L, Vass JA, Kereskai L, et al. Silent Philadelphia chromosome: a distinct developmental stage in a Philadelphia chromosome-positive chronic myeloproliferation? *Cancer Genet Cytogenet* 2000;118:14–19.

Morphologic Subtypes

1. Gardais J, Suraniti S, Fressinaud P. Polycythaemia after myeloid metaplasia with fibrosis: an unusual sequence. *Haematologica* 1992;77:433–434.

2. Higuchi T, Oba R, Endo M, et al. Transition of polycythemia vera to chronic neutrophilic leukemia. *Leuk Lymphoma* 1999;33: 203–206.

3. Jantunen R, Juvonen E, Ikkala E, et al. Development of erythrocytosis in the course of essential thrombocythemia. *Ann Hematol* 1999;78:219–222.

4. Johansson P, Safai-Kutti S, Lindstedt G, et al. Red cell mass, spleen size and plasma erythropoietin in polycythaemia vera and apparent polycythaemia. *Acta Haematol* 2002;108:1–7.

5. Kelly NP, Alkan S, Nand S. Hairy cell leukemia variant developing in a background of polycythemia vera. *Arch Pathol Lab Med* 2003;127:e209–e211.

6. Kreft A, Nolde C, Busche G, et al. Polycythaemia vera: bone marrow histopathology under treatment with interferon, hydroxyurea and busulphan. *Eur J Haematol* 2000;64:32–41.

7. Kurosawa M, Iwasaki H. Megakaryoblastic transformation of polycythemia vera with hypercalcemia. *Ann Hematol* 2002;81: 668–671.

8. Mavrogianni D, Viniou N, Michali E, et al. Leukemogenic risk of hydroxyurea therapy as a single agent in polycythemia vera and essential thrombocythemia: N- and K-ras mutations and microsatellite instability in chromosomes 5 and 7 in 69 patients. *Int J Hematol* 2002;75:394–400.

9. Pearson TC. Evaluation of diagnostic criteria in polycythemia vera. *Semin Hematol* 2001;38[1 Suppl 2]:21–24.

10. Randi ML, Tison T, Zelante A, et al. Polycythemia vera and essential thrombocythemia with monoclonal gammopathy: experience of a single institution. *Haematologica* 2001;86:769–770.

11. Saba NF, Warth JA, Ross DG. Simultaneous occurrence of polycythemia vera and Waldenstrom macroglobulinemia: a case report and review of the literature. *Haematologia (Budap)* 2002; 32:17–23.

12. Shih LY, Wang ML, Fu JF. Simultaneous occurrence of multiple aetiologies of polycythaemia: renal cell carcinoma, sleep apnoea syndrome, and relative polycythaemia in a smoker with masked polycythaemia rubra vera. *J Clin Pathol* 2000;53:561–564.

13. Streiff MB, Smith B, Spivak JL. The diagnosis and management of polycythemia vera in the era since the Polycythemia Vera Study Group: a survey of American Society of Hematology members' practice patterns. *Blood* 2002;99:1144–1149.

14. Suzuki K, Konishi N, Tokura Y, et al. Telangiectasia macularis eruptiva perstans in polycythemia rubra vera. *Eur J Dermatol* 2002;12:201–203.

15. Talarico L, Wolf BC, Kumar A, et al. Reversal of bone marrow fibrosis and subsequent development of polycythemia in patients with myeloproliferative disorders. *Am J Hematol* 1989;30: 248–253.

16. Thiele J, Kvasnicka HM, Muehlhausen K, et al. Polycythemia rubra vera versus secondary polycythemias. A clinicopathological evaluation of distinctive features in 199 patients. *Pathol Res Pract* 2001;197:77–84.

17. Thiele J, Kvasnicka HM, Zankovich R, et al. The value of bone marrow histology in differentiating between early stage polycythemia vera and secondary (reactive) polycythemias. *Haematologica* 2001;86:368–374.

18. Turker M, Ozer EA, Oniz H, et al. Polycythemia vera in a 12-year-old girl: a case report. *Pediatr Hematol Oncol* 2002;19: 263–266.

19. Westwood NB, Gruszka-Westwood AM, Atkinson S, et al. Polycythemia vera: analysis of DNA from blood granulocytes using comparative genomic hybridization. *Haematologica* 2001;86:464–469.

20. Westwood NB, Gruszka-Westwood AM, Pearson CE, et al. The incidences of trisomy 8, trisomy 9 and D20S108 deletion in polycythaemia vera: an analysis of blood granulocytes using interphase fluorescence *in situ* hybridization. *Br J Haematol* 2000;110:839–846.

21. Andersson PO, Ridell B, Wadenvik H, et al. Leukemic transformation of essential thrombocythemia without previous cytoreductive treatment. *Ann Hematol* 2000;79:40–42.

22. Annaloro C, Lambertenghi Deliliers G, Oriani A, et al. Prognostic significance of bone marrow biopsy in essential thrombocythemia. *Haematologica* 1999;84:17–21.

23. Bizzaro N. Chronic lymphocytic leukaemia in a patient with essential thrombocythaemia. *Clin Lab Haematol* 1998;20: 377–379.

24. Ciaudo M, Hadjez JM, Teyssandier I, et al. Prognostic and diagnostic value of endogenous erythroid colony formation in essential thrombocythemia. *Hematol Cell Ther* 1998;40: 171–174.

25. Dror Y, Zipursky A, Blanchette VS. Essential thrombocythemia in children. *J Pediatr Hematol Oncol* 1999;21:356–363.

26. Finazzi G, Ruggeri M, Rodeghiero F, et al. Second malignancies in patients with essential thrombocythaemia treated with busulphan and hydroxyurea: long-term follow-up of a randomized clinical trial. *Br J Haematol* 2000;110:577–583.

27. Gupta R, Abdalla SH, Bain BJ. Thrombocytosis with sideroblastic erythropoiesis: a mixed myeloproliferative myelodysplastic syndrome. *Leuk Lymphoma* 1999;34:615–619.

28. Hejlova N, Gaja A, Frankova H. Pulmonary sarcoidosis in a patient with essential thrombocythemia treated with interferon alfa: a short case report. *Med Sci Monit* 2000;6:380–382.

29. Hernandez-Boluda JC, Cervantes F, Alvarez A, et al. Non-Hodgkin's lymphoma following untreated essential thrombocythemia. *Leuk Lymphoma* 2000;36:421–423.

30. Hirose Y, Masaki Y, Sugai S. Leukemic transformation with trisomy 8 in essential thrombocythemia: a report of four cases. *Eur J Haematol* 2002;68:112–116.

31. Hou M, Carneskog J, Mellqvist UH, et al. Impact of endogenous thrombopoietin levels on the differential diagnosis of essential thrombocythaemia and reactive thrombocytosis. *Eur J Haematol* 1998;61:119–122.

32. Jantunen R, Juvonen E, Ikkala E, et al. Essential thrombocythemia at diagnosis: causes of diagnostic evaluation and presence of positive diagnostic findings. *Ann Hematol* 1998;77: 101–106.

33. Jensen MK, de Nully Brown P, Nielsen OJ, et al. Incidence,

clinical features and outcome of essential thrombocythaemia in a well defined geographical area. *Eur J Haematol* 2000;65: 132–139.

34. Khoury H, Adkins D, Zehnbauer B, et al. Essential thrombocythemia after allogeneic bone marrow transplantation for chronic myelogenous leukemia. *Bone Marrow Transplant* 1998; 22:107–109.

35. Kikawa Y, Fukumoto Y, Obata K, et al. Successful treatment of essential thrombocytemia evolving into agnogenic myeloid metaplasia with interferon-alpha. *J Pediatr Hematol Oncol* 1998;20:463–466.

36. Koike T, Uesugi Y, Toba K, et al. 5q-syndrome presenting as essential thrombocythemia: myelodysplastic syndrome or chronic myeloproliferative disorders? *Leukemia* 1995;9:517–518.

37. Lengfelder E, Hochhaus A, Kronawitter U, et al. Should a platelet limit of 600 × 10(9)/l be used as a diagnostic criterion in essential thrombocythaemia? An analysis of the natural course including early stages. *Br J Haematol* 1998;100:15–23.

38. Lewis S, Oscier D, Boultwood J, et al. Hematological features of patients with myelodysplastic syndromes associated with a chromosome 5q deletion. *Am J Hematol* 1995;49:194–200.

39. Lichtman SM, Wasil T, Ahmad M, et al. Development of essential thrombocythemia in a patient treated with interferon alfa and pentostatin for hairy cell leukemia. *Leuk Lymphoma* 1998;28:423–427.

40. Mesa RA, Hanson CA, Li CY, et al. Diagnostic and prognostic value of bone marrow angiogenesis and megakaryocyte c-Mpl expression in essential thrombocythemia. *Blood* 2002;99:4131–4137.

41. Munro LR, Stevenson DA, Culligan DJ. Translocation (X;5) (q13;q33) in essential thrombocythemia. *Cancer Genet Cytogenet* 1999;114:78–79.

42. Murphy S, Peterson P, Iland H, et al. Experience of the Polycythemia Vera Study Group with essential thrombocythemia: a final report on diagnostic criteria, survival, and leukemic transition by treatment. *Semin Hematol* 1997;34:29–39.

43. Randi ML, Fabris F, Girolami A. Leukemia and myelodysplasia effect of multiple cytotoxic therapy in essential thrombocythemia. *Leuk Lymphoma* 2000;37:379–385.

44. Randi ML, Putti MC, Fabris F, et al. Features of essential thrombocythaemia in childhood: a study of five children. *Br J Haematol* 2000;108:86–89.

45. Regev A, Stark P, Blickstein D, et al. Thrombotic complications in essential thrombocythemia with relatively low platelet counts. *Am J Hematol* 1997;56:168–172.

46. Sacchi S, Vinci G, Gugliotta L, et al. Diagnosis of essential thrombocythemia at platelet counts between 400 and 600 × 10(9)/L. Gruppo Italiano Malattie Mieloproliferative Croniche (GIMMC). *Haematologica* 2000;85:492–495.

47. Sterkers Y, Preudhomme C, Lai JL, et al. Acute myeloid leukemia and myelodysplastic syndromes following essential thrombocythemia treated with hydroxyurea: high proportion of cases with 17p deletion. *Blood* 1998;91:616–622.

48. Takahashi H, Furukawa T, Hashimoto S, et al. 5q- syndrome presenting chronic myeloproliferative disorders-like manifestation: a case report. *Am J Hematol* 2000;64:120–123.

49. Tefferi A. Recent progress in the pathogenesis and management of essential thrombocythemia. *Leuk Res* 2001;25:369–377.

50. Tefferi A, Fonseca R, Pereira DL, et al. A long-term retrospective study of young women with essential thrombocythemia. *Mayo Clin Proc* 2001;76:22–28.

51. Thiele J, Kvasnicka HM, Zankovich R, et al. Relevance of bone marrow features in the differential diagnosis between essential thrombocythemia and early stage idiopathic myelofibrosis. *Haematologica* 2000;85:1126–1134.

52. Uozumi K, Ohno N, Shimotakahara S, et al. Trisomy 8 in essential thrombocythemia in leukemic transformation. *Cancer Genet Cytogenet* 2000;116:84–86.

53. Yang RC, Qian LS. Essential thrombocythaemia in children: a report of nine cases. *Br J Haematol* 2000;110:1009–1010.

54. Akpek G, McAneny D, Weintraub L. Risks and benefits of splenectomy in myelofibrosis with myeloid metaplasia: a retrospective analysis of 26 cases. *J Surg Oncol* 2001;77:42–48.

55. Barosi G. Myelofibrosis with myeloid metaplasia: diagnostic definition and prognostic classification for clinical studies and treatment guidelines. *J Clin Oncol* 1999;17:2954–2970.

56. Barosi G, Ambrosetti A, Centra A, et al. Splenectomy and risk of blast transformation in myelofibrosis with myeloid metaplasia. Italian Cooperative Study Group on Myeloid with Myeloid Metaplasia. *Blood* 1998;91:3630–3636.

57. Barosi G, Ambrosetti A, Finelli C, et al. The Italian Consensus Conference on diagnostic criteria for myelofibrosis with myeloid metaplasia. *Br J Haematol* 1999;104:730–737.

58. Bohm J, Schmitt-Graff A. Gelatinous bone marrow transformation in a case of idiopathic myelofibrosis: a morphological paradox. *Pathol Res Pract* 2000;196:775–779.

59. Chan KW, Ho CP. Amyloidosis complicating idiopathic myelofibrosis. *Am J Kidney Dis* 1999;34:E27.

60. Cervantes F. Prognostic factors and current practice in treatment of myelofibrosis with myeloid metaplasia: an update anno 2000. *Pathol Biol (Paris)* 2001;49:148–152.

61. Cervantes F, Barosi G, Hernandez-Boluda JC, et al. Myelofibrosis with myeloid metaplasia in adult individuals 30 years old or younger: presenting features, evolution and survival. *Eur J Haematol* 2001;66:324–327.

62. Cervantes F, Pereira A, Esteve J, et al. The changing profile of idiopathic myelofibrosis: a comparison of the presenting features of patients diagnosed in two different decades. *Eur J Haematol* 1998;60:101–105.

63. Le Bousse-Kerdiles MC, Martyre MC. Dual implication of fibrogenic cytokines in the pathogenesis of fibrosis and myeloproliferation in myeloid metaplasia with myelofibrosis. *Ann Hematol* 1999;78:437–444.

64. Liu K, Coogan AC, Mann KP. Fine-needle aspiration of large cell lymphoma in a patient with agnogenic myeloid metaplasia: a case report and review of the literature. *Diagn Cytopathol* 1998;19:205–209.

65. Mallouh AA, Sa'di AR. Agnogenic myeloid metaplasia in children. *Am J Dis Child* 1992;146:965–967.

66. Mesa RA, Elliott MA, Tefferi A. Splenectomy in chronic myeloid leukemia and myelofibrosis with myeloid metaplasia. *Blood Rev* 2000;14:121–129.

67. Mesa RA, Hanson CA, Rajkumar SV, et al. Evaluation and clinical correlations of bone marrow angiogenesis in myelofibrosis with myeloid metaplasia. *Blood* 2000;96:3374–3380.

68. Nieto LH, Raya Sanchez JM, Arguelles HA, et al. A case of chronic lymphocytic leukemia overwhelmed by rapidly progressive idiopathic myelofibrosis. *Haematologica* 2000;85: 973–977.

69. Ragni MV, Shreiner DP. Spontaneous "remission" of agnogenic myeloid metaplasia and termination in acute myeloid leukemia. *Arch Intern Med* 1981;141:1481–1484.

70. Reich JM. Sarcoidosis and agnogenic myeloid metaplasia. *J Intern Med* 1994;235:175–178.

71. Shimizu K, Hotta T. Spontaneous remission of agnogenic myeloid metaplasia in a splenectomized patient: a case report with erythrokinetic studies. *Acta Haematol* 1990;83:45–48.

72. Shreiner DP. Spontaneous hematologic remission in agnogenic myeloid metaplasia. *Am J Med* 1976;60:1014–1018.

73. Subramanian VP, Gomez GA, Han T, et al. Coexistence of myeloid metaplasia with myelofibrosis and hairy-cell leukemia. *Arch Intern Med* 1985;145:164–166.

74. Tefferi A. Myelofibrosis with myeloid metaplasia. *N Engl J Med* 2000;342:1255–1265.

75. Tefferi A, Mesa RA, Schroeder G, et al. Cytogenetic findings and their clinical relevance in myelofibrosis with myeloid metaplasia. *Br J Haematol* 2001;113:763–771.

76. Thiele J, Kvasnicka HM, Zankovich R, et al. Clinical and morphological criteria for the diagnosis of prefibrotic idiopathic (primary) myelofibrosis. *Ann Hematol* 2001;80:160–165.

77. Vukelja SJ, Krishnan J, Ward FT, et al. Synchronous Hodgkin's disease and myelofibrosis terminating with granulocytic sarcoma and acute megakaryocytic leukemia. *South Med J* 1990;83:1317–1320.

78. Basara N, Markova J, Schmetzer B, et al. Chronic eosinophilic leukemia: successful treatment with an unrelated bone marrow transplantation. *Leuk Lymphoma* 1998;32:189–193.

79. Bigoni R, Cuneo A, Roberti MG, et al. Cytogenetic and molecular cytogenetic characterization of 6 new cases of idiopathic hypereosinophilic syndrome. *Haematologica* 2000;85:486–491.

80. Chang HW, Leong KH, Koh DR, et al. Clonality of isolated eosinophils in the hypereosinophilic syndrome. *Blood* 1999;93:1651–1657.

81. Darbyshire PJ, Shortland D, Swansbury GJ, et al. A myeloproliferative disease in two infants associated with eosinophilia and chromosome t(1;5) translocation. *Br J Haematol* 1987;66: 483–486.

82. Duell T, Mittermuller J, Schmetzer HM, et al. Chronic myeloid leukemia associated hypereosinophilic syndrome with a clonal t(4;7)(q11;q32). *Cancer Genet Cytogenet* 1997;94:91–94.

83. Dvilansky A, Alkan ML, Ho W, et al. Chronic eosinophilic leukemia complicated by epidural myeloblastoma. *Acta Haematol* 1975;53:356–361.

84. Egesten A, Hagerstrand I, Kristoffersson U, et al. Hypereosinophilic syndrome in a child mosaic for a congenital triplication of the short arm of chromosome 8. *Br J Haematol* 1997;96: 369–373.

85. Ellman L, Hammond D, Atkins L. Eosinophilia, chloromas and a chromosome abnormality in a patient with a myeloproliferative syndrome. *Cancer* 1979;43:2410–2413.

86. Fukushima T, Kuriyama K, Ito H, et al. Successful bone marrow transplantation for idiopathic hypereosinophilic syndrome. *Br J Haematol* 1995;90:213–215.

87. Fureder W, Streubel B, Jordan JH, et al. Reciprocal translocation (3;5)(q26;q22) and possible BCHE gene involvement in an unusual myelogenous disorder with both myeloproliferative and dysplastic features. *Cancer Genet Cytogenet* 2000;121: 133–138.

88. Granjo E, Lima M, Lopes JM, et al. Chronic eosinophilic leukaemia presenting with erythroderma, mild eosinophilia and hyper-IgE: clinical, immunological and cytogenetic features and therapeutic approach. A case report. *Acta Haematol* 2002; 107:108–112.

89. Hermida G, Manjon R, Rodriguez-Salazar M, et al. Hypereosinophilia associated with dysplastic features and a constitutional translocation previously not described. *Haematologica* 2000;85:997–998.

90. Huang CS, Gomez GA, Kohno SI, et al. Chromosomes and causation of human cancer and leukemia. XXXIV. A case of "hypereosinophilic syndrome" with unusual cytogenetic findings in a chloroma, terminating in blastic transformation and CNS leukemia. *Cancer* 1979;44:1284–1289.

91. Juneja S, Stewart J, McKenzie A, et al. Hypereosinophilic syndrome or chronic eosinophilic leukemia: report of a case with a lytic bone lesion. *Leukemia* 1997;11:765–766.

92. Keung YK, Beaty M, Steward W, et al. Chronic myelocytic leukemia with eosinophilia, t(9;12)(q34;p13), and ETV6-ABL gene rearrangement: case report and review of the literature. *Cancer Genet Cytogenet* 2002;138:139–142.

93. Kueck BD, Smith RE, Parkin J, et al. Eosinophilic leukemia: a myeloproliferative disorder distinct from the hypereosinophilic syndrome. *Hematol Pathol* 1991;5:195–205.

94. Kusanagi Y, Ochi H, Matsubara K, et al. Hypereosinophilic syndrome in a trisomy 21 fetus. *Obstet Gynecol* 1998;92:701–702.

95. Lepretre S, Jardin F, Buchonnet G, et al. Eosinophilic leukemia associated with t(2;5)(p23;q31). Eosinophilic leukemia associated with t(2;5)(p23;q31). *Cancer Genet Cytogenet* 2002;133: 164–167.

96. Luciano L, Catalano L, Sarrantonio C, et al. AlphaIFN-induced hematologic and cytogenetic remission in chronic eosinophilic leukemia with t(1;5). *Haematologica* 1999;84:651–653.

97. Ma SK, Kwong YL, Shek TW, et al. The role of trisomy 8 in the pathogenesis of chronic eosinophilic leukemia. *Hum Pathol* 1999;30:864–868.

98. Malbrain ML, Van den Bergh H, Zachee P. Further evidence for the clonal nature of the idiopathic hypereosinophilic syndrome: complete haematological and cytogenetic remission induced by interferon-alpha in a case with a unique chromosomal abnormality. *Br J Haematol* 1996;92:176–183.

99. Maubach PA, Bauchinger M, Emmerich B, et al. Trisomy 7 and 8 in Ph-negative chronic eosinophilic leukemia. *Cancer Genet Cytogenet* 1985;17:159–164.

100. Michel G, Thuret I, Capodano AM, et al. Myelofibrosis in a child suffering from a hypereosinophilic syndrome with trisomy 8: response to corticotherapy. *Med Pediatr Oncol* 1991;19:62–65.

101. Needleman SW, Mane SM, Gutheil JC, et al. Hypereosinophilic syndrome with evolution to myeloproliferative disorder: temporal relationship to loss of Y chromosome and c-N-ras activation. *Hematol Pathol* 1990;4:149–155.

102. Oliver JW, Deol I, Morgan DL, et al. Chronic eosinophilic leukemia and hypereosinophilic syndromes. Proposal for classification, literature review, and report of a case with a unique chromosomal abnormality. *Cancer Genet Cytogenet* 1998;107: 111–117.

103. Ribeiro I, Carvalho IR, Fontes M, et al. Eosinophilic leukaemia with trisomy 8 and double gammopathy. *J Clin Pathol* 1993;46: 672–673.

104. Sato H, Saito H, Ikebuchi K, et al. Biological characteristics of chronic eosinophilic leukemia cells with a t(2;5)(p23;q35) translocation. *Leuk Lymphoma* 1995;19:499–505.

105. Schoffski P, Ganser A, Pascheberg U, et al. Complete haematological and cytogenetic response to interferon alpha-2a of a myeloproliferative disorder with eosinophilia associated with a unique t(4;7) aberration. *Ann Hematol* 2000;79:95–98.

106. Shanske AL, Kalman A, Grunwald H. A myeloproliferative disorder with eosinophilia associated with a unique translocation (3;5). *Br J Haematol* 1996;95:524–526.

107. Suzuki S, Chiba K, Toyoshima N, et al. Chronic eosinophilic leukemia with t(6;11)(q27;q23) translocation. *Ann Hematol* 2001;80:553–556.

108. Takimoto Y, Imanaka F, Hayashi Y, et al. A patient with basophilic-eosinophilic myeloproliferative disorder showing monosomy 7 and hyperhistaminemia. *Acta Haematol* 1997;98: 37–41.

109. Vazquez L, Caballero D, Canizo CD, et al. Allogeneic peripheral blood cell transplantation for hypereosinophilic syndrome with myelofibrosis. *Bone Marrow Transplant* 2000;25:217–218.

110. Viniou N, Yataganas X, Abazis D, et al. Hypereosinophilia associated with monosomy 7. *Cancer Genet Cytogenet* 1995;80:68–71.

111. Weide R, Rieder H, Mehraein Y, et al. Chronic eosinophilic leukaemia (CEL): a distinct myeloproliferative disease. *Br J Haematol* 1997;96:117–123.

112. Yakushijin K, Murayama T, Mizuno I, et al. Chronic eosinophilic leukemia with unique chromosomal abnormality, t(5;12) (q33;q22). *Am J Hematol* 2001;68:301–302.

113. Yamada O, Kitahara K, Imamura K, et al. Clinical and cytogenetic remission induced by interferon-alpha in a patient with chronic eosinophilic leukemia associated with a unique t(3;9;5) translocation. *Am J Hematol* 1998;58:137–141.

114. Lertprasertsuke N, Tsutsumi Y. An unusual form of chronic myeloproliferative disorder. Aleukemic basophilic leukemia. *Acta Pathol Jpn* 1991;41:73–81.

115. Pardanani AD, Morice WG, Hoyer JD, et al. Chronic basophilic leukemia: a distinct clinico-pathologic entity? *Eur J Haematol* 2003;71:18–22.

116. Akin C, Jaffe ES, Raffeld M, et al. An immunohistochemical study of the bone marrow lesions of systemic mastocytosis: expression of stem cell factor by lesional mast cells. *Am J Clin Pathol* 2002;118:242–247.

117. Akin C, Scott LM, Metcalfe DD. Slowly progressive systemic mastocytosis with high mast-cell burden and no evidence of a non-mast-cell hematologic disorder: an example of a smoldering case? *Leuk Res* 2001;25:635–638.

118. Athanassiadou F, Fidani L, Papageorgiou T, et al. Acute lymphoblastic leukemia and urticaria pigmentosa in an infant. *Med Pediatr Oncol* 2000;34:368–369.

119. Brinkley AB Jr, O'Brien MW. Case report 320. Localized eosinophilic fibrohistiocytic lesion of bone (tibia)—a localized form of mastocytosis. *Skeletal Radiol* 1985;14:68–72.

120. Brockow K, Akin C, Huber M, et al. Assessment of the extent of cutaneous involvement in children and adults with mastocytosis: relationship to symptomatology, tryptase levels, and bone marrow pathology. *J Am Acad Dermatol* 2003;48:508–516.

121. Brockow K, Scott LM, Worobec AS, et al. Regression of urticaria pigmentosa in adult patients with systemic mastocytosis: correlation with clinical patterns of disease. *Arch Dermatol* 2002; 138:785–790.

122. Buttner C, Henz BM, Welker P, et al. Identification of activating c-kit mutations in adult-, but not in childhood-onset indolent mastocytosis: a possible explanation for divergent clinical behavior. *J Invest Dermatol* 1998;111:1227–1231.

123. Cox JV, Balaban EP, Demian SE, et al. An eosinophilic fibrohistiocytic lesion of bone marrow in a patient with Hodgkin's disease. A potential for morphologic confusion. *Cancer* 1991;68:1824–1827.

124. Escribano L, Akin C, Castells M, et al. Mastocytosis: current concepts in diagnosis and treatment. *Ann Hematol* 2002;81: 677–690.

125. Escribano L, Diaz-Agustin B, Bellas C, et al. Utility of flow cytometric analysis of mast cells in the diagnosis and classification of adult mastocytosis. *Leuk Res* 2001;25:563–570.

126. Fearfield LA, Francis N, Henry K, et al. Bone marrow involvement in cutaneous mastocytosis. *Br J Dermatol* 2001;144: 561–566.

127. Feger F, Ribadeau Dumas A, Leriche L, et al. Kit and c-kit mutations in mastocytosis: a short overview with special reference to novel molecular and diagnostic concepts. *Int Arch Allergy Immunol* 2002;127:110–114.

128. Fritsche-Polanz R, Jordan JH, Feix A, et al. Mutation analysis of C-KIT in patients with myelodysplastic syndromes without mastocytosis and cases of systemic mastocytosis. *Br J Haematol* 2001;113:357–364.

129. Gupta R, Bain BJ, Knight CL. Cytogenetic and molecular genetic abnormalities in systemic mastocytosis. *Acta Haematol* 2002;107:123–128.

130. Hartmann K, Henz BM. Cutaneous mastocytosis—clinical heterogeneity. *Int Arch Allergy Immunol* 2002;127:143–146.

131. Hauswirth AW, Sperr WR, Ghannadan M, et al. A case of smouldering mastocytosis with peripheral blood eosinophilia and lymphadenopathy. *Leuk Res* 2002;26:601–606.

132. Horny HP, Greschniok A, Jordan JH, et al. Chymase expressing bone marrow mast cells in mastocytosis and myelodysplastic syndromes: an immunohistochemical and morphometric study. *J Clin Pathol* 2003;56:103–106.

133. Horny HP, Valent P. Histopathological and immunohistochemical aspects of mastocytosis. *Int Arch Allergy Immunol* 2002;127: 115–117.

134. Jordan JH, Fritsche-Polanz R, Sperr WR, et al. A case of 'smouldering' mastocytosis with high mast cell burden, monoclonal myeloid cells, and C-KIT mutation Asp-816-Val. *Leuk Res* 2001;25:627–634.

135. Jordan JH, Schernthaner GH, Fritsche-Polanz R, et al. Stem cell factor-induced bone marrow mast cell hyperplasia mimicking systemic mastocytosis (SM): histopathologic and morphologic evaluation with special reference to recently established SM-criteria. *Leuk Lymphoma* 2002;43:575–582.

136. Jordan JH, Walchshofer S, Jurecka W, et al. Immunohistochemical properties of bone marrow mast cells in systemic mastocytosis: evidence for expression of CD2, CD117/Kit, and bcl-x(L). *Hum Pathol* 2001;32:545–552.

137. Jost E, Michaux L, Vanden Abeele M, et al. Complex karyotype and absence of mutation in the c-kit receptor in aggressive mastocytosis presenting with pelvic osteolysis, eosinophilia and brain damage. *Ann Hematol* 2001;80:302–307.

138. Kuint J, Bielorai B, Gilat D, et al. C-kit activating mutation in a neonate with *in-utero* presentation of systemic mastocytosis associated with myeloproliferative disorder. *Br J Haematol* 1999; 106:838–839.

139. Li CY. Diagnosis of mastocytosis: value of cytochemistry and immunohistochemistry. *Leuk Res* 2001;25:537–541.

140. Longley BJ, Metcalfe DD. A proposed classification of mastocytosis incorporating molecular genetics. *Hematol Oncol Clin North Am* 2000;14:697–701.

141. Longley BJ Jr, Metcalfe DD, Tharp M, et al. Activating and dominant inactivating c-KIT catalytic domain mutations in distinct clinical forms of human mastocytosis. *Proc Natl Acad Sci U S A* 1999;96:1609–1614.

142. Longley BJ, Reguera MJ, Ma Y. Classes of c-KIT activating mutations: proposed mechanisms of action and implications for disease classification and therapy. *Leuk Res* 2001;25:571–576.

143. Nagler A, Ben-Arieh Y, Brenner B, et al. Eosinophilic fibrohistiocytic lesion of bone marrow associated with monoclonal gammopathy and osteolytic lesions. *Am J Hematol* 1986;23: 277–281.

144. Natkunam Y, Rouse RV. Utility of paraffin section immunohistochemistry for C-KIT (CD117) in the differential diagnosis of systemic mast cell disease involving the bone marrow. *Am J Surg Pathol* 2000;24:81–91.

145. Noack F, Escribano L, Sotlar K, et al. Evolution of urticaria pigmentosa into indolent systemic mastocytosis: abnormal immunophenotype of mast cells without evidence of c-kit mutation ASP-816-VAL. *Leuk Lymphoma* 2003;44:313–319.

146. Pardanani A, Baek JY, Li CY, et al. Systemic mast cell disease without associated hematologic disorder: a combined retrospective and prospective study. *Mayo Clin Proc* 2002;77:1169–1175.

147. Parker RI. Hematologic aspects of systemic mastocytosis. *Hematol Oncol Clin North Am* 2000;14:557–568.

148. Pullarkat VA, Pullarkat ST, Calverley DC, et al. Mast cell disease associated with acute myeloid leukemia: detection of a new c-kit mutation Asp816His. *Am J Hematol* 2000;65:307–309.

149. Rywlin AM, Hoffman EP, Ortega RS. Eosinophilic fibrohistiocytic lesion of bone marrow: a distinctive new morphologic

finding, probably related to drug hypersensitivity. *Blood* 1972;40: 464–472.

150. Sotlar K, Fridrich C, Mall A, et al. Detection of c-kit point mutation Asp-816 → Val in microdissected pooled single mast cells and leukemic cells in a patient with systemic mastocytosis and concomitant chronic myelomonocytic leukemia. *Leuk Res* 2002;26:979–984.

151. Sperr WR, Escribano L, Jordan JH, et al. Morphologic properties of neoplastic mast cells: delineation of stages of maturation and implication for cytological grading of mastocytosis. *Leuk Res* 2001;25:529–536.

152. Sperr WR, Horny HP, Lechner K, et al. Clinical and biologic diversity of leukemias occurring in patients with mastocytosis. *Leuk Lymphoma* 2000;37:473–486.

153. Sperr WR, Horny HP, Valent P. Spectrum of associated clonal hematologic non-mast cell lineage disorders occurring in patients with systemic mastocytosis. *Int Arch Allergy Immunol* 2002;127:140–142.

154. Valent P, Akin C, Sperr WR, et al. Smouldering mastocytosis: a novel subtype of systemic mastocytosis with slow progression. *Int Arch Allergy Immunol* 2002;127:137–139.

155. Valent P, Horny HP, Escribano L, et al. Diagnostic criteria and classification of mastocytosis: a consensus proposal. *Leuk Res* 2001;25:603–625.

156. Valent P, Samorapoompichit P, Sperr WR, et al. Myelomastocytic leukemia: myeloid neoplasm characterized by partial differentiation of mast cell-lineage cells. *Hematol J* 2002;3:90–94.

157. Valent P, Sperr WR, Samorapoompichit P, et al. Myelomastocytic overlap syndromes: biology, criteria, and relationship to mastocytosis. *Leuk Res* 2001;25:595–602.

158. Waxtein LM, Vega-Memije ME, Cortes-Franco R, et al. Diffuse cutaneous mastocytosis with bone marrow infiltration in a child: a case report. *Pediatr Dermatol* 2000;17:198–201.

159. Wimazal F, Sperr WR, Horny HP, et al. Hyperfibrinolysis in a case of myelodysplastic syndrome with leukemic spread of mast cells. *Am J Hematol* 1999;61:66–77.

160. Yang F, Tran TA, Carlson JA, et al. Paraffin section immunophenotype of cutaneous and extracutaneous mast cell disease: comparison to other hematopoietic neoplasms. *Am J Surg Pathol* 2000;24:703–709.

161. Yavuz AS, Lipsky PE, Yavuz S, et al. Evidence for the involvement of a hematopoietic progenitor cell in systemic mastocytosis from single-cell analysis of mutations in the c-kit gene. *Blood* 2002;100:661–665.

Genotypic Subtypes

1. Lee SJ. Chronic myelogenous leukaemia. *Br J Haematol* 2000; 111:993–1009.

2. Mauro MJ, Druker BJ. Chronic myelogenous leukemia. *Curr Opin Oncol* 2001;13:3–7.

3. Roth AD, Oral A, Przepiorka D, et al. Chronic myelogenous leukemia and acute lymphoblastic leukemia occurring in the course of polycythemia vera. *Am J Hematol* 1993;43:123–128.

4. Waller CF, Fetscher S, Lange W. Treatment-related chronic myelogenous leukemia. *Ann Hematol* 1999;78:341–354.

5. Campo MC, Fortun A, Travieso J. Chronic myeloid leukemia with progression to polycythemia vera. *Sangre (Barc)* 1992;37: 207–208.

6. Kubota K, Arai T, Shirakura T, et al. Erythrocytosis and complex Ph translocation 46,XY,t(9;11;22) in a patient with chronic myelogenous leukemia. *Cancer Genet Cytogenet* 1987;24: 359–362.

7. Shenkenberg TD, Waddell CC, Rice L. Erythrocytosis and marked leukocytosis in overlapping myeloproliferative diseases. *South Med J* 1982;75:868–869.

8. Cagirgan S, Sencan M, Tombuloglu M, et al. Two consecutive spontaneous regressions to chronic phase in a patient with blastic transformation of chronic myelogenous leukemia. *Leuk Lymphoma* 1998;29:423–425.

9. Smadja N, Krulik M, Audebert AA, et al. Spontaneous regression of cytogenetic and haematologic anomalies in Ph1-positive chronic myelogenous leukaemia. *Br J Haematol* 1986;63: 257–262.

10. Yamauchi K, Ide A. Spontaneous remission with cyclic leukocytosis in chronic myelogenous leukemia. *Acta Haematol* 1992;88: 136–138.

11. Acar H, Ecirli S, Gundogan F, et al. Simultaneous occurrence of chronic myelogenous leukemia and non-Hodgkin lymphoma at diagnosis. *Cancer Genet Cytogenet* 1999;108:171–174.

12. al-Amin A, Lennartz K, Runde V, et al. Frequency of clonal B lymphocytes in chronic myelogenous leukemia evaluated by fluorescence in situ hybridization. *Cancer Genet Cytogenet* 1998; 104:45–47.

13. Alvarez-Larran A, Rozman M, Cervantes F. Simultaneous occurrence of multiple myeloma and chronic myeloid leukemia. *Haematologica* 2001;86:894.

14. Blonk MC, van der Valk P, Beverstock GC, et al. Sequential development of peripheral T-cell lymphoma in the course of chronic myelogenous leukemia. *Cancer* 1990;66:1198–1203.

15. Ichinohasama R, Miura I, Takahashi N, et al. Ph-negative non-Hodgkin's lymphoma occurring in chronic phase of Ph-positive chronic myelogenous leukemia is defined as a genetically different neoplasm from extramedullary localized blast crisis: report of two cases and review of the literature. *Leukemia* 2000;14:169–182.

16. Mossafa H, Fourcade C, Pulic M, et al. Chronic lymphocytic leukemia associated with myelodysplastic syndrome and/or chronic myeloid leukemia: evidence for independent clonal chromosomal evolution. *Leuk Lymphoma* 2001;41:337–341.

17. Reeves JE, Robbins BA, Pankey LR, et al. The simultaneous occurrence of variant hairy cell leukemia and chronic-phase chronic myelogenous leukemia. A case report. *Cancer* 1995;75:2089–2092.

18. Sigal Nahum M, Rostoker G, Gaulier A, et al. A combination of mycosis fungoides and chronic myeloid leukemia. A propos of a case. *Ann Dermatol Venereol* 1988;115:159–166.

19. Tanaka M, Kimura R, Matsutani A, et al. Coexistence of chronic myelogenous leukemia and multiple myeloma. Case report and review of the literature. *Acta Haematol* 1998;99:221–223.

20. Wandroo FA, Bareford D, el-Jehani F. Chronic myeloid leukaemia occurring in a patient with hairy cell leukaemia. *J Clin Pathol* 2000;53:940–941.

21. Cervantes F, Villamor N, Esteve J, et al. 'Lymphoid' blast crisis of chronic myeloid leukaemia is associated with distinct clinicohaematological features. *Br J Haematol* 1998;100:123–128.

22. Kahl C, Pelz AF, Bartsch R, et al. Myeloid/natural killer cell precursor blast crisis of chronic myelogenous leukemia with two Philadelphia (Ph-1) chromosomes. *Ann Hematol* 2001;80: 58–61.

23. Khalidi HS, Brynes RK, Medeiros LJ, et al. The immunophenotype of blast transformation of chronic myelogenous leukemia: a high frequency of mixed lineage phenotype in "lymphoid" blasts and a comparison of morphologic, immunophenotypic, and molecular findings. *Mod Pathol* 1998;11:1211–1221.

24. Marinone G, Rossi G, Verzura P. Eosinophilic blast crisis in a case of chronic myeloid leukaemia. *Br J Haematol* 1983;55:251–256.

25. Narita A, Aoki K, Hata S, et al. Basophilic crisis of chronic myeloid leukemia with a novel chromosomal aberration. *Cancer Genet Cytogenet* 1999;114:83–84.

26. Oren H, Duzovali O, Yuksel E, et al. Development of acute promyelocytic leukemia with isochromosome 17q after BCR/ABL positive chronic myeloid leukemia. *Cancer Genet Cytogenet* 1999;109:141–143.

27. Pelloso LA, Baiocchi OC, Chauffaille ML, et al. Megakaryocytic blast crisis as a first presentation of chronic myeloid leukemia. *Eur J Haematol* 2002;69:58–61.

28. Piccinini L, Bonacorsi G, Artusi T. Blast crisis of Ph1-CML, with the prevalent features of malignant histiocytosis. *Haematologica* 1998;83:187–188.

29. Valent P, Spanblochl E, Bankl HC, et al. Kit ligand/mast cell growth factor-independent differentiation of mast cells in myelodysplasia and chronic myeloid leukemic blast crisis. *Blood* 1994;84:4322–4332.

30. Warzynski MJ, White C, Golightly MG, et al. Natural killer lymphocyte blast crisis of chronic myelogenous leukemia. *Am J Hematol* 1989;32:279–286.

31. Winter SS, Greene JM, McConnell TS, et al. Pre-B acute lymphoblastic leukemia with b3a2 (p210) and e1a2 (p190) BCR-ABL fusion transcripts relapsing as chronic myelogenous leukemia with a less differentiated b3a2 (p210) clone. *Leukemia* 1999;13:2007–2011.

32. Ye CC, Echeverri C, Anderson JE, et al. T-cell blast crisis of chronic myelogenous leukemia manifesting as a large mediastinal tumor. *Hum Pathol* 2002;33:770–773.

33. Spiers AS, Bain BJ, Turner JE. The peripheral blood in chronic granulocytic leukaemia. Study of 50 untreated Philadelphia-positive cases. *Scand J Haematol* 1977;18:25–38.

34. Borregaard N, Kjeldsen L, Sengelov H. Mobilization of granules in neutrophils from patients with myeloproliferative disorders. *Eur J Haematol* 1993;50:189–199.

35. Dotti G, Garattini E, Borleri G, et al. Leucocyte alkaline phosphatase identifies terminally differentiated normal neutrophils and its lack in chronic myelogenous leukaemia is not dependent on p210 tyrosine kinase activity. *Br J Haematol* 1999;105:163–172.

36. Farhi DC, Luckey CN, Siddiqui AM. Breakpoint cluster region, immunoglobulin, and T-cell receptor gene rearrangement analysis in juvenile chronic myelogenous leukemia. *Mod Pathol* 1995;8:389–393.

37. Jaffe JP, Gertner E, Miller W. Absent neutrophil alkaline phosphatase in the eosinophilia myalgia syndrome associated with L-tryptophan use. *Am J Hematol* 1991;36:280–281.

38. Saitoh H, Shibata A. Levels of serum granulocyte colony-stimulating factor in patients with chronic myeloid leukemia. *Leuk Lymphoma* 1993;11:443–446.

39. Stagno F, Guglielmo P, Consoli U, et al. All-trans-retinoic-acid- and growth-factor-mediated induction of alkaline phosphatase activity in freshly isolated chronic myeloid leukemia cells. *Acta Haematol* 1999;102:61–65.

40. Taylor DL, Kerwick AM, Elliott SL, et al. Discordant neutrophil alkaline phosphatase activity and cytogenetic response in chronic myeloid leukemia treated with alpha-interferon. *Pathology* 1993;25:363–366.

41. Schmidt U, Mlynek ML, Leder LD. Electron-microscopic characterization of mixed granulated (hybridoid) leucocytes of chronic myeloid leukemia. *Br J Haematol* 1988;68:175–180.

42. Takemori N, Saito N, Tachibana N, et al. Hybrid eosinophilic-basophilic granulocytes in chronic myeloid leukemia. *Am J Clin Pathol* 1988;89:702–703.

43. Aviram A, Blickstein D, Stark P, et al. Significance of BCR-ABL transcripts in bone marrow aspirates of Philadelphia-negative essential thrombocythemia patients. *Leuk Lymphoma* 1999;33:77–82.

44. Cervantes F, Colomer D, Vives-Corrons JL, et al. Chronic myeloid leukemia of thrombocythemic onset: a CML subtype with distinct hematological and molecular features? *Leukemia* 1996;10:1241–1243.

45. Emilia G, Luppi M, Ferrari MG, et al. Chronic myeloid leukemia with thrombocythemic onset may be associated with different BCR/ABL variant transcripts. *Cancer Genet Cytogenet* 1998;101:75–77.

46. Fadilah SA, Cheong SK. BCR-ABL positive essential thrombocythaemia: a variant of chronic myelogenous leukaemia or a distinct clinical entity: a special case report. *Singapore Med J* 2000;41:595–598.

47. Lee JJ, Kim HJ, Chung IJ, et al. Portal, mesenteric, and splenic vein thromboses after splenectomy in a patient with chronic myeloid leukemia variant with thrombocythemic onset. *Am J Hematol* 1999;61:212–215.

48. Trapp OM, Beykirch MK, Petrides PE. Anagrelide for treatment of patients with chronic myelogenous leukemia and a high platelet count. *Blood Cells Mol Dis* 1998;24:9–13.

49. Yamagata T, Mitani K, Kanda Y, et al. Elevated platelet count features the variant type of BCR/ABL junction in chronic myelogenous leukaemia. *Br J Haematol* 1996;94:370–372.

50. Jacobsson S, Wadenvik H, Kutti J, et al. Low megakaryocyte ploidy in Ph-positive chronic myelogenous leukemia measured by flow cytometry. *Am J Clin Pathol* 1999;111:185–190.

51. Sokal JE, Sheerin KA. Decreased stainable marrow iron in chronic granulocytic leukemia. *Am J Med* 1986;81:395–399.

52. Welborn JL, Lewis JP. Correlation of marrow iron patterns with disease status of chronic myelogenous leukemia. *Leuk Lymphoma* 1993;10:469–475.

53. Facchetti F, Tironi A, Marocolo D, et al. Histopathological changes in bone marrow biopsies from patients with chronic myeloid leukaemia after treatment with recombinant alpha-interferon. *Histopathology* 1997;31:3–11.

54. Hirri HM, Green PJ. Pure red cell aplasia in a patient with chronic granulocytic leukaemia treated with interferon-alpha. *Clin Lab Haematol* 2000;22:53–54.

55. Mijovic A, Rolovic Z, Novak A, et al. Chronic myeloid leukemia associated with pure red cell aplasia and terminating in promyelocytic transformation. *Am J Hematol* 1989;31:128–130.

56. Nowell PC, Kant JA, Finan JB, et al. Marrow fibrosis associated with a Philadelphia chromosome. *Cancer Genet Cytogenet* 1992;59:89–92.

57. Thiele J, Kvasnicka HM, Beelen DW, et al. Megakaryopoiesis and myelofibrosis in chronic myeloid leukemia after allogeneic bone marrow transplantation: an immunohistochemical study of 127 patients. *Mod Pathol* 2001;14:129–138.

58. Thiele J, Kvasnicka HM, Schmitt-Graeff A, et al. Changing patterns of histological subgroups during therapy of Ph1+ chronic myelogenous leukaemia. *Histopathology* 2000;37:355–362.

59. Thiele J, Kvasnicka HM, Schmitt-Graeff A, et al. Effects of interferon and hydroxyurea on bone marrow fibrosis in chronic myelogenous leukaemia: a comparative retrospective multicentre histological and clinical study. *Br J Haematol* 2000;108:64–71.

60. Anastasi J, Musvee T, Roulston D, et al. Pseudo-Gaucher histiocytes identified up to 1 year after transplantation for CML are BCR/ABL-positive. *Leukemia* 1998;12:233–237.

61. Roche-Lestienne C, Soenen-Cornu V, Grardel-Duflos N, et al. Several types of mutations of the Abl gene can be found in chronic myeloid leukemia patients resistant to STI571, and they can pre-exist to the onset of treatment. *Blood* 2002;100:1014–1018.

62. Sessarego M, Fugazza G, Bruzzone R, et al. Complex chromosome rearrangements may locate the bcr/abl fusion gene sites other than 22q11. *Haematologica* 2000;85:35–39.

63. Takahashi N, Miura I, Saitoh K, et al. Lineage involvement of stem cells bearing the Philadelphia chromosome in chronic

myeloid leukemia in the chronic phase as shown by a combination of fluorescence-activated cell sorting and fluorescence in situ hybridization. *Blood* 1998;92:4758–4763.

64. Thiele J, Schmitz B, Fuchs R, et al. Detection of the bcr/abl gene in bone marrow macrophages in CML and alterations during interferon therapy—a fluorescence in situ hybridization study on trephine biopsies. *J Pathol* 1998;186:331–335.

65. Wilson GA, Vandenberghe EA, Pollitt RC, et al. Are aberrant *BCR-ABL* transcripts more common than previously thought? *Br J Hematol* 2000;111:1109–1111.

66. Deininger MW, Goldman JM, Melo JV. The molecular biology of chronic myeloid leukemia. *Blood* 2000;96:3343–3356.

67. Lichty BD, Keating A, Callum J, et al. Expression of p210 and p190 BCR-ABL due to alternative splicing in chronic myelogenous leukaemia. *Br J Haematol* 1998;103:711–715.

68. Maru Y. Molecular biology of chronic myeloid leukemia. *Int J Hematol* 2001;73:308–322.

69. Saglio G, Pane F, Gottardi E, et al. Consistent amounts of acute leukemia-associated P190BCR/ABL transcripts are expressed by chronic myelogenous leukemia patients at diagnosis. *Blood* 1996;87:1075–1080.

70. Serrano J, Roman J, Sanchez J, et al. Molecular analysis of lineage-specific chimerism and minimal residual disease by RT-PCR of p210(BCR-ABL) and p190(BCR-ABL) after allogeneic bone marrow transplantation for chronic myeloid leukemia: increasing mixed myeloid chimerism and p190(BCR-ABL) detection precede cytogenetic relapse. *Blood* 2000;95:2659–2665.

71. Witte O. The role of Bcr-Abl in chronic myeloid leukemia and stem cell biology. *Semin Hematol* 2001;38:3–8.

72. Yokohama A, Karasawa M, Okamoto K, et al. ALL- and CML-type BCR/ABL mRNA transcripts in chronic myelogenous leukemia and related disorders. *Leuk Res* 1999;23:477–481.

73. Ohsaka A, Hoshino S, Kobayashi M, et al. Blast crisis of Philadelphia chromosome-positive chronic myeloid leukaemia carrying micro-bcr breakpoint (e19a2 and e191a). *Br J Haematol* 2002;118:251–254.

74. Wada H, Mizutani S, Nishimura J, et al. Establishment and molecular characterization of a novel leukemic cell line with Philadelphia chromosome expressing p230 BCR/ABL fusion protein. *Cancer Res* 1995;55:3192–3196.

75. Bennett JM, Catovsky D, Daniel MT, et al. The chronic myeloid leukaemias: guidelines for distinguishing chronic granulocytic, atypical chronic myeloid, and chronic myelomonocytic leukaemia: proposals by the French-American-British Cooperative Leukaemia Group. *Br J Haematol* 1994;87:746–754.

76. Chan LC, Kwong YL, Lie AK, et al. A case of Philadelphia-negative, M-BCR rearranged eosinophilic leukaemia with trisomy 8 localized by in situ hybridization. *Leukemia* 1994;8:195–198.

77. Costello R, Sainty D, Lafage-Pochitaloff M, et al. Clinical and biological aspects of Philadelphia-negative/BCR-negative chronic myeloid leukemia. *Leuk Lymphoma* 1997;25:225–232.

78. Mahon FX, Labouyrie E, Aurich-Costa J, et al. Philadelphia negative BCR-ABL positive chronic myeloid leukemia mimicking juvenile chronic myeloid leukemia in a 2-year-old child. *Leuk Lymphoma* 1997;26:615–619.

79. Martiat P, Michaux JL, Rodhain J. Philadelphia-negative (Ph-) chronic myeloid leukemia (CML): comparison with Ph+ CML and chronic myelomonocytic leukemia. *Blood* 1991;78:205–211.

80. Berger R. Differences between blastic chronic myeloid leukemia and Ph-positive acute leukemia. *Leuk Lymphoma* 1993;11:235–237.

81. Dawson L, Slater R, Hagemeijer A, et al. Secondary T-acute lymphoblastic leukaemia mimicking blast crisis in chronic myeloid leukaemia. *Br J Haematol* 1999;106:104–106.

82. Harder L, Gesk S, Martin-Subero JI, et al. Cytogenetic and molecular characterization of simultaneous chronic and acute myelocytic leukemia. *Cancer Genet Cytogenet* 2003;142:80–82.

83. Kroschinsky F, Friedrich K, Hanel M, et al. Extramedullary blast crisis of chronic myeloid leukemia after allogeneic hematopoietic stem cell transplantation mimicking aggressive, translocation t(14;18)-positive B-cell lymphoma. *Ann Hematol* 2003;82:47–52.

84. Lim LC, Heng KK, Vellupillai M, et al. Molecular and phenotypic spectrum of *de novo* Philadelphia positive acute leukemia. *Int J Mol Med* 1999;4:665–667.

85. Manley R, Cochrane J, McDonald M, et al. Clonally unrelated BCR-ABL-negative acute myeloblastic leukemia masquerading as blast crisis after busulphan and interferon therapy for BCR-ABL-positive chronic myeloid leukemia. *Leukemia* 1999;13:126–129.

86. Costello RT, Gabert J, Brunel V, et al. Minor breakpoint cluster region (m-BCR) positive chronic myeloid leukaemia with an acute lymphoblastic leukaemia onset: a case report. *Br J Haematol* 1995;91:428–430.

87. Lemes A, Gomez Casares MT, de la Iglesia S, et al. p190 BCR-ABL rearrangement in chronic myeloid leukemia and acute lymphoblastic leukemia. *Cancer Genet Cytogenet* 1999;113:100–102.

88. Dautel MM, Francois S, Bertheas MF, et al. Successive transformation of chronic myelomonocytic leukemia into acute myeloblastic then lymphoblastic leukemia, both with minor-bcr rearrangement. *Br J Haematol* 1997;98:210–212.

89. Hur M, Song EY, Kang SH, et al. Lymphoid preponderance and the absence of basophilia and splenomegaly are frequent in m-bcr-positive chronic myelogenous leukemia. *Ann Hematol* 2002;81:219–223.

90. Ohno T, Hada S, Sugiyama T, et al. Chronic myeloid leukemia with minor-bcr breakpoint developed hybrid type of blast crisis. *Am J Hematol* 1998;57:320–325.

91. Ohsaka A, Shiina S, Kobayashi M, et al. Philadelphia chromosome-positive chronic myeloid leukemia expressing p190(BCR-ABL). *Intern Med* 2002;41:1183–1187.

92. Ravandi F, Cortes J, Albitar M, et al. Chronic myelogenous leukaemia with p185(BCR/ABL) expression: characteristics and clinical significance. *Br J Haematol* 1999;107:581–586.

93. Roumier C, Daudignon A, Soenen V, et al. p190 bcr-abl rearrangement: a secondary cytogenetic event in some chronic myeloid disorders? *Haematologica* 1999;84:1075–1080.

94. Solves P, Bolufer P, Lopez JA, et al. Chronic myeloid leukemia with expression of ALL-type BCR/ABL transcript: a case-report and review of the literature. *Leuk Res* 1999;23:851–854.

95. Yamaguchi H, Inokuchi K, Shinohara T, et al. Extramedullary presentation of chronic myelogenous leukemia with p190 BCR/ABL transcripts. *Cancer Genet Cytogenet* 1998;102:74–77.

96. Christopoulos C, Kottoris K, Mikraki V, et al. Presence of the bcr/abl rearrangement in a patient with chronic neutrophilic leukaemia. *J Clin Pathol* 1996;49:1013–1015.

97. Cioc AM, Nuovo GJ. Expression of mu-BCR-ADL transcripts in chronic neutrophilic leukemia. *Am J Clin Pathol* 2002;118:842–847.

98. Pane F, Frigeri F, Sindona M, et al. Neutrophilic-chronic myeloid leukemia: a distinct disease with a specific molecular marker. *Blood* 1996;88:2410–2414.

99. Quackenbush RC, Reuther GW, Miller JP, et al. Analysis of the biologic properties of p230 Bcr-Abl reveals unique and

overlapping properties with the oncogenic p185 and p210 Bcr-Abl tyrosine kinases. *Blood* 2000;95:2913–2921.

100. Verstovsek S, Lin H, Kantarjian H, et al. Neutrophilic-chronic myeloid leukemia: low levels of p230 BCR/ABL mRNA and undetectable BCR/ABL protein may predict an indolent course. *Cancer* 2002;94:2416–2425.

101. Dincol G, Nalcaci M, Dogan O, et al. Coexistence of chronic neutrophilic leukemia with multiple myeloma. *Leuk Lymphoma* 2002;43:649–651.

102. Ito K, Usuki K, Iki S, et al. Chronic neutrophilic leukemia associated with chronic lymphocytic leukemia. *Int J Hematol* 1998;68:87–94.

103. Stevenson JP, Schwarting R, Schuster SJ. Analysis of clonality using X-linked polymorphisms in a patient with multiple myeloma and myelofibrosis. *Am J Hematol* 1998;59:79–82.

104. Usuda H, Naito M, Ohyach K, et al. A case of multiple myeloma producing granulocyte colony-stimulating factor. *Pathol Int* 1997;47:866–869.

105. Billio A, Venturi R, Morello E, et al. Chronic neutrophilic leukemia evolving from polycythemia vera with multiple chromosome rearrangements: a case report. *Haematologica* 2001;86:1225–1226.

106. Boggs DR, Kaplan SS. Cytobiologic and clinical aspects in a patient with chronic neutrophilic leukemia after Thorotrast exposure. *Am J Med* 1986;81:905–910.

107. Elliott MA, Dewald GW, Tefferi A, et al. Chronic neutrophilic leukemia (CNL): a clinical, pathologic and cytogenetic study. *Leukemia* 2001;15:35–40.

108. Foa P, Iurlo A, Saglio G, et al. Chronic neutrophilic leukaemia associated with polycythemia vera: pathogenetic implications and therapeutic approach. *Br J Haematol* 1991;78:286–288.

109. Froberg MK, Brunning RD, Dorion P, et al. Demonstration of clonality in neutrophils using FISH in a case of chronic neutrophilic leukemia. *Leukemia* 1998;12:623–626.

110. Frank MB, Norwood TH, Willerford DM. Chimeric del20q in a case of chronic neutrophilic leukemia. *Am J Hematol* 2000;64:229–231.

111. Hasle H, Olesen G, Kerndrup G, et al. Chronic neutrophil leukaemia in adolescence and young adulthood. *Br J Haematol* 1996;94:628–630.

112. Higuchi T, Oba R, Endo M, et al. Transition of polycythemia vera to chronic neutrophilic leukemia. *Leuk Lymphoma* 1999;33:203–206.

113. Iurlo A, Foa P, Maiolo AT, et al. Polycythemia vera terminating in chronic neutrophilic leukemia: report of a case. *Am J Hematol* 1990;35:139–140.

114. Katsuki K, Shinohara K, Takeda K, et al. Chronic neutrophilic leukemia with acute myeloblastic transformation. *Jpn J Clin Oncol* 2000;30:362–365.

115. Kojima K, Yasukawa M, Hara M, et al. Familial occurrence of chronic neutrophilic leukaemia. *Br J Haematol* 1999;105:428–430.

116. Matano S, Nakamura S, Kobayashi K, et al. Deletion of the long arm of chromosome 20 in a patient with chronic neutrophilic leukemia: cytogenetic findings in chronic neutrophilic leukemia. *Am J Hematol* 1997;54:72–75.

117. Orazi A, Cattoretti G, Sozzi G. A case of chronic neutrophilic leukemia with trisomy 8. *Acta Haematol* 1989;81:148–151.

118. Ota S, Tanaka J, Kobayashi S, et al. Evolution to acute myeloblastic leukemia from chronic neutrophilic leukemia with dysplastic features in granulocytic lineage. *Acta Haematol* 2000;104:207–211.

119. Pascucci M, Dorion P, Makary A, et al. Chronic neutrophilic leukemia evolving from a myelodysplastic syndrome. *Acta Haematol* 1997;98:163–166.

120. Takamatsu Y, Kondo S, Inoue M, et al. Chronic neutrophilic leukemia with dysplastic features mimicking myelodysplastic syndromes. *Int J Hematol* 1996;63:65–69.

121. Terre C, Garcia I, Bastie JN, et al. A case of chronic neutrophilic leukemia with deletion (11)(q23). *Cancer Genet Cytogenet* 1999;110:70–71.

122. Yamamoto K, Nagata K, Kida A, et al. Acquired gain of an X chromosome as the sole abnormality in the blast crisis of chronic neutrophilic leukemia. *Cancer Genet Cytogenet* 2002;134:84–87.

123. Yanagisawa K, Ohminami H, Sato M, et al. Neoplastic involvement of granulocytic lineage, not granulocytic-monocytic, monocytic, or erythrocytic lineage, in a patient with chronic neutrophilic leukemia. *Am J Hematol* 1998;57:221–224.

124. Zittoun R, Rea D, Ngoc LH, et al. Chronic neutrophilic leukemia. A study of four cases. *Ann Hematol* 1994;68:55–60.

125. Zoumbos NC, Symeonidis A, Kourakli-Symeonidis A. Chronic neutrophilic leukemia with dysplastic features. A new variant of the myelodysplastic syndromes. *Acta Haematol* 1989;82:156–160.

126. Haskovec C, Ponzetto C, Polak J, et al. P230 BCR/ABL protein may be associated with an acute leukaemia phenotype. *Br J Haematol* 1998;103:1104–1108.

127. Melo JV. BCR-ABL gene variants. *Baillieres Clin Haematol* 1997;10:203–222.

128. Yamagata T, Mitani K, Kanda Y, et al. Elevated platelet count features the variant type of BCR/ABL junction in chronic myelogenous leukaemia. *Br J Haematol* 1996;94:370–372.

129. Aguiar RC, Chase A, Coulthard S, et al. Abnormalities of chromosome band 8p11 in leukemia: two clinical syndromes can be distinguished on the basis of MOZ involvement. *Blood* 1997;90:3130–3135.

130. Chaffanet M, Popovici C, Leroux D, et al. t(6;8), t(8;9) and t(8;13) translocations associated with stem cell myeloproliferative disorders have close or identical breakpoints in chromosome region 8p11-12. *Oncogene* 1998;16:945–949.

131. Demiroglu A, Steer EJ, Heath C, et al. The t(8;22) in chronic myeloid leukemia fuses BCR to FGFR1: transforming activity and specific inhibition of FGFR1 fusion proteins. *Blood* 2001;98:3778–3783.

132. Fioretos T, Panagopoulos I, Lassen C, et al. Fusion of the BCR and the fibroblast growth factor receptor-1 (FGFR1) genes as a result of t(8;22)(p11;q11) in a myeloproliferative disorder: the first fusion gene involving BCR but not ABL. *Genes Chromosomes Cancer* 2001;32:302–310.

133. Jabbar Al-Obaidi M, Rymes N, White P, et al. A fourth case of 8p11 myeloproliferative disorder transforming to B-lineage acute lymphoblastic leukemia. A case report. *Acta Haematol* 2002;107:98–100.

134. Kulkarni S, Reiter A, Smedley D, et al. The genomic structure of ZNF198 and location of breakpoints in the t(8;13) myeloproliferative syndrome. *Genomics* 1999;55:118–121.

135. Macdonald D, Reiter A, Cross NC. The 8p11 myeloproliferative syndrome: a distinct clinical entity caused by constitutive activation of FGFR1. *Acta Haematol* 2002;107:101–107.

136. Martinez-Climent JA, Vizcarra E, Benet I, et al. Cytogenetic response induced by interferon alpha in the myeloproliferative disorder with eosinophilia, T cell lymphoma and the chromosomal translocation t(8;13). *Leukemia* 1998;12:999–1000.

137. Matsumoto K, Morita K, Takada S, et al. A chronic myelogenous leukemia-like myeloproliferative disorder accompanied by T-cell lymphoblastic lymphoma with chromosome translocation t(8;13)(p11;q12): a Japanese case. *Int J Hematol* 1999;70:278–282.

138. Popovici C, Adelaide J, Ollendorff V, et al. Fibroblast growth factor receptor 1 is fused to FIM in stem-cell myeloproliferative

disorder with t(8;13). *Proc Natl Acad Sci U S A* 1998;95:5712–5717.

139. Popovici C, Zhang B, Gregoire MJ, et al. The t(6;8)(q27;p11) translocation in a stem cell myeloproliferative disorder fuses a novel gene, FOP, to fibroblast growth factor receptor 1. *Blood* 1999;93:1381–1389.

140. Reiter A, Sohal J, Kulkarni S, et al. Consistent fusion of ZNF198 to the fibroblast growth factor receptor-1 in the t(8;13)(p11;q12) myeloproliferative syndrome. *Blood* 1998;92:1735–1742.

141. Roy S, Szer J, Campbell LJ, et al. Sequential transformation of t(8;13)-related disease: a case report. *Acta Haematol* 2002;107:95–97.

142. Sohal J, Chase A, Mould S, et al. Identification of four new translocations involving FGFR1 in myeloid disorders. *Genes Chromosomes Cancer* 2001;32:155–163.

143. Still IH, Cowell JK. The t(8;13) atypical myeloproliferative disorder: further analysis of the ZNF198 gene and lack of evidence for multiple genes disrupted on chromosome 13. *Blood* 1998;92:1456–1458.

144. Xiao S, Nalabolu SR, Aster JC, et al. FGFR1 is fused with a novel zinc-finger gene, ZNF198, in the t(8;13) leukaemia/lymphoma syndrome. *Nat Genet* 1998;18:84–87.

Unclassified Myeloproliferative Disorders

1. Baxter EJ, Kulkarni S, Vizmanos JL, et al. Novel translocations that disrupt the platelet-derived growth factor receptor beta (PDGFRB) gene in BCR-ABL-negative chronic myeloproliferative disorders. *Br J Haematol* 2003;120:251–256.

2. Duell T, Mittermuller J, Schmetzer HM, et al. Chronic myeloid leukemia associated hypereosinophilic syndrome with a clonal t(4;7)(q11;q32). *Cancer Genet Cytogenet* 1997;94:91–94.

3. Myint H, Chacko J, Mould S, et al. Karyotypic evolution in a granulocytic sarcoma developing in a myeloproliferative disorder with a novel (3;4) translocation. *Br J Haematol* 1995;90:462–464.

4. Steer EJ, Cross NC. Myeloproliferative disorders with translocations of chromosome 5q31-35: role of the platelet-derived growth factor receptor beta. *Acta Haematol* 2002;107:113–122.

5. Lertprasertsuke N, Tsutsumi Y. An unusual form of chronic myeloproliferative disorder. Aleukemic basophilic leukemia. *Acta Pathol Jpn* 1991;41:73–81.

6. Takimoto Y, Imanaka F, Hayashi Y, et al. A patient with basophilic-eosinophilic myeloproliferative disorder showing monosomy 7 and hyperhistaminemia. *Acta Haematol* 1997;98:37–41.

HISTIOCYTIC NEOPLASMS

Clonal histiocyte disorders are rare (Tables 23-1 and 23-2). They are, in effect, the developmentally mature counterparts of the clonal myeloid disorders, showing similar risk factors and a propensity for coexisting lymphoplasmacytic disease. In some cases, these disorders are difficult to distinguish from one another (Table 23-3).

LANGERHANS CELL HISTIOCYTOSIS

Langerhans cell histiocytosis (LCH) is a clonal disease of epithelial dendritic cells (1–9) (Figs. 23-1 and 23-2). Slightly more common in male patients, LCH may present at any age but is usually seen in the first two decades of life. LCH is more common in patients with a history of acute lymphoblastic leukemia and possibly germ cell tumors. LCH may be localized or generalized. Disseminated disease is characterized by involvement of bone marrow, bone, liver, spleen, lymph nodes, and visceral organs. The course of the disease is often indolent, even spontaneously regressing, but may occasionally show aggressive or even malignant clinicopathologic features (Langerhans cell sarcoma).

The peripheral blood usually shows nonspecific findings including eosinophilia, monocytosis, and/or thrombocytopenia. Circulating Langerhans cells are rarely found (5). Marrow aspirate smears show ovoid to elongated histiocytes containing a bland, eccentric nucleus and moderately abundant pale-staining cytoplasm. The nucleus shows a central linear groove, indentation, or twist; a small distinct nucleolus; and finely granular chromatin. Electron microscopy

TABLE 23-1. CLASSIFICATION OF HISTIOCYTIC AND DENDRITIC CELL NEOPLASMS ACCORDING TO THE WORLD HEALTH ORGANIZATION

Macrophage/histiocytic neoplasm
  Histiocytic sarcoma

Dendritic cell neoplasms
  Langerhans cell histiocytosis
  Langerhans cell sarcoma
  Interdigitating dendritic cell sarcoma/tumor
  Follicular dendritic cell sarcoma/tumor
  Dendritic cell sarcoma, not otherwise specified

TABLE 23-2. ORGANIZATION OF HISTIOCYTIC NEOPLASMS IN THIS CHAPTER

Langerhans cell histiocytosis
Histiocytic sarcoma
Malignant histiocytosis
Erdheim-Chester disease
Xanthomatous disease

TABLE 23-3. DIFFERENTIAL FEATURES OF HISTIOCYTIC NEOPLASMS INVOLVING THE BONE MARROW

	Blasts	Foam Cells	GC	BG	CD1a	CD68	S100
AMoL	+	−	−	−	−	+/−	−
ECD	−	+	+	−	−	+	+/−
LCH	−	+/−	+/−	+	+	+	+
MH	−/+	−	−	−	−	+	+/−
HS	−	−	−	−	−	+	+/−
XD	−	+	+	−	−	−	

AMoL, acute monocytic leukemia; BG, Birbeck granules; ECD, Erdheim-Chester disease; GC, giant cells; HS, histiocytic sarcoma; LCH, Langerhans cell histiocytosis; MH, malignant histiocytosis; XD, xanthomatous disease; +, positive; −, negative; +/−, usually positive, sometimes negative.

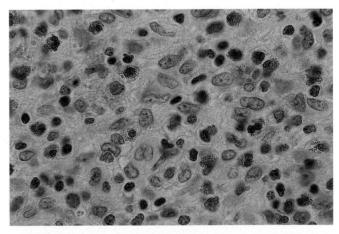

FIGURE 23-1. Bone biopsy specimen, Langerhans cell histiocytosis. Numerous typical Langerhans cells are present, admixed with eosinophils and lymphocytes, in this specimen from a patient with eosinophilic granuloma of the skull.

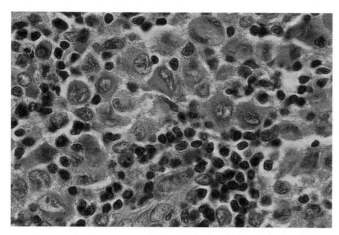

FIGURE 23-2. Bone biopsy specimen, Langerhans cell histiocytosis. The Langerhans cells are larger and more pleomorphic than those in Figure 23-1, in this vertebral specimen from a patient with multifocal disease.

shows Birbeck granules. Histologic sections of the bone marrow show interstitial clusters or sheets of histiocytes, admixed with variable numbers of eosinophils and lymphocytes. Other findings may include fibrosis and dysplastic hematopoiesis (10). Hemophagocytosis is often prominent, and hemophagocytic syndrome may be the presenting disorder in LCH (11–13).

Flow cytometry and immunostains show expression of CD1a, CD4, CD11c, CD25, CD68, HLA-DR, bcl-2 protein, p53 protein, S100 protein, and vimentin. CD2, CD11a, and CD11b may also be expressed. CD3, CD5, CD14, CD15, CD45, and lysozyme are not expressed. Genetic studies have demonstrated clonal X inactivation and numerous chromosomal gains and losses (14–16).

LCH may be accompanied or followed by lymphoblastic malignancy and has often been reported with B-cell and plasma cell malignancies (17–22). The coexistence of LCH and Erdheim-Chester disease suggests a spectrum of disease encompassing both disorders (23–25).

The differential diagnosis includes other reactive and clonal histiocytoses. However, no other disorders show the elongated, grooved nuclei and Birbeck granules seen in LCH.

HISTIOCYTIC SARCOMA

Histiocytic sarcoma, or true histiocytic lymphoma, is a tumor of phenotypically mature, morphologically atypical histiocytes. Histiocytic sarcoma may involve the bone marrow as a primary site or as a secondary site after discovery of a solid tumor in the gastrointestinal tract or elsewhere (1–7). It has been reported as a *de novo* tumor and as a transformation of B-cell chronic lymphocytic leukemia (8).

The peripheral blood is typically not involved, although in some cases a terminal leukemic phase resembling acute monocytic leukemia has been reported. Bone marrow aspi-

rate smears and sections show a diffuse proliferation of large, pleomorphic cells with bizarre nuclei, prominent nucleoli, and abundant, sometimes vacuolated cytoplasm. Multinuclearity, spindled cells, foam cells, and a high mitotic rate have been described. Cytochemical stains show strong positivity for nonspecific esterase and acid phosphatase.

Immunophenotyping shows expression of CD4 (variable), CD11b and 11c (variable), CD13 (variable), CD14 (variable), CD15 (variable), CD30, CD45 (variable), CD56, CD68, α_1-antitrypsin, lysozyme, p53 protein, and S100 protein (variable). CD1a is not expressed. Genetic studies have rarely, if ever, been successful in histiocytic sarcoma.

The differential diagnosis includes malignant histiocytosis, which tends to present with prominent systemic symptoms and widespread bone marrow disease, and other histiocytic lesions.

MALIGNANT HISTIOCYTOSIS

Malignant histiocytosis is a leukemia-like disorder of histiocytes, presenting as widespread disease with bone marrow involvement (1–16) (Figs. 23-3 through 23-8). Patients typically present with fever, wasting, and hepatosplenomegaly. Malignant histiocytosis has been reported as a *de novo* malignancy and as a terminal event in true histiocytic lymphoma and chronic myeloid leukemia (17–19).

The peripheral blood often shows cytopenias. Neutrophilia owing to tumor production of macrophage colony-stimulating factor has been reported (20). The bone marrow shows a diffuse infiltrate of pleomorphic cells with irregular nuclei, multinuclearity, nucleoli, and clear to granular, periodic acid-Schiff–positive cytoplasm. Hemophagocytosis may be present within malignant cells and/or reactive histiocytes. Cytochemical stains are intensely positive for fluoride-inhibitable nonspecific esterase and tartrate-resistant acid phosphatase and negative for myeloperoxidase.

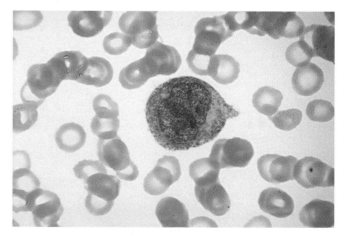

FIGURE 23-3. Peripheral blood smear, malignant histiocytosis. A large cell with a pleomorphic nucleus, of uncertain lineage without additional studies, is seen.

24. Kambouchner M, Colby TV, Domenge C, et al. Erdheim-Chester disease with prominent pulmonary involvement associated with eosinophilic granuloma of mandibular bone. *Histopathology* 1997;30:353–358.
25. Vital C, Bioulac-Sage P, Tison F, et al. Brain stem infiltration by mixed Langerhans cell histiocytosis and Chester-Erdheim disease: more than just an isolated case? *Clin Exp Pathol* 1999;47:71–76.

Histiocytic Sarcoma

1. Alexandrakis MG, Chatzivasili A, Stefanaki K, et al. Co-existence of cutaneous true histiocytic lymphoma with refractory anaemia: report of a case. *Haematologia (Budap)* 2000;30:61–67.
2. Chin NW, Gangi M, Fani K, et al. Colonic histiocytic neoplasm mimicking malignant histiocytosis and presenting as intussusception. *Hum Pathol* 1995;26:682–687.
3. Copie-Bergman C, Wotherspoon AC, Norton AJ, et al. True histiocytic lymphoma: a morphologic, immunohistochemical, and molecular genetic study of 13 cases. *Am J Surg Pathol* 1998;22:1386–1392.
4. Esteve J, Rozman M, Campo E, et al. Leukemia after true histiocytic lymphoma: another type of acute monocytic leukemia with histiocytic differentiation (AML-M5c)? *Leukemia* 1995;9:1389–1391.
5. Hull DR, Alexander HD, Markey GM, et al. Histiocytic lymphoma presenting as a testicular tumour and terminating in acute monoblastic leukaemia. *J Clin Pathol* 2000;53:788–790.
6. Osborne BM, Mackay B. True histiocytic lymphoma with multiple skin nodules. *Ultrastruct Pathol* 1994;18:241–246.
7. Seo IS, Henley JD, Min KW, et al. True histiocytic lymphoma of the esophagus in an HIV-positive patient: an ultrastructural study. *Ultrastruct Pathol* 1999;23:333–339.
8. Wetzler M, Kurzrock R, Goodacre AM, et al. Transformation of chronic lymphocytic leukemia to lymphoma of true histiocytic type. *Cancer* 1995;76:609–617.

Malignant Histiocytosis

1. Bucsky P, Favara B, Feller AC, et al. Malignant histiocytosis and large cell anaplastic (Ki-1) lymphoma in childhood: guidelines for differential diagnosis—report of the Histiocyte Society. *Med Pediatr Oncol* 1994;22:200–203.
2. Egeler RM, Schmitz L, Sonneveld P, et al. Malignant histiocytosis: a reassessment of cases formerly classified as histiocytic neoplasms and review of the literature. *Med Pediatr Oncol* 1995;25:1–7.
3. Esteve J, Rozman M, Campo E, et al. Leukemia after true histiocytic lymphoma: another type of acute monocytic leukemia with histiocytic differentiation (AML-M5c)? *Leukemia* 1995;9:1389–1391.
4. Ferster A, Corazza F, Heimann P, et al. Anaplastic large cell lymphoma of true histiocytic origin in an infant: unusual clinical, hematological, and cytogenetic features. *Med Pediatr Oncol* 1994;22:147–152.
5. Fine KD, Solano M, Polter DE, et al. Malignant histiocytosis in a patient presenting with hepatic dysfunction and peliosis hepatis. *Am J Gastroenterol* 1995;90:485–488.
6. Gogusev J, Nezelof C. Malignant histiocytosis. histologic, cytochemical, chromosomal, and molecular data with a nosologic discussion. *Hematol Oncol Clin North Am* 1998;12:445–463.
7. Jain M, Nangia A, Bajaj P. Malignant histiocytosis in childhood: a case report. *Diagn Cytopathol* 1999;21:359–361.
8. Kobari S, Ohshima K, Sumiyoshi Y, et al. Analysis of the Epstein-Barr viral genome in so-called malignant histiocytosis syndrome. *Pathol Int* 1996;46:355–363.
9. Laurencet FM, Chapuis B, Roux-Lombard P, et al. Malignant histiocytosis in the leukaemic stage: a new entity (M5c-AML) in the FAB classification? *Leukemia* 1994;8:502–506.
10. Lima M, Orfao A, Coutinho J, et al. An unusual acute myeloid leukemia associated with hyper IgE: another case of AML-M5c? *Haematologica* 2001;86:216–217.
11. Mongkonsritragoon W, Li CY, Phyliky RL. True malignant histiocytosis. *Mayo Clin Proc* 1998;73:520–528.
12. Ohno T, Sugiyama T, Furukawa H, et al. Malignant histiocytosis associated with autoimmune thrombocytopenia. *Am J Hematol* 1994;45:244–247.
13. Ohshima K, Fujisaki T, Nagafuchi S, et al. Malignant histiocytosis derived from a common histiocyte clone in a patient with chronic Epstein-Barr virus infection. *Leuk Lymphoma* 1995;17:355–360.
14. Sasou S, Nakamura SI, Habano W, et al. True malignant histiocytosis developed during chemotherapy for mediastinal immature teratoma. *Hum Pathol* 1996;27:1099–1103.
15. Sato T, Terui T, Kogawa K, et al. A case of true malignant histiocytosis: identification of histiocytic origin with use of immunohistochemical and immunocytogenetic methods. *Ann Hematol* 2002;81:285–288.
16. Schmidt D. Malignant histiocytosis. *Curr Opin Hematol* 2001;8:1–4.
17. Srichaikul T, Sonakul D, Meekungwal P, et al. Pleomorphic large cell hemato-lymphoma (the so-called "malignant histiocytosis"): clinicopathological and immunophenotypic studies in 35 cases. *J Med Assoc Thai* 1994;77:588–598.
18. Takahashi S, Asamoto M, Nakazawa T, et al. Robb-Smith type malignant histiocytosis associated with a mediastinal germ cell tumor. *Jpn J Clin Oncol* 1994;24:327–330.
19. Piccinini L, Bonacorsi G, Artusi T. Blast crisis of Ph1-CML, with the prevalent features of malignant histiocytosis. *Haematologica* 1998;83:187–188.
20. Ozaki S, Matsushita T, Ide M, et al. Macrophage colony-stimulating factor-producing malignant histiocytosis. *Br J Haematol* 1995;90:453–456.
21. Ohshima K, Kikuchi M, Mizuno S, et al. Hepatosinusoidal leukaemia/lymphoma consisting of Epstein-Barr virus-containing natural killer cell leukaemia/lymphoma and T-cell lymphoma; mimicking malignant histiocytosis. *Hematol Oncol* 1995;13:83–97.
22. Tsutsumi Y, Tang X, Yamada T. Epstein-Barr virus (EBV)-induced CD30+ natural killer cell-type malignancy resembling malignant histiocytosis: malignant transformation in chronic active EBV infection associating hypogammaglobulinemia. *Pathol Int* 1997;47:384–392.

Erdheim-Chester Disease

1. Gupta A, Kelly B, McGuigan JE. Erdheim-Chester disease with prominent pericardial involvement: clinical, radiologic, and histologic findings. *Am J Med Sci* 2002;324:96–100.
2. Kim NR, Ko YH, Choe YH, et al. Erdheim-Chester disease with extensive marrow necrosis: a case report and literature review. *Int J Surg Pathol* 2001;9:73–79.
3. Kenn W, Eck M, Allolio B, et al. Erdheim-Chester disease: evidence for a disease entity different from Langerhans cell histiocytosis? Three cases with detailed radiological and immunohistochemical analysis. *Hum Pathol* 2000;31:734–739.
4. Murray D, Marshall M, England E, et al. Erdheim-Chester disease. *Clin Radiol* 2001;56:481–484.
5. Ono K, Oshiro M, Uemura K, et al. Erdheim-Chester disease: a case report with immunohistochemical and biochemical examination. *Hum Pathol* 1996;27:91–95.

6. Reithmeier T, Trost HA, Wolf S, et al. Xanthogranuloma of the Erdheim-Chester type within the sellar region: case report. *Clin Neuropathol* 2002;21:24–28.

7. Rush WL, Andriko JA, Galateau-Salle F, et al. Pulmonary pathology of Erdheim-Chester disease. *Mod Pathol* 2000;13: 747–754.

8. Serratrice J, Granel B, De Roux C, et al. "Coated aorta": a new sign of Erdheim-Chester disease. *J Rheumatol* 2000;27:1550–1553.

9. Veyssier-Belot C, Cacoub P, Caparros-Lefebvre D, et al. Erdheim-Chester disease. Clinical and radiologic characteristics of 59 cases. *Medicine (Baltimore)* 1996;75:157–169.

10. Al-Quran S, Reith J, Bradley J, et al. Erdheim-Chester disease: case report, PCR-based analysis of clonality, and review of literature. *Mod Pathol* 2002;15:666–672.

11. Chetritt J, Paradis V, Dargere D, et al. Chester-Erdheim disease: a neoplastic disorder. *Hum Pathol* 1999;30:1093–1096.

12. Adle-Biassette H, Chetritt J, Bergemer-Fouquet AM, et al. Pathology of the central nervous system in Chester-Erdheim disease: report of three cases. *J Neuropathol Exp Neurol* 1997;56:1207–1216.

13. Kambouchner M, Colby TV, Domenge C, et al. Erdheim-Chester disease with prominent pulmonary involvement associated with eosinophilic granuloma of mandibular bone. *Histopathology* 1997;30:353–358.

14. Vital C, Bioulac-Sage P, Tison F, et al. Brain stem infiltration by mixed Langerhans cell histiocytosis and Chester-Erdheim disease: more than just an isolated case? *Clin Exp Pathol* 1999;47: 71–76.

Xanthomatous Disease

1. Boisgard S, Bringer O, Aufauvre B, et al. Intraosseous xanthoma without lipid disorders. Case-report and literature review. *Joint Bone Spine* 2000;67:71–74.

2. Friedman O, Hockstein N, Willcox TO Jr, et al. Xanthoma of the temporal bone: a unique case of this rare condition. *Ear Nose Throat J* 2000;79:433–436.

3. Hamada T, Ito H, Araki Y, et al. Benign fibrous histiocytoma of the femur: review of three cases. *Skeletal Radiol* 1996;25:25–29.

4. Huang CF, Cheng SN, Hung CH, et al. Xanthoma of bone in a normolipidemic child: report of one case. *Acta Paediatr Taiwan* 2000;41:158–160.

5. Kuroiwa T, Ohta T, Tsutsumi A. Xanthoma of the temporal bone: case report. *Neurosurgery* 2000;46:996–998.

6. Calverly DC, Wismer J, Rosenthal D, et al. Xanthoma disseminatum in an infant with skeletal and marrow involvement. *J Pediatr Hematol Oncol* 1995;17:61–65.

7. Maize JC, Ahmed AR, Provost TT. Xanthoma disseminatum and multiple myeloma. *Arch Dermatol* 1974;110:758–761.

8. Mishkel MA, Cockshott WP, Nazir DJ, et al. Xanthoma disseminatum. Clinical, metabolic, pathologic, and radiologic aspects. *Arch Dermatol* 1977;113:1094–1100.

9. Odell WD, Doggett RS. Xanthoma disseminatum, a rare cause of diabetes insipidus. *J Clin Endocrinol Metab* 1993;76:777–780.

10. Szekeres E, Tiba A, Korom I. Xanthoma disseminatum: a rare condition with non-X, non-lipid cutaneous histiocytopathy. *J Dermatol Surg Oncol* 1988;14:1021–1024.

24

B-CELL NEOPLASMS

B-cell neoplasms are a heterogeneous group of clinicopathologic entities, ranging from indolent to highly aggressive (Table 24-1). The useful category of high-grade B-cell lymphoma is not included in the World Health Organization classification but is discussed at the end of this chapter. Neoplasms composed predominantly of mature small B-cells may be difficult to distinguish from one another in the bone marrow (Table 24-2).

PRECURSOR B-CELL NEOPLASM

B-Cell Lymphoblastic Lymphoma

B-cell lymphoblastic lymphoma is essentially identical to acute lymphoblastic leukemia of precursor B-cell phenotype, except that it presents predominantly as a mass lesion rather than as leukemia (1–5). Lymphoblastic malignancy presenting as a lytic bone lesion may be interpreted as either B-cell lymphoblastic lymphoma or acute lymphoblastic leukemia. B-cell lymphoblastic lymphoma usually occurs as a *de novo* tumor but has also been reported as a terminal phase of chronic lymphocytic leukemia (CLL) (6).

Bone marrow aspirate smears and histologic sections show, in the rare involved case, less than 25% blasts. The tumor cells are small to moderate-sized cells with round, sometimes cleaved or convoluted, nuclei and scant cytoplasm.

Flow cytometry and immunostains show expression of CD10, CD19, CD20 (dim), CD22, CD43, CD79a, CD99, HLA-DR, terminal deoxynucleotidyltransferase, and clonal cytoplasmic immunoglobulin light chain. CD34 expression is variable. CD45 expression is dim to negative. Occasional cases show expression of CD3, CD14, CD56, or surface immunoglobulin light chain or lack expression of CD10 (7–10).

Genetic studies show rearrangement of *IgH,* the immunoglobulin heavy chain gene. Rearrangements of T-cell receptor genes may also be present. Translocation (8;22) has rarely been reported (11).

The differential diagnosis includes other high-grade hematolymphoid neoplasms, especially the blastoid variant of mantle cell lymphoma (MCL), T-cell lymphoblastic lymphoma and myeloid sarcoma (extramedullary myeloid tumor); and nonhematopoietic malignancies (12–15).

MATURE B-CELL NEOPLASMS

Chronic Lymphocytic Leukemia/Small Lymphocytic Lymphoma

CLL and small lymphocytic lymphoma (SLL) are essentially identical, except that CLL is leukemic by definition (1,2) (Figs. 24-1 through 24-7). CLL is found in approximately 80% of cases of SLL. CLL/SLL usually arises *de novo* but occasionally occurs as a transformation of monoclonal gammopathy of undetermined significance (3). Hybrid cases with features of CLL/SLL and lymphoplasmacytic lymphoma (LPL), hairy cell leukemia (HCL), follicular lymphoma (FL), MCL, and multiple myeloma have been reported (4–10).

The peripheral blood shows an absolute lymphocyte count of 5×10^9 cells/L or greater; however, this criterion is arbitrary. Immune-mediated cytopenias, cold agglutinin disease, and neutrophilic leukemoid reactions have been reported (12,13). The neoplastic lymphocytes are slightly larger than normal lymphocytes. At low magnification, they may appear triangular, polygonal, or tapered. At high

TABLE 24-1. CLASSIFICATION OF B-CELL NEOPLASMS ACCORDING TO THE WORLD HEALTH ORGANIZATION

Precursor B-cell neoplasm
  B-cell lymphoblastic lymphoma

Mature B-cell neoplasms
  Chronic lymphocytic leukemia/small lymphocytic lymphoma
  B-cell prolymphocytic leukemia
  Lymphoplasmacytic lymphoma
  Marginal zone lymphoma
  Hairy cell leukemia
  Follicular lymphoma
  Mantle cell lymphoma
  Diffuse large B-cell lymphoma
  Primary effusion lymphoma
  Burkitt lymphoma/leukemia
  High-grade B-cell lymphoma[a]

[a]Included in this chapter but not in the World Health Organization classification.

TABLE 24-2. DIFFERENTIAL FEATURES OF MATURE SMALL B-CELL NEOPLASMS

	CLL	LPL	MZL	HCL	FL	MCL
Nucleus	Round	Round	Round	Irregular	Irregular	Irregular
Nucleolus	−	−/+	+	+	+	+
Infiltrate	D,N	D,N,P	D,I,N	D	D,N,P	D,N,P
CD5	+	−	−	−	−	+
CD10	−	−	−	−	+	−
CD23	+	−	−	+	+/−	−
CD103	−	−	−	+	−	−
FMC7	−/+	+	+	+	+	+

CLL, chronic lymphocytic leukemia/small lymphocytic lymphoma; D, diffuse; FL, follicular lymphoma; HCL, hairy cell leukemia; I, intrasinusoidal/intravascular; LPL, lymphoplasmacytic lymphoma; MCL, mantle cell lymphoma; MZL, marginal zone lymphoma; N, nodular; P, paratrabecular; +, positive; −, negative; +/−, usually positive, sometimes negative; −/+, usually negative, sometimes positive.

magnification, they show ovoid nuclei with coarsely clumped chromatin and no nucleoli. The cytoplasm is scanty to moderate in amount and agranular. Disrupted cells are common and usually appear as smudged nuclei devoid of cytoplasm (smudge cells) or ballooned skeins of chromatin (basket cells). Smudge cells are accurately counted as lymphocytes by automated blood analyzers but are routinely excluded from a manual white blood cell differential. This practice may lead to an artefactual increase in manually calculated absolute neutrophil counts (14).

Bone marrow aspirate smears and histologic sections show approximately 20% to 90% neoplastic lymphocytes. The infiltrates may be nodular, interstitial, diffuse, and/or interfollicular (15,16). In sections, the neoplastic cells appear as closely packed, dark-staining nuclei with scant cytoplasm. Proliferation centers and/or germinal centers may be present. The lymphoid infiltrates also contain T cells and dendritic cells (17). Other findings include erythroid and/or megakaryocytic hyperplasia owing to immune-mediated cytopenias, pure red cell aplasia, reactive mastocytosis, amyloidosis, and immunoglobulin deposition disease (18,19).

Immunoglobulin M (IgM) production in CLL/SLL is associated with μ-heavy-chain disease, pseudonuclear immunoglobulin inclusions (Dutcher bodies), spherical cytoplasmic accumulations of immunoglobulin (Russell bodies), cytoplasmic vacuolation with signet-ring morphology, and immunoglobulin crystals (20–22). The nucleus may be displaced or obscured by multiple Russell bodies (Mott cell).

Morphologic variants of CLL/SLL have been described. The paraimmunoblastic variant of CLL/SLL is composed of larger cells with more basophilic cytoplasm (23). A binucleated variant has been reported (24). CLL/SLL with prolymphocytic transformation shows 10% or more prolymphocytes (25). Atypical CLL/SLL is a general term used for cases with unusual clinical, morphologic, immunophenotypic, and/or genetic characteristics (26–31). These include more than 10% prolymphocytes; bright CD20, CD23, and/or surface immunoglobulin light chain expression; clonal karyotypic anomalies; and a more aggressive clinical course. Some cases of atypical CLL/SLL may be indistinguishable from the leukemic phase of MCL.

Discordant morphology between bone marrow and lymph node biopsies sometimes occurs, with CLL/SLL in the bone marrow and LPL or marginal zone lymphoma (MZL) in the lymph node or other extramedullary site (32).

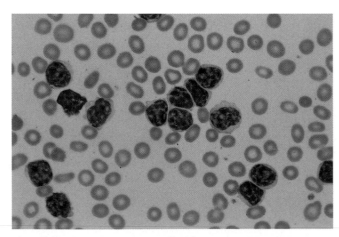

FIGURE 24-1. Peripheral blood smear, B-cell chronic lymphocytic leukemia. The lymphocytes are small and monomorphous, with round nuclei and condensed chromatin.

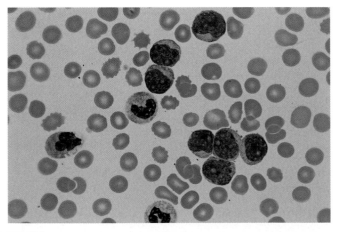

FIGURE 24-2. Peripheral blood smear, B-cell chronic lymphocytic leukemia in prolymphocytic transformation. Numerous prolymphocytes are present in this specimen from a patient with long-standing B-cell chronic lymphocytic leukemia.

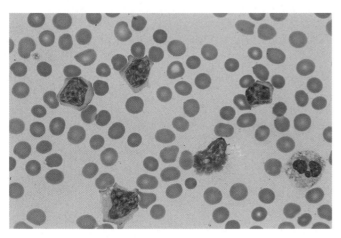

FIGURE 24-3. Peripheral blood smear, atypical B-cell chronic lymphocytic leukemia. The lymphocytes are relatively small and monomorphous but show plasmacytoid features.

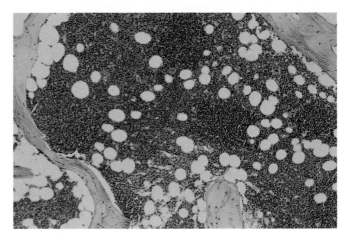

FIGURE 24-5. Bone marrow biopsy specimen, B-cell chronic lymphocytic leukemia/small lymphocytic lymphoma. The hematopoietic tissue is displaced by nodular and interstitial aggregates of clonal B cells.

Flow cytometry and immunostains show expression of CD5, CD11c, CD19, CD20, CD23, CD43, CD45, HLA-DR, and clonal surface immunoglobulin light chain (dim to moderate) (33–52). CD23 is positive, ranging from dim to bright. CD11c, CD38, FMC7, bcl-1, and bcl-2 are variably expressed. Occasional cases show expression of CD2, CD8, CD10, CD13, CD14, CD33, CD138, or FMC7 or lack expression of surface immunoglobulin light chain. Weak (dim) CD5 expression must be carefully distinguished from true CD5 negativity because CD5-negative B-cell neoplasms likely represent disorders other than CLL/SLL.

Genetic studies show anomalies in more than 80% of cases (53–59). The most common abnormalities are trisomy 12 and abnormalities involving *IgH, p53,* and chromosome bands 11q23 and 13q14. Translocations (11;14) and (14;18) have been reported. Most of these anomalies are evidence of clonal evolution and thus associated with poor survival.

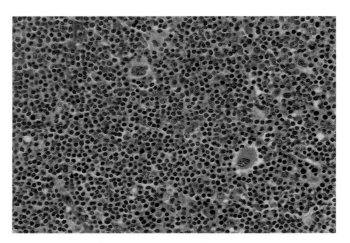

FIGURE 24-6. Bone marrow biopsy specimen, B-cell chronic lymphocytic leukemia/small lymphocytic lymphoma. A diffuse interstitial infiltrate of small round lymphocytes is present.

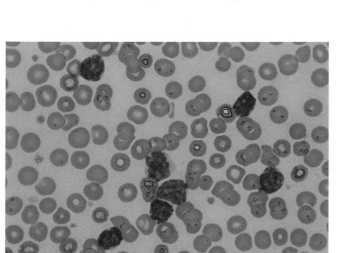

FIGURE 24-4. Peripheral blood smear, atypical B-cell chronic lymphocytic leukemia. The lymphocytes are relatively small and monomorphous but show irregular nuclear contours.

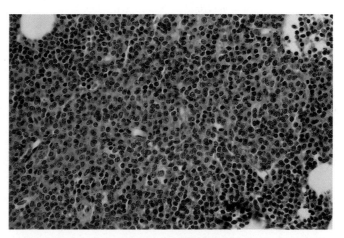

FIGURE 24-7. Bone marrow biopsy specimen, B-cell chronic lymphocytic leukemia/small lymphocytic lymphoma. A poorly defined zone of larger cells is present, constituting a proliferation center.

Transformation to a higher-grade neoplasm occurs in approximately 10% of cases. The most common type is prolymphocytic transformation, in which prolymphocytes exceed 10% of nucleated cells; CD5 and CD23 expression is typically retained (60–62). Other transformations are characterized by large cells (Richter transformation), Reed-Sternberg cells (Hodgkin lymphoma), or Burkitt-like, lymphoblastic, plasmacytoid, or histiocytic differentiation (63–70). Spontaneous remission has occasionally been reported (71–73).

Other hematolymphoid diseases reported in CLL/SLL, which appear to be clonally unrelated, include myeloproliferative disorders, myelodysplastic syndromes, acute myeloid leukemia, histiocytic neoplasms, other B-cell lymphomas, solitary plasmacytoma and multiple myeloma, and clonal T-cell disorders (74–94).

The differential diagnosis includes benign lymphoid aggregates, persistent polyclonal lymphocytosis, hepatitis C–related oligoclonal B-cell proliferation, and other neoplasms of mature B cells (95,96).

B-Cell Prolymphocytic Leukemia

B-cell prolymphocytic leukemia is a relatively rare *de novo* disease (97–103) (Figs. 24-8 and 24-9). The peripheral blood shows marked leukocytosis, with white blood cell counts often exceeding 100×10^9/L and prolymphocytes exceeding 55% of nucleated cells. Prolymphocytes are large cells with ovoid nuclei containing moderately condensed chromatin and a single, prominent, centrally located nucleolus. The pale blue cytoplasm is moderately abundant.

Bone marrow aspirate smears and histologic sections show abundant prolymphocytes. The neoplastic infiltrate is interstitial or diffuse. Reticulin fibrosis may be present.

Flow cytometry shows expression of CD11c, CD19, CD20, CD22, CD79b, HLA-DR, and clonal surface

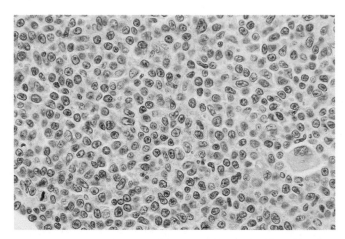

FIGURE 24-9. Bone marrow biopsy specimen, B-cell prolymphocytic leukemia. A diffuse interstitial infiltrate of monomorphous lymphocytes is present, the majority of cells showing a single nucleolus.

immunoglobulin light chain (bright). CD5 and FMC7 expression is variable. Occasional cases show CD11b or CD13 expression. Genetic studies frequently show deletions involving chromosome bands 11q23 and 13q14.

The differential diagnosis includes various B-cell neoplasms (CLL/SLL, HCL, MCL) in prolymphocytic transformation, large B-cell lymphoma in leukemic phase, T-cell prolymphocytic leukemia, and acute leukemia. The distinction between *de novo* B prolymphocytic leukemia and prolymphocytic transformation of CLL/SLL is often blurred, but is not critical because outcomes are similar.

Lymphoplasmacytic Lymphoma

LPL (immunocytoma, small lymphocytic lymphoma with plasmacytoid features) occurs *de novo,* as a complication of chronic hepatitis C virus infection, as a posttransplantation lymphoproliferative disorder, and as a transformation of other B-cell neoplasms (104–107) (Figs. 24-10 and 24-11). LPL with IgM secretion seems to be genetically different from multiple myeloma with IgM secretion (108); however, a clear distinction between LPL and other lymphoplasmacytic disorders is not always apparent. Hybrid cases with features of LPL and CLL, HCL, multiple myeloma, and μ-heavy-chain disease have been reported (109–111).

The relationships among LPL, Waldenström macroglobulinemia, clonal IgM production, and immunoglobulin-related hyperviscosity are intricate (112). LPL often produces IgM but may also produce IgG, IgA, IgE, or more than one immunoglobulin (113–115). Some cases of LPL are accompanied by Waldenström macroglobulinemia, a clinical syndrome characterized by an increased serum clonal IgM level and immunoglobulin-related hyperviscosity (116,117). Waldenström macroglobulinemia is found not only in LPL but also in some cases of MZL and other B-cell neoplasms (118–120). Increased serum clonal IgM levels are

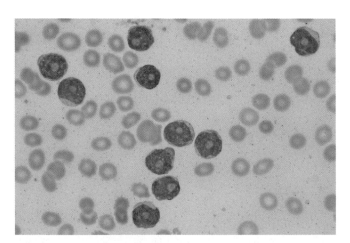

FIGURE 24-8. Peripheral blood smear, B-cell prolymphocytic leukemia. A monomorphous population of large lymphocytes is present, each cell containing a single large nucleolus.

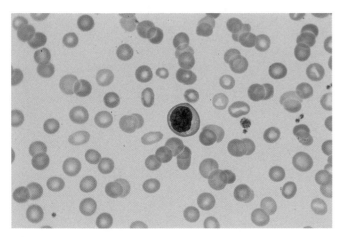

FIGURE 24-10. Peripheral blood smear, lymphoplasmacytic lymphoma. A plasmacytoid lymphocyte is surrounded by rouleaux in this specimen from a patient with lymphoplasmacytic lymphoma and Waldenström macroglobulinemia.

found not only in LPL but also in CLL, multiple myeloma, and other lymphoplasmacytic neoplasms. Immunoglobulin-related hyperviscosity is seen not only in LPL with clonal IgM but also in multiple myeloma and in association with polyclonal hypergammaglobulinemia, cryoglobulinemia, and clonal IgG, IgA, and IgD production (121–125).

The peripheral blood often shows anemia, which may be immune-mediated (126). Other findings may include leukocytosis or leukopenia, thrombocytopenia, and cryoglobulinemia. Monocytosis may be present (127). A definite leukemic phase is uncommon.

Bone marrow aspirate smears and histologic sections show a mixed population of small lymphocytes, plasmacytoid lymphocytes, and plasma cells. The neoplastic infiltrate may be diffuse, interstitial, nodular, and/or paratrabecular. Dutcher bodies, Russell bodies, Mott cells, and vacuolated or signet-ring cells may be present (128). Cerebriform nuclei

have been reported (128). Admixed cells include dendritic cells, histiocytes, and T cells. Other reported findings include pure red cell aplasia, reactive mastocytosis, storage histiocytes (pseudo-Gaucher cells), crystal-storing histiocytosis, fibrosis, and sarcoidosis (17,18,128–132).

Discordant morphology between bone marrow and lymph node biopsies sometimes occurs, with LPL in the bone marrow and mixed small cleaved and large cell lymphoma in the lymph node (133).

Flow cytometry shows expression of CD19, CD20 (bright), CD38, CD45, FMC7, HLA-DR, and clonal surface immunoglobulin light chain (moderate to bright). CD23 expression is variable. Rare cases show expression of CD5.

Genetic studies frequently demonstrate gain of chromosome 3 or 3q and deletion of chromosome 6q (134,135).

Transformation to large B-cell lymphoma, Hodgkin lymphoma, and light chain amyloidosis has been reported (136–140).

Other hematolymphoid diseases reported in LPL, which appear to be clonally unrelated, include myeloproliferative disorders, myelodysplastic syndromes, acute myeloid leukemia, multiple myeloma, and cutaneous T-cell lymphoma (81,141–147).

The differential diagnosis includes other neoplasms of mature B cells and plasma cells.

Marginal Zone Lymphoma

MZL is composed of morphologically similar but clinically distinct tumors, including nodal MZL, extranodal marginal zone B-cell lymphoma of mucosa-associated lymphoid tissue (MALToma), and splenic marginal cell lymphoma (or splenic lymphoma with circulating villous lymphocytes) (1,148–151) (Fig. 24-12). MZL occurs as a *de novo* disease and as a

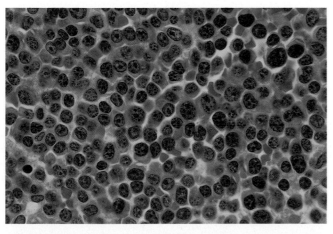

FIGURE 24-11. Bone marrow biopsy specimen, lymphoplasmacytic lymphoma. A diffuse infiltrate of lymphocytes, plasmacytoid lymphocytes, and plasma cells is present in this specimen from a patient with Waldenström macroglobulinemia.

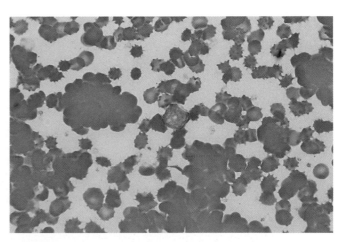

FIGURE 24-12. Peripheral blood smear, marginal zone lymphoma. The lymphocyte in the center is small and shows slightly dispersed chromatin and a small nucleolus. It is nearly obscured by agglutinated red blood cells in this specimen from a patient with splenic lymphoma with villous lymphocytes and marked cold agglutinin disease.

complication of chronic hepatitis C virus infection (152). Hybrid cases with features of MZL and HCL, MCL, LPL, and Waldenström macroglobulinemia have been reported (117–120,153,154).

Peripheral blood and bone marrow involvement occurs in approximately 70% of cases with primary splenic disease and 15% to 20% of cases with primary salivary gland or skin disease but is uncommon in cases with primary nodal disease. Circulating neoplastic cells may show villous cytoplasmic projections. Other findings include immune-mediated cytopenias and cold agglutinin disease. Laboratory studies may demonstrate clonal serum immunoglobulin, usually IgM.

Bone marrow aspirate smears and histologic sections show neoplastic lymphocytes, plasmacytoid lymphocytes, and plasma cells. The neoplastic infiltrate may be intrasinusoidal, intravascular, nodular, and/or diffuse (155–157). The intrasinusoidal pattern is not specific for MZL but may also be seen in large granular lymphocytic leukemia, hepatosplenic T-cell lymphoma, anaplastic large cell lymphoma, and intravascular B-cell lymphoma. The nuclei range from round to irregular or even Sézary-like (158). The cytoplasm is moderately abundant and agranular. Dutcher bodies and reactive germinal centers may be present.

Morphologic variants of MZL include cases with larger cells, blastlike morphology, and cerebriform nuclei (159, 160).

Discordant morphology between bone marrow and lymph node biopsies sometimes occurs, with MZL in the bone marrow and HCL in the lymph node or other extramedullary site (32).

Flow cytometry and immunostains typically show expression of CD11c, CD19, CD20, CD45, CD79b, FMC7, HLA-DR, clonal surface immunoglobulin light chain (moderate to bright), and bcl-2. Rare cases show expression of CD5, CD10, CD23, or CD43 or lack expression of surface immunoglobulin light chain (42,161,162).

Genetic studies characteristically show t(11;18) and other rearrangements involving the immunoglobulin genes and, in some cases, T-cell receptor genes (163–165).

Transformation of MZL to blastic and large cell variants has been reported (166–168).

The differential diagnosis includes other mature B-cell neoplasms, especially LPL.

Hairy Cell Leukemia

HCL occurs as a *de novo* malignancy and, interestingly, as a transformation of chronic myeloid leukemia (169) (Figs. 24-13 through 24-16). Hybrid cases with features of HCL and CLL, LPL, MZL, multiple myeloma, and acute lymphoblastic leukemia have been reported (4,109, 170–172).

The peripheral blood typically shows cytopenias, especially leukopenia. Monocytes and dendritic cells are markedly decreased, which accounts for the unusual susceptibility

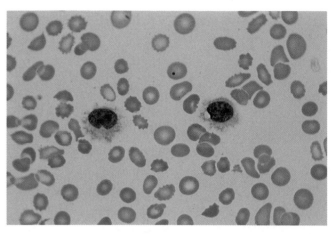

FIGURE 24-13. Peripheral blood smear, hairy cell leukemia. The lymphocytes are slightly enlarged and show indented nuclei, dispersed chromatin, and irregular, ruffled cytoplasmic membranes with peripheral projections (hairs).

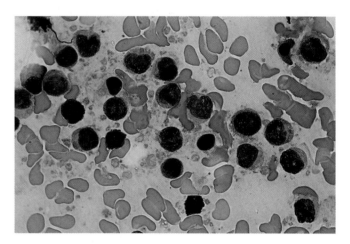

FIGURE 24-14. Bone marrow aspirate smear, hairy cell leukemia. Numerous hairy lymphocytes are present.

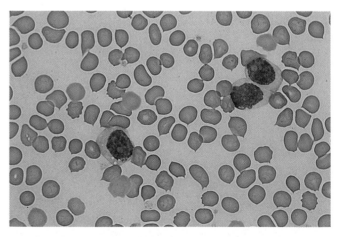

FIGURE 24-15. Peripheral blood smear, variant hairy cell leukemia. The neoplastic lymphocytes contain a single small nucleolus and lack peripheral cytoplasmic projections (hairs).

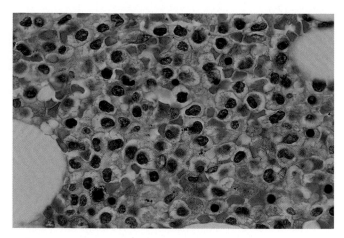

FIGURE 24-16. Bone marrow biopsy specimen, hairy cell leukemia. Small reniform and cleaved nuclei are present, surrounded by ample amounts of clear cytoplasm.

to mycobacterial and fungal infections associated with HCL (173,174). Immune-mediated hemolytic anemia and thrombocytopenia may be severe (175,176).

The peripheral blood typically shows few circulating hairy cells, although cases with absolute lymphocyte counts of $100 \times 10^9/L$ and more have been reported (177). Hairy cells are medium-sized lymphoid cells with an eccentric, flattened to reniform or bilobed nucleus. Nuclei may also be multilobated, cerebriform, or ring-shaped (178–180). The chromatin is evenly condensed, not clumped as in a mature lymphocyte, and may show a small, centrally located nucleolus. The cytoplasm is pale blue with Wright stain and shows short, fine peripheral projections ("hairs"). The cytoplasm may show sparse, indistinct granules. Tartrate-resistant acid phosphatase (TRAP) is usually detectable within the cytoplasm by enzymatic or immunologic methods; however, TRAP positivity is neither completely sensitive nor specific for HCL (181–184).

Bone marrow aspirate smears are often poor because of fibrosis (dry tap); thus, touch imprints of the core biopsy are especially valuable in HCL (185–192). The neoplastic infiltrate is interstitial and/or diffuse. Hairy cells appear in histologic sections as small, reniform or monocytoid nuclei surrounded by clear cytoplasm and a well-defined cell membrane. Hematopoiesis is typically decreased, and aplasia may be present. Reticulin fibrosis and osteosclerosis are common. Other findings include reactive mastocytosis, myelodysplastic changes, necrosis, amyloidosis, and granulomas (193–199).

Morphologic variants of HCL have been described. The Japanese variant is characterized by moderate leukocytosis, a round nucleus with condensed chromatin and inconspicuous nucleolus, and weak to absent expression of TRAP, CD25, and surface immunoglobulin light chain (200). The blastic variant shows a round to oval nucleus, scant basophilic cytoplasm containing large azurophilic granules,

lack of marrow fibrosis, and no expression of TRAP, CD11c, or CD25 (201). The prolymphocytic variant is characterized by larger cells containing a single prominent nucleolus (202). A variant with cerebriform nuclei has also been reported (160).

Flow cytometry and immunostains typically show expression of CD11c (bright), CD19, CD20, CD22 (bright), CD25, CD45 (bright), CD103, FMC7, HLA-DR, and clonal surface immunoglobulin light chain (bright) (203). CD23 is variably expressed. Rare cases show expression of CD2, CD5, or CD10 or lack expression of CD11c, CD25, or CD103 (41,204–207).

Genetic studies have demonstrated numerous anomalies, most involving the immunoglobulin genes (208,209).

Transformation to the blastic variant, large B-cell lymphoma, and multiple myeloma have been reported (210–213).

Other hematolymphoid diseases reported with HCL, which appear to be clonally unrelated, include myeloproliferative disorders, myelodysplastic syndromes, a second occurrence of HCL, FL, Hodgkin lymphoma, monoclonal gammopathy, cutaneous T-cell lymphoma, and T-cell large granular lymphocytic leukemia (214–225).

The differential diagnosis includes polyclonal B-cell lymphocytosis, reactive marrow fibrosis, MZL, and T-cell neoplasms with pancytopenia and/or "hairy" cytoplasmic projections (226–229).

Follicular Lymphoma

FL occurs predominantly as a *de novo* malignancy (Figs. 24-17 through 24-20). Hybrid cases with features of FL and CLL have been reported (8,9)

The peripheral blood often contains clonal cells but shows overt leukemia in only 5% of cases with bone marrow involvement. The neoplastic cells are slightly larger than normal lymphocytes, with irregular to cleaved nuclei, condensed

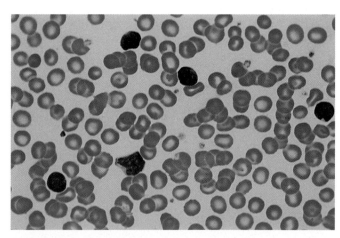

FIGURE 24-17. Peripheral blood smear, follicular lymphoma. The cells are small, with irregular to cleaved nuclei and condensed chromatin.

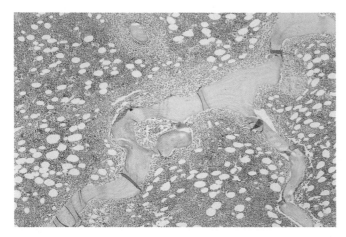

FIGURE 24-18. Bone marrow biopsy specimen, follicular lymphoma. The malignant infiltrate hugs the contours of the trabecular bone.

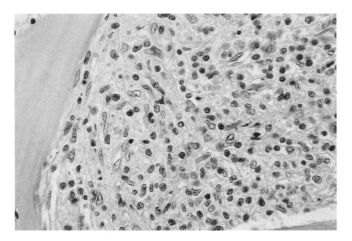

FIGURE 24-19. Bone marrow biopsy specimen, follicular lymphoma. A paratrabecular infiltrate is composed predominantly of small irregular, elongated, and cleaved lymphocytes.

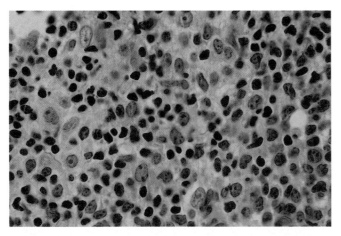

FIGURE 24-20. Bone marrow biopsy specimen, follicular lymphoma. The infiltrate is composed of both small cleaved and large lymphocytes.

chromatin, indistinct nucleoli, and scant agranular cytoplasm. Auer rod–like inclusions have rarely been reported (230).

Bone marrow aspirate smears and histologic sections show FL in approximately 50% of cases initially diagnosed in a lymph node or other site. The neoplastic infiltrate may be nodular, follicular, interstitial, and/or diffuse (231). The neoplastic cells preferentially migrate to sites closely apposed to the trabecular bone and extend along the bony surface, entrapped in reticulin fibers. They often appear as dark, angular, compressed nuclei. Small cleaved cells usually predominate, admixed with reactive T-cells, dendritic cells, and mast cells (17–19). Storage histiocytes (pseudo-Gaucher cells) may be present (232). Anti-CD20 (rituximab) therapy eliminates the neoplastic B-cells, but T-cells persist and may be mistaken for residual tumor (233).

Morphologic variants of FL have been described, including cases with abundant T-cells (T-cell–rich FL) or epithelioid histiocytes, signet-ring morphology, and cells with cerebriform nuclei (234–238).

Discordant morphology between bone marrow and lymph node biopsies sometimes occurs, with FL in the bone marrow and MCL in the lymph node (32). In some cases, FL is found in both sites, but the histologic grade is higher in the lymph node than in the bone marrow (32,239, 240).

Flow cytometry and immunohistochemistry show expression of CD10, CD19, CD20 (bright), CD45, clonal surface immunoglobulin light chain (bright), and bcl-2 (36,241–243). CD11c, CD22, CD23, and FMC7 are variably expressed. Rare cases show expression of CD2 or CD5, or lack expression of CD10 or surface immunoglobulin light chain.

Genetic studies have demonstrated numerous clonal anomalies, usually involving the immunoglobulin genes.

Discordance among morphology, flow cytometry, and genetic analysis is not unusual in bone marrow samples with FL because of focal involvement by FL and entrapment of neoplastic cells by reticulin fibers (244,245).

Transformation to lymphoblastic malignancy, large B-cell lymphoma, and Burkitt lymphoma/leukemia (BLL) have been reported (246–248).

Other lymphoid neoplasms have been reported with FL, which appear to be clonally unrelated (221,300).

The differential diagnosis includes benign lymphoid aggregates, CLL, MZL, and MCL. Location, fibrosis, and molecular analysis (but not bcl-2 immunostaining) may be helpful in distinguishing reactive from clonal lymphoid infiltrates (250–253).

Mantle Cell Lymphoma

MCL occurs predominantly as a *de novo* disease (254) (Figs. 24-21 through 24-24). Hybrid cases with features

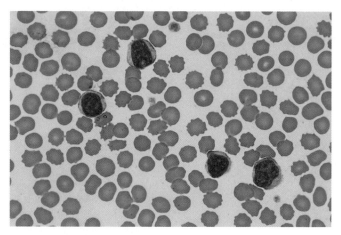

FIGURE 24-21. Peripheral blood smear, mantle cell lymphoma. The cells are predominantly small, with round to irregular nuclear contours and condensed chromatin.

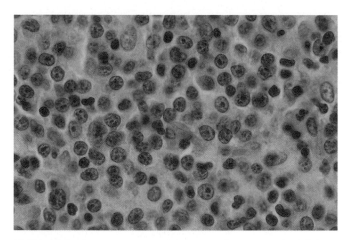

FIGURE 24-24. Bone marrow biopsy specimen, mantle cell lymphoma, blastoid variant. A diffuse infiltrate is present, composed of monomorphous medium-sized lymphocytes with dispersed chromatin and small nucleoli.

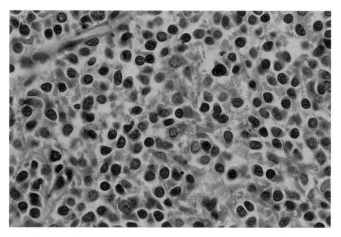

FIGURE 24-22. Bone marrow biopsy specimen, mantle cell lymphoma. A diffuse infiltrate is present, composed of small, slightly irregular lymphocytes with condensed chromatin.

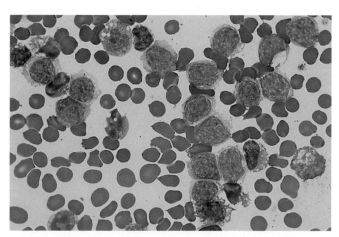

FIGURE 24-23. Peripheral blood smear, mantle cell lymphoma, blastoid variant. The cells are monomorphous and medium to large in size and show dispersed chromatin.

of MCL and CLL, MZL, and HCL have been reported (5,6,8,153,154).

The peripheral blood shows a leukemic phase in more than 75% of cases at some point during the disease (255–258). The neoplastic cells are slightly larger than normal lymphocytes, with irregular, folded or indented nuclei and scant, agranular cytoplasm. Anemia and platelet satellitism around the malignant cells have been reported as presenting signs of MCL (259,260).

Bone marrow aspirate smears and histologic sections often show involvement by MCL. The neoplastic infiltrate may be paratrabecular, intratrabecular, nodular, interstitial, and/or diffuse. The lymphocytes are small, with irregular nuclei and scant cytoplasm.

Morphologic variants of MCL have been described. The blastic (or blastoid) variant is characterized by intermediate to large, blastlike cells with round nuclei and finely dispersed chromatin, a high mitotic rate, abnormalities of chromosome band 8q24, and a particularly aggressive clinical course (261–263). The prolymphocytic (or nucleolated) variant is composed of prolymphocytes as well as more typical small, irregular cells (264–266). Variants composed of large cells, giant cells, and cells with cerebriform nuclei have also been reported (267–269). Each of these variants shows the immunophenotype and genotype of usual MCL.

Flow cytometry and immunostains show expression of CD5, CD19, CD20 (bright), CD43, CD45, CD79b, FMC7, HLA-DR, clonal surface immunoglobulin light chain (bright), bcl-1, and bcl-2. CD10 and CD25 are variably expressed. CD23 expression is usually dim to negative (39). Rare cases show moderate expression of CD10 or CD23 or lack expression of CD5 (48,270,271). Expression of bcl-1 is not specific for MCL.

Genetic studies typically show t(11;14), involving *BCL-1* at 11q13 and *IgH* at 14q32; however, this anomaly is not specific for MCL (272). Other reported anomalies include trisomy 12 and deletion of chromosome band 13q. These anomalies are also common in atypical CLL, suggesting a close relationship between the two disorders.

Transformation to the prolymphocytic variant of MCL has been reported.

The differential diagnosis includes other mature B-cell neoplasms and, in the case of the blastic variant of MCL, lymphoblastic malignancies. It is important to distinguish MCL from other mature B-cell neoplasms because it has a much more aggressive course. Immunophenotype and genetic analysis help to distinguish the blastic variant of MCL from lymphoblastic lymphoma (273). In CD5-negative cases, characteristic morphology, bcl-1 overexpression, and the presence of t(11;14) help to establish a diagnosis of MCL.

Diffuse Large B-Cell Lymphoma

Diffuse large B-cell lymphoma (DLBCL) occurs as a *de novo* disease and as a transformation of CLL, LPL, MZL, FL, and monoclonal gammopathy of undetermined significance (63,136–140,168,210,211,274) (Figs. 24-25 and 24-26).

The peripheral blood shows cytopenias. A definite leukemic phase is seen in less than 5% of cases. The neoplastic cells range from small cleaved to large lymphocytes with ovoid nuclei, coarsely clumped chromatin, nucleoli, and variable amounts of agranular cytoplasm.

Bone marrow aspirate smears and histologic sections may show DLBCL as an extension of a primary tumor in another site or as a primary tumor of the bone marrow (275–279). The neoplastic infiltrate may be paratrabecular, nodular, interstitial, diffuse, intrasinusoidal, or intravascular (155). The cells are large and generally round to ovoid, with ovoid to cleaved and irregular nuclei and prominent nucleoli. Some cases show immunoblastic, anaplastic, signet-ring, or histiocytic features (280–284). Admixed cells include dendritic

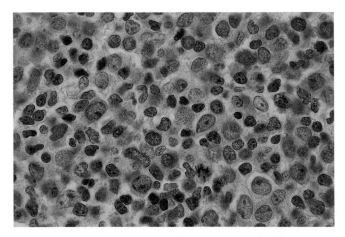

FIGURE 24-26. Bone marrow biopsy specimen, diffuse large B-cell lymphoma. An infiltrate of large, pleomorphic cells is present; elsewhere, the biopsy showed large areas of necrotic tumor.

cells, histiocytes, and reactive T-cells. Other findings include necrosis, fibrosis, bony changes, storage histiocytes (pseudo-Gaucher cells), and hemophagocytic syndrome (285–288).

Morphologic variants of DLBCL include cases with abundant T-cells (T-cell–rich DLBCL) and cases with nuclear multilobation (289–290). Cases with c-*myc* rearrangement may be difficult to distinguish from cases of BLL.

Discordant morphology between bone marrow and lymph node biopsies sometimes occurs, with DLBCL in the bone marrow and either low-grade lymphoma or Burkitt-like lymphoma in the lymph node or other extramedullary site (32).

Flow cytometry and immunostains usually show expression of CD10, CD19, CD20 (bright), CD45, and clonal surface immunoglobulin light chain. CD10, CD23, FMC7, and bcl-2 expression are variable (242). Cases with anaplastic morphology may express CD30 and CD68. Occasional cases show expression of CD2, CD5, CD7, CD14, or CD56 or lack expression of CD10 or surface immunoglobulin light chain (36,42,291–297).

Genetic studies have demonstrated a variety of clonal karyotypic anomalies, including c-*myc* rearrangement (298).

Hematopoietic disorders reported with LCL, which appear to be clonally unrelated, include myeloproliferative disorders and myelodysplastic syndrome (299–306).

The differential diagnosis includes Hodgkin lymphoma, large T-cell lymphoma, acute leukemia, malignant histiocytosis, multiple myeloma, and nonhematolymphoid tumors.

Primary Effusion Lymphoma

Primary effusion lymphoma occurs as a complication of infection with human herpesvirus 8 or hepatitis C virus, usually in a setting of human immunodeficiency virus infection or other immunocompromised state (307–311). The peripheral blood and bone marrow are very seldom involved.

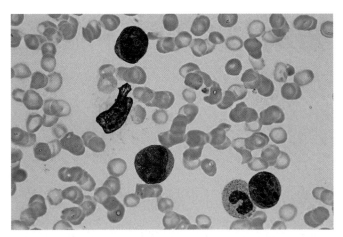

FIGURE 24-25. Peripheral blood smear, diffuse large B-cell lymphoma. The abnormal lymphocytes are large, with round to irregular nuclei.

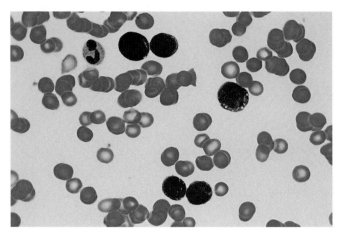

FIGURE 24-27. Peripheral blood smear, Burkitt lymphoma/leukemia. The lymphocytes are small to medium in size and monomorphous, with evenly dispersed chromatin and scant basophilic cytoplasm containing a few vacuoles.

Burkitt Lymphoma/Leukemia

BLL may present as a mass, with secondary involvement of the peripheral blood and bone marrow, or as a leukemia, with primary peripheral blood and bone marrow disease and secondary development of a mass (312) (Figs. 24-27 through 24-30). BLL occurs as a *de novo* malignancy, especially in immunocompromised patients, and as a transformation of various B-cell lymphomas, acute lymphoblastic leukemia, and chronic myeloid leukemia (313–319). Hybrid cases with features of BLL and precursor B-cell acute lymphoblastic leukemia have been reported (320–322).

The peripheral blood shows, in the leukemic phase, medium-sized cells with round to folded nuclei and moderately abundant basophilic cytoplasm with prominent vacuolation. The chromatin is dispersed but not as evenly as

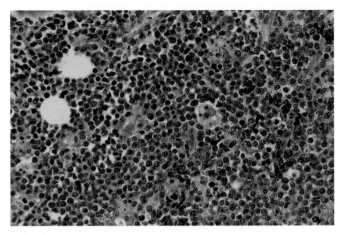

FIGURE 24-29. Bone marrow biopsy specimen, Burkitt lymphoma/leukemia. The hematopoietic tissue is replaced by a diffuse, monomorphous infiltrate with a "starry-sky" pattern, imparted by histiocytes containing ingested cellular remnants.

in true blasts. The tumor cells show round nuclei, multiple small nucleoli, and numerous mitoses.

Bone marrow aspirate smears and histologic sections are often involved by tumor. The neoplastic infiltrate is usually diffuse and may show a "starry-sky" appearance imparted by numerous macrophages containing ingested nuclear debris. Other findings may include eosinophilic hyperplasia and myelodysplastic changes (323,324).

Discordant morphology between bone marrow and lymph node biopsies has been reported with BLL in the bone marrow and Burkitt-like lymphoma in the lymph node (32); these distinctions may not be biologically significant.

Flow cytometry and immunostains show expression of CD10, CD19, CD20, CD22, CD45, FMC-7, HLA-DR, clonal surface immunoglobulin light chain, and bcl-6 (42,298,325,326). Rare cases show expression of CD5 or lack expression of CD20 or surface immunoglobulin light chain.

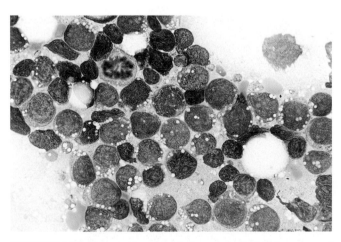

FIGURE 24-28. Bone marrow aspirate smear, Burkitt lymphoma/leukemia. The malignant cells are large and monomorphous, with round nuclei, dispersed chromatin, and prominently vacuolated basophilic cytoplasm.

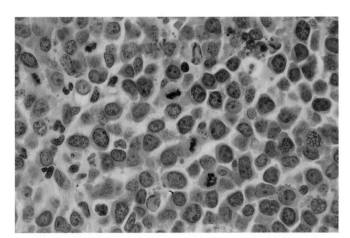

FIGURE 24-30. Bone marrow biopsy specimen, Burkitt lymphoma/leukemia. The infiltrate is composed of monomorphous cells with round nuclei containing nucleoli and dispersed chromatin; the mitotic rate is high.

Genetic studies usually show reciprocal translocation of c-*myc* and an immunoglobulin gene. The most common finding is t(8;14)(q24;q32), involving c-*myc* and *IgH,* followed by t(8;22)(q24;q11), involving the λ-light-chain gene, and t(2;8)(p12;q24), involving the κ-light-chain gene (327,328). Clonal evolution is accompanied by trisomy 12, 17p anomalies, and *p53* mutation. Translocation (14;18) is relatively common in adult cases (329). Molecular studies usually show clonal integration of Epstein-Barr virus genome into tumor cells. Translocation of c-*myc* and an immunoglobulin gene are not pathognomonic of BLL but have also been reported in a variety of B-cell and plasma cell malignancies (330–335).

The differential diagnosis includes acute myeloid leukemia, lymphoblastic malignancy, the blastic variant of MCL, other high-grade B-cell and T-cell lymphomas, and small round cell tumors of nonhematolymphoid origin (336,337).

High-Grade B-Cell Lymphoma

High-grade B-cell lymphoma is not included in the World Health Organization classification but is nevertheless a useful diagnosis for aggressive, otherwise unclassifiable B-cell lymphomas (Figs. 24-31 through 24-33). High-grade B-cell lymphoma may occur as an extramedullary or bone marrow *de novo* malignancy, usually in an immunocompromised patient, or as a transformation of a lower grade B-cell lymphoma (314,325,336,338).

The peripheral blood shows, in the leukemic phase, a heterogeneous population of moderate-sized cells. The nuclei are round to irregular, with finely clumped chromatin and one or more indistinct nucleoli. The cytoplasm is moderately abundant and ampho- to basophilic.

Bone marrow aspirate smears and histologic sections often show involvement by tumor. The neoplastic infiltrate may be

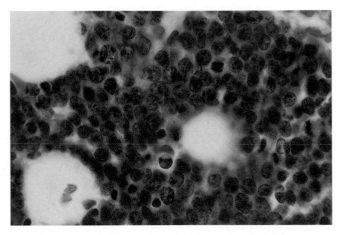

FIGURE 24-32. Bone marrow biopsy specimen, high-grade B-cell lymphoma. A diffuse infiltrate of relatively monomorphous cells is present in this specimen from a patient infected with human immunodeficiency virus.

nodular, interstitial, and/or diffuse. The tumor cells usually show a high mitotic rate. Necrosis may be the dominant finding (339–341).

Flow cytometry and immunostains show expression of CD10, CD19, CD20 (bright), CD45, clonal surface immunoglobulin, bcl-2, bcl-6, and c-myc. Occasional cases show expression of CD5.

Genetic studies show immunoglobulin heavy chain gene rearrangement and, in some cases, c-*myc* rearrangement.

Another hematologic disorder reported with high-grade B-cell lymphoma, which appears to be clonally unrelated, is polycythemia vera (342).

The differential diagnosis includes BLL, acute leukemia, lymphoblastic malignancy, and high-grade nonhematolymphoid malignancies.

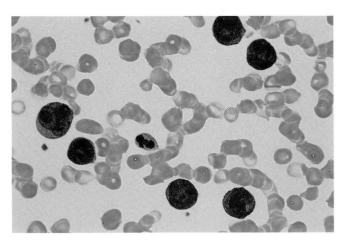

FIGURE 24-31. Peripheral blood smear, high-grade B-cell lymphoma. The cells resemble those of Burkitt lymphoma/leukemia but lack cytoplasmic vacuoles in this specimen from a patient with human immunodeficiency virus infection.

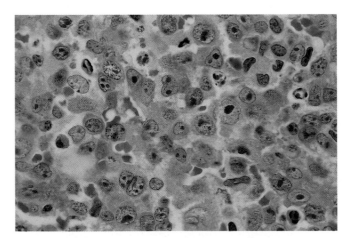

FIGURE 24-33. Bone marrow biopsy specimen, high-grade B-cell lymphoma. A diffuse infiltrate of pleomorphic large cells is seen in this specimen from a patient infected with human immunodeficiency virus.

REFERENCES

Precursor B-Cell Neoplasm

1. Jaffe ES, Harris NL, Stein H, et al., eds. *Pathology and genetics of haematopoietic and lymphoid tissues.* Lyon: IARC Press, 2001.
2. Chimenti S, Fink-Puches R, Peris K, et al. Cutaneous involvement in lymphoblastic lymphoma. *J Cutan Pathol* 1999;26: 379–385.
3. Iravani S, Singleton TP, Ross CW, et al. Precursor B lymphoblastic lymphoma presenting as lytic bone lesions. *Am J Clin Pathol* 1999;112:836–843.
4. Lin P, Jones D, Dorfman DM, et al. Precursor B-cell lymphoblastic lymphoma: a predominantly extranodal tumor with low propensity for leukemic involvement. *Am J Surg Pathol* 2000;24: 1480–1490.
5. Neth O, Seidemann K, Jansen P, et al. Precursor B-cell lymphoblastic lymphoma in childhood and adolescence: clinical features, treatment, and results in trials NHL-BFM 86 and 90. *Med Pediatr Oncol* 2000;35:20–27.
6. Pistoia V, Roncella S, Di Celle PF, et al. Emergence of a B-cell lymphoblastic lymphoma in a patient with B-cell chronic lymphocytic leukemia: evidence for the single-cell origin of the two tumors. *Blood* 1991;78:797–804.
7. Amo Y, Yonemoto K, Ohkawa T, et al. CD56 and terminal deoxynucleotidyl transferase positive cutaneous lymphoblastic lymphoma. *Br J Dermatol* 2000;143:666–667.
8. Pilozzi E, Pulford K, Jones M, et al. Co-expression of CD79a (JCB117) and CD3 by lymphoblastic lymphoma. *J Pathol* 1998; 186:140–143.
9. Soslow RA, Bhargava V, Warnke RA. MIC2, TdT, bcl-2, and CD34 expression in paraffin-embedded high-grade lymphoma/ acute lymphoblastic leukemia distinguishes between distinct clinicopathologic entities. *Hum Pathol* 1997;28:1158–1165.
10. Stroup R, Sheibani K, Misset JL, et al. Surface immunoglobulin-positive lymphoblastic lymphoma. A report of three cases. *Cancer* 1990;65:2559–2563.
11. Slavutsky I, Andreoli G, Gutierrez M, et al. Variant (8;22) translocation in lymphoblastic lymphoma. *Leuk Lymphoma* 1996;21:169–172.
12. Lucas DR, Bentley G, Dan ME, et al. Ewing sarcoma vs lymphoblastic lymphoma. A comparative immunohistochemical study. *Am J Clin Pathol* 2001;115:11–17.
13. Quintanilla-Martinez L, Zukerberg LR, Ferry JA, et al. Extramedullary tumors of lymphoid or myeloid blasts. The role of immunohistology in diagnosis and classification. *Am J Clin Pathol* 1995;104:431–443.
14. Soslow RA, Baergen RN, Warnke RA. B-lineage lymphoblastic lymphoma is a clinicopathologic entity distinct from other histologically similar aggressive lymphomas with blastic morphology. *Cancer* 1999;85:2648–2654.
15. Soslow RA, Zukerberg LR, Harris NL, et al. BCL-1 (PRAD-1/cyclin D-1) overexpression distinguishes the blastoid variant of mantle cell lymphoma from B-lineage lymphoblastic lymphoma. *Mod Pathol* 1997;10:810–817.

Mature B-Cell Neoplasms

1. Jaffe ES, Harris NL, Stein H, et al., eds. *Pathology and genetics of haematopoietic and lymphoid tissues.* Lyon: IARC Press, 2001.
2. Pangalis GA, Angelopoulou MK, Vassilakopoulos TP, et al. B-chronic lymphocytic leukemia, small lymphocytic lymphoma, and lymphoplasmacytic lymphoma, including Waldenstrom's macroglobulinemia: a clinical, morphologic, and biologic spectrum of similar disorders. *Semin Hematol* 1999;36:104–114.

3. Kyle RA, Rajkumar SV. Monoclonal gammopathies of undetermined significance. *Hematol Oncol Clin North Am* 1999;13: 1181–1202.
4. Aljurf M, Cornbleet PJ, Michel F. CD5+ chronic B-cell leukemia with features intermediate to chronic lymphocytic leukemia and hairy cell leukemia. *Hematol Pathol* 1994;8:99–109.
5. Bentz M, Plesch A, Bullinger L, et al. t(11;14)-positive mantle cell lymphomas exhibit complex karyotypes and share similarities with B-cell chronic lymphocytic leukemia. *Genes Chromosomes Cancer* 2000;27:285–294.
6. De Angeli C, Gandini D, Cuneo A, et al. BCL-1 rearrangements and p53 mutations in atypical chronic lymphocytic leukemia with t(11;14)(q13;q32). *Haematologica* 2000;85:913–921.
7. Dunphy CH, Oza YV, Skelly ME. Previously undescribed form of B-cell chronic lymphoid leukemia with IgA expression/secretion and lytic bone lesions. *Am J Hematol* 1997;55: 208–211.
8. Nelson BP, Variakojis D, Peterson LC. Leukemic phase of B-cell lymphomas mimicking chronic lymphocytic leukemia and variants at presentation. *Mod Pathol* 2002;15:1111–1120.
9. Sen F, Lai R, Albitar M. Chronic lymphocytic leukemia with t(14;18) and trisomy 12. *Arch Pathol Lab Med* 2002;126:1543–1546.
10. Stefanidou MP, Kanavaros PE, Tosca AD. Chronic lymphocytic leukemia presenting as cutaneous and bone involvement. *Int J Dermatol* 2001;40:50–52.
11. Yasui O, Tukamoto F, Sasaki N, et al. Malignant lymphoma of the transverse colon associated with macroglobulinemia. *Am J Gastroenterol* 1997;92:2299–2301.
12. Ito K, Usuki K, Iki S, et al. Chronic neutrophilic leukemia associated with chronic lymphocytic leukemia. *Int J Hematol* 1998;68:87–94.
13. Seipelt G, Bohme A, Koschmieder S, et al. Effective treatment with rituximab in a patient with refractory prolymphocytoid transformed B-chronic lymphocytic leukemia and Evans syndrome. *Ann Hematol* 2001;80:170–173.
14. Macdonald D, Richardson H, Raby A. Practice guidelines on the reporting of smudge cells in the white blood cell differential count. *Arch Pathol Lab Med* 2003;127:105.
15. Zengin N, Kars A, Sungur A, et al. The significance of the bone marrow biopsy pattern in chronic lymphocytic leukemia: a prognostic dilemma. *Am J Hematol* 1999;62:208–211.
16. Kim YS, Ford RJ Jr, Faber JA, et al. B-cell chronic lymphocytic leukemia/small lymphocytic lymphoma involving bone marrow with an interfollicular pattern. *Am J Clin Pathol* 2000;114: 41–46.
17. Meuge-Moraw C, Delacretaz F, Baur AS. Follicular dendritic cells in bone marrow lymphoproliferative diseases: an immunohistochemical study including a new paraffin-resistant monoclonal antibody, DR53. *Histopathology* 1996;28:341–347.
18. Prokocimer M, Polliack A. Increased bone marrow mast cells in preleukemic syndromes, acute leukemia, and lymphoproliferative disorders. *Am J Clin Pathol* 1981;75:34–38.
19. Yoo D, Lessin LS, Jensen WN. Bone-marrow mast cells in lymphoproliferative disorders. *Ann Intern Med* 1978;88: 753–757.
20. Clark C, Rydell RE, Kaplan ME. Frequent association of IgM with crystalline inclusions in chronic lymphatic leukemic lymphocytes. *N Engl J Med* 1973;289:113–117.
21. Preud'homme JL, Bauwens M, Dumont G, et al. Cast nephropathy in mu heavy chain disease. *Clin Nephrol* 1997;48: 118–121.
22. Ramnani D, Lindberg G, Gokaslan ST, et al. Signet-ring cell variant of small lymphocytic lymphoma with a prominent sinusoidal pattern. *Ann Diagn Pathol* 1999;3:220–226.

23. Espinet B, Larriba I, Salido M, et al. Genetic characterization of the paraimmunoblastic variant of small lymphocytic lymphoma/chronic lymphocytic leukemia: a case report and review of the literature. *Hum Pathol* 2002;33:1145–1148.

24. Amouroux I, Mossafa H, Gentilhomme O, et al. Chronic lymphocytic leukaemia with binucleated lymphocytes. *Leuk Lymphoma* 1997;27:533–537.

25. Bennett JM, Catovsky D, Daniel MT, et al. Proposals for the classification of chronic (mature) B and T lymphoid leukaemias. French-American-British (FAB) Cooperative Group. *J Clin Pathol* 1989;42:567–584.

26. Bentz M, Plesch A, Bullinger L, et al. t(11;14)-positive mantle cell lymphomas exhibit complex karyotypes and share similarities with B-cell chronic lymphocytic leukemia. *Genes Chromosomes Cancer* 2000;27:285–294.

27. Criel A, Verhoef G, Vlietinck R, et al. Further characterization of morphologically defined typical and atypical CLL: a clinical, immunophenotypic, cytogenetic and prognostic study on 390 cases. *Br J Haematol* 1997;97:383–391.

28. Frater JL, McCarron KF, Hammel JP, et al. Typical and atypical chronic lymphocytic leukemia differ clinically and immunophenotypically. *Am J Clin Pathol* 2001;116:655–664.

29. Matutes E, Carrara P, Coignet L, et al. FISH analysis for BCL-1 rearrangements and trisomy 12 helps the diagnosis of atypical B cell leukaemias. *Leukemia* 1999;13:1721–1726.

30. O'Connor SJ, Su'ut L, Morgan GJ, et al. The relationship between typical and atypical B-cell chronic lymphocytic leukemia. A comparative genomic hybridization-based study. *Am J Clin Pathol* 2000;114:448–458.

31. Oscier DG, Matutes E, Copplestone A, et al. Atypical lymphocyte morphology: an adverse prognostic factor for disease progression in stage A CLL independent of trisomy 12. *Br J Haematol* 1997;98:934–939.

32. Buhr T, Langer F, Schlue J, et al. Reliability of lymphoma classification in bone marrow trephines. *Br J Haematol* 2002;118:470–476.

33. Callea V, Morabito F, Oliva BM, et al. Surface CD14 positivity in B-cell chronic lymphocytic leukaemia is related to clinical outcome. *Br J Haematol* 1999;107:347–352.

34. Chen CC, Raikow RB, Sonmez-Alpan E, et al. Classification of small B-cell lymphoid neoplasms using a paraffin section immunohistochemical panel. *Appl Immunohistochem Mol Morphol* 2000;8:1–11.

35. D'Arena G, Musto P, Cascavilla N, et al. CD38 expression correlates with adverse biological features and predicts poor clinical outcome in B-cell chronic lymphocytic leukemia. *Leuk Lymphoma* 2001;42:109–114.

36. Delmer A, Ajchenbaum-Cymbalista F, Tang R, et al. Overexpression of cyclin D2 in chronic B-cell malignancies. *Blood* 1995;85:2870–2876.

37. Dong HY, Gorczyca W, Liu Z, et al. B-cell lymphomas with coexpression of CD5 and CD10. *Am J Clin Pathol* 2003;119:218–230.

38. Garcia DP, Rooney MT, Ahmad E, et al. Diagnostic usefulness of CD23 and FMC-7 antigen expression patterns in B-cell lymphoma classification. *Am J Clin Pathol* 2000;115:258–265.

39. Gong JZ, Lagoo AS, Peters D, et al. Value of CD23 determination by flow cytometry in differentiating mantle cell lymphoma from chronic lymphocytic leukemia/small lymphocytic lymphoma. *Am J Clin Pathol* 2001;116:893–897.

40. Huang JC, Finn WG, Goolsby CL, et al. CD5- small B-cell leukemias are rarely classifiable as chronic lymphocytic leukemia. *Am J Clin Pathol* 1999;111:123–130.

41. Huh YO, Pugh WC, Kantarjian HM, et al. Detection of sub-groups of chronic B-cell leukemias by FMC7 monoclonal antibody. *Am J Clin Pathol* 1994;101:283–289.

42. Islam A, Vladutiu AO, Donahue T, et al. CD8 expression on B cells in chronic lymphocytic leukemia: a case report and review of the literature. *Arch Pathol Lab Med* 2000;124:1361–1363.

43. Kaleem Z, White G, Zutter MM. Aberrant expression of T-cell-associated antigens on B-cell non-Hodgkin lymphomas. *Am J Clin Pathol* 2001;115:396–403.

44. Kingma DW, Imus P, Xie XY, et al. CD2 is expressed by a sub-population of normal B cells and is frequently present in mature B-cell neoplasms. *Cytometry* 2002;50:243–248.

45. Li S, Eshleman JR, Borowitz MJ. Lack of surface immunoglobulin light chain expression by flow cytometric immunophenotyping can help diagnose peripheral B-cell lymphoma. *Am J Clin Pathol* 2002;118:229–234.

46. Marotta G, Raspadori D, Sestigiani C, et al. Expression of the CD11c antigen in B-cell chronic lymphoproliferative disorders. *Leuk Lymphoma* 2000;37:145–149.

47. Marschitz I, Tinhofer I, Hittmair A, et al. Analysis of Bcl-2 protein expression in chronic lymphocytic leukemia. A comparison of three semiquantitation techniques. *Am J Clin Pathol* 2000;113:219–229.

48. Nakase K, Kita K, Shiku H, et al. Myeloid antigen, CD13, CD14, and/or CD33 expression is restricted to certain lymphoid neoplasms. *Am J Clin Pathol* 1996;105:761–768.

49. Shapiro JL, Miller ML, Pohlman B, et al. CD5- B-cell lymphoproliferative disorders presenting in blood and bone marrow. A clinicopathologic study of 40 patients. *Am J Clin Pathol* 1999;111:477–487.

50. Thunberg U, Johnson A, Roos G, et al. CD38 expression is a poor predictor for VH gene mutational status and prognosis in chronic lymphocytic leukemia. *Blood* 2001;97:1892–1894.

51. Tworek JA, Singleton TP, Schnitzer B, et al. Flow cytometric and immunohistochemical analysis of small lymphocytic lymphoma, mantle cell lymphoma, and plasmacytoid small lymphocytic lymphoma. *Am J Clin Pathol* 1998;110:582–589.

52. Witzig TE, Kimlinger T, Stenson M, et al. Syndecan-1 expression on malignant cells from the blood and marrow of patients with plasma cell proliferative disorders and B-cell chronic lymphocytic leukemia. *Leuk Lymphoma* 1998;31:167–175.

53. Barnabas N, Shurafa M, Van Dyke DL, et al. Significance of p53 mutations in patients with chronic lymphocytic leukemia. *Cancer* 2001;91:285–293.

54. Dohner H, Stilgenbauer S, Benner A, et al. Genomic aberrations and survival in chronic lymphocytic leukemia. *N Engl J Med* 2000;343:1910–1916.

55. Doneda L, Castorina P, Tedeschi A, et al. Multicolor FISH in chronic lymphocytic leukemia. An interphase study of patients with early-onset disease. *Cancer Genet Cytogenet* 2001;125:63–69.

56. Hogan WJ, Tefferi A, Borell TJ, et al. Prognostic relevance of monosomy at the 13q14 locus detected by fluorescence *in situ* hybridization in B-cell chronic lymphocytic leukemia. *Cancer Genet Cytogenet* 1999;110:77–81.

57. Kojima K, Taniwaki M, Yoshino T, et al. Trisomy 12 and t(14;18) in B-cell chronic lymphocytic leukemia. *Int J Hematol* 1998;67:199–203.

58. Koski T, Karhu R, Visakorpi T, et al. Complex chromosomal aberrations in chronic lymphocytic leukemia are associated with cellular drug and irradiation resistance. *Eur J Haematol* 2000;65:32–39.

59. Shaw GR, Kronberger DL. TP53 deletions but not trisomy 12 are adverse in B-cell lymphoproliferative disorders. *Cancer Genet Cytogenet* 2000;119:146–154.

60. Enno A, Catovsky D, O'Brien M, et al. 'Prolymphocytoid' transformation of chronic lymphocytic leukaemia. *Br J Haematol* 1979;41:9–18.

61. Kjeldsberg CR, Marty J. Prolymphocytic transformation of chronic lymphocytic leukemia. *Cancer* 1981;48:2447–2457.

62. Dunphy CH, Wheaton SE, Perkins SL. CD23 expression in transformed small lymphocytic lymphomas/chronic lymphocytic leukemias and blastic transformations of mantle cell lymphoma. *Mod Pathol* 1997;10:818–822.

63. Kroft SH, Dawson DB, McKenna RW. Large cell lymphoma transformation of chronic lymphocytic leukemia/small lymphocytic lymphoma. A flow cytometric analysis of seven cases. *Am J Clin Pathol* 2001;115:385–395.

64. Mohamed AN, Compean R, Dan ME, et al. Clonal evolution of chronic lymphocytic leukemia to acute lymphoblastic leukemia. *Cancer Genet Cytogenet* 1996;86:143–146.

65. Paietta E, Tudoriu CD, Goldstein M, et al. Plasmacytoid blast crisis in B-cell chronic lymphocytic leukemia: effect of estradiol on growth and differentiation *in vitro. Leuk Res* 1985;9:19–29.

66. Pistoia V, Roncella S, Di Celle PF, et al. Emergence of a B-cell lymphoblastic lymphoma in a patient with B-cell chronic lymphocytic leukemia: evidence for the single-cell origin of the two tumors. *Blood* 1991;78:797–804.

67. Spath-Schwalbe E, Flath B, Kaufmann O, et al. An unusual case of leukemic non-Hodgkin's lymphoma with blastic transformation. *Ann Hematol* 2000;79:217–221.

68. Kanzler H, Kuppers R, Helmes S, et al. Hodgkin and Reed-Sternberg-like cells in B-cell chronic lymphocytic leukemia represent the outgrowth of single germinal-center B-cell-derived clones: potential precursors of Hodgkin and Reed-Sternberg cells in Hodgkin's disease. *Blood* 2000;95:1023–1031.

69. O'Sullivan MJ, Kaleem Z, Bolger MJ, et al. Composite prolymphocytoid and Hodgkin transformation of chronic lymphocytic leukemia. *Arch Pathol Lab Med* 2000;124:907–909.

70. Wetzler M, Kurzrock R, Goodacre AM, et al. Transformation of chronic lymphocytic leukemia to lymphoma of true histiocytic type. *Cancer* 1995;76:609–617.

71. Thomas R, Ribeiro I, Shepherd P, et al. Spontaneous clinical regression in chronic lymphocytic leukaemia. *Br J Haematol* 2002;116:341–345.

72. Upshaw JD Jr, Callihan TR. Spontaneous remission of B-cell chronic lymphocytic leukemia associated with T lymphocytic hyperplasia in bone marrow. *South Med J* 2002;95:647–649.

73. Wajima T. Spontaneous regression of chronic lymphocytic leukemia and simultaneous development of autoimmune hemolytic anemia and autoimmune thrombocytopenia. *Am J Hematol* 2000;65:88–89.

74. Ballard HS, Kouri Y. The association of erythrocytosis and chronic lymphocytic leukemia. *Cancer* 1992;70:2431–2435.

75. Bizzaro N. Chronic lymphocytic leukaemia in a patient with essential thrombocythaemia. *Clin Lab Haematol* 1998;20:377–379.

76. Nieto LH, Raya Sanchez JM, Arguelles HA, et al. A case of chronic lymphocytic leukemia overwhelmed by rapidly progressive idiopathic myelofibrosis. *Haematologica* 2000;85:973–977.

77. Sanz MA, Valcarcel D, Sureda A, et al. Systemic mast cell disease associated with B-chronic lymphocytic leukemia. *Haematologica* 2001;86:1106–1107.

78. Esteve J, Cervantes F, Rives S, et al. Simultaneous occurrence of B-cell chronic lymphocytic leukemia and chronic myeloid leukemia with further evolution to lymphoid blast crisis. *Haematologica* 1997;82:596–599.

79. Lai R, Arber DA, Brynes RK, et al. Untreated chronic lymphocytic leukemia concurrent with or followed by acute myelogenous leukemia or myelodysplastic syndrome. A report of five cases and review of the literature. *Am J Clin Pathol* 1999;111:373–378.

80. Okada M, Okamoto T, Takemoto Y, et al. Function and X chromosome inactivation analysis of B lymphocytes in myelodysplastic syndromes with immunological abnormalities. *Acta Haematol* 2000;102:124–130.

81. Florensa L, Vallespi T, Woessner S, et al. Incidence and characteristics of lymphoid malignancies in untreated myelodysplastic syndromes. *Leuk Lymphoma* 1996;23:609–612.

82. Xie XY, Filie AC, Jasper GA, et al. Diagnosis of unexpected acute myeloid leukemia and chronic lymphocytic leukemia: a case report demonstrating the perils of restricted panels in flow cytometric immunophenotyping. *Cytometry* 2000;42:114–117.

83. Yenerel MN, Hatemi I, Keskin H. Concomitant chronic lymphocytic leukemia and acute myeloid leukemia diagnosed by two color flow cytometric analysis. *Haematologica* 1999;84:766–767.

84. Bonetti F, Knowles DM 2nd, Chilosi M, et al. A distinctive cutaneous malignant neoplasm expressing the Langerhans cell phenotype. Synchronous occurrence with B-chronic lymphocytic leukemia. *Cancer* 1985;55:2417–2425.

85. Vasef MA, Zaatari GS, Chan WC, et al. Dendritic cell tumors associated with low-grade B-cell malignancies. Report of three cases. *Am J Clin Pathol* 1995;104:696–701.

86. Gine E, Bosch F, Villamor N, et al. Simultaneous diagnosis of hairy cell leukemia and chronic lymphocytic leukemia/small lymphocytic lymphoma: a frequent association? *Leukemia* 2002;16:1454–1459.

87. Nakamura N, Kuze T, Hashimoto Y, et al. Analysis of the immunoglobulin heavy chain gene of secondary diffuse large B-cell lymphoma that subsequently developed in four cases with B-cell chronic lymphocytic leukemia or lymphoplasmacytoid lymphoma (Richter syndrome). *Pathol Int* 2000;50:636–643.

88. Yahata N, Iwase O, Iwama H, et al. Chronic lymphocytic leukemia complicated by plasmacytoma originating from different clones. *Leuk Lymphoma* 2000;39:203–207.

89. Patriarca F, Gaidano G, Capello D, et al. Occurrence of multiple myeloma after fludarabine treatment of a chronic lymphocytic leukemia: evidence of a biclonal derivation and clinical response to autologous stem cell transplantation. *Haematologica* 2000;85:982–985.

90. Goolsby CL, Kuchnio M, Finn WG, et al. Expansions of clonal and oligoclonal T cells in B-cell chronic lymphocytic leukemia are primarily restricted to the CD3(+)CD8(+) T-cell population. *Cytometry* 2000;42:188–195.

91. Lesesve JF, Feugier P, Lamy T, et al. Association of B-chronic lymphocytic leukaemia and T-large granular lymphocyte leukaemia. *Clin Lab Haematol* 2000;22:121–122.

92. Hull PR, Saxena A. Mycosis fungoides and chronic lymphocytic leukaemia—composite T-cell and B-cell lymphomas presenting in the skin. *Br J Dermatol* 2000;143:439–444.

93. Konstantopoulos K, Kapsimalis V, Vaiopoulos G, et al. Simultaneous appearance of mycosis fungoides and chronic lymphocytic leukemia in the same patient. *Haematologia (Budap)* 2000;30:41–43.

94. Novogrudsky A, Amorosi EL, Gottesman SR. High-grade T-cell lymphoma complicating B-cell chronic lymphocytic leukemia: an unusual manifestation of "Richter's syndrome." *Am J Hematol* 2001;66:203–206.

95. Reimer P, Weissinger F, Tony HP, et al. Persistent polyclonal B-cell lymphocytosis—an important differential diagnosis of B-cell chronic lymphocytic leukemia. *Ann Hematol* 2000;79:327–331.

96. De Vita S, De Re V, Gasparotto D, et al. Oligoclonal non-neoplastic B cell expansion is the key feature of type II mixed

cryoglobulinemia: clinical and molecular findings do not support a bone marrow pathologic diagnosis of indolent B cell lymphoma. *Arthritis Rheum* 2000;43:94–102.

97. Hercher C, Robain M, Davi F, et al. A multicentric study of 41 cases of B-prolymphocytic leukemia: two evolutive forms. *Leuk Lymphoma* 2001;42:981–987.

98. Schlette E, Bueso-Ramos C, Giles F, et al. Mature B-cell leukemias with more than 55% prolymphocytes. A heterogeneous group that includes an unusual variant of mantle cell lymphoma. *Am J Clin Pathol* 2001;115:571–581.

99. Sole F, Woessner S, Espinet B, et al. Cytogenetic abnormalities in three patients with B-cell prolymphocytic leukemia. *Cancer Genet Cytogenet* 1998;103:43–45.

100. Nieto LH, Lampert IA, Catovsky D. Bone marrow histological patterns in B-cell and T-cell prolymphocytic leukemia. *Hematol Pathol* 1989;3:79–84.

101. Emery CL, Cleveland RP. B-cell prolymphocytic leukemia expressing discordant myeloid-associated antigens in simultaneous specimens from bone marrow and peripheral blood. *Cytometry* 1995;22:243–249.

102. Matsushita A, Nagai K, Ishikawa T, et al. B-cell prolymphocytic leukemia expressing CD13 antigen. *Int J Hematol* 1994;60: 157–161.

103. Lens D, Matutes E, Catovsky D, et al. Frequent deletions at 11q23 and 13q14 in B cell prolymphocytic leukemia (B-PLL). *Leukemia* 2000;14:427–430.

104. Fischer T, Miller M, Bott-Silverman C, et al. Posttransplant lymphoproliferative disease after cardiac transplantation. Two unusual variants with predominantly plasmacytoid features. *Transplantation* 1996;62:1687–1690.

105. Silvestri F, Barillari G, Fanin R, et al. Impact of hepatitis C virus infection on clinical features, quality of life and survival of patients with lymphoplasmacytoid lymphoma/immunocytoma. *Ann Oncol* 1998;9:499–504.

106. Ogmundsdottir HM, Haraldsdottir VM, Johannesson G, et al. Monoclonal gammopathy in Iceland: a population-based registry and follow-up. *Br J Haematol* 2002;118:166–173.

107. Owen RG, Barrans SL, Richards SJ, et al. Waldenstrom macroglobulinemia. Development of diagnostic criteria and identification of prognostic factors. *Am J Clin Pathol* 2001;116: 420–428.

108. Sahota SS, Forconi F, Ottensmeier CH, et al. Typical Waldenstrom macroglobulinemia is derived from a B-cell arrested after cessation of somatic mutation but prior to isotype switch events. *Blood* 2002;100:1505–1507.

109. Aboul-Nasr R, O'Brien S, Freireich EJ, et al. "T-cell-rich B-cell lymphoproliferative disorder" of the bone marrow. *Leuk Lymphoma* 2001;42:1023–1031.

110. Iwasaki T, Hamano T, Kobayashi K, et al. A case of mu-heavy chain disease: combined features of mu-chain disease and macroglobulinemia. *Int J Hematol* 1997;66:359–365.

111. Kondo H, Yokoyama K. IgM myeloma: different features from multiple myeloma and macroglobulinaemia. *Eur J Haematol* 1999;63:366–368.

112. Kraus MD. Lymphoplasmacytic lymphoma/Waldenstrom macroglobulinemia. One disease or three? *Am J Clin Pathol* 2001; 116:799–801.

113. Garand R, Sahota SS, Avet-Loiseau H, et al. IgG-secreting lymphoplasmacytoid leukaemia: a B-cell disorder with extensively mutated VH genes undergoing Ig isotype-switching frequently associated with trisomy 12. *Br J Haematol* 2000;109: 71–80.

114. Barnard DL, Worman CP, Boldersen I, et al. IgE lambda paraproteinaemia associated with a pleomorphic lymphoproliferative disorder. *Clin Lab Haematol* 1981;3:129–136.

115. Hara T, Ozaki S, Kosaka M, et al. Biclonal lymphoplasmacytic immunocytoma associated with Crohn's disease. *Intern Med* 1999;38:500–503.

116. Garcia-Sanz R, Montoto S, Torrequebrada A, et al. Waldenstrom macroglobulinaemia: presenting features and outcome in a series with 217 cases. *Br J Haematol* 2001;115:575–582.

117. Kyrtsonis MC, Vassilakopoulos TP, Angelopoulou MK, et al. Waldenstrom's macroglobulinemia: clinical course and prognostic factors in 60 patients. Experience from a single hematology unit. *Ann Hematol* 2001;80:722–727.

118. Allez M, Mariette X, Linares G, et al. Low-grade MALT lymphoma mimicking Waldenstrom's macroglobulinemia. *Leukemia* 1999;13:484–485.

119. Sekikawa T, Takahara S, Kawano T, et al. No V(H) somatic hypermutation was detected in B-cells of a patient with macroglobulinemia due to splenic marginal zone lymphoma. *Int J Hematol* 2002;76:453–459.

120. Valdez R, Finn WG, Ross CW, et al. Waldenstrom macroglobulinemia caused by extranodal marginal zone B-cell lymphoma: a report of six cases. *Am J Clin Pathol* 2001;116:683–690.

121. Zakzook SI, Yunus MB, Mulconrey DS. Hyperviscosity syndrome in rheumatoid arthritis with Felty's syndrome: case report and review of the literature. *Clin Rheumatol* 2002;21:82–85.

122. Della Rossa A, Tavoni A, Baldini C, et al. Treatment of chronic hepatitis C infection with cryoglobulinemia. *Curr Opin Rheumatol* 2002;14:231–237.

123. Jin DK, Nowakowski M, Kramer M, et al. Hyperviscosity syndrome secondary to a myeloma-associated IgG(1)kappa paraprotein strongly reactive against the HIV-1 p24 gag antigen. *Am J Hematol* 2000;64:210–213.

124. Magro CM, Crowson AN. A clinical and histologic study of 37 cases of immunoglobulin A-associated vasculitis. *Am J Dermatopathol* 1999;21:234–240.

125. Kes P, Pecanic Z, Getaldic B, et al. Treatment of hyperviscosity syndrome in the patients with plasma cell dyscrasias. *Acta Med Croatica* 1996;50:173–177.

126. Tetreault SA, Saven A. Delayed onset of autoimmune hemolytic anemia complicating cladribine therapy for Waldenstrom macroglobulinemia. *Leuk Lymphoma* 2000;37:125–130.

127. Nakajima H, Mori S, Takeuchi T, et al. Monocytosis and high serum macrophage colony-stimulating factor in Waldenstrom's macroglobulinemia. *Blood* 1995;86:2863–2864.

128. Molero T, De La Iglesia S, Santana C, et al. Signet-ring cells in a Waldenstrom's macroglobulinaemia. *Leuk Lymphoma* 1998;32:175–177.

129. Jones D, Bhatia VK, Krausz T, et al. Crystal-storing histiocytosis: a disorder occurring in plasmacytic tumors expressing immunoglobulin kappa light chain. *Hum Pathol* 1999;30:1441–1448.

130. Karakantza M, Matutes E, MacLennan K, et al. Association between sarcoidosis and lymphoma revisited. *J Clin Pathol* 1996;49:208–212.

131. Karmochkine M, Oksenhendler E, Leruez-Ville M, et al. Persistent parvovirus B19 infection and pure red cell aplasia in Waldenstrom's macroglobulinemia: successful treatment with high-dose intravenous immunoglobulin. *Am J Hematol* 1995;50: 227–228.

132. Padmalatha C, Warner TF, Hafez GR. Pseudo-Gaucher cell in IgMk plasmacytoid lymphoma. *Am J Surg Pathol* 1981;5: 501–505.

133. Bartl R, Hansmann ML, Frisch B, et al. Comparative histology of malignant lymphomas in lymph node and bone marrow. *Br J Haematol* 1988;69:229–237.

134. Schop RF, Kuehl WM, Van Wier SA, et al. Waldenstrom macroglobulinemia neoplastic cells lack immunoglobulin heavy

chain locus translocations but have frequent 6q deletions. *Blood* 2002;100:2996–3001.

135. Wong KF, So CC, Chan JC, et al. Gain of chromosome 3/3q in B-cell chronic lymphoproliferative disorder is associated with plasmacytoid differentiation with or without IgM overproduction. *Cancer Genet Cytogenet* 2002;136:82–85.

136. Gertz MA, Kyle RA, Noel P. Primary systemic amyloidosis: a rare complication of immunoglobulin M monoclonal gammopathies and Waldenstrom's macroglobulinemia. *J Clin Oncol* 1993;11:914–920.

137. Hamada T, Ishizuka H, Asai Y, et al. A case of anaplastic large cell (Ki-1) lymphoma of B-cell phenotype, occurring in Waldenstrom's macroglobulinemia. *Pathol Int* 1999;49:913–917.

138. Nakamura N, Kuze T, Hashimoto Y, et al. Analysis of the immunoglobulin heavy chain gene of secondary diffuse large B-cell lymphoma that subsequently developed in four cases with B-cell chronic lymphocytic leukemia or lymphoplasmacytoid lymphoma (Richter syndrome). *Pathol Int* 2000;50: 636–643.

139. Rosales CM, Lin P, Mansoor A, et al. Lymphoplasmacytic lymphoma/Waldenstrom macroglobulinemia associated with Hodgkin disease. A report of two cases. *Am J Clin Pathol* 2001; 116:34–40.

140. Rosique P, Majado MJ, Bas A. Unusual evolution to immunoblastic lymphoma of a case of Waldenstrom macroglobulinemia presenting with thrombocytopenia. *Haematologica* 1997;82: 509–510.

141. Saba NF, Warth JA, Ross DG. Simultaneous occurrence of polycythemia vera and Waldenstrom macroglobulinemia: a case report and review of the literature. *Haematologia (Budap)* 2002; 32:17–23.

142. Schulze R, Schlimok G, Renner D. Coincidence of primary myelodysplastic syndrome and non-Hodgkin lymphoma. *Clin Invest* 1992;70:1082–1084.

143. Murashige N, Tabanda R, Zalusky R. Occurrence of acute monocytic leukemia in a case of untreated Waldenstrom's macroglobulinemia. *Am J Hematol* 2002;71:94–97.

144. Pagano L, Larocca LM. Simultaneous presentation of Waldenstrom's macroglobulinemia and acute myeloid leukemia. *Haematologica* 2002;87:EIM07.

145. Rodriguez JN, Fernandez-Jurado A, Martino ML, et al. Waldenstrom's macroglobulinemia complicated with acute myeloid leukemia. Report of a case and review of the literature. *Haematologica* 1998;83:91–92.

146. Fine JM, Gorin NC, Gendre JP, et al. Simultaneous occurrence of clinical manifestations of myeloma and Waldenstrom's macroglobulinemia with monoclonal IgG lambda and IgM kappa in a single patient. *Acta Med Scand* 1981;209: 229–234.

147. Geerts ML, Hamers J, Schwarze EW, et al. Mycosis fungoides and lymphoplasmacytoid immunocytoma in the same patient. A case report. *Cancer* 1984;54:2294–2299.

148. Berger F, Felman P, Thieblemont C, et al. Non-MALT marginal zone B-cell lymphomas: a description of clinical presentation and outcome in 124 patients. *Blood* 2000;95:1950–1956.

149. Campo E, Miquel R, Krenacs L, et al. Primary nodal marginal zone lymphomas of splenic and MALT type. *Am J Surg Pathol* 1999;23:59–68.

150. Graziadei G, Pruneri G, Carboni N, et al. Low-grade MALT lymphoma involving multiple mucosal sites and bone marrow. *Ann Hematol* 1998;76:81–83.

151. Thieblemont C, Felman P, Callet-Bauchu E, et al. Splenic marginal-zone lymphoma: a distinct clinical and pathological entity. *Lancet Oncol* 2003;4:95–103.

152. Hermine O, Lefrere F, Bronowicki JP, et al. Regression of splenic lymphoma with villous lymphocytes after treatment of hepatitis C virus infection. *N Engl J Med* 2002;347:89–94.

153. Leith CP, Mangalik A, Foucar K. A B-cell "chameleon": striking clinical, morphological, and immunophenotypic diversity of a single low-grade B cell clone. *Hum Pathol* 1997;28:104–108.

154. Shibata K, Shimamoto Y, Nakano S, et al. Mantle cell lymphoma with the features of mucosa-associated lymphoid tissue (MALT) lymphoma in an HTLV-I-seropositive patient. *Ann Hematol* 1995;70:47–51.

155. Costes V, Duchayne E, Taib J, et al. Intrasinusoidal bone marrow infiltration: a common growth pattern for different lymphoma subtypes. *Br J Haematol* 2002;119:916–922.

156. Franco V, Florena AM, Stella M, et al. Splenectomy influences bone marrow infiltration in patients with splenic marginal zone cell lymphoma with or without villous lymphocytes. *Cancer* 2001;91:294–301.

157. Kent SA, Variakojis D, Peterson LC. Comparative study of marginal zone lymphoma involving bone marrow. *Am J Clin Pathol* 2002;117:698–708.

158. Woessner S, Domingo A, Guma J, et al. Lymphocytes with cerebriform nuclei in chronic B-cell lymphoproliferative diseases. *Leuk Res* 1997;21:893–895.

159. Batanian JR, Dunphy CH, Richart JM, et al. Simultaneous presence of t(2;8)(p12;q24) and t(14;18)(q32;q21) in a B-cell lymphoproliferative disorder with features suggestive of an aggressive variant of splenic marginal-zone lymphoma. *Cancer Genet Cytogenet* 2000;120:136–140.

160. Woessner S, Domingo A, Guma J, et al. Lymphocytes with cerebriform nuclei in chronic B-cell lymphoproliferative disorders. *Leuk Res* 1997;21:893–895.

161. Ballesteros E, Osborne BM, Matsushima AY. CD5+ low-grade marginal zone B-cell lymphomas with localized presentation. *Am J Surg Pathol* 1998;22:201–207.

162. Miyawaki S, Machii T, Hirabayashi H, et al. Splenic lymphoma with villous lymphocytes with CD5+, CD11c+ B-cell phenotype. *Intern Med* 1993;32:472–475.

163. Akagi T, Motegi M, Tamura A, et al. A novel gene, MALT1 at 18q21, is involved in t(11;18) (q21;q21) found in low-grade B-cell lymphoma of mucosa-associated lymphoid tissue. *Oncogene* 1999;18:5785–5794.

164. Dierlamm J, Baens M, Stefanova-Ouzounova M, et al. Detection of t(11;18)(q21;q21) by interphase fluorescence in situ hybridization using API2 and MLT specific probes. *Blood* 2000;96:2215–2218.

165. Hanawa H, Abo J, Inokuchi K, et al. Dual rearrangement of immunoglobulin and T-cell receptor genes in a case of splenic lymphoma with villous lymphocytes. *Leuk Lymphoma* 1995;18:357–360.

166. Cualing H, Steele P, Zellner D. Blastic transformation of splenic marginal zone B-cell lymphoma. *Arch Pathol Lab Med* 2000;124:748–752.

167. Kuwayama M, Machii T, Yamaguchi M, et al. Blastic transformation of splenic lymphoma with villous lymphocytes after a well-controlled chronic phase of more than 10 years. *Int J Hematol* 2000;71:167–171.

168. Thorson P, Hess JL. Transformation of monocytoid B-cell lymphoma to large cell lymphoma associated with crystal-storing histiocytes. *Arch Pathol Lab Med* 2000;124:460–462.

169. Pajor L, Kereskai L, Tamaska P, et al. Coexistence of chronic myeloid leukemia and hairy cell leukemia of common clonal origin. *Cancer Genet Cytogenet* 2002;134:114–117.

170. Adami F, Chilosi M, Lestani M, et al. A CD5+ leukemic lymphoma with monocytoid features: an unusual B-cell lymphoma mimicking hairy-cell leukemia. *Acta Haematol* 1993;89: 94–99.

171. Algino KM, Hendrix LE, Henderson CA, et al. Multiple myeloma with hairy cell-like features. *Am J Clin Pathol* 1997;107: 665–671.

172. Yetgin S, Olcay L, Yel L, et al. T-ALL with monoclonal gammopathy and hairy cell features. *Am J Hematol* 2000;65:166–170.

173. Bourguin-Plonquet A, Rouard H, Roudot-Thoraval F, et al. Severe decrease in peripheral blood dendritic cells in hairy cell leukaemia. *Br J Haematol* 2002;116:595–597.

174. Janckila AJ, Wallace JH, Yam LT. Generalized monocyte deficiency in leukaemic reticuloendotheliosis. *Scand J Haematol* 1982;29:153–160.

175. Cesana C, Brando B, Boiani E, et al. Effective treatment of autoimmune hemolytic anemia and hairy cell leukemia with interferon-alpha. *Eur J Haematol* 2002;68:120–121.

176. Mainwaring CJ, Walewska R, Snowden J, et al. Fatal cold anti-i autoimmune haemolytic anaemia complicating hairy cell leukaemia. *Br J Haematol* 2000;109:641–643.

177. Ardley BP, Sun X, Shaw JM, et al. Hairy cell leukemia with marked lymphocytosis. *Arch Pathol Lab Med* 2003;127: 253–254.

178. Hanson CA, Ward PC, Schnitzer B. A multilobular variant of hairy cell leukemia with morphologic similarities to T-cell lymphoma. *Am J Surg Pathol* 1989;13:671–679.

179. Lemez P, Friedmann B, Vanasek J, et al. Hairy cell leukemia with ring-shaped nuclei. *Blut* 1990;61:251.

180. Woessner S, Domingo A, Guma J, et al. Lymphocytes with cerebriform nuclei in chronic B-cell lymphoproliferative diseases. *Leuk Res* 1997;21:893–895.

181. Drexler HG, Gaedicke G, Minowada J. Occurrence of particular isoenzymes in fresh and cultured leukemia-lymphoma cells. I. Tartrate-resistant acid phosphatase isoenzyme. *Cancer* 1986;57:1776–1782.

182. Hoyer JD, Li CY, Yam LT, et al. Immunohistochemical demonstration of acid phosphatase isoenzyme 5 (tartrate-resistant) in paraffin sections of hairy cell leukemia and other hematologic disorders. *Am J Clin Pathol* 1997;108:308–315.

183. Usui T, Konishi H, Sawada H, et al. Existence of tartrate-resistant acid phosphatase activity in differentiated lymphoid leukemic cells. *Am J Hematol* 1982;12:47–54.

184. Yam LT, Janckila AJ, Li CY, et al. Cytochemistry of tartrate-resistant acid phosphatase: 15 years' experience. *Leukemia* 1987; 1:285–288.

185. Katayama I. Bone marrow in hairy cell leukemia. *Hematol Oncol Clin North Am* 1988;2:585–602.

186. Laughlin M, Islam A, Barcos M, et al. Effect of alpha-interferon therapy on bone marrow fibrosis in hairy cell leukemia. *Blood* 1988;72:936–939.

187. Lembersky BC, Ratain MJ, Golomb HM. Skeletal complications in hairy cell leukemia: diagnosis and therapy. *J Clin Oncol* 1988;6:1280–1284.

188. Marinone GM, Roncoli B. Selective myeloid aplasia: a long-lasting presentation of an unusual hairy cell leukemia variant? *Haematologica* 1993;78:239–241.

189. Osterholz J, Wohlleber M, Kahnt C, et al. The use of interferon-alpha and granulocyte colony-stimulating factor in hairy cell leukaemia with aplastic marrow. *Eur J Haematol* 1995;55: 140–142.

190. Podzimek K, Kerekes Z, Chrobak L, et al. The value of bone marrow biopsy in the prognosis of hairy cell leukemia (HCL). *Neoplasma* 1994;41:325–330.

191. VanderMolen LA, Urba WJ, Longo DL, et al. Diffuse osteosclerosis in hairy cell leukemia. *Blood* 1989;74:2066–2069.

192. Verhoef GE, De Wolf-Peeters C, Zachee P, et al. Regression of diffuse osteosclerosis in hairy cell leukaemia after treatment with interferon. *Br J Haematol* 1990;76:150–151.

193. Franco V, Florena AM, Quintini G, et al. Bone marrow granulomas in hairy cell leukaemia following 2-chlorodeoxyadenosine therapy. *Histopathology* 1994;24:271–273.

194. Hudson J, Cobby M, Yates P, et al. Extensive infiltration of bone with marrow necrosis in a case of hairy cell leukaemia. *Skeletal Radiol* 1995;24:228–231.

195. Linder J, Silberman HR, Croker BP. Amyloidosis complicating hairy cell leukemia. *Am J Clin Pathol* 1982;78:864–867.

196. Macon WR, Kinney MC, Glick AD, et al. Marrow mast cell hyperplasia in hairy cell leukemia. *Mod Pathol* 1993;6:695–698.

197. Marisavljevic D, Rolovic Z, Vuckovic S, et al. Hairy cell leukemia associated with congenital dyserythropoietic anemia type II (HEMPAS). *Haematologia (Budap)* 1994;26:39–43.

198. Psiachou-Leonard E, Bain BJ. Persistent bone marrow failure with dysplastic features following pentostatin therapy for hairy cell leukaemia. *Clin Lab Haematol* 1998;20:195–197.

199. Zak P, Chrobak L, Podzimek K, et al. Dyserythropoietic changes and sideroblastic anemia in patients with hairy cell leukemia before and after therapy with 2-chlorodeoxyadenosine. *Neoplasma* 1998;45:261–265.

200. Shibayama H, Machii T, Tokumine Y, et al. Establishment of a new cell line from a patient with hairy cell leukemia-Japanese variant. *Leuk Lymphoma* 1997;25:373–380.

201. Diez Martin JL, Li CY, Banks PM. Blastic variant of hairy-cell leukemia. *Am J Clin Pathol* 1987;87:576–583.

202. Dunphy CH, Petruska PJ. Atypical prolymphocytic variant of hairy-cell leukemia: case report and review of the literature. *Am J Hematol* 1996;53:121–125.

203. Tytherleigh L, Taparia M, Leahy MF. Detection of hairy cell leukaemia in blood and bone marrow using multidimensional flow cytometry with CD45-PECy5 and SS gating. *Clin Lab Haematol* 2001;23:385–390.

204. de Totero D, Tazzari PL, Lauria F, et al. Phenotypic analysis of hairy cell leukemia: "variant" cases express the interleukin-2 receptor beta chain, but not the alpha chain (CD25). *Blood* 1993;82:528–535.

205. Dunphy CH, Oza YV, Skelly ME. An otherwise typical case of non-Japanese hairy cell leukemia with CD10 and CDw75 expression: response to cladribine phosphate therapy. *J Clin Lab Anal* 1999;13:141–144.

206. Usha L, Bradlow B, Stock W, et al. CD5+ immunophenotype in the bone marrow but not in the peripheral blood in a patient with hairy cell leukemia. *Acta Haematol* 2000;103:210–213.

207. Wu ML, Kwaan HC, Goolsby CL. Atypical hairy cell leukemia. *Arch Pathol Lab Med* 2000;124:171–173.

208. Sambani C, Trafalis DT, Mitsoulis-Mentzikoff C, et al. Clonal chromosome rearrangements in hairy cell leukemia: personal experience and review of literature. *Cancer Genet Cytogenet* 2001; 129:138–144.

209. Wong KF, Kwong YL, Hui PK. Hairy cell leukemia variant with t(2;8)(p12;q24) abnormality. *Cancer Genet Cytogenet* 1997;98:102–105.

210. Arnalich F, Camacho J, Jimenez C, et al. Occurrence of immunoblastic B-cell lymphoma in hairy cell leukemia. *Cancer* 1987;59:1161–1164.

211. Huang AT, Silverstein L, Gonias SL, et al. Transformation of hairy cell leukemia to EBV genome-containing aggressive B-cell lymphoma. *Leukemia* 1987;1:369–372.

212. Nazeer T, Burkart P, Dunn H, et al. Blastic transformation of hairy cell leukemia. *Arch Pathol Lab Med* 1997;121:707–713.

213. Saif MW, Greenberg BR. Multiple myeloma and hairy cell leukemia: a rare association or coincidence? *Leuk Lymphoma* 2001;42:1043–1048.

214. Mufti GJ, Hamblin TJ, Stevenson FK, et al. Polycythemia rubra vera and hairy cell leukemia. *Acta Haematol* 1985;73:189.

215. Lichtman SM, Wasil T, Ahmad M, et al. Development of essential thrombocythemia in a patient treated with interferon alfa and pentostatin for hairy cell leukemia. *Leuk Lymphoma* 1998;28:423–427.

216. Petrella T, Depret O, Arnould L, et al. Systemic mast cell disease associated with hairy cell leukaemia. *Leuk Lymphoma* 1997;25:593–595.

217. Reeves JE, Robbins BA, Pankey LR, et al. The simultaneous occurrence of variant hairy cell leukemia and chronic-phase chronic myelogenous leukemia. A case report. *Cancer* 1995;75:2089–2092.

218. Wandroo FA, Bareford D, el-Jehani F. Chronic myeloid leukaemia occurring in a patient with hairy cell leukaemia. *J Clin Pathol* 2000;53:940–941.

219. Lorand-Metze I, Lima CS, Cardinalli IA, et al. Association of a myelodysplastic syndrome with hairy cell leukaemia. *Eur J Haematol* 1995;55:341–343.

220. Schirmer M, Haun M, Grunewald K, et al. New rearrangement pattern after treatment of hairy-cell leukemia with 2-chlorodeoxyadenosine. *Acta Haematol* 2000;103:109–111.

221. Diaz-Pavon JR, Pugh W, Cabanillas F. Simultaneous presentation of hairy cell leukemia and follicular small cleaved cell lymphoma in a patient with previous diagnosis of renal cell carcinoma. *Hematol Oncol* 1995;13:63–67.

222. Nakamine H, Okamoto Y, Tsuda T, et al. Hodgkin's disease in hairy cell leukemia. Phenotypic characterization of neoplastic cells. *Cancer* 1987;60:1751–1756.

223. Copeland AR, Bueso-Ramos C, Liu FJ, et al. Molecular study of hairy cell leukemia variant with biclonal paraproteinemia. *Arch Pathol Lab Med* 1997;121:150–154.

224. Paolini R, Poletti A, Ramazzina E, et al. Co-existence of cutaneous T-cell lymphoma and B hairy cell leukemia. *Am J Hematol* 2000;64:197–202.

225. Airo P, Rossi G, Facchetti F, et al. Monoclonal expansion of large granular lymphocytes with a CD4+ CD8dim+/− phenotype associated with hairy cell leukemia. *Haematologica* 1995;80:146–149.

226. Machii T, Yamaguchi M, Inoue R, et al. Polyclonal B-cell lymphocytosis with features resembling hairy cell leukemia-Japanese variant. *Blood* 1997;89:2008–2014.

227. Hasselbalch H, Jans H, Nielsen PL. A distinct subtype of idiopathic myelofibrosis with bone marrow features mimicking hairy cell leukemia: evidence of an autoimmune pathogenesis. *Am J Hematol* 1987;25:225–229.

228. Nair CN, Shinde S, Kumar A, et al. Sezary cells with hairy projections. *Leuk Res* 1999;23:195–197.

229. Palumbo AP, Corradini P, Battaglio S, et al. Dual rearrangement of immunoglobulin and T-cell receptor gene in a case of T-cell hairy-cell leukemia. *Eur J Haematol* 1991;46:71–76.

230. Groom DA, Wong D, Brynes RK, et al. Auer rod-like inclusions in circulating lymphoma cells. *Am J Clin Pathol* 1991;96:111–115.

231. Torlakovic E, Torlakovic G, Brunning RD. Follicular pattern of bone marrow involvement by follicular lymphoma. *Am J Clin Pathol* 2002;118:780–786.

232. Alterini R, Rigacci L, Stefanacci S. Pseudo-Gaucher cells in the bone marrow of a patient with centrocytic nodular non-Hodgkin's lymphoma. *Haematologica* 1996;81:282–283.

233. Douglas VK, Gordon LI, Goolsby CL, et al. Lymphoid aggregates in bone marrow mimic residual lymphoma after rituximab therapy for non-Hodgkin lymphoma. *Am J Clin Pathol* 1999;112:844–853.

234. Dunphy CH, Lattuada CP Jr. Follicular center cell lymphoma with an extremely high content of T cells: case report with useful diagnostic techniques. *Arch Pathol Lab Med* 1998;122:936–938.

235. Kojima M, Nakamura S, Ichimura K, et al. Centroblastic and centroblastic/centrocytic lymphoma associated with a prominent epithelioid granulomatous response: a clinicopathologic study of 50 cases. *Mod Pathol* 2002;15:750–758.

236. Chim CS, Ma SK, Lam CK, et al. Two uncommon lymphomas. Case 2: signet ring lymphoma of the bone marrow. *J Clin Oncol* 1999;17:728–729.

237. Nathwani BN, Sheibani K, Winberg CD, et al. Neoplastic B cells with cerebriform nuclei in follicular lymphomas. *Hum Pathol* 1985;16:173–180.

238. O'Briain DS, Lawlor E, Sarsfield P, et al. Circulating cerebriform lymphoid cells (Sezary-type cells) in a B-cell malignant lymphoma. *Cancer* 1988;61:1587–1593.

239. Conlan MG, Bast M, Armitage JO, et al. Bone marrow involvement by non-Hodgkin's lymphoma: the clinical significance of morphologic discordance between the lymph node and bone marrow. Nebraska Lymphoma Study Group. *J Clin Oncol* 1990;8:1163–1172.

240. Robertson LE, Redman JR, Butler JJ, et al. Discordant bone marrow involvement in diffuse large-cell lymphoma: a distinct clinical-pathologic entity associated with a continuous risk of relapse. *J Clin Oncol* 1991;9:236–242.

241. Barry TS, Jaffe ES, Kingma DW, et al. CD5+ follicular lymphoma: a clinicopathologic study of three cases. *Am J Clin Pathol* 2002;118:589–598.

242. Cook JR, Craig FE, Swerdlow SH. Bcl-2 expression by multicolor flow cytometric analysis assists in the diagnosis of follicular lymphoma in lymph node and bone marrow. *Am J Clin Pathol* 2003;119:145–151.

243. Tiesinga JJ, Wu CD, Inghirami G. CD5+ follicle center lymphoma: immunophenotyping detects a unique subset of "floral" follicular lymphoma. *Am J Clin Pathol* 2000;114:912–921.

244. Coad JE, Olson DJ, Christensen DR, et al. Correlation of PCR-detected clonal gene rearrangements with bone marrow morphology in patients with B-lineage lymphomas. *Am J Surg Pathol* 1997;21:1047–1056.

245. Hanson CA, Kurtin PJ, Katzmann JA, et al. Immunophenotypic analysis of peripheral blood and bone marrow in the staging of B-cell malignant lymphoma. *Blood* 1999;94:3889–3896.

246. Karsan A, Gascoyne RD, Coupland RW, et al. Combination of t(14;18) and a Burkitt's type translocation in B-cell malignancies. *Leuk Lymphoma* 1993;10:433–441.

247. Kroft SH, Domiati-Saad R, Finn WG, et al. Precursor B-lymphoblastic transformation of grade I follicle center lymphoma. *Am J Clin Pathol* 2000;113:411–418.

248. Sun X, Gordon LI, Peterson LC. Transformation of follicular lymphoma to acute lymphoblastic leukemia. *Arch Pathol Lab Med* 2002;126:997–998.

249. Siebert JD, Mulvaney DA, Vukov AM, et al. Utility of flow cytometry in subtyping composite and sequential lymphoma. *J Clin Lab Anal* 1999;13:199–204.

250. Thiele J, Zirbes TK, Kvasnicka HM, et al. Focal lymphoid aggregates (nodules) in bone marrow biopsies: differentiation between benign hyperplasia and malignant lymphoma—a practical guideline. *J Clin Pathol* 1999;52:294–300.

251. Ben-Ezra J, Hazelgrove K, Ferreira-Gonzalez A, et al. Can polymerase chain reaction help distinguish benign from malignant lymphoid aggregates in bone marrow aspirates? *Arch Pathol Lab Med* 2000;124:511–515.

252. Kremer M, Cabras AD, Fend F, et al. PCR analysis of IgH-gene rearrangements in small lymphoid infiltrates microdissected from

sections of paraffin-embedded bone marrow biopsy specimens. *Hum Pathol* 2000;31:847–853.

253. Fakan F, Skalova A, Kuntscherova J. Expression of bcl-2 protein in distinguishing benign from malignant lymphoid aggregates in bone marrow biopsies. *Gen Diagn Pathol* 1996;141:359–363.

254. Campo E, Raffeld M, Jaffe ES. Mantle-cell lymphoma. *Semin Hematol* 1999;36:115–127.

255. Cohen PL, Kurtin PJ, Donovan KA, et al. Bone marrow and peripheral blood involvement in mantle cell lymphoma. *Br J Haematol* 1998;101:302–310.

256. Schlette E, Lai R, Onciu M, et al. Leukemic mantle cell lymphoma: clinical and pathologic spectrum of twenty-three cases. *Mod Pathol* 2001;14:1133–1140.

257. Wasman J, Rosenthal NS, Farhi DC. Mantle cell lymphoma. Morphologic findings in bone marrow involvement. *Am J Clin Pathol* 1996;106:196–200.

258. Wong KF, Chan JK, So JC, et al. Mantle cell lymphoma in leukemic phase: characterization of its broad cytologic spectrum with emphasis on the importance of distinction from other chronic lymphoproliferative disorders. *Cancer* 1999;86:850–857.

259. Brink DS, Grosso LE, Dunphy CH. Leukemic phase of mantle cell lymphoma presenting as anemia: diagnosis by combining flow cytometry and cytomorphology. *Arch Pathol Lab Med* 1998;122:1018–1022.

260. Cesca C, Ben-Ezra J, Riley RS. Platelet satellitism as presenting finding in mantle cell lymphoma. A case report. *Am J Clin Pathol* 2001;115:567–570.

261. Hao S, Sanger W, Onciu M, et al. Mantle cell lymphoma with 8q24 chromosomal abnormalities: a report of 5 cases with blastoid features. *Mod Pathol* 2002;15:1266–1272.

262. Singleton TP, Anderson MM, Ross CW, et al. Leukemic phase of mantle cell lymphoma, blastoid variant. *Am J Clin Pathol* 1999;111:495–500.

263. Viswanatha DS, Foucar K, Berry BR, et al. Blastic mantle cell leukemia: an unusual presentation of blastic mantle cell lymphoma. *Mod Pathol* 2000;13:825–833.

264. Dunphy CH, Perkins SL. Mantle cell leukemia, prolymphocytoid type: a rarely described form. *Leuk Lymphoma* 2001;41:683–687.

265. Schlette E, Bueso-Ramos C, Giles F, et al. Mature B-cell leukemias with more than 55% prolymphocytes. A heterogeneous group that includes an unusual variant of mantle cell lymphoma. *Am J Clin Pathol* 2001;115:571–581.

266. Wong KF, So CC, Chan JK. Nucleolated variant of mantle cell lymphoma with leukemic manifestations mimicking prolymphocytic leukemia. *Am J Clin Pathol* 2002;117:246–251.

267. Burke JS, Warnke RA, Connors JM, et al. Diffuse malignant lymphoma with cerebriform nuclei: a B-cell lymphoma studied with monoclonal antibodies. *Am J Clin Pathol* 1985;83:753–759.

268. Carbone A, Manconi R, Poletti A, et al. B-cell malignant lymphoma with cerebriform nuclei showing mantle-zone phenotype. *Am J Clin Pathol* 1986;86:552–554.

269. Wong KF, Chan JK, So JC, et al. Mantle cell lymphoma in leukemic phase: characterization of its broad cytologic spectrum with emphasis on the importance of distinction from other chronic lymphoproliferative disorders. *Cancer* 1999;86:850–857.

270. Liu Z, Dong HY, Gorczyca W, et al. CD5- mantle cell lymphoma. *Am J Clin Pathol* 2002;118:216–224.

271. Xu Y, McKenna RW, Asplund SL, et al. Comparison of immunophenotypes of small B-cell neoplasms in primary lymph nodes and concurrent blood or marrow samples. *Am J Clin Pathol* 2002;118:758–764.

272. Onciu M, Schlette E, Medeiros LJ, et al. Cytogenetic findings in mantle cell lymphoma cases with a high level of peripheral blood involvement have a distinct pattern of abnormalities. *Am J Clin Pathol* 2001;116:886–892.

273. Soslow RA, Zukerberg LR, Harris NL, et al. BCL-1 (PRAD-1/cyclin D-1) overexpression distinguishes the blastoid variant of mantle cell lymphoma from B-lineage lymphoblastic lymphoma. *Mod Pathol* 1997;10:810–817.

274. van de Poel MH, Coebergh JW, Hillen HF. Malignant transformation of monoclonal gammopathy of undetermined significance among out-patients of a community hospital in southeastern Netherlands. *Br J Haematol* 1995;91:121–125.

275. Dufau JP, Le Tourneau A, Molina T, et al. Intravascular large B-cell lymphoma with bone marrow involvement at presentation and haemophagocytic syndrome: two Western cases in favour of a specific variant. *Histopathology* 2000;37:509–512.

276. Estalilla OC, Koo CH, Brynes RK, et al. Intravascular large B-cell lymphoma. A report of five cases initially diagnosed by bone marrow biopsy. *Am J Clin Pathol* 1999;112:248–255.

277. Murase T, Nakamura S. An Asian variant of intravascular lymphomatosis: an updated review of malignant histiocytosis-like B-cell lymphoma. *Leuk Lymphoma* 1999;33:459–473.

278. Tucker TJ, Bardales RH, Miranda RN. Intravascular lymphomatosis with bone marrow involvement. *Arch Pathol Lab Med* 1999;123:952–956.

279. Wong KF, Chan JK, Ng CS, et al. Large cell lymphoma with initial presentation in the bone marrow. *Hematol Oncol* 1992;10:261–271.

280. Carbone A, Gloghini A, Volpe R, et al. KP1 (CD68)-positive large cell lymphomas: a histopathologic and immunophenotypic characterization of 12 cases. *Hum Pathol* 1993;24:886–896.

281. Haralambieva E, Pulford KA, Lamant L, et al. Anaplastic large-cell lymphomas of B-cell phenotype are anaplastic lymphoma kinase (ALK) negative and belong to the spectrum of diffuse large B-cell lymphomas. *Br J Haematol* 2000;109:584–591.

282. Lai R, Medeiros LJ, Dabbagh L, et al. Sinusoidal CD30-positive large B-cell lymphoma: a morphologic mimic of anaplastic large cell lymphoma. *Mod Pathol* 2000;13:223–228.

283. McCluggage WG, Bharucha H, el-Agnaf M, et al. B cell signet-ring cell lymphoma of bone marrow. *J Clin Pathol* 1995;48:275–278.

284. Wong KF, Chan JK, Ng CS, et al. Anaplastic large cell Ki-1 lymphoma involving bone marrow: marrow findings and association with reactive hemophagocytosis. *Am J Hematol* 1991;37:112–119.

285. Miyahara M, Sano M, Shibata K, et al. B-cell lymphoma-associated hemophagocytic syndrome: clinicopathological characteristics. *Ann Hematol* 2000;79:378–388.

286. Papadimitriou JC, Chakravarthy A, Heyman MR. Pseudo-Gaucher cells preceding the appearance of immunoblastic lymphoma. *Am J Clin Pathol* 1988;90:454–458.

287. Shimazaki C, Inaba T, Nakagawa M. B-cell lymphoma-associated hemophagocytic syndrome. *Leuk Lymphoma* 2000;38:121–130.

288. Skinnider BF, Connors JM, Gascoyne RD. Bone marrow involvement in T-cell-rich B-cell lymphoma. *Am J Clin Pathol* 1997;108:570–578.

289. Sun T, Susin M, Tomao FA, et al. Histiocyte-rich B-cell lymphoma. *Hum Pathol* 1997;28:1321–1324.

290. Weinberg DS, Pinkus GS. Non-Hodgkin's lymphoma of large multilobated cell type. A clinicopathologic study of ten cases. *Am J Clin Pathol* 1981;76:190–196.

291. Harada S, Suzuki R, Uehira K, et al. Molecular and immunological dissection of diffuse large B cell lymphoma: CD5+, and CD5- with CD10+ groups may constitute clinically relevant subtypes. *Leukemia* 1999;13:1441–1447.

292. Inaba T, Shimazaki C, Sumikuma T, et al. Expression of T-cell-associated antigens in B-cell non-Hodgkin's lymphoma. *Br J Haematol* 2000;109:592–599.

293. Khalidi HS, Brynes RK, Browne P, et al. Intravascular large B-cell lymphoma: the CD5 antigen is expressed by a subset of cases. *Mod Pathol* 1998;11:983–988.

294. Kroft SH, Howard MS, Picker LJ, et al. *De novo* CD5+ diffuse large B-cell lymphomas. A heterogeneous group containing an unusual form of splenic lymphoma. *Am J Clin Pathol* 2000;114:523–533.

295. Nakase K, Kita K, Shiku H, et al. Myeloid antigen, CD13, CD14, and/or CD33 expression is restricted to certain lymphoid neoplasms. *Am J Clin Pathol* 1996;105:761–768.

296. Sekita T, Tamaru JI, Isobe K, et al. Diffuse large B cell lymphoma expressing the natural killer cell marker CD56. *Pathol Int* 1999;49:752–758.

297. Uherova P, Ross CW, Schnitzer B, et al. The clinical significance of CD10 antigen expression in diffuse large B-cell lymphoma. *Am J Clin Pathol* 2001;115:582–588.

298. Nakamura N, Nakamine H, Tamaru J, et al. The distinction between Burkitt lymphoma and diffuse large B-cell lymphoma with c-myc rearrangement. *Mod Pathol* 2002;15:771–776.

299. Acar H, Ecirli S, Gundogan F, et al. Simultaneous occurrence of chronic myelogenous leukemia and non-Hodgkin lymphoma at diagnosis. *Cancer Genet Cytogenet* 1999;108:171–174.

300. Hutchinson RM. Mastocytosis and co-existent non-Hodgkin's lymphoma and myeloproliferative disorders. *Leuk Lymphoma* 1992;7:29–36.

301. Ichinohasama R, Miura I, Takahashi N, et al. Ph-negative non-Hodgkin's lymphoma occurring in chronic phase of Ph-positive chronic myelogenous leukemia is defined as a genetically different neoplasm from extramedullary localized blast crisis: report of two cases and review of the literature. *Leukemia* 2000;14:169 182.

302. Liu K, Coogan AC, Mann KP. Fine-needle aspiration of large cell lymphoma in a patient with agnogenic myeloid metaplasia: a case report and review of the literature. *Diagn Cytopathol* 1998;19:205–209.

303. Steinberg E, Ben-Dor D, Lugassy G. Anaplastic B-cell (Ki-1) lymphoma developing in a patient with polycythemia vera. *Leuk Lymphoma* 1995;19:507–509.

304. Jaalouk G, Avvisati G, Latagliata R, et al. Simultaneous occurrence of large B-cell non-Hodgkin lymphoma and myelodysplastic syndrome rapidly evolving into acute myeloblastic leukemia. *Leuk Lymphoma* 1996;21:339–341.

305. Mori A, Hashino S, Imamura M, et al. Bone marrow dysplasia with basophilic cells in a patient with angiocentric lymphoma. *Acta Haematol* 1998;99:98–101.

306. Uematsu M, Ochi H, Ueda Y, et al. Coexistent myelodysplastic syndrome and non-Hodgkin lymphoma. Report of a case and review of the literature. *Int J Hematol* 1995;62:45–51.

307. Ascoli V, Lo Coco F, Mecucci C. Herpesvirus 8-negative primary effusion lymphoma associated with hepatitis C virus. *Am J Surg Pathol* 2000;24:157–158.

308. Boulanger E, Agbalika F, Maarek O, et al. A clinical, molecular and cytogenetic study of 12 cases of human herpesvirus 8 associated primary effusion lymphoma in HIV-infected patients. *Hematol J* 2001;2:172–179.

309. Hara T, Nishi S, Horimoto A, et al. Primary effusion lymphoma in a patient with hepatitis C virus-related liver cirrhosis. *J Gastroenterol Hepatol* 2001;16:948–949.

310. Hong S, Krafft AE. Primary effusion lymphoma with herpesvirus 8 DNA in patients coinfected with HIV and hepatitis C virus: a report of 2 cases. *AIDS Read* 2001;11:418–422.

311. Wakely PE Jr, Menezes G, Nuovo GJ. Primary effusion lymphoma: cytopathologic diagnosis using in situ molecular genetic analysis for human herpesvirus 8. *Mod Pathol* 2002;15:944–950.

312. Fenaux P, Bourhis JH, Ribrag V. Burkitt's acute lymphocytic leukemia (L3ALL) in adults. *Hematol Oncol Clin North Am* 2001;15:37–50.

313. Colovic M, Jankovic G, Lazrevic V. Burkitt-like blast crisis in chronic myeloid leukemia. *Med Oncol* 1996;13:119–120.

314. Davi F, Delecluse HJ, Guiet P, et al. Burkitt-like lymphomas in AIDS patients: characterization within a series of 103 human immunodeficiency virus-associated non-Hodgkin's lymphomas. Burkitt's Lymphoma Study Group. *J Clin Oncol* 1998;16:3788–3795.

315. Masauzi N, Kasai M, Suzuki G, et al. A translocation t(8;14) and c-myc gene rearrangement associated with the histological transformation of B-cell acute lymphocytic leukemia (FAB-L2) into Burkitt's type (FAB-L3) leukemia. *Leuk Lymphoma* 1997;27:357–363.

316. Mohamed AN, Compean R, Dan ME, et al. Clonal evolution of chronic lymphocytic leukemia to acute lymphoblastic leukemia. *Cancer Genet Cytogenet* 1996;86:143–146.

317. Rana I, Pinto RM, Caniglia M, et al. Reciprocal bone marrow transplantation between brother and sister. *Bone Marrow Transplant* 2002;29:705–707.

318. Salloum E, Tallini G, Levy A, et al. Burkitt's lymphoma-leukemia in patients treated for Hodgkin's disease. *Cancer Invest* 1996;14:527–533.

319. Tweddle DA, Gennery AR, Reid MM, et al. Posttransplantation B lymphoblastic leukemia with Burkitt-like features. *Transplantation* 1999;67:1379–1380.

320. Mangan KF, Rauch AE, Bishop M, et al. Acute lymphoblastic leukemia of Burkitt's type (L-3 ALL) lacking surface immunoglobulin and the 8;14 translocation. *Am J Clin Pathol* 1985;83:121–126.

321. Navid F, Mosijczuk AD, Head DR, et al. Acute lymphoblastic leukemia with the (8;14)(q24;q32) translocation and FAB L3 morphology associated with a B-precursor immunophenotype: the Pediatric Oncology Group experience. *Leukemia* 1999;13:135–141.

322. Troussard X, Rimokh R, Valensi F, et al. Heterogeneity of t(1;19)(q23;p13) acute leukaemias. *Br J Haematol* 1995;89:516–526.

323. Lim EJ, Peh SC. Bone marrow and peripheral blood changes in non-Hodgkin's lymphoma. *Singapore Med J* 2000;41:279–285.

324. Sham RL, Bennett JM. Burkitt cell leukemia with myelodysplasia as a presentation of HIV infection. *Hematol Pathol* 1992;6:95–98.

325. Hutchison RE, Finch C, Kepner J, et al. Burkitt lymphoma is immunophenotypically different from Burkitt-like lymphoma in young persons. *Ann Oncol* 2000;11[Suppl 1]:35–38.

326. Lin CW, O'Brien S, Faber J, et al. *De novo* CD5+ Burkitt lymphoma/leukemia. *Am J Clin Pathol* 1999;112:828–835.

327. Kornblau SM, Goodacre A, Cabanillas F. Chromosomal abnormalities in adult non-endemic Burkitt's lymphoma and leukemia: 22 new reports and a review of 148 cases from the literature. *Hematol Oncol* 1991;9:63–78.

328. Nomdedeu JF, Lete I, Baiget M, et al. Mutational analysis of p53 in 16 cases of acute lymphoblastic leukemia and Burkitt's lymphoma. *Haematologica* 1997;82:550–554.

329. Velangi MR, Reid MM, Bown N, et al. Acute lymphoblastic leukaemia of the L3 subtype in adults in the Northern health region of England 1983–99. *J Clin Pathol* 2002;55:591–595.

330. Busschots AM, Geerts ML, Mecucci C, et al. A translocation (8;14) in a cutaneous large B-cell lymphoma. *Am J Clin Pathol* 1993;99:615–621.

331. Chong YY, Lau LC, Lui WO, et al. A case of t(8;14) with total and partial trisomy 3 in Waldenstrom macroglobulinemia. *Cancer Genet Cytogenet* 1998;103:65–67.

332. Copplestone JA, Oscier DG, Johnson S. An 8;14 translocation in a case of plasma cell leukemia. *Leuk Res* 1987;11:655–659.

333. Karsan A, Gascoyne RD, Coupland RW, et al. Combination of t(14;18) and a Burkitt's type translocation in B-cell malignancies. *Leuk Lymphoma* 1993;10:433–441.

334. Kubonishi I, Daibata M, Yano S, et al. Establishment of a new Epstein-Barr virus nuclear antigen-positive B-cell line, BALL-2, with t(8;14) (q24;q32) chromosome abnormality from B-cell acute lymphoblastic leukemia, L2. *Am J Hematol* 1991;37: 179–185.

335. Slavutsky I, Andreoli G, Gutierrez M, et al. Variant (8;22) translocation in lymphoblastic lymphoma. *Leuk Lymphoma* 1996;21:169–172.

336. Dayton VD, Arthur DC, Gajl-Peczalska KJ, et al. L3 acute lymphoblastic leukemia. Comparison with small noncleaved cell lymphoma involving the bone marrow. *Am J Clin Pathol* 1994;101:130–139.

337. Shimamoto Y, Matsuzaki M, Yamaguchi M. Vacuolated Burkitt-like cells in adult T-cell leukaemia/lymphoma. *Clin Lab Haematol* 1992;14:155–157.

338. Bernell P, Arvidsson I, Jacobsson B. Gain of chromosome 7, which marks the progression from indolent to aggressive follicle centre lymphomas, is restricted to the B-lymphoid cell lineage: a study by FISH in combination with morphology and immunocytochemistry. *Br J Haematol* 1999;105:1140–1144.

339. Majumdar G. Massive bone marrow necrosis as the presenting feature in a case of primary bone marrow high grade non-Hodgkin's lymphoma. *Leuk Lymphoma* 1997;26: 409–412.

340. Murphy PT, Sivakumaran M, Casey MC, et al. Lymphoma associated bone marrow necrosis with raised anticardiolipin antibody. *J Clin Pathol* 1998;51:407–409.

341. Schwonzen M, Pohl C, Steinmetz T, et al. Bone marrow involvement in non-Hodgkin's lymphoma: increased diagnostic sensitivity by combination of immunocytology, cytomorphology and trephine histology. *Br J Haematol* 1992;81:362–369.

342. Schlaifer D, Dastugue N, Brousset P, et al. B-cell lymphoma following polycythemia vera: evidence for the involvement of two different clones. *Leukemia* 1994;8:895–896.

25

HODGKIN LYMPHOMA

Hodgkin lymphoma (HL) is a B-cell neoplasm characterized by neoplastic cells in a prominent inflammatory and fibrous background (1–5). Different morphologic subtypes are recognized (Table 25-1). HL occurs as a *de novo* disease and as a transformation of other B-cell neoplasms, especially B-cell chronic lymphocytic leukemia/small lymphocytic lymphoma.

The peripheral blood often shows anemia and eosinophilia (6–10). Other findings include immune-mediated and cyclic cytopenias, thalassemia-like microcytic anemia, and large granular lymphocytosis.

Bone marrow aspirate smears and histologic sections may show involvement by HL, hematopoietic changes, and other findings (Figs. 25-1 through 25-7).

Bone marrow involvement by HL occurs most often in mixed cellularity and rarely in lymphocyte predominant disease (11–17). The neoplastic infiltrate may be focal or diffuse and is composed of lymphocytes, eosinophils, plasma cells, and Reed-Sternberg (RS) cells and variants, embedded in fibrous stroma. Extensive fibrosis may dominate the morphologic findings and preclude adequate aspiration. Necrosis has also been reported. RS cells and variants are found in cellular areas of the infiltrate and not among hematopoietic cells. Careful examination of multiple sections may be required to identify RS cells and variants. If the diagnosis of HL has been previously established in a lymph node or other site, an RS variant is sufficient for the diagnosis of HL in the bone marrow; if not, a diagnostic RS cell should be sought (18).

Bone marrow involvement by HL in the setting of human immunodeficiency virus (HIV) infection has distinctive characteristics (19–22). Such cases are much more likely to present with bone marrow disease as the initial or only site of disease. The bone marrow in HIV–related HL typically shows abundant RS cells and variants, numerous fibrohistiocytoid stromal cells, and relatively few lymphocytes.

Hematopoietic changes in the uninvolved bone marrow are common and usually consist of neutrophilic hyperplasia, megakaryocytic hyperplasia, eosinophilia, and reactive plasmacytosis (23–25). Other findings include dyserythropoiesis, pure red cell aplasia benign lymphoid aggregates, granulomas, reactive histiocytosis with increased hemophagocytosis, overt hemophagocytic syndrome, pseudo-Gaucher cells, eosinophilic fibrohistiocytic lesion, necrosis, and sarcoidosis (26–31).

Flow cytometry shows no diagnostic findings. Immunostains may show, in RS cells, expression of CD15, CD20, CD21, CD30, CD68, CD138, fascin, S100 protein, epithelial membrane antigen, and/or Epstein-Barr virus latent membrane protein (32,33).

Genetic studies may show, in RS cells, deletions of 1p, 4q, 6q, and/or 7q; clonal immunoglobulin gene and T-cell

TABLE 25-1. CLASSIFICATION OF HODGKIN LYMPHOMA ACCORDING TO THE WORLD HEALTH ORGANIZATION

Nodular lymphocyte predominant Hodgkin lymphoma
Classical Hodgkin lymphoma
   Nodular sclerosis classical Hodgkin lymphoma
   Mixed cellularity classical Hodgkin lymphoma
   Lymphocyte-rich classical Hodgkin lymphoma
   Lymphocyte-depleted classical Hodgkin lymphoma

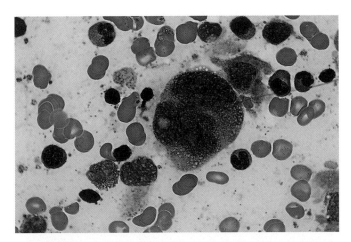

FIGURE 25-1. Bone marrow aspirate smear, Hodgkin lymphoma. A diagnostic Reed-Sternberg cell is illustrated, showing three nuclear lobes and prominent nucleoli within two of the lobes. The Reed-Sternberg cell is approximately the size of a megakaryocyte but has a less abundant cytoplasm, a larger nucleus, nuclear lobation, and prominent nuclei.

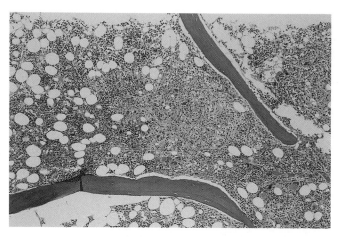

FIGURE 25-2. Bone marrow biopsy specimen, Hodgkin lymphoma. Hodgkin lymphoma typically occurs as a focal lesion of the intratrabecular space, sometimes abutting trabecular bone. The cell population is nonhematopoietic and heterogeneous.

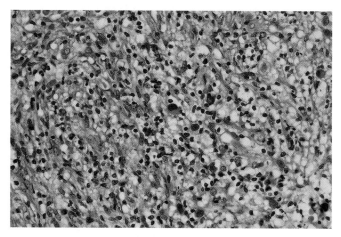

FIGURE 25-3. Bone marrow biopsy specimen, Hodgkin lymphoma. At higher power, Hodgkin lymphoma can be seen to be composed of small lymphocytes and fibrous tissue in which are entrapped occasional much larger cells.

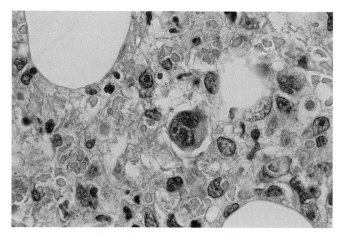

FIGURE 25-4. Bone marrow biopsy specimen, Hodgkin lymphoma. A single diagnostic Reed-Sternberg cell is seen, surrounded by inflammatory cells in a fibrohistiocytic background.

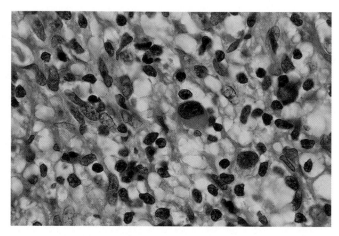

FIGURE 25-5. Bone marrow biopsy specimen, Hodgkin lymphoma. A single variant Reed-Sternberg cell is seen, surrounded by inflammatory cells in a fibrohistiocytic background.

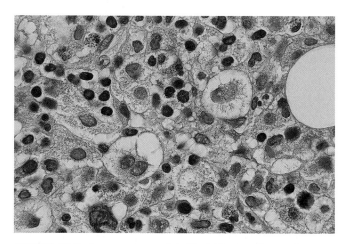

FIGURE 25-6. Bone marrow clot, Hodgkin lymphoma. Lacunar Reed-Sternberg cells are seen in this case of nodular sclerosis Hodgkin lymphoma.

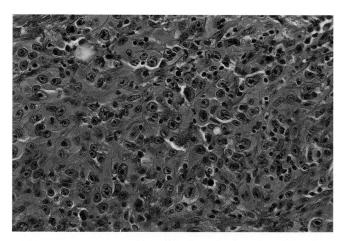

FIGURE 25-7. Bone marrow biopsy specimen, Hodgkin lymphoma. A nearly solid sheet of Reed-Sternberg cells and variants is seen. This appearance is typical of Hodgkin lymphoma in patients infected with human immunodeficiency virus, which often presents as primary bone marrow disease without accompanying lymphadenopathy.

receptor gene rearrangements; and clonal integration of Epstein-Barr viral DNA (1–4,34,35).

Other hematolymphoid disorders reported with HL, some of which may be clonally related, include myeloproliferative disorders, myelodysplastic syndromes, acute leukemia, and neoplasms of B cells, T cells, and histiocytes (36–51).

The differential diagnosis includes other causes of marrow fibrosis and granulomatous inflammation, eosinophilic fibrohistiocytic lesion, other B-cell neoplasms, and T-cell and histiocytic neoplasms (52–60).

REFERENCES

1. Jox A, Zander T, Kornacker M, et al. Detection of identical Hodgkin-Reed Sternberg cell specific immunoglobulin gene rearrangements in a patient with Hodgkin's disease of mixed cellularity subtype at primary diagnosis and in relapse two and a half years later. *Ann Oncol* 1998;9:283–287.
2. Kanzler H, Kuppers R, Helmes S, et al. Hodgkin and Reed-Sternberg-like cells in B-cell chronic lymphocytic leukemia represent the outgrowth of single germinal-center B-cell-derived clones: potential precursors of Hodgkin and Reed-Sternberg cells in Hodgkin's disease. *Blood* 2000;95:1023–1031.
3. Marafioti T, Hummel M, Foss HD, et al. Hodgkin and Reed-Sternberg cells represent an expansion of a single clone originating from a germinal center B-cell with functional immunoglobulin gene rearrangements but defective immunoglobulin transcription. *Blood* 2000;95:1443–1450.
4. Pescarmona E, Pignoloni P, Mauro FR, et al. Hodgkin/Reed-Sternberg cells and Hodgkin's disease in patients with B-cell chronic lymphocytic leukaemia: an immunohistological, molecular and clinical study of four cases suggesting a heterogeneous pathogenetic background. *Virchows Arch* 2000;437:129–132.
5. Uherova P, Valdez R, Ross CW, et al. Nodular lymphocyte predominant Hodgkin lymphoma. An immunophenotypic reappraisal based on a single-institution experience. *Am J Clin Pathol* 2003; 119:192–198.
6. Di Biagio E, Sanchez-Borges M, Desenne JJ, et al. Eosinophilia in Hodgkin's disease: a role for interleukin 5. *Int Arch Allergy Immunol* 1996;110:244–251.
7. Fahey JL, Rahbar S, Farbstein MJ, et al. Microcytosis in Hodgkin disease associated with unbalanced globin chain synthesis. *Am J Hematol* 1986;23:123–129.
8. Ertem M, Uysal Z, Yavuz G, et al. Immune thrombocytopenia and hemolytic anemia as a presenting manifestation of Hodgkin disease. *Pediatr Hematol Oncol* 2000;17:181–185.
9. Kingreen D, Dalal BI, Heyman M, et al. Lymphocytosis of large granular lymphocytes in patients with Hodgkin's disease. *Am J Hematol* 1995;50:234–236.
10. Schoengen A, Fembacher PM, Schulz PC. Immunoglobulin therapy for autoimmune neutropenia in Hodgkin's disease. *Acta Haematol* 1995;94:36–38.
11. Chang KL, Kamel OW, Arber DA, et al. Pathologic features of nodular lymphocyte predominance Hodgkin's disease in extranodal sites. *Am J Surg Pathol* 1995;19:1313–1324.
12. Mahoney DH Jr, Schreuders LC, Gresik MV, et al. Role of staging bone marrow examination in children with Hodgkin disease. *Med Pediatr Oncol* 1998;30:175–177.
13. Meadows LM, Rosse WR, Moore JO, et al. Hodgkin's disease presenting as myelofibrosis. *Cancer* 1989;64:1720–1726.
14. Munker R, Hasenclever D, Brosteanu O, et al. Bone marrow involvement in Hodgkin's disease: an analysis of 135 consecutive cases. German Hodgkin's Lymphoma Study Group. *J Clin Oncol* 1995;13:403–409.
15. O'Carroll DI, McKenna RW, Brunning RD. Bone marrow manifestations of Hodgkin's disease. *Cancer* 1976;38:1717–1728.
16. Paydas S, Ergin M, Baslamisli F, et al. Bone marrow necrosis: clinicopathologic analysis of 20 cases and review of the literature. *Am J Hematol* 2002;70:300–305.
17. Siebert JD, Stuckey JH, Kurtin PJ, et al. Extranodal lymphocyte predominance Hodgkin's disease. Clinical and pathologic features. *Am J Clin Pathol* 1995;103:485–491.
18. Lukes RJ. Criteria for involvement of lymph node, bone marrow, spleen, and liver in Hodgkin's disease. *Cancer Res* 1971;31:1755–1767.
19. Karcher DS. Clinically unsuspected Hodgkin disease presenting initially in the bone marrow of patients infected with the human immunodeficiency virus. *Cancer* 1993;71:1235–1238.
20. Levine AM. Hodgkin's disease in the setting of human immunodeficiency virus infection. *J Natl Cancer Inst Monogr* 1998;:37–42.
21. Ponzoni M, Fumagalli L, Bossi G, et al. Isolated bone marrow manifestation of HIV-associated Hodgkin lymphoma. *Mod Pathol* 2002;15:1273–1278.
22. Ree HJ, Strauchen JA, Khan AA, et al. Human immunodeficiency virus-associated Hodgkin's disease. Clinicopathologic studies of 24 cases and preponderance of mixed cellularity type characterized by the occurrence of fibrohistiocytoid stromal cells. *Cancer* 1991; 67:1614–1621.
23. Kass L, Votaw ML. Eosinophilia and plasmacytosis of the bone marrow in Hodgkin's disease. *Am J Clin Pathol* 1975;64: 248–250.
24. Macintyre EA, Vaughan Hudson B, Vaughan Hudson G, et al. Incidence and clinical importance of bone marrow eosinophilia in Hodgkin's disease (BNLI report no.29). British National Lymphoma Investigation. *J Clin Pathol* 1987;40:245–246.
25. Te Velde J, Den Ottolander GJ, Spaander PJ, et al. The bone marrow in Hodgkin's disease: the non-involved marrow. *Histopathology* 1978;2:31–46.
26. Cox JV, Balaban EP, Demian SE, et al. An eosinophilic fibrohistiocytic lesion of bone marrow in a patient with Hodgkin's disease. A potential for morphologic confusion. *Cancer* 1991;68:1824–1827.
27. Dawson L, den Ottolander GJ, Kluin PM, et al. Reactive hemophagocytic syndrome as a presenting feature of Hodgkin's disease. *Ann Hematol* 2000;79:322–326.
28. Karakantza M, Matutes E, MacLennan K, et al. Association between sarcoidosis and lymphoma revisited. *J Clin Pathol* 1996;49: 208–212.
29. Penchansky L, Krause JR. Phagocytic macrophages in the bone marrow biopsies of children with Hodgkin's disease. *Pediatr Pathol* 1986;6:369–375.
30. Reid TJ 3rd, Mullaney M, Burrell LM, et al. Pure red cell aplasia after chemotherapy for Hodgkin's lymphoma: in vitro evidence for T cell mediated suppression of erythropoiesis and response to sequential cyclosporin and erythropoietin. *Am J Hematol* 1994; 46:48–53.
31. Zidar BL, Hartsock RJ, Lee RE, et al. Pseudo-Gaucher cells in the bone marrow of a patient with Hodgkin's disease. *Am J Clin Pathol* 1987;87:533–536.
32. Carbone A, Gloghini A, Gattei V, et al. Reed-Sternberg cells of classical Hodgkin's disease react with the plasma cell-specific monoclonal antibody B-B4 and express human syndecan-1. *Blood* 1997;89:3787–3794.
33. Nakamura S, Nagahama M, Kagami Y, et al. Hodgkin's disease expressing follicular dendritic cell marker CD21 without any other

B-cell marker: a clinicopathologic study of nine cases. *Am J Surg Pathol* 1999;23:363–376.

34. Atkin NB. Cytogenetics of Hodgkin's disease. *Cytogenet Cell Genet* 1998;80:23–27.

35. Seitz V, Hummel M, Marafioti T, et al. Detection of clonal T-cell receptor gamma-chain gene rearrangements in Reed-Sternberg cells of classic Hodgkin disease. *Blood* 2000;95: 3020–3024.

36. Alpers CE, Beckstead JH, Newman AB. Malignant fibrous histiocytoma, myelomonocytic leukemia, and Hodgkin's disease arising in an elderly man. *Cancer* 1984;53:1943–1947.

37. Di Benedetto G, Cataldi A, Verde A, et al. Gamma heavy chain disease associated with Hodgkin's disease. Clinical, pathologic, and immunologic features of one case. *Cancer* 1989;63:1804–1809.

38. Elghetany MT. Hodgkin's disease coexisting with myelodysplastic syndrome prior to therapy: a case report and a review of the association of Hodgkin's disease with stem cell disorders. *Ann Hematol* 1997;75:231–234.

39. Hancock JC, Wells A, Halling KC, et al. Composite B-cell and T-cell lymphoma arising 24 years after nodular lymphocyte predominant Hodgkin's disease. *Ann Diagn Pathol* 1999;3:23–34.

40. Ibarrola de Andres C, Toscano R, Lahuerta JJ, et al. Simultaneous occurrence of Hodgkin's disease, nodal Langerhans' cell histiocytosis and multiple myeloma IgA(kappa). *Virchows Arch* 1999; 434:259–262.

41. Kremer M, Sandherr M, Geist B, et al. Epstein-Barr virus-negative Hodgkin's lymphoma after mycosis fungoides: molecular evidence for distinct clonal origin. *Mod Pathol* 2001;14:91–97.

42. Lalayanni C, Theodoridou S, Athanasiadou A, et al. Simultaneous occurrence of multiple myeloma and Hodgkin's disease. A case report. *Haematologica* 2000;85:772–773.

43. Miyata A, Kojima K, Yoshino T, et al. Concurrent Hodgkin's disease (mixed cellularity type) and T-cell chronic lymphocytic leukemia/prolymphocytic leukemia. *Int J Hematol* 2001;73: 230–235.

44. Mohrmann RL, Arber DA. CD20-Positive peripheral T-cell lymphoma: report of a case after nodular sclerosis Hodgkin's disease and review of the literature. *Mod Pathol* 2000;13:1244–1252.

45. Roufosse C, Lespagnard L, Sales F, et al. Langerhans' cell histiocytosis associated with simultaneous lymphocyte predominance Hodgkin's disease and malignant melanoma. *Hum Pathol* 1998; 29:200–201.

46. Saletti P, Ghielmini M, Scali G, et al. Hodgkin's and Castleman's disease in a patient with systemic mastocytosis. *Ann Hematol* 1999;78:97–100.

47. Stolinsky DC. Twelve-year remission of polycythemia vera following Hodgkin's disease and chemotherapy. *CA Cancer J Clin* 1981; 31:57–60.

48. Suh YK, Shin SS, Koo CH. Synchronous Hodgkin's disease and granulocytic sarcoma with no prior therapy. *Hum Pathol* 1996;27: 1103–1106.

49. Takimoto Y, Tanabe O, Kuramoto A, et al. Hodgkin's disease associated with chronic myeloid leukemia. Determination of bcr-abl rearrangement in paraffin-embedded tumors using the polymerase chain reaction. *Acta Haematol* 1994;92:97–100.

50. Vukelja SJ, Krishnan J, Ward FT, et al. Synchronous Hodgkin's disease and myelofibrosis terminating with granulocytic sarcoma and acute megakaryocytic leukemia. *South Med J* 1990;83: 1317–1320.

51. Zarate-Osorno A, Medeiros J, Jaffe ES. Hodgkin's disease coexistent with plasma cell dyscrasia. *Arch Pathol Lab Med* 1992;116: 969–972.

52. Cazals-Hatem D, Andre M, Mounier N, et al. Pathologic and clinical features of 77 Hodgkin's lymphoma patients treated in a lymphoma protocol (LNH87): a GELA study. *Am J Surg Pathol* 2001; 25:297–306.

53. Colon-Otero G, McClure SP, Phyliky RL, et al. Peripheral T-cell lymphoma simulating Hodgkin's disease with initial bone marrow involvement. *Mayo Clin Proc* 1986;61:68–71.

54. Filippa DA, Ladanyi M, Wollner N, et al. CD30 (Ki-1)-positive malignant lymphomas: clinical, immunophenotypic, histologic, and genetic characteristics and differences with Hodgkin's disease. *Blood* 1996;87:2905–2917.

55. Gottlieb CA, Maeda K, Hawley RC, et al. Myelodysplasia with bone marrow lymphocytosis and fibrosis mimicking recurrent Hodgkin's disease. *Am J Clin Pathol* 1989;91:6–11.

56. McBride JA, Rodriguez J, Luthra R, et al. T-cell-rich B large-cell lymphoma simulating lymphocyte-rich Hodgkin's disease. *Am J Surg Pathol* 1996;20:193–201.

57. McKenna RW, Brunning RD. Reed-Sternberg-like cells in nodular lymphoma involving the bone marrow. *Am J Clin Pathol* 1975;63: 779–785.

58. Nakanuma Y, Kurumaya H, Kurashima K. An autopsy case of malignant histiocytosis with Reed-Sternberg-like cells. *Acta Pathol Jpn* 1989;39:79–83.

59. Skinnider BF, Connors JM, Gascoyne RD. Bone marrow involvement in T-cell-rich B-cell lymphoma. *Am J Clin Pathol* 1997; 108:570–578.

60. Sun T, Susin M, Tomao FA, et al. Histiocyte-rich B-cell lymphoma. *Hum Pathol* 1997;28:1321–1324.

PLASMA CELL NEOPLASMS

Plasma cell neoplasms (or dyscrasias) comprise a wide spectrum of disease (Tables 26-1 and 26-2). These entities differ widely in tumor burden and clinical aggressiveness (Tables 26-3 and 26-4).

The clonal immunoglobulin disorders are essentially a by-product of clonal plasma cell disorders, in which the main signs and symptoms are caused by immunoglobulin deposition; the neoplastic plasma cells may or may not be detectable.

Clinicopathologic syndromes are also included in this chapter (Table 26-5). Although the underlying disease is essentially a clonal plasma cell disorder, evidence of neoplastic plasma cells or immunoglobulin deposition may be difficult to find.

PLASMA CELL NEOPLASMS

Heavy Chain Disease

Heavy chain disease (HCD) is characterized by the presence of free clonal immunoglobulin heavy chains in the serum or urine or by the presence of clonal heavy chains (without detectable light chains) in plasma cell cytoplasm (1,2).

α-HCD is typically characterized by low to absent serum and urine clonal immunoglobulin levels and abnormally truncated α heavy chains within plasma cells (3–7). The underlying disorder is usually intestinal lymphoma of mucosa-associated lymphoid tissue (immunoproliferative small intestinal disease), but other types of lymphoma and multiple myeloma (MM) have also been reported. The peripheral blood rarely shows leukemic dissemination. The bone marrow is involved only in the presence of a histologically high-grade component. Complications include clonal amyloidosis. The differential diagnosis includes other plasma cell disorders producing intact immunoglobulin molecules

TABLE 26-1. CLASSIFICATION OF PLASMA CELL NEOPLASMS ACCORDING TO THE WORLD HEALTH ORGANIZATION

Plasma cell myeloma
Solitary plasmacytoma of bone
Extraosseous plasmacytoma

TABLE 26-2. ORGANIZATION OF PLASMA CELL NEOPLASMS IN THIS CHAPTER

Plasma cell neoplasms
  Heavy chain disease
  Light chain disease
  Monoclonal gammopathy of undetermined significance
  Multiple myeloma
  Plasmablastic lymphoma
  Plasma cell leukemia
  Solitary plasmacytoma of bone

Clonal immunoglobulin disorders
  Heavy chain amyloidosis
  Light chain amyloidosis
  Heavy chain deposition disease
  Light chain deposition disease

Clinicopathologic syndromes
  POEMS syndrome
  Schnitzler syndrome

but giving false-negative test results for serum or urine light chains, with a resulting erroneous diagnosis of α-HCD.

γ-HCD may involve any of the γ-chain classes (8–14). The γ chain is typically truncated and/or dimerized. The underlying disorder may be Franklin disease, a syndrome characterized by fever, hepatosplenomegaly, autoimmunity, acquired immunodeficiency, and variable serum levels of free γ chains. Other associated disorders include autoimmune disease, malignant lymphoma (including

TABLE 26-3. DIFFERENTIAL FEATURES OF PLASMA CELL NEOPLASMS

	HCD	LCD	LPL	MGUS	MM	PCL
Serum Ig	+/−	−/+	+	<30 g/L	>30 g/L	+/−
Urine Ig	+/−	+	+	−/+	+/−	+/−
Lytic lesions	−	+	−	−	+	+/−
BM PCs	−/+	>10%	+/−	<10%	>10%	+
IgH rearr	−	+	−/+	+	+	+

BM PCs, bone marrow plasma cells; HCD, heavy chain disease; Ig, clonal immunoglobulin; *IgH* rearr, immunoglobulin heavy chain gene rearrangement; LCD, light chain disease; LPL, lymphoplasmacytic lymphoma; MGUS, monoclonal gammopathy of undetermined significance; MM, multiple myeloma; PCL, plasma cell leukemia; +, positive; −, negative; +/−, usually positive, sometimes negative; −/+, usually negative, sometimes positive.

TABLE 26-4. DIFFERENTIAL FEATURES OF CLONAL IMMUNOGLOBULIN DISORDERS

Immunoglobulin Chain	Amyloid	IDD	Crystals
κ light chain	AL	LCDD	+
λ light chain	AL	LCDD	−/+
α heavy chain	AH	HCDDV	−
δ heavy chain	−	HCDD	−
γ heavy chain	AH	HCDD	−
μ heavy chain	AH	HCDD	−

AH, heavy chain amyloidosis; AL, light chain amyloidosis; HCDD, heavy chain deposition disease; IDD, immunoglobulin deposition disease; LCDD, light chain deposition disease; +, positive; −, negative; −/+, usually negative, sometimes positive.

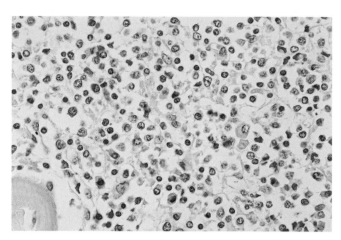

FIGURE 26-1. Bone marrow biopsy specimen, μ-heavy-chain disease. A diffuse lymphoplasmacytoid infiltrate replaces the hematopoietic tissue.

Hodgkin lymphoma), MM, and clonal myeloid disease. Peripheral blood findings include pancytopenia, atypical lymphocytosis, and eosinophilia. The bone marrow usually fails to show a lymphoplasmacytic disorder; when present, the plasma cells are often vacuolated. Complications include γ-heavy-chain deposition disease and clonal amyloidosis. The differential diagnosis includes the detection of normal urine γ-chain fragments, which may lead to an erroneous diagnosis of γ-HCD (15).

δ-HCD occurs in immunoglobulin D (IgD)–λ MM owing to dissociation of immunoglobulin heavy and light chains; in such cases, λ light chains are also detected (16–18). δ-HCD has also been reported in IgM MM, possibly attributable to clonal heavy chain switching followed by dissociation of immunoglobulin heavy and light chains.

μ-HCD is characterized by low serum and urine levels of free μ chains, sometimes accompanied by intact IgM-κ, free κ chains, or κ-chain urinary casts (19–25). The μ chain is abnormally truncated. The underlying disorder may be chronic lymphocytic leukemia, monoclonal gammopathy of undetermined significance (MGUS), or MM. In some cases, no definite morphologic diagnosis can be rendered. When involved, the bone marrow shows an infiltrate of lymphocytes and vacuolated plasma cells expressing IgM-κ (Fig. 26-1).

Light Chain Disease

Light chain disease is characterized by the presence of free clonal immunoglobulin light chains in the serum and/or urine. Clonal light chain excretion, or Bence Jones proteinuria, occurs in B-cell chronic lymphocytic leukemia/small lymphocytic lymphoma, lymphoplasmacytic lymphoma, hairy cell leukemia, large B-cell lymphoma, MGUS, MM, solitary plasmacytoma of bone, and light chain amyloidosis (AL amyloidosis) (26–28). The peripheral blood and bone marrow show findings characteristic of the underlying disorder. In some cases, no underlying disorder can be identified. Complications include AL amyloidosis and light chain deposition disease (LCDD). The differential diagnosis includes urinary excretion of polyclonal light chains, which has been reported in acute myeloid leukemia and acute lymphoid leukemia.

Monoclonal Gammopathy of Undetermined Significance

MGUS is a common condition, occurring in 3% of individuals older than 70 years of age (29). It is usually characterized by a serum clonal immunoglobulin level of less than 30 g/L, minimal to absent urinary clonal immunoglobulin level, bone marrow plasmacytosis less than 10%, and no evidence of systemic disease (lytic bone lesions, anemia, hypercalcemia, and/or renal failure).

Laboratory studies demonstrate clonal serum and/or urine immunoglobulin, which is composed of IgG in more than 70% of cases. IgM MGUS, accounting for 16% of cases, is associated with polyneuropathy, POEMS (polyneuropathy, organomegaly, endocrinopathy, monoclonal gammopathy, and skin changes) syndrome, and cold agglutinin disease (30–32). IgA MGUS, seen in approximately 10% of cases, may be associated with a higher risk of transformation to MM. IgD, IgE, and light chain MGUS are rare and have been reported to show minimal bone marrow disease and no evidence of progression (33,34). Serum studies demonstrate biclonality in 2% of cases, usually a combination of IgG with IgA, IgM, or a second IgG (35).

TABLE 26-5. DIFFERENTIAL FEATURES OF CLINICOPATHOLOGIC SYNDROMES ASSOCIATED WITH PLASMA CELL NEOPLASMS

POEMS Syndrome	Schnitzler Syndrome
Polyneuropathy	Fever
Organomegaly	Urticaria
Endocrinopathy	Bone and joint pain
Monoclonal gammopathy	Osteosclerosis
Skin changes	Lymphadenopathy

The peripheral blood rarely shows morphologically identifiable clonal cells. A neutrophilic leukemoid reaction may be present, caused by clonal plasma cell production of granulocyte colony-stimulating factor; this finding may be mistaken for chronic neutrophilic leukemia (36,37).

Bone marrow aspirate smears show both clonal and reactive plasmacytosis in almost all cases, usually comprising no more than 10% of nucleated cells. Although usually larger, clonal cells are not always morphologically indistinguishable from reactive cells (38). Histologic sections of the bone marrow show scattered, minimally atypical plasma cells without discrete aggregates. Other findings may include pure red cell aplasia, erythroid and megakaryocytic hyperplasia caused by immune-mediated cytopenias, storage histiocytes, and immunoglobulin crystals (39–41).

Flow cytometry usually shows clonal populations in both the peripheral blood and bone marrow (42–44). Clonal circulating cells are identifiable by bright CD38 and little or no CD45 expression. Clonal bone marrow cells are accompanied by reactive plasma cells in almost all cases. Reactive cells tend to express CD19 and bright CD38 but not CD56; clonal cells tend to express weaker CD38 and CD56 but not CD19. Compared with MM, MGUS cells more often co-express B-cell and plasma cell antigens, including CD10, CD11, CD20, CD22, CD138, and surface immunoglobulin. CD5 and CD23 may not be expressed. Immunostains show positive reactions for CD38, CD138, and bcl-2 and negative to faintly positive reactions for CD45 in both reactive and clonal cells (45,46).

Genetic studies show clonal anomalies of chromosomes 6, 9, 13, and 17 in more than 50% of cases, with more than one clone occurring in 67% of cases (47–50). The most common translocations are t(11;14)(q13;q32) and t(4;14)(p16;q32). Monosomy 13 is linked to transformation to MM.

MGUS transforms to a more aggressive disorder in approximately 40% of cases within 25 years of diagnosis (51,52). MGUS usually converts to MM but may also progress to lymphoplasmacytic lymphoma, systemic amyloidosis, immunoglobulin deposition disease, or other lymphoplasmacytic disorders. A higher number of bone marrow plasma cells (10% to 30% of nucleated cells) is associated with a greater risk of transformation.

Many lymphoid and myeloid disorders have been reported with MGUS, including Hodgkin lymphoma, Sézary syndrome, myeloproliferative disorders, myelodysplastic syndromes, histiocytic disorders, and acute myeloid leukemia (53–63). These may be clonally related or unrelated to coexisting MGUS.

The differential diagnosis consists primarily of lymphoplasmacytic lymphoma and MM.

Multiple Myeloma

MM is characterized by a serum clonal immunoglobulin level of more than 30 g/L, the presence of serum and/or

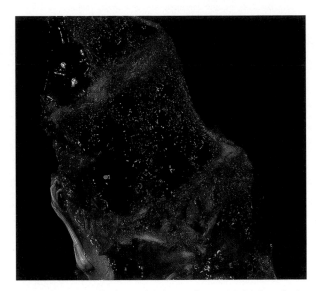

FIGURE 26-2. Vertebrae, multiple myeloma. Multiple soft, hemorrhagic masses have excavated the hematopoietic bone marrow; this appearance accounts for the term multiple myeloma.

urine clonal immunoglobulin, bone marrow plasmacytosis of more than 10%, and evidence of systemic disease (lytic bone lesions, anemia, hypercalcemia, and/or renal failure) (64) (Figs. 26-2 through 26-14). Cases with findings intermediate between MGUS and MM may be considered "smoldering" MM and may or may not progress to overt MM. MM occurs as a *de novo* disease, as a complication of Gaucher disease, and as a transformation of MGUS, AL amyloidosis, immunoglobulin deposition disease, and possibly hairy cell leukemia (65–68).

Laboratory studies demonstrate clonal serum and/or urine immunoglobulin, which is composed of IgG in most cases. IgA MM is next in order of frequency; IgA-λ disease, the predominant form, is associated with tumor-related neutrophilia, POEMS syndrome, osteosclerosis, anaplastic

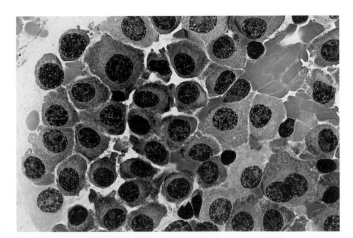

FIGURE 26-3. Bone marrow aspirate, multiple myeloma. The clonal plasma cells are larger than normal plasma cells and show more abundant cytoplasm.

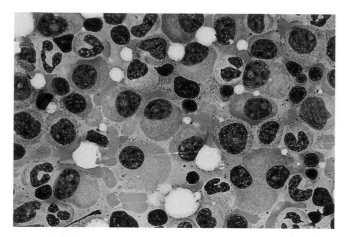

FIGURE 26-4. Bone marrow aspirate, multiple myeloma. The clonal plasma cells show a single prominent nucleolus within each nucleus; an occasional binucleated plasma cell is present.

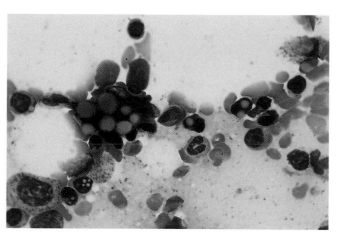

FIGURE 26-7. Bone marrow aspirate, multiple myeloma with Russell bodies. The clonal plasma cells are virtually replaced by spherical globules of immunoglobulin.

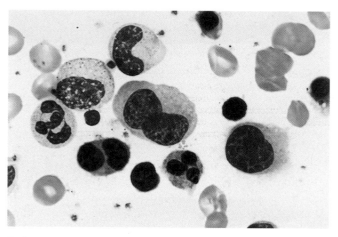

FIGURE 26-5. Bone marrow aspirate, multiple myeloma with multinuclearity. The clonal plasma cells show deep clefts or overt binucleation.

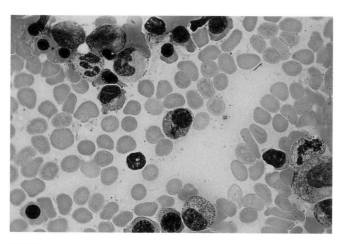

FIGURE 26-8. Bone marrow aspirate, multiple myeloma with immunoglobulin crystals. The plasma cell contains deep red, needle-like immunoglobulin inclusions, which may be mistaken for Auer rods.

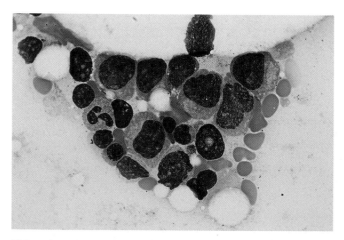

FIGURE 26-6. Bone marrow aspirate, anaplastic multiple myeloma. The clonal plasma cells show little or no resemblance to normal plasma cells and can easily be mistaken for malignant lymphoma or carcinoma cells.

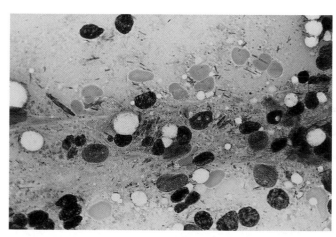

FIGURE 26-9. Bone marrow aspirate, multiple myeloma with immunoglobulin crystals. Numerous free crystals are present in the background.

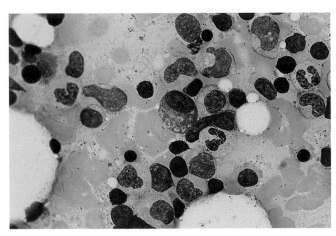

FIGURE 26-10. Bone marrow aspirate, multiple myeloma with phagocytosis. A clonal plasma cell contains ingested platelets.

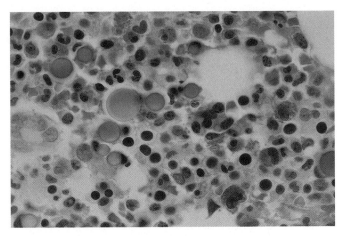

FIGURE 26-12. Bone marrow biopsy specimen, multiple myeloma with Russell bodies. Prominent Russell bodies appear among the plasma cells and hematopoietic cells.

morphology, and a poor prognosis. Light chain MM accounts for 12% of cases and is associated with a poor prognosis (69). IgD MM is rare and often nonsecretory. IgD-λ is the predominant form and has been associated with anaplastic or plasmablastic morphology, plasma cell leukemia (PCL), and a poor prognosis (70–72). IgE MM is associated with t(11;14) and leukemic transformation (73–75). IgM MM may show features reminiscent of lymphoplasmacytic lymphoma and is associated with t(11;14) (75–77). Biclonal MM accounts for approximately 1% of cases and usually shows a combination of IgG with IgA, IgM, or a second IgG (78,79). Nonsecretory MM accounts for 2% to 3% of cases and is associated with t(11;14) (75). Most cases are IgD-committed plasma cell neoplasms with impaired synthesis or secretion of intact IgD.

The peripheral blood shows anemia and, in cases with at least 9.0 gm/L of serum protein, rouleau formation. PCL may be present. Other findings include neutrophilic leukemoid reaction (usually reported as chronic neutrophilic

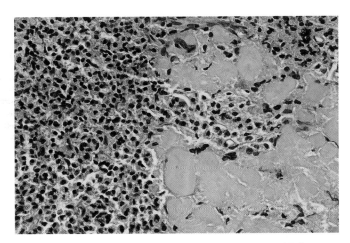

FIGURE 26-13. Bone marrow biopsy specimen, multiple myeloma with amyloidosis. A massive amyloid deposit is present, adjacent to a diffuse infiltrate of abnormal plasma cells.

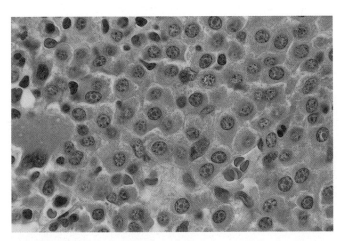

FIGURE 26-11. Bone marrow biopsy specimen, multiple myeloma. A sheet of atypical plasma cells replaces the hematopoietic tissue.

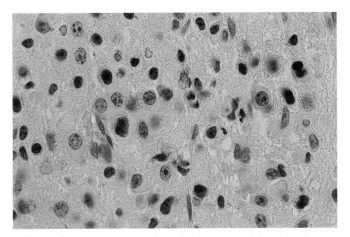

FIGURE 26-14. Bone marrow biopsy specimen, multiple myeloma with fibrosis. Abnormal plasma cells are widely separated by fibrous tissue.

leukemia) and eosinophilia, caused by plasma cell production of granulocyte colony-stimulating factor and interleukin-3, respectively (80,81).

Bone marrow aspirate smears and/or histologic sections taken from the iliac crest show evidence of disease in approximately 85% of cases (82,83). Although usually larger and more pleomorphic, clonal cells are not always clearly distinguishable from reactive plasma cells. Clues to neoplastic origin include a large nucleus with more dispersed chromatin and a single prominent nucleolus.

Morphologic variants of MM cells are numerous (84–90). The nucleus may be lymphoplasmacytic, cleaved, multilobated, or multiple. The cytoplasm may appear clear, hairy, oncocytic, monocytoid, or signet ring–like. The term plasmablastic has been applied to large MM cells with a high nuclear:cytoplasmic ratio (91) (see also Plasmablastic Lymphoma section below). Other plasma cell abnormalities include nuclear pseudoinclusions (Dutcher bodies), cytoplasmic vacuoles, and dense, spherical cytoplasmic immunoglobulin inclusions (Russell bodies), which may transform the plasma cell into an unrecognizable mass of spheres (Mott cell). Immunoglobulin crystals may be present in the cytoplasm of neoplastic cells and in the peripheral blood smear, bone marrow histiocytes, renal tubular cells, and blood vessels (92–95). Plasma cells may cluster around histiocytes or show phagocytic activity, possibly facilitated by opsonic properties of the clonal immunoglobulin (96–98).

Histologic sections of the bone marrow show interstitial, nodular, and/or diffuse plasma cell infiltrates. The neoplastic plasma cells may resemble myelocytes but show more abundant, amphophilic to eosinophilic cytoplasm and an eccentric nucleus with a prominent nuclear membrane, clumped chromatin, and a distinct eosinophilic nucleolus.

Other bone marrow findings include reactive mastocytosis, storage histiocytosis, sarcoidosis, AL amyloidosis, immunoglobulin deposition disease, hypervascularity, fibrosis, osteomalacia, osteoporosis, and osteosclerosis (99–103). Fibrotic MM is characterized by severe anemia, often with leukopenia and thrombocytopenia and focal megakaryocytic hyperplasia resembling a myeloproliferative disorder (104,105). Osteosclerotic MM is characterized by hepatosplenomegaly and lymphadenopathy rather than lytic bone lesions, and is associated with IgA secretion, POEMS syndrome, and polyneuropathy (106,107). Osteosclerosis may be focal or diffuse and may be accompanied by bone marrow fibrosis.

Flow cytometry of the peripheral blood often shows two plasma cell populations, the majority polyclonal (108–110). The polyclonal cells usually express CD38 (dim), CD45, CD56 (dim), CD138 (dim), and cytoplasmic immunoglobulin. The clonal cells usually express CD22, CD138 (moderate), and cytoplasmic immunoglobulin but not CD10, CD20, CD23, or HLA-DR. Expression of CD19, CD38, CD56, CD117, and surface immunoglobulin is variable.

Flow cytometry of the bone marrow may also show two plasma cell populations, but the majority are clonal (111–

113). The polyclonal cells usually express CD19, CD38 (bright), CD45, and cytoplasmic immunoglobulin but not CD117. The clonal cells usually express CD38 (dim to moderate), CD45 (dim to negative), CD56 (bright), CD117, CD138 (bright), HLA-DR (dim), and cytoplasmic immunoglobulin but not CD10, CD19, CD22, CD23, or surface immunoglobulin. Neoplastic plasma cells occasionally express CD10, CD14, CD15, CD19, CD20, CD33, and/or surface immunoglobulin or lack expression of CD38, CD56, or CD117. CD138 may be lost during apoptosis (114). In addition to these markers, immunostains may show expression of epithelial membrane antigen and cytokeratin and overexpression of p53 protein, cyclin D1 mRNA, and cyclin D1 protein (115–117).

Genetic studies show karyotypic anomalies in approximately 50% and molecular anomalies in virtually 100% of MM cases. Translocation of *IgH*, located at chromosome 14q32, is consistently present (118–120).

Transformation to PCL occurs in 1% to 3% of cases. Transformation to the anaplastic variant or plasmablastic lymphoma has also been reported.

Other hematolymphoid disorders reported with MM include myeloproliferative disorders, myelodysplastic syndromes, histiocytic disorders, acute myeloid leukemia, and a variety of B-cell and T-cell malignancies (121–138). A common clonal origin of MM and myeloid disease has been demonstrated in some cases.

The differential diagnosis includes reactive plasmacytosis, lymphoplasmacytic lymphoma, plasmablastic lymphoma, B-cell lymphoma with lytic bone lesions, granulocytic sarcoma, and undifferentiated carcinoma (139–141).

Plasmablastic Lymphoma

Plasmablastic lymphoma is a rare disorder, characterized by prominent tumor masses in soft tissue and viscera rather than bony disease (142–153). It shows overlapping features with anaplastic myeloma and primary effusion lymphoma. Plasmablastic lymphoma occurs *de novo,* as a complication of human immunodeficiency virus (HIV) infection and other immunosuppressed states, and as a terminal phase of MM.

The peripheral blood may show a leukemic phase. The tumor cells are large and bizarre and resemble high-grade lymphoma cells. The mitotic rate is high. Genetic anomalies are numerous and complex. Tumor cells from immunosuppressed patients show clonal integration of Epstein-Barr virus DNA. Tumor cells from patients infected with HIV show immunoglobulin specificity for HIV–encoded proteins.

Plasma Cell Leukemia

PCL is defined as the presence of circulating clonal plasma cells, at a minimum absolute count of approximately 2×10^9

2. Witzig TE, Wahner-Roedler DL. Heavy chain disease. *Curr Treat Options Oncol* 2002;3:247–254.

3. Fine KD, Stone MJ. Alpha-heavy chain disease, Mediterranean lymphoma, and immunoproliferative small intestinal disease: a review of clinicopathological features, pathogenesis, and differential diagnosis. *Am J Gastroenterol* 1999;94:1139–1152.

4. Ghevaert C, Fournier M, Bernardi F, et al. Non-secretory multiple myeloma with multinucleated giant plasma cells. *Leuk Lymphoma* 1997;27:185–189.

5. Hubmann R, Kaiser W, Radaszkiewicz T, et al. Malabsorption associated with a high-grade-malignant non-Hodgkin's lymphoma, alpha-heavy-chain disease and immunoproliferative small intestinal disease. *Z Gastroenterol* 1995;33:209–213.

6. Su L, Keren DF, Warren JS. Failure of anti-lambda immunofixation reagent mimics alpha heavy-chain disease. *Clin Chem* 1995;41:121–123.

7. Zamir A, Parasher G, Moukarzel AA, et al. Immunoproliferative small intestinal disease in a 16-year-old boy presenting as severe malabsorption with excellent response to tetracycline treatment. *J Clin Gastroenterol* 1998;27:85–89.

8. Hudnall SD, Alperin JB, Petersen JR. Composite nodular lymphocyte-predominance Hodgkin disease and gamma-heavy-chain disease: a case report and review of the literature. *Arch Pathol Lab Med* 2001;125:803–807.

9. Husby G, Blichfeldt P, Brinch L, et al. Chronic arthritis and gamma heavy chain disease: coincidence or pathogenic link? *Scand J Rheumatol* 1998;27:257–264.

10. Prelli F, Frangione B. Franklin's disease: Ig gamma 2 H chain mutant BUR. *J Immunol* 1992;148:949–952.

11. Takatani T, Morita K, Takaoka N, et al. Gamma heavy chain disease screening showing a discrepancy between electrophoretic and nephelometric determinations of serum gamma globulin concentration. *Ann Clin Biochem* 2002;39:531–533.

12. Teng MH, Rosen S, Gorny MK, et al. Gamma heavy chain disease in man: independent structural abnormalities and reduced transcription of a functionally rearranged lambda L-chain gene result in the absence of L-chains. *Blood Cells Mol Dis* 2000;26:177–185.

13. Tichy M, Stulik J, Osanec J, et al. Electrophoretic characterization of a gamma-1-heavy chain disease. *Neoplasma* 2000;47:118–121.

14. Tissot JD, Tridon A, Ruivard M, et al. Electrophoretic analyses in a case of monoclonal gamma chain disease. *Electrophoresis* 1998;19:1771–1773.

15. Charles EZ, Valdes AJ. Free fragments of gamma chain in the urine. A possible source of confusion with gamma heavy-chain disease. *Am J Clin Pathol* 1994;101:462–464.

16. Blade J, Kyle RA. Nonsecretory myeloma, immunoglobulin D myeloma, and plasma cell leukemia. *Hematol Oncol Clin North Am* 1999;13:1259–1272.

17. Rabhi H, Ghaffor M, Abbadi MC. Spontaneous enzymatic cleavage of IgD myeloma protein giving a pattern of delta heavy chain disease. *Arch Inst Pasteur Alger* 1989;57:135–140.

18. Virella G, Monteiro JM, Lopes-Virella MF, et al. Asynchronous development of two monoclonal proteins (IgM lambda and delta 1 chains) in a patient with abdominal lymphoma. *Cancer* 1977;39:2247–2253.

19. Cogne M, Aucouturier P, Brizard A, et al. Complete variable region deletion in a mu heavy chain disease protein (ROUL). Correlation with light chain secretion. *Leuk Res* 1993;17:527–532.

20. Franklin EC. Mu-chain disease. *Arch Intern Med* 1975;135:71–72.

21. Iwasaki T, Hamano T, Kobayashi K, et al. A case of mu-heavy chain disease: combined features of mu-chain disease and macroglobulinemia. *Int J Hematol* 1997;66:359–365.

22. Preud'homme JL, Bauwens M, Dumont G, et al. Cast nephropathy in mu heavy chain disease. *Clin Nephrol* 1997;48:118–121.

23. Pruzanski W, Hasselback R, Katz A, et al. Multiple myeloma (light chain disease) with rheumatoid-like amyloid arthropathy and mu-heavy chain fragment in the serum. *Am J Med* 1978;65:334–341.

24. Wahner-Roedler DL, Kyle RA. Mu-heavy chain disease: presentation as a benign monoclonal gammopathy. *Am J Hematol* 1992;40:56–60.

25. Witzens M, Egerer G, Stahl D, et al. A case of mu heavy-chain disease associated with hyperglobulinemia, anemia, and a positive Coombs test. *Ann Hematol* 1998;77:231–234.

26. Pascali E, Pezzoli A. The clinical spectrum of pure Bence Jones proteinuria. A study of 66 patients. *Cancer* 1988;62:2408–2415.

27. Pezzoli A, Pascali E. The clinical significance of pure Bence Jones proteinuria at low concentration. *Am J Clin Pathol* 1989;91:473–475.

28. Solling K, Nielsen JL, Solling J, et al. Free light chains of immunoglobulins in serum from patients with leukaemias and multiple myeloma. *Scand J Haematol* 1982;28:309–318.

29. Kyle RA, Rajkumar SV. Monoclonal gammopathies of undetermined significance. *Rev Clin Exp Hematol* 2002;6:225–252.

30. Ciejka JZ, Cook EB, Lawler D, et al. Severe cold agglutinin disease and cryoglobulinemia secondary to a monoclonal anti-Pr2 IgM lambda cryoagglutinin. *Clin Exp Rheumatol* 1999,17:227–231.

31. Pujol M, Ribera JM, Jimenez C, et al. Essential monoclonal gammopathy with an IgM paraprotein that is a cryoglobulin with cold agglutinin and EDTA-dependent platelet antibody properties. *Br J Haematol* 1998;100:603–604.

32. Ponsford S, Willison H, Veitch J, et al. Long-term clinical and neurophysiological follow-up of patients with peripheral, neuropathy associated with benign monoclonal gammopathy. *Muscle Nerve* 2000;23:164–174.

33. Kinoshita T, Nagai H, Murate T, et al. IgD monoclonal gammopathy of undetermined significance. *Int J Hematol* 1997;65:169–172.

34. Ludwig H, Vormittag W. "Benign" monoclonal IgE gammopathy. *BMJ* 1980;281:539–540.

35. Nilsson T, Norberg B, Rudolphi O, et al. Double gammopathies: incidence and clinical course of 20 patients. *Scand J Haematol* 1986;36:103–106.

36. Florensa L, Woessner S, Vicente P, et al. Chronic neutrophilic leukemia associated with monoclonal gammopathy of undetermined significance. A multimethod study. *Ann Hematol* 1993;67:129–131.

37. Ito T, Kojima H, Otani K, et al. Chronic neutrophilic leukemia associated with monoclonal gammopathy of undetermined significance. *Acta Haematol* 1996;95:140–143.

38. Milla F, Oriol A, Aguilar J, et al. Usefulness and reproducibility of cytomorphologic evaluations to differentiate myeloma from monoclonal gammopathies of unknown significance. *Am J Clin Pathol* 2001;115:127–135.

39. Goteri G, Lorenzini P, Morroni M, et al. Bone marrow extracellular large geometric crystals in IgG/lambda MGUS. *Pathol Res Pract* 2002;198:299–302.

40. Jonsson V, Svendsen B, Vorstrup S, et al. Multiple autoimmune manifestations in monoclonal gammopathy of undetermined significance and chronic lymphocytic leukemia. *Leukemia* 1996;10:327–332.

41. Regazzoli A, Pozzi A, Rossi G. Pseudo-Gaucher plasma cells in the bone marrow of a patient with monoclonal gammopathy of undetermined significance. *Haematologica* 1997;82:727.

42. Ocqueteau M, Orfao A, Almeida J, et al. Immunophenotypic characterization of plasma cells from monoclonal gammopathy

of undetermined significance patients. Implications for the differential diagnosis between MGUS and multiple myeloma. *Am J Pathol* 1998;152:1655–1665.

43. Wang C, Amato D, Fernandes B. CD5-negative phenotype of monoclonal B-lymphocytosis of undetermined significance (MLUS). *Am J Hematol* 2002;69:147–149.

44. Zandecki M, Facon T, Bernardi F, et al. CD19 and immunophenotype of bone marrow plasma cells in monoclonal gammopathy of undetermined significance. *J Clin Pathol* 1995;48:548–552.

45. Chilosi M, Adami F, Lestani M, et al. CD138/syndecan-1: a useful immunohistochemical marker of normal and neoplastic plasma cells on routine trephine bone marrow biopsies. *Mod Pathol* 1999;12:1101–1106.

46. Miguel-Garcia A, Orero T, Matutes E, et al. bcl-2 expression in plasma cells from neoplastic gammopathies and reactive plasmacytosis: a comparative study. *Haematologica* 1998;83:298–304.

47. Avet-Loiseau H, Li JY, Morineau N, et al. Monosomy 13 is associated with the transition of monoclonal gammopathy of undetermined significance to multiple myeloma. Intergroupe Francophone du Myelome. *Blood* 1999;94:2583–2589.

48. Konigsberg R, Ackermann J, Kaufmann H, et al. Deletions of chromosome 13q in monoclonal gammopathy of undetermined significance. *Leukemia* 2000;14:1975–1979.

49. Lloveras E, Sole F, Florensa L, et al. Contribution of cytogenetics and *in situ* hybridization to the study of monoclonal gammopathies of undetermined significance. *Cancer Genet Cytogenet* 2002;132:25–29.

50. Rasillo A, Tabernero MD, Sanchez ML, et al. Fluorescence *in situ* hybridization analysis of aneuploidization patterns in monoclonal gammopathy of undetermined significance versus multiple myeloma and plasma cell leukemia. *Cancer* 2003;97:601–609.

51. Morra E, Cesana C, Klersy C, et al. Predictive variables for malignant transformation in 452 patients with asymptomatic IgM monoclonal gammopathy. *Semin Oncol* 2003;30:172–177.

52. Pasqualetti P, Festuccia V, Collacciani A, et al. The natural history of monoclonal gammopathy of undetermined significance. A 5- to 20-year follow-up of 263 cases. *Acta Haematol* 1997;97:174–179.

53. Borish L, Dishuck J, Cox L, et al. Sezary syndrome with elevated serum IgE and hypereosinophilia: role of dysregulated cytokine production. *J Allergy Clin Immunol* 1993;92:123–131.

54. Economopoulos T, Economidou J, Papageorgiou E, et al. Monoclonal gammopathy in chronic myeloproliferative disorders. *Blut* 1989;58:7–9.

55. Ribeiro I, Carvalho IR, Fontes M, et al. Eosinophilic leukaemia with trisomy 8 and double gammopathy. *J Clin Pathol* 1993;46:672–673.

56. Lindner PS, Pardanani B, Angadi C, et al. Acute nonlymphocytic leukemia in systemic mastocytosis with biclonal gammopathy. *J Allergy Clin Immunol* 1992;90:410–412.

57. Nitta M, Tsuboi K, Yamashita S, et al. Multiple myeloma preceding the development of chronic myelogenous leukemia. *Int J Hematol* 1999;69:170–173.

58. Copplestone JA, Mufti GJ, Hamblin TJ, et al. Immunological abnormalities in myelodysplastic syndromes. II. Coexistent lymphoid or plasma cell neoplasms: a report of 20 cases unrelated to chemotherapy. *Br J Haematol* 1986;63:149–159.

59. Itoh K, Kashimura T, Kobayashi Y, et al. Atypical chronic myeloid leukemia presenting with trilineage dysplasia and IgG (lambda) type monoclonal gammopathy. *Rinsho Ketsueki* 1999;40:129–134.

60. Mufti GJ, Figes A, Hamblin TJ, et al. Immunological abnormalities in myelodysplastic syndromes. I. Serum immunoglobulins and autoantibodies. *Br J Haematol* 1986;63:143–147.

61. Marcoval J, Moreno A, Bordas X, et al. Diffuse plane xanthoma: clinicopathologic study of 8 cases. *J Am Acad Dermatol* 1998;39:439–442.

62. Allen EL, Metz EN, Balcerzak SP. Acute myelomonocytic leukemia with macroglobulinemia, Bence Jones proteinuria, and hypercalcemia. *Cancer* 1973;32:121–129.

63. Atkins H, Drouin J, Izaguirre CA, et al. Acute promyelocytic leukemia associated with a paraprotein that reacts with leukemic cells. *Cancer* 1989;63:1750–1751.

64. Kyle RA. Diagnosis of multiple myeloma. *Semin Oncol* 2002;29 [Suppl 17]:2–4.

65. Rajkumar SV, Gertz MA, Kyle RA. Primary systemic amyloidosis with delayed progression to multiple myeloma. *Cancer* 1998;82:1501–1505.

66. Daliani D, Weber D, Alexanian R. Light-heavy chain deposition disease progressing to multiple myeloma. *Am J Hematol* 1995;50:296–298.

67. Saif MW, Greenberg BR. Multiple myeloma and hairy cell leukemia: a rare association or coincidence? *Leuk Lymphoma* 2001;42:1043–1048.

68. Harder H, Eucker J, Zang C, et al. Coincidence of Gaucher's disease due to a 1226G/1448C mutation and of an immunoglobulin G lambda multiple myeloma with Bence-Jones proteinuria. *Ann Hematol* 2000;79:640–643.

69. Wisloff F, Andersen P, Andersson TR, et al. Incidence and follow-up of asymptomatic multiple myeloma. The myeloma project of health region I in Norway. II. *Eur J Haematol* 1991;47:338–341.

70. Blade J, Kyle RA. Nonsecretory myeloma, immunoglobulin D myeloma, and plasma cell leukemia. *Hematol Oncol Clin North Am* 1999;13:1259–1272.

71. Fujishima M, Komatsuda A, Imai H, et al. Amyloid arthropathy resembling seronegative rheumatoid arthritis in a patient with IgD-kappa multiple myeloma. *Intern Med* 2003;42:121–124.

72. Iwasaki T, Hamano T, Ogata A, et al. IgD multiple myeloma preceding the development of extensive extramedullary disease without medullary involvement. *Acta Haematol* 2000;104:42–45.

73. Macro M, Andre I, Comby E, et al. IgE multiple myeloma. *Leuk Lymphoma* 1999;32:597–603.

74. Bakkus MH, Schots R, Gomez La, Fuente PB, et al. Clonally related IgA- and IgE-secreting plasma cells in a myeloma patient. *Eur J Haematol* 2000;65:348–355.

75. Avet-Loiseau H, Garand R, Lode L, et al. Translocation t(11;14)(q13;q32) is the hallmark of IgM, IgE, and nonsecretory multiple myeloma variants. *Blood* 2003;101:1570–1571.

76. Dierlamm T, Laack E, Dierlamm J, et al. IgM myeloma: a report of four cases. *Ann Hematol* 2002;81:136–139.

77. Kondo H, Yokoyama K. IgM myeloma: different features from multiple myeloma and macroglobulinemia. *Eur J Haematol* 1999;63:366–368.

78. Pizzolato M, Bragantini G, Bresciani P, et al. IgG1-kappa biclonal gammopathy associated with multiple myeloma suggests a regulatory mechanism. *Br J Haematol* 1998;102:503–508.

79. Zent CS, Wilson CS, Tricot G, et al. Oligoclonal protein bands and Ig isotype switching in multiple myeloma treated with high-dose therapy and hematopoietic cell transplantation. *Blood* 1998;91:3518–3523.

80. Usuda H, Naito M, Ohyach K, et al. A case of multiple myeloma producing granulocyte colony-stimulating factor. *Pathol Int* 1997;47:866–869.

81. Glantz L, Rintels P, Samoszuk M, et al. Plasma cell myeloma associated with eosinophilia. *Am J Clin Pathol* 1995;103:583–587.

82. Buss DH, Prichard RW, Hartz JW, et al. Comparison of the usefulness of bone marrow sections and smears in diagnosis of multiple myeloma. *Hematol Pathol* 1987;1:35–43.

83. Terpstra WE, Lokhorst HM, Blomjous F, et al. Comparison of plasma cell infiltration in bone marrow biopsies and aspirates in patients with multiple myeloma. *Br J Haematol* 1992;82:46–49.

84. Algino KM, Hendrix LE, Henderson CA, et al. Multiple myeloma with hairy cell-like features. *Am J Clin Pathol* 1997;107:665–671.

85. Bosman C, Fusilli S, Bisceglia M, et al. Oncocytic nonsecretory multiple myeloma. A clinicopathologic study of a case and review of the literature. *Acta Haematol* 1996;96:50–56.

86. Caenazzo A, Sartori D, Poletti A. Bence Jones myeloma with signet-ring-like plasma cells. *Haematologica* 1997;82:122.

87. Chen KT, Ma CK, Nelson JW, et al. Clear cell myeloma. *Am J Surg Pathol* 1985;9:149–154.

88. Ghevaert C, Fournier M, Bernardi F, et al. Non-secretory multiple myeloma with multinucleated giant plasma cells. *Leuk Lymphoma* 1997;27:185–189.

89. Sun NC, Fishkin BG, Nies KM, et al. Lymphoplasmacytic myeloma: an immunological, immunohistochemical and electron microscopic study. *Cancer* 1979;43:2268–2278.

90. Yeh YA, Pappas AA, Flick JT, et al. A case of aggressive multiple myeloma with cleaved, multilobated, and monocytoid nuclei, and no serum monoclonal gammopathy. *Ann Clin Lab Sci* 2000;30:283–288.

91. Greipp PR, Leong T, Bennett JM, et al. Plasmablastic morphology—an independent prognostic factor with clinical and laboratory correlates: Eastern Cooperative Oncology Group (ECOG) myeloma trial E9486 report by the ECOG Myeloma Laboratory Group. *Blood* 1998;91:2501–2507.

92. Castoldi G, Piva N, Tomasi P. Multiple myeloma with Auer-rod-like inclusions. *Haematologica* 1999;84:859–860.

93. Gardais J, Genevieve F, Foussard C, et al. Is there any significance for intracellular crystals in plasma cells from patients with monoclonal gammopathies? *Eur J Haematol* 2001;67:119–122.

94. Gruszecki AC, Vishnu VVB. Plasma cell crystalline inclusions. *Arch Pathol Lab Med* 2002;126:755.

95. Lajoie G, Leung R, Bargman JM. Clinical, biochemical, and pathological features in a patient with plasma cell dyscrasia and Fanconi syndrome. *Ultrastruct Pathol* 2000;24:221–226.

96. Pillay TS, Sayers G, Bird AR, et al. Plasmacyte-reticulum cell satellitism in multiple myeloma associated with amyloidosis. *J Clin Pathol* 1992;45:623–624.

97. Invernizzi R, Pecci A. A case of phagocytic multiple myeloma. *Haematologica* 2000;85:318.

98. Kanoh T, Fujii H. Phagocytic myeloma cells. Report of a case and review of the literature. *Am J Clin Pathol* 1985;84:121–124.

99. Kapadia SB. Multiple myeloma: a clinicopathologic study of 62 consecutively autopsied cases. *Medicine (Baltimore)* 1980;59:380–392.

100. Ribatti D, Vacca A, Nico B, et al. Bone marrow angiogenesis and mast cell density increase simultaneously with progression of human multiple myeloma. *Br J Cancer* 1999;79:451–455.

101. Schreiber S, Ackermann J, Obermair A, et al. Multiple myeloma with deletion of chromosome 13q is characterized by increased bone marrow neovascularization. *Br J Haematol* 2000;110:605–609.

102. Scullin DC Jr, Shelburne JD, Cohen HJ. Pseudo-Gaucher cells in multiple myeloma. *Am J Med* 1979;67:347–352.

103. Sen F, Mann KP, Medeiros LJ. Multiple myeloma in association with sarcoidosis. *Arch Pathol Lab Med* 2002;365–368.

104. McCluggage WG, Jones FG, Hull D, et al. Sclerosing IgA multiple myeloma. *Acta Haematol* 1995;94:98–101.

105. Vandermolen L, Rice L, Lynch EC. Plasma cell dyscrasia with marrow fibrosis. Clinicopathologic syndrome. *Am J Med* 1985;79:297–302.

106. Lacy MQ, Gertz MA, Hanson CA, et al. Multiple myeloma associated with diffuse osteosclerotic bone lesions: a clinical entity distinct from osteosclerotic myeloma (POEMS syndrome). *Am J Hematol* 1997;56:288–293.

107. Schey S. Osteosclerotic myeloma and 'POEMS' syndrome. *Blood Rev* 1996;10:75–80.

108. Luque R, Brieva JA, Moreno A, et al. Normal and clonal B lineage cells can be distinguished by their differential expression of B cell antigens and adhesion molecules in peripheral blood from multiple myeloma (MM) patients—diagnostic and clinical implications. *Clin Exp Immunol* 1998;112:410–418.

109. Ocqueteau M, Orfao A, Almeida J, et al. Immunophenotypic characterization of plasma cells from monoclonal gammopathy of undetermined significance patients. Implications for the differential diagnosis between MGUS and multiple myeloma. *Am J Pathol* 1998;152:1655–1665.

110. Schneider U, van Lessen A, Huhn D, et al. Two subsets of peripheral blood plasma cells defined by differential expression of CD45 antigen. *Br J Haematol* 1997;97:56–64.

111. Leo R, Boeker M, Peest D, et al. Multiparameter analyses of normal and malignant human plasma cells: CD38++, CD56+, CD54+, cIg+ is the common phenotype of myeloma cells. *Ann Hematol* 1992;64:132–139.

112. Kucukkaya RD, Hacihanefioglu A, Yenerel MN, et al. CD15-expressing phagocytic plasma cells in a patient with multiple myeloma. *Blood* 2001;97:581–583.

113. Pellat-Deceunynck C, Barille S, Jego G, et al. The absence of CD56 (NCAM) on malignant plasma cells is a hallmark of plasma cell leukemia and of a special subset of multiple myeloma. *Leukemia* 1998;12:1977–1982.

114. Jourdan M, Ferlin M, Legouffe E, et al. The myeloma cell antigen syndecan-1 is lost by apoptotic myeloma cells. *Br J Haematol* 1998;100:637–646.

115. Pileri S, Poggi S, Baglioni P, et al. Histology and immunohistology of bone marrow biopsy in multiple myeloma. *Eur J Haematol Suppl* 1989;51:52–59.

116. Kanavaros P, Stefanaki K, Vlachonikolis J, et al. Immunohistochemical expression of the p53, p21/Waf-1, Rb, p16 and Ki67 proteins in multiple myeloma. *Anticancer Res* 2000;20:4619–4625.

117. Athanasiou E, Kaloutsi V, Kotoula V, et al. Cyclin D1 overexpression in multiple myeloma. A morphologic, immunohistochemical, and in situ hybridization study of 71 paraffin-embedded bone marrow biopsy specimens. *Am J Clin Pathol* 2001;116:535–542.

118. Avet-Loiseau H, Brigaudeau C, Morineau N, et al. High incidence of cryptic translocations involving the Ig heavy chain gene in multiple myeloma, as shown by fluorescence *in situ* hybridization. *Genes Chromosomes Cancer* 1999;24:9–15.

119. Avet-Louseau H, Daviet A, Sauner S, et al. Chromosome 13 abnormalities in multiple myeloma are mostly monosomy 13. *Br J Haematol* 2000;111:1116–1117.

120. Drach J, Ackermann J, Fritz E, et al. Presence of a p53 gene deletion in patients with multiple myeloma predicts for short survival after conventional-dose chemotherapy. *Blood* 1998;92:802–809.

121. Schoevaerdts D, Mineur P, Hennaux V, et al. Hypercalcemia, chronic lymphocytic leukemia and multiple myeloma: uncommon association. *Acta Clin Belg* 1999;54:217–219.

122. Fine JM, Gorin NC, Gendre JP, et al. Simultaneous occurrence of clinical manifestations of myeloma and Waldenstrom's macroglobulinemia with monoclonal IgG lambda and IgM kappa in a single patient. *Acta Med Scand* 1981;209:229–234.

123. Lalayanni C, Theodoridou S, Athanasiadou A, et al. Simultaneous occurrence of multiple myeloma and Hodgkin's disease. A case report. *Haematologica* 2000;85:772–773.

124. Zech L, Hammarstrom L, Smith CI. Chromosomal aberrations

in a case of T-cell CLL with concomitant IgA myeloma. *Int J Cancer* 1983;32:431–435.

125. Cartron G, Roingeard P, Benboubker L, et al. Sezary syndrome in a patient with multiple myeloma: demonstration of a clonally distinct second malignancy. *Eur J Haematol* 1999;63:354–357.

126. Wickenhauser C, Borchmann P, Diehl V, et al. Development of IgG lambda multiple myeloma in a patient with cutaneous CD30+ anaplastic T-cell lymphoma. *Leuk Lymphoma* 1999;35:201–206.

127. Fink L, Bauer F, Perry JJ. Coincidental polycythemia vera and multiple myeloma: case report and review. *Am J Hematol* 1993;44:196–200.

128. Cobo F, Cervantes F, Martinez C, et al. Multiple myeloma following essential thrombocythemia. *Leuk Lymphoma* 1995;20:177–179.

129. Duhrsen U, Uppenkamp M, Meusers P, et al. Frequent association of idiopathic myelofibrosis with plasma cell dyscrasias. *Blut* 1988;56:97–102.

130. Hagen W, Schwarzmeier J, Walchshofer S, et al. A case of bone marrow mastocytosis associated with multiple myeloma. *Ann Hematol* 1998;76:167–174.

131. Nitta M, Tsuboi K, Yamashita S, et al. Multiple myeloma preceding the development of chronic myelogenous leukemia. *Int J Hematol* 1999;69:170–173.

132. Tanaka M, Kimura R, Matsutani A, et al. Coexistence of chronic myelogenous leukemia and multiple myeloma. Case report and review of the literature. *Acta Haematol* 1998;99:221–223.

133. Anderson CM, Bueso-Ramos CE, Wallner SA, et al. Primary myeloid leukemia presenting concomitantly with primary multiple myeloma: two cases and an update of the literature. *Leuk Lymphoma* 1999;32:385–390.

134. Hall R, Hopkinson N, Hamblin T. Relapsing polychondritis, smouldering non-secretory myeloma and early myelodysplastic syndrome in the same patient: three difficult diagnoses produce a life threatening illness. *Leuk Res* 2000;24:91–93.

135. Ng MH, Kan A, Chung YF, et al. Combined morphological and interphase fluorescence *in situ* hybridization study in multiple myeloma of Chinese patients. *Am J Pathol* 1999;154:15–22.

136. Rios R, Sole F, Gascon F. Simultaneous occurrence of the 5q- syndrome and multiple myeloma. *Clin Lab Haematol* 2000;22:49–53.

137. Schmetzer HM, Mittermuller J, Duell T, et al. Development of myeloma and secondary myelodysplastic syndrome from a common clone. *Cancer Genet Cytogenet* 1998;100:31–35.

138. Tsiara S, Economou G, Panteli A, et al. Coexistence of myelodysplastic syndrome and multiple myeloma. *J Exp Clin Cancer Res* 1999;18:565–566.

139. Chim CS, Ma SK, Leung CY. Malignant lymphoma masquerading as multiple myeloma. *Leuk Lymphoma* 1998;28:607–611.

140. Carmichael GP, Lee YT. Granulocytic sarcoma simulating "nonsecretory" multiple myeloma. *Hum Pathol* 1977;8:697–700.

141. Rossi JF, Bataille R, Chappard D, et al. B cell malignancies presenting with unusual bone involvement and mimicking multiple myeloma. Study of nine cases. *Am J Med* 1987;83:10–16.

142. Butler RC, Thomas SM, Thompson JM, et al. Anaplastic myeloma in systemic lupus erythematosus. *Ann Rheum Dis* 1984;43:653–655.

143. Fassas AB, Muwalla F, Berryman T, et al. Myeloma of the central nervous system: association with high-risk chromosomal abnormalities, plasmablastic morphology and extramedullary manifestations. *Br J Haematol* 2002;117:103–108.

144. Flaitz CM, Nichols CM, Walling DM, et al. Plasmablastic lymphoma: an HIV-associated entity with primary oral manifestations. *Oral Oncol* 2002;38:96–102.

145. Gaidano G, Cerri M, Capello D, et al. Molecular histogenesis of plasmablastic lymphoma of the oral cavity. *Br J Haematol* 2002;119:622–628.

146. Goh J, Otridge B, Brady H, et al. Aggressive multiple myeloma presenting as mesenteric panniculitis. *Am J Gastroenterol* 2001;96:238–241.

147. Jin DK, Nowakowski M, Kramer M, et al. Hyperviscosity syndrome secondary to a myeloma-associated IgG(1)kappa paraprotein strongly reactive against the HIV-1 p24 gag antigen. *Am J Hematol* 2000;64:210–213.

148. Lin Y, Rodrigues GD, Turner JF, et al. Plasmablastic lymphoma of the lung. *Arch Pathol Lab Med* 2001;125:282–285.

149. Maslovsky I, Lugassy G, Blumental R, et al. Multiple chromosomal abnormalities in fulminant anaplastic myeloma. *Clin Lab Haematol* 1999;21:207–210.

150. Oksenhendler E, Boulanger E, Galicier L, et al. High incidence of Kaposi sarcoma-associated herpesvirus-related non-Hodgkin lymphoma in patients with HIV infection and multicentric Castleman disease. *Blood* 2002;99:2331–2336.

151. Papadaki HA, Stefanaki K, Kanavaros P, et al. Epstein-Barr virus-associated high-grade anaplastic plasmacytoma in a renal transplant patient. *Leuk Lymphoma* 2000;36:411–415.

152. Robak T, Urbanska-Rys H, Strzelecka B, et al. Plasmablastic lymphoma in a patient with chronic lymphocytic leukemia heavily pretreated with cladribine (2-CdA): an unusual variant of Richter's syndrome. *Eur J Haematol* 2001;67:322–327.

153. Strand WR, Banks PM, Kyle RA. Anaplastic plasma cell myeloma and immunoblastic lymphoma. Clinical, pathologic, and immunologic comparison. *Am J Med* 1984;76:861–867.

154. Blade J, Kyle RA. Nonsecretory myeloma, immunoglobulin D myeloma, and plasma cell leukemia. *Hematol Oncol Clin North Am* 1999;13:1259–1272.

155. Garcia-Sanz R, Orfao A, Gonzalez M, et al. Primary plasma cell leukemia: clinical, immunophenotypic, DNA ploidy, and cytogenetic characteristics. *Blood* 1999;93:1032–1037.

156. Alonso ML, Rubiol E, Mateu R, et al. cCD79a expression in a case of plasma cell leukemia. *Leuk Res* 1998;22:649–653.

157. Avet-Loiseau H, Daviet A, Brigaudeau C, et al. Cytogenetic, interphase, and multicolor fluorescence *in situ* hybridization analyses in primary plasma cell leukemia: a study of 40 patients at diagnosis. *Blood* 2001;97:822–825.

158. Hermouet S, Corre I, Gassin M, et al. Hepatitis C virus, human herpesvirus 8, and the development of plasma cell leukemia. *N Engl J Med* 2003;348:178–179.

159. Kawada E, Shinonome S, Saitoh T, et al. Primary nonsecretory plasma cell leukemia: a rare variant of multiple myeloma. *Ann Hematol* 1999;78:25–27.

160. Kuo MC, Shih LY. Primary plasma cell leukemia with extensive dense osteosclerosis: complete remission following combination chemotherapy. *Ann Hematol* 1995;71:147–151.

161. Lloveras E, Sole F, Espinet B, et al. Cytogenetic and fluorescence *in situ* hybridization studies in four cases of plasma cell leukemia. *Cancer Genet Cytogenet* 2000;121:163–166.

162. Ohsaka A, Sato N, Imai Y, et al. Multiple gastric involvement by myeloid antigen CD13-positive non-secretory plasma cell leukaemia. *Br J Haematol* 1996;92:134–136.

163. Pasqualetti P, Casale R. Monoclonal gammopathy of undetermined significance evolving directly in primary plasma cell leukemia. *Biomed Pharmacother* 1997;51:284–285.

164. Pellat-Deceunynck C, Barille S, Jego G, et al. The absence of CD56 (NCAM) on malignant plasma cells is a hallmark of plasma cell leukemia and of a special subset of multiple myeloma. *Leukemia* 1998;12:1977–1982.

165. Richter J, Swedin A, Olofsson T, et al. Aggressive course of primary plasma cell leukemia with unusual morphological and cytogenetic features. *Ann Hematol* 1995;71:307–310.

166. Robak T, Urbanska-Rys H, Robak E, et al. Aggressive primary plasma cell leukemia with skin manifestations, trisomy 8 and molecular oligoclonal features. *Leuk Lymphoma* 2002;43:1067–1073.

167. Sajeva MR, Greco MM, Cascavilla N, et al. Effective autologous peripheral blood stem cell transplantation in plasma cell leukemia followed by T-large granular lymphocyte expansion: a case report. *Bone Marrow Transplant* 1996;18:225–227.

168. Singh VP, Rai M, Shukla J, et al. Chronic lymphocytic leukaemia terminating into plasma cell leukaemia. *J Assoc Physicians India* 2002;50:840–841.

169. Toth Z, Sipos J. Biclonal primary plasma cell leukemia. *Pathol Oncol Res* 1998;4:48–51.

170. Bertoni-Salateo R, de Camargo B, Soares F, et al. Solitary plasmocytoma of bone in an adolescent. *J Pediatr Hematol Oncol* 1998;20:574–576.

171. Dimopoulos MA, Moulopoulos LA, Maniatis A, et al. Solitary plasmacytoma of bone and asymptomatic multiple myeloma. *Blood* 2000;96:2037–2044.

172. Franchi F, De Rosa F, Seminara P, et al. Hypereosinophilic syndrome and plasmocytoma. Report of a case and review of the literature. *Acta Haematol* 1984;72:14–20.

173. Karasick D, Schweitzer ME, Miettinen M, et al. Osseous metaplasia associated with amyloid-producing plasmacytoma of bone: a report of two cases. *Skeletal Radiol* 1996;25:263–267.

174. Kyle RA. Monoclonal gammopathy of undetermined significance and solitary plasmacytoma. Implications for progression to overt multiple myeloma. *Hematol Oncol Clin North Am* 1997;11:71–87.

175. Pambuccian SE, Horyd ID, Cawte T, et al. Amyloidoma of bone, a plasma cell/plasmacytoid neoplasm. Report of three cases and review of the literature. *Am J Surg Pathol* 1997;21:179–186.

176. Sakai A, Fujii T, Noda M, et al. Plasma cells composing plasmacytoma have phenotypes different from those of myeloma cells. *Am J Hematol* 1996;53:251–253.

Clonal Immunoglobulin Disorders

1. Buxbaum J. Mechanisms of disease: monoclonal immunoglobulin deposition. Amyloidosis, light chain deposition disease, and light and heavy chain deposition disease. *Hematol Oncol Clin North Am* 1992;6:323–346.

2. Eulitz M, Weiss DT, Solomon A. Immunoglobulin heavy-chain-associated amyloidosis. *Proc Natl Acad Sci U S A* 1990;87:6542–6546.

3. Liapis H, Papadakis I, Nakopoulou L. Nodular glomerulosclerosis secondary to mu heavy chain deposits. *Hum Pathol* 2000;31:122–125.

4. Sakka T, Meknini B, Ayed K, et al. An unusual case of heavy alpha chain disease associated with amyloidosis. *Tunis Med* 1986;64:161–164.

5. Solomon A, Weiss DT, Murphy C. Primary amyloidosis associated with a novel heavy-chain fragment (AH amyloidosis). *Am J Hematol* 1994;45:171–176.

6. Kyle RA. Clinical aspects of multiple myeloma and related disorders including amyloidosis. *Pathol Biol (Paris)* 1999;47:148–157.

7. Sezer O, Eucker J, Jakob C, et al. Diagnosis and treatment of AL amyloidosis. *Clin Nephrol* 2000;53:417–423.

8. Mohr A, Miehlke S, Klauck S, et al. Hepatomegaly and cholestasis as primary clinical manifestations of an AL-kappa amyloidosis. *Eur J Gastroenterol Hepatol* 1999;11:921–925.

9. Nowak G, Westermark P, Wernerson A, et al. Liver transplantation as rescue treatment in a patient with primary AL kappa amyloidosis. *Transpl Int* 2000;13:92–97.

10. Choufani EB, Sanchorawala V, Ernst T, et al. Acquired factor X deficiency in patients with amyloid light-chain amyloidosis: incidence, bleeding manifestations, and response to high-dose chemotherapy. *Blood* 2001;97:1885–1887.

11. Mumford AD, O'Donnell J, Gillmore JD, et al. Bleeding symptoms and coagulation abnormalities in 337 patients with AL-amyloidosis. *Br J Haematol* 2000;110:454–460.

12. Casiraghi MA, De Paoli A, Assi A, et al. Hepatic amyloidosis with light chain deposition disease. A rare association. *Dig Liver Dis* 2000;32:795–798.

13. Kaloterakis A, Filiotou A, Koskinas J, et al. Systemic AL amyloidosis in Gaucher disease. A case report and review of the literature. *J Intern Med* 1999;246:587–590.

14. Stather D, Ford S, Kisilevsky R. Sarcoid, amyloid, and acute myocardial failure. *Mod Pathol* 1998;11:901–904.

15. Zhou H, Linke RP, Schaefer HE, et al. Progressive liver failure in a patient with adult Niemann-Pick disease associated with generalized AL amyloidosis. *Virchows Arch* 1995;426:635–639.

16. Fonseca R, Ahmann GJ, Jalal SM, et al. Chromosomal abnormalities in systemic amyloidosis. *Br J Haematol* 1998;103:704–710.

17. Amparo E, Kaplan L, Rosenbloom B, et al. T-gamma-lymphoproliferative disorder arising in a background of autoimmune disease and terminating in plasma cell dyscrasia with primary amyloidosis. *Arch Pathol Lab Med* 1991;115:74–77.

18. Chan KW, Ho CP. Amyloidosis complicating idiopathic myelofibrosis. *Am J Kidney Dis* 1999;34:E27.

19. Gold JE, Louis-Charles A, Ghali V, et al. T-cell chronic lymphocytic leukemia. Unusual morphologic, phenotypic, and karyotypic features in association with light chain amyloidosis. *Cancer* 1992;70:86–93.

20. Kilpatrick SE, Wenger DE, Gilchrist GS, et al. Langerhans' cell histiocytosis (histiocytosis X) of bone. A clinicopathologic analysis of 263 pediatric and adult cases. *Cancer* 1995;76:2471–2484.

21. Lanjewar DN, Raghuwanshi SR, Gupta D, et al. Systemic amyloidosis in Hodgkin's disease. *Indian J Pathol Microbiol* 1998;41:169–171.

22. Laudet J, Baumelou E, Chaignon M, et al. Amyloidosis and polycythemia vera. *Semin Hop* 1981;57:1951–1954.

23. Morschhauser F, Wattel E, Pagniez D, et al. Glomerular injury in chronic myelomonocytic leukemia. *Leuk Lymphoma* 1995;18:479–483.

24. Shimm DS, Logue GL, Rohlfing MB, et al. Primary amyloidosis, pure red cell aplasia, and Kaposi's sarcoma in a single patient. *Cancer* 1979;44:1501–1503.

25. Lachmann HJ, Booth DR, Booth SE, et al. Misdiagnosis of hereditary amyloidosis as AL (primary) amyloidosis. *N Engl J Med* 2002;346:1786–1791.

26. Buxbaum J, Gallo G. Nonamyloidotic monoclonal immunoglobulin deposition disease. Light-chain, heavy-chain, and light- and heavy-chain deposition diseases. *Hematol Oncol Clin North Am* 1999;13:1235–1248.

27. Lin J, Markowitz GS, Valeri AM, et al. Renal monoclonal immunoglobulin deposition disease: the disease spectrum. *J Am Soc Nephrol* 2001;12:1482–1492.

28. Preud'homme JL, Aucouturier P, Touchard G, et al. Monoclonal immunoglobulin deposition disease: a review of immunoglobulin chain alterations. *Int J Immunopharmacol* 1994;16:425–431.

29. Cheng IK, Ho SK, Chan DT, et al. Crescentic nodular glomerulosclerosis secondary to truncated immunoglobulin alpha heavy chain deposition. *Am J Kidney Dis* 1996;28:283–288.

30. Daliani D, Weber D, Alexanian R. Light-heavy chain deposition disease progressing to multiple myeloma. *Am J Hematol* 1995;50:296–298.

31. Danevad M, Sletten K, Gaarder PI, et al. The amino acid sequence of a monoclonal gamma 3-heavy chain from a patient

with articular gamma-heavy chain deposition disease. *Scand J Immunol* 2000;51:602–606.

32. Tichy M, Stulik J, Osanec J, et al. Electrophoretic characterization of a gamma-1-heavy chain disease. *Neoplasma* 2000;47:118–121.

33. Kubo Y, Morita T, Koda Y, et al. Two types of glomerular lesion in non-amyloid immunoglobulin deposition disease: a case report of IgD-lambda myeloma. *Clin Nephrol* 1990;33:259–263.

34. Rabhi H, Ghaffor M, Abbadi MC. Spontaneous enzymatic cleavage of IgD myeloma protein giving a pattern of delta heavy chain disease. *Arch Inst Pasteur Alger* 1989;57:135–140.

35. Da'as N, Kleinman Y, Polliack A, et al. Immunotactoid glomerulopathy with massive bone marrow deposits in a patient with IgM kappa monoclonal gammopathy and hypocomplementemia. *Am J Kidney Dis* 2001;38:395–399.

36. Liapis H, Papadakis I, Nakopoulou L. Nodular glomerulosclerosis secondary to mu heavy chain deposits. *Hum Pathol* 2000;31:122–125.

37. Wahner-Roedler DL, Kyle RA. Mu-heavy chain disease: presentation as a benign monoclonal gammopathy. *Am J Hematol* 1992;40:56–60.

38. Baur A, Stabler A, Lamerz R, et al. Light chain deposition disease in multiple myeloma: MR imaging features correlated with histopathological findings. *Skeletal Radiol* 1998;27:173–176.

39. Buxbaum JN, Genega EM, Lazowski P, et al. Infiltrative non-amyloidotic monoclonal immunoglobulin light chain cardiomyopathy: an underappreciated manifestation of plasma cell dyscrasias. *Cardiology* 2000;93:220–228.

40. Casiraghi MA, De Paoli A, Assi A, et al. Hepatic amyloidosis with light chain deposition disease. A rare association. *Dig Liver Dis* 2000;32:795–798.

41. de Lajarte-Thirouard AS, Molina T, Audouin J, et al. Spleen localization of light chain deposition disease associated with sea blue histiocytosis, revealed by spontaneous rupture. *Virchows Arch* 1999;434:463–465.

42. Grassi MP, Clerici F, Perin C, et al. Light chain deposition disease neuropathy resembling amyloid neuropathy in a multiple myeloma patient. *Ital J Neurol Sci* 1998;19:229–233.

43. Gu X, Barrios R, Cartwright J, et al. Light chain crystal deposition as a manifestation of plasma cell dyscrasias: the role of immunoelectron microscopy. *Hum Pathol* 2003;34:270–277.

44. Jones D, Bhatia VK, Krausz T, et al. Crystal-storing histiocytosis: a disorder occurring in plasmacytic tumors expressing immunoglobulin kappa light chain. *Hum Pathol* 1999;30:1441–1448.

45. Rostagno A, Frizzera G, Ylagan L, et al. Tumoral non-amyloidotic monoclonal immunoglobulin light chain deposits ('aggregoma'):

presenting feature of B-cell dyscrasia in three cases with immunohistochemical and biochemical analyses. *Br J Haematol* 2002;119:62–69.

46. Vidal R, Goni F, Stevens F, et al. Somatic mutations of the L12a gene in V-kappa(1) light chain deposition disease: potential effects on aberrant protein conformation and deposition. *Am J Pathol* 1999;155:2009–2017.

Clinicopathologic Syndromes

1. Jaccard A, Royer B, Bordessoule D, et al. High-dose therapy and autologous blood stem cell transplantation in POEMS syndrome. *Blood* 2002;99:3057–3059.

2. Jackson A, Burton IE. A case of POEMS syndrome associated with essential thrombocythaemia and dermal mastocytosis. *Postgrad Med J* 1990;66:761–767.

3. Kihara Y, Hori H, Murakami H, et al. A case of POEMS syndrome associated with reactive amyloidosis and Waldenstrom's macroglobulinaemia. *J Intern Med* 2002;252:255–258.

4. Lipsker D, Rondeau M, Massard G, et al. The AESOP (adenopathy and extensive skin patch overlying a plasmacytoma) syndrome: report of 4 cases of a new syndrome revealing POEMS (polyneuropathy, organomegaly, endocrinopathy, monoclonal protein, and skin changes) syndrome at a curable stage. *Medicine (Baltimore)* 2003;82:51–59.

5. Murphy PT, Ahmed N, Hassan HT. Chronic myeloid leukemia and acromegaly in POEMS syndrome. *Leuk Res* 2002;26:1135–1137.

6. Pavord SR, Murphy PT, Mitchell VE. POEMS syndrome and Waldenstrom's macroglobulinaemia. *J Clin Pathol* 1996;49:181–182.

7. Rose C, Zandecki M, Copin MC, et al. POEMS syndrome: report on six patients with unusual clinical signs, elevated levels of cytokines, macrophage involvement and chromosomal aberrations of bone marrow plasma cells. *Leukemia* 1997;11:1318–1323.

8. Schulz W, Domenico D, Nand S. POEMS syndrome associated with polycythemia vera. *Cancer* 1989;63:1175–1178.

9. Weichenthal M, Stemm AV, Ramsauer J, et al. POEMS syndrome: cicatricial alopecia as an unusual cutaneous manifestation associated with an underlying plasmacytoma. *J Am Acad Dermatol* 1999;40:808–812.

10. Zenone T, Bastion Y, Salles G, et al. POEMS syndrome, arterial thrombosis and thrombocythaemia. *J Intern Med* 1996;240:107–109.

11. Lipsker D, Veran Y, Grunenberger F, et al. The Schnitzler syndrome. Four new cases and review of the literature. *Medicine (Baltimore)* 2001;80:37–44.

27

T-CELL NEOPLASMS

The T-cell neoplasms are a heterogeneous group, and their terminology is still evolving. This chapter uses a simplified version of the World Health Organization classification (Tables 27-1 and 27-2). Neoplasms composed predominantly of mature small to medium-sized T-cells may be difficult to distinguish from one another in the bone marrow (Table 27-3).

PRECURSOR T-CELL NEOPLASM

T-Cell Lymphoblastic Lymphoma

T-cell lymphoblastic lymphoma is found predominantly in young male patients, who often present with involvement of the mediastinum, pleural and pericardial cavities, lymph nodes, and central nervous system (1–31) (Fig. 27-1). Cases with prominent peripheral blood and bone marrow disease at the outset are better classified as precursor T-cell acute lymphoblastic leukemia. T-cell lymphoblastic lymphoma arises *de novo,* as a therapy-related malignancy, and as a blast crisis of chronic myeloid leukemia. It typically has an aggressive course, with eventual development of disseminated disease and a leukemic phase.

The peripheral blood and bone marrow may show blasts, comprising less than 25% of nucleated cells. Histologic sections of the bone marrow may show focal or patchy disease,

as opposed to the uniform involvement usually seen in acute lymphoblastic leukemia.

Immunophenotyping usually shows expression of CD1, CD2, CD3, CD4, CD5, CD7, CD8, CD38, CD43, CD45, CD57, CD99, T-cell receptor (TCR) α/β, and terminal deoxynucleotidyl transferase (TdT). Compared with normal T-cells, expression of pan–T-cell markers (CD2, CD3, CD5, CD7) may be decreased. CD10 is expressed in more than 50% of cases. Occasional cases fail to express CD2, CD4, CD5, CD8, and/or TdT. Some cases express TCR γ/δ instead of TCR α/β. CD13, CD33, CD19, CD20, CD34, CD56, and CD79a are variably expressed. In some cases, coexpression of myeloid or B-cell antigens may warrant interpretation as biphenotypic lymphoblastic lymphoma. In a few instances, conversion from T-cell to myeloid, histiocytic, or B-cell lineage has been documented (11,16,26).

Genetic studies have demonstrated various clonal karyotypic anomalies, often involving the TCR γ-chain gene at chromosome 7p15, the TCR β-chain gene at chromosome 7q35, and the TCR α- and δ-chain genes at 14q11. TCR gene rearrangements are found in approximately 75% to 80% of cases, involving (in decreasing order) the TCR δ-, γ-, and β-chain genes. Concomitant immunoglobulin H (IgH) gene rearrangement is found in approximately 10% of cases. Detection of *BCR/ABL* rearrangement helps to classify a case of T-cell lymphoblastic lymphoma as a blast crisis of chronic myeloid leukemia.

TABLE 27-1. CLASSIFICATION OF T-CELL NEOPLASMS ACCORDING TO THE WORLD HEALTH ORGANIZATION

Precursor T-cell neoplasm
  T-cell lymphoblastic lymphoma

Mature T-cell neoplasms
  T-cell prolymphocytic leukemia
  T-cell large granular lymphocytic leukemia
  Adult T-cell leukemia/lymphoma
  Extranodal natural killer cell/T-cell lymphoma, nasal type
  Enteropathy-type T-cell lymphoma
  Hepatosplenic T-cell lymphoma
  Subcutaneous panniculitis-like T-cell lymphoma
  Mycosis fungoides/Sézary syndrome
  Primary cutaneous CD30+ T-cell lymphoproliferative disorders
  Angioimmunoblastic T-cell lymphoma
  Peripheral T-cell lymphoma, unspecified
  Anaplastic large cell lymphoma

TABLE 27-2. ORGANIZATION OF T-CELL NEOPLASMS IN THIS CHAPTER

Precursor T-cell neoplasm
  T-cell lymphoblastic lymphoma

Mature T-cell neoplasms
  CD4+ T-cell chronic lymphocytic leukemia
  CD8+ T-cell chronic lymphocytic leukemia*
  T-cell prolymphocytic leukemia
  Adult T-cell leukemia/lymphoma
  Hepatosplenic T-cell lymphoma
  Mycosis fungoides/Sézary syndrome
  Peripheral T-cell lymphoma
  Anaplastic large T-cell lymphoma

*T-cell large granular lymphocytic leukemia.

TABLE 27-3. DIFFERENTIAL FEATURES OF MATURE, SMALL TO MEDIUM-SIZED T-CELL NEOPLASMS

	CD4 CLL	CD8 CLL	PLL	ATLL	HSTL	MF/SS	PTCL
Leukemia	+	+	+	+	+/−	+/−	+/−
Cyto gran	Rare	+	−	+/−	Rare	−	Rare
CD4	+	Rare	+/−	+/−	−	+	+/−
CD8	Rare	+	−/+	−/+	+/−	−	−/+
TCR α/β	+	+/−	+/−	+	Rare	+	+/−
TCR γ/δ	−	−/+	−/+	−	+	−	−/+

ATLL, adult T-cell leukemia/lymphoma; CD4 CLL, CD4+ T-cell chronic lymphocytic leukemia; CD8 CLL, CD8+ T-cell chronic lymphocytic leukemia or T-cell large granular lymphocytic leukemia; cyto gran, cytoplasmic granules; HSTL, hepatosplenic T-cell lymphoma; MF, mycosis fungoides/Sézary syndrome; PLL, T-cell prolymphocytic leukemia; PTCL, peripheral T-cell lymphoma; TCR α/β, T-cell receptor α/β; TCR γ/δ, T-cell receptor γ/δ; +, positive; −, negative; +/−, usually positive, sometimes negative; −/+, usually negative, sometimes positive.

The differential diagnosis includes 8p11 myeloproliferative disorder; other high-grade clonal T-cell, B-cell, and natural killer cell neoplasms; and nonhematolymphoid small round cell tumors, such as Ewing sarcoma.

MATURE T-CELL NEOPLASMS

CD4+ T-Cell Chronic Lymphocytic Leukemia

CD4+ T-cell chronic lymphocytic leukemia (TCLL) is a rare disorder that predominates in male patients, who may present with modest lymphadenopathy, hepatosplenomegaly, and skin lesions (1–28) (Fig. 27-2). CD4+ TCLL occurs *de novo* and as a complication of ataxia telangiectasia. It has a variable course, ranging from indolent to aggressive. CD4+ TCLL may undergo morphologic transformation to T-cell prolymphocytic leukemia (TPLL).

The peripheral blood shows cytopenias and absolute lymphocytosis from 4 to more than 800×10^9 cells/L. The lymphocytes are mainly small, with less than 10% larger cells.

The nuclei are predominantly round to oval, occasionally irregular or "knobby." The chromatin is condensed, and nucleoli are inconspicuous or absent. The cytoplasm is scant and usually agranular; however, rare cases have been reported showing granular cytoplasm (13,25). Eosinophilia may be present.

Bone marrow aspirate smears show small atypical lymphocytes, as described above. Histologic sections of the bone marrow may show an interstitial infiltrate of small lymphocytes. Other disorders reported with CD4+ TCLL include multiple myeloma and clonal amyloidosis.

Immunophenotyping usually shows expression of CD2, CD3, CD4, CD5, CD25, CD45, and TCR α/β. CD8 (15) and CD57 may be coexpressed. TdT is not expressed.

Genetic studies have shown various clonal karyotypic anomalies, frequently involving the TCR α-chain gene at chromosome 14q11. Concomitant immunoglobulin gene rearrangements have also been reported.

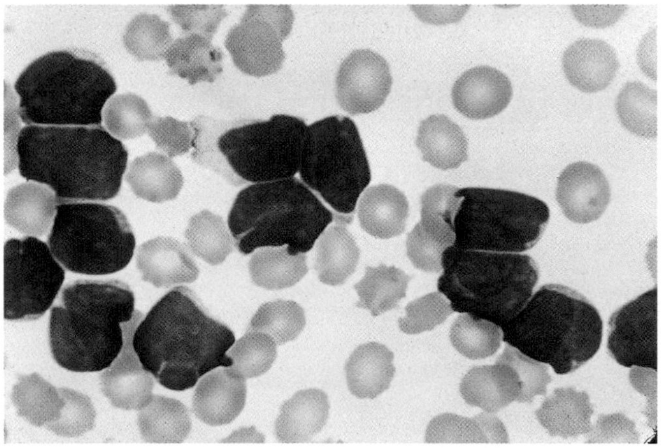

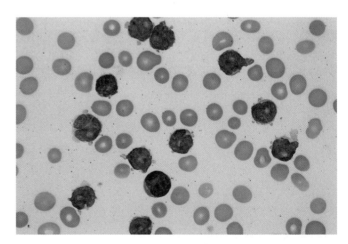

FIGURE 27-2. Peripheral blood smear, CD4+ T-cell chronic lymphocytic leukemia. Small, atypical lymphocytes show irregular nuclear contours, condensed chromatin, and a single nucleolus in this specimen from a 70-year-old man with chronic leukemia. The neoplastic cells showed a characteristic pericentric inversion of chromosome 14, involving bands q11.2 and q32, as well as other clonal karyotypic anomalies.

FIGURE 27-1. Peripheral blood smear, T-cell lymphoblastic lymphoma. Numerous blasts, many with deep nuclear cleaves, are present in this specimen from a patient with leukemic spread of a mediastinal tumor.

The differential diagnosis includes reactive T-cell lymphocytosis (which may be clonal although clinically nonmalignant), CD8+ TCLL with CD4 coexpression, CD4+ TPLL, and other clonal T-cell disorders.

CD8+ T-Cell Chronic Lymphocytic Leukemia (T-Cell Large Granular Lymphocytic Leukemia)

CD8+ TCLL accounts for approximately 90% of cases of large granular cell lymphocytic leukemia (1,7,9,29–68) (Figs. 27-3 through 27-5). Although commonly termed large granular lymphocytic leukemia, it should be kept in mind that large granular cell morphology is also seen in natural killer cell lymphocytosis and rarely in CD4+ TCLL (13,25).

Presenting features of CD8+ TCLL include splenomegaly, recurrent infections caused by neutropenia, autoimmune disorders, and skin lesions. CD8+ TCLL occurs *de novo,* as a complication of rheumatoid arthritis and other autoimmune disorders, and possibly as a result of human T-cell lymphotropic virus type II (HTLV-II) infection (49,59). Approximately one-third of CD8+ TCLL cases occur in patients with a prior diagnosis of rheumatoid arthritis and Felty syndrome; conversely, approximately one-third of patients with rheumatoid arthritis and Felty syndrome have large granular lymphocytosis. CD8+ TCLL usually has an indolent, slowly progressive course and may show spontaneous regression. Clinically aggressive cases are characterized by marked lymphocytosis, splenomegaly, hypercalcemia, and CD56 expression (38,57,66,67). Transformation from indolent disease to high-grade large T-cell lymphoma has been reported (51).

The peripheral blood shows macrocytic or normocytic anemia, neutropenia, and variable numbers of large granular lymphocytes, with absolute lymphocyte counts ranging from 0.75 to 24 × 10⁹ cells/L. In some cases, lymphocytosis

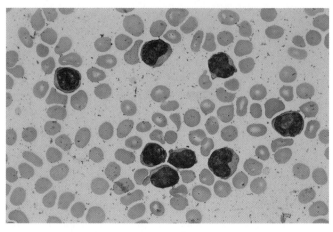

FIGURE 27-4. Peripheral blood smear, CD8+ T-cell chronic lymphocytic leukemia (T-cell large granular lymphocytic leukemia). Compared with those in Figure 27-3, the clonal cells are slightly larger and show more irregular nuclei, less abundant cytoplasm, and almost no granules. This specimen is from a patient with co-existing follicular lymphoma.

is initially absent. The lymphocytes show variable nuclear morphology and moderately abundant cytoplasm with dispersed reddish granules. Rare cases show hairy cell–like morphology and/or fail to show cytoplasmic granules (34,52,58). Concomitant reactive natural killer cell lymphocytosis may be present (44,64).

Bone marrow aspirate smears show variable numbers of large granular lymphocytes. Histologic sections of the bone marrow show hypercellularity, with variable amounts of hematopoietic tissue. Large granular lymphocytes may be present as a diffuse interstitial infiltrate, in aggregates, and/or in an intrasinusoidal pattern. Lymphocytic infiltration is subtle or morphologically undetectable in some cases. The hematopoietic tissue may show a decreased myeloid:erythroid ratio, megaloblastic change, and a shift in myelopoiesis

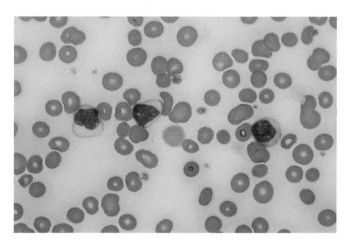

FIGURE 27-3. Peripheral blood smear, CD8+ T-cell chronic lymphocytic leukemia (T-cell large granular lymphocytic leukemia). The clonal cells resemble normal T-cell large granular lymphocytes.

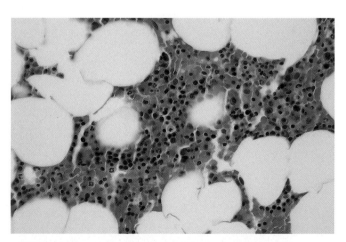

FIGURE 27-5. Bone marrow biopsy specimen, CD8+ T-cell chronic lymphocytic leukemia (T-cell large granular lymphocytic leukemia). Granulocytes are virtually absent in this specimen from a patient with rheumatoid arthritis and Felty syndrome.

toward immature forms. Other findings may include pure red cell aplasia, amegakaryocytosis, fibrosis, and sarcoidosis. Other disorders reported with CD8+ TCLL include myeloid diseases, B-cell neoplasms, Hodgkin lymphoma, and plasma cell proliferations.

Immunophenotyping usually shows expression of CD2, CD3, CD5, CD7, CD8, CD11b, CD16, CD38, CD45, HLA-DR, granzyme B, TIA-1, and TCR α/β. Compared with normal T cells, expression of pan–T-cell antigens (CD2, CD3, CD5, CD7) may be reduced or absent. Some cases express TCR γ/δ rather than TCR α/β. CD57 is usually, but not always, expressed. CD4, CD20, and CD56 may be expressed. CD25 is typically not expressed. Rare cases lack CD8 expression (43,62,63). TdT is not expressed.

Genetic studies have shown various clonal karyotypic anomalies, including abnormalities involving chromosomes 7p14-15, the site of the TCR γ-chain gene; and chromosome 14q11, the site of the TCR α- and δ-chain genes. Concomitant immunoglobulin gene rearrangement has also been reported.

The differential diagnosis includes reactive T-cell lymphocytosis (which may be clonal although clinically nonmalignant), CD4+ TCLL with large granular lymphocyte morphology or CD8 coexpression, CD8+ TPLL, other clonal T-cell disorders, and reactive and neoplastic natural killer cell proliferations.

T-Cell Prolymphocytic Leukemia

TPLL occurs predominantly in male patients, who often present with marked hepatosplenomegaly, lymphadenopathy, effusions, skin lesions, and/or thrombosis (1,9,15,69–110) (Fig. 27-6). TPLL occurs *de novo,* as a complication of ataxia telangiectasia and HTLV-I infection, and as a transformation of TCLL and hepatosplenic T-cell lymphoma. It has a variable course, ranging from indolent (or spontaneously remitting) to aggressive. Transformations to large T-cell lymphoma and myeloid/T-cell lymphoblastic lymphoma have been reported (79,80,87).

The peripheral blood typically shows anemia, thrombocytopenia, and lymphocytosis, sometimes exceeding 900 × 10^9 cells/L. Cases with leukopenia may resemble hairy cell leukemia (101). Prolymphocytes are larger than normal lymphocytes and have a round to oval nucleus, moderately condensed chromatin, and a single, prominent nucleolus. The cytoplasm is variable in quantity and typically agranular. Morphologic variants may show nuclei that are small, large, irregular, carrot shaped, or Sézary-like/cerebriform (72,73,77,81,86,89,90,95,96,100).

Bone marrow aspirate smears show a variable number of T-prolymphocytes. Histologic sections of the bone marrow show an interstitial, diffuse, and/or nodular prolymphocytic infiltrate, sometimes with fibrosis. Other disorders reported with TPLL include large B-cell lymphoma and Hodgkin lymphoma.

Immunophenotyping usually shows expression of CD2, CD3, CD5, and CD7. Compared with normal T-cells, expression of pan–T-cell antigens (CD2, CD3, CD5, CD7) may be reduced or absent (39). TPLL cells also express (in decreasing order) CD4 only, CD4 and CD8, CD8 only, or neither CD4 nor CD8. Either TCR α/β or γ/δ may be expressed. CD16, CD20, CD56, TIA-1, and perforin may be expressed. CD1 and TdT are not expressed.

Genetic studies have shown various clonal karyotypic abnormalities, especially involving chromosome band Xq28; chromosome band 14q11, the site of the TCR α- and δ-chain genes; chromosome band 14q32, the site of *IgH;* and chromosome band 11q23, the site of *ATM* (ataxia telangiectasia mutated gene) (104,105,110).

The differential diagnosis includes reactive T-cell lymphocytosis (which may be clonal although clinically nonmalignant), TCLL, B-cell PLL, and acute leukemia.

Adult T-Cell Leukemia/Lymphoma

Adult T-cell leukemia/lymphoma (ATLL) is a clonal T-cell disorder usually caused by HTLV-I or, less often, by HTLV-II infection (39,111–144) (Figs. 27-7 and 27-8). ATLL often presents with hypercalcemia and disseminated disease involving skin, lymph nodes, liver, spleen, peripheral blood, and bone marrow. The clinical course is usually aggressive, and the prognosis is poor. Spontaneous remission occurs but may be transient (118,121,137,138).

The peripheral blood shows cytopenias and absolute lymphocytosis. The abnormal lymphocytes are typically heterogeneous, consisting of a range of small and large cells. Nuclei range from small and irregular to large and prominently lobated. Nucleoli may be present. The cytoplasm is scant to moderately abundant and basophilic and may contain inclusions, vacuoles, and/or granules, and may display

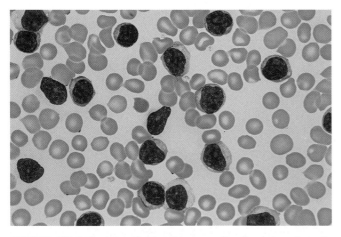

FIGURE 27-6. Peripheral blood smear, T-cell prolymphocytic leukemia. The neoplastic cells are larger than normal T-cell large granular lymphocytes and show a prominent nucleolus.

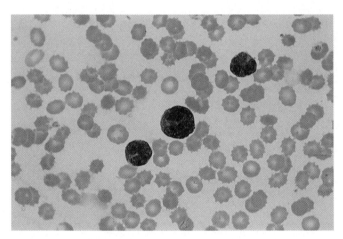

FIGURE 27-7. Peripheral blood smear, adult T-cell leukemia/lymphoma. The neoplastic cells vary in size and show pleomorphic nuclei in this specimen from a patient with positive serology for human T-cell lymphotropic virus type II.

tartrate-resistant acid phosphatase activity. Many morphologic variants are recognized. ATLL may resemble Burkitt lymphoma, lymphoblastic lymphoma, TCLL, anaplastic large cell lymphoma, or mycosis fungoides/Sézary syndrome.

Bone marrow aspirate smears show variable numbers of abnormal lymphocytes. Histologic sections of the bone marrow show a patchy to diffuse interstitial infiltrate composed of abnormal lymphocytes. Other findings include hemophagocytic syndrome and osteitis fibrosa cystica owing to tumor cell secretion of parathormone-related protein (114,142). Other disorders reported with ATLL and/or HTLV-I infection include myeloid diseases and B-cell neoplasms.

Immunophenotyping usually shows expression of CD2, CD3, CD4, CD7, CD25, and TCR α/β. Compared with

normal T cells, expression of pan–T-cell antigens (CD2, CD3, CD5, CD7) may be reduced or absent. Some cases express both CD4 and CD8 (15,125), CD8 only (126), or neither CD4 nor CD8 (132). In CD8+ cases, granzyme B and TIA-1 (but not perforin) may be expressed (126). CD20, CD30, CD56, epithelial membrane antigen, and S100 protein are expressed in some cases.

Genetic studies have shown various clonal karyotypic anomalies, especially del(6q) and TCR gene rearrangements and deletions. Clonal integration of HTLV-I proviral DNA into tumor cells is consistently found.

The differential diagnosis includes other T-cell neoplasms, clonal B-cell and natural killer cell disorders, and acute leukemia.

Hepatosplenic T-Cell Lymphoma

Hepatosplenic T-cell lymphoma is rare disorder, often occurring in young male patients and immunosuppressed patients with a history of solid organ transplantation (37,74,145–167) (Figs. 27-9 and 27-10). The predominant finding is hepatosplenomegaly, with peripheral blood and bone marrow disease occurring at any time during the clinical course. Transformation to prolymphocytic and blastlike morphology has been reported (151,157,160).

The peripheral blood may show cytopenias, sometimes immune-mediated, and lymphocytosis. The abnormal lymphocytes are typically monomorphic, medium-sized cells, with round to folded nuclei, condensed chromatin, and agranular cytoplasm. Occasional cases have been described showing larger, more pleomorphic cells or granular cytoplasm (153,166).

Bone marrow aspirate smears show abnormal lymphocytes. Histologic sections of the bone marrow show interstitial and/or sinusoidal infiltration by abnormal lymphocytes

FIGURE 27-8. Bone marrow biopsy specimen, adult T-cell leukemia/lymphoma. The hematopoietic tissue is replaced by neoplastic cells of variable size and shape embedded in fibrous tissue in this specimen from a patient with positive serology for human T-cell lymphotropic virus type II.

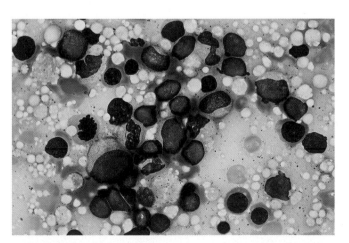

FIGURE 27-9. Touch imprint of bone marrow biopsy specimen, hepatosplenic T-cell lymphoma. Small and large neoplastic cells with condensed chromatin and agranular cytoplasm are present. The cells were positive by flow cytometry for T-cell receptor γ/δ and negative for T-cell receptor α/β.

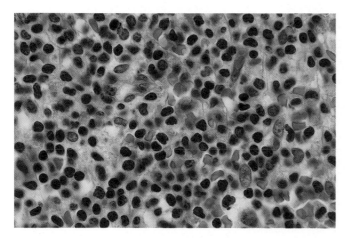

FIGURE 27-10. Bone marrow biopsy specimen, hepatosplenic T-cell lymphoma. The hematopoietic tissue is replaced by a diffuse infiltrate of small lymphocytes with clear cytoplasm. The cells were positive by flow cytometry for T-cell receptor γ/δ and negative for T-cell receptor α/β.

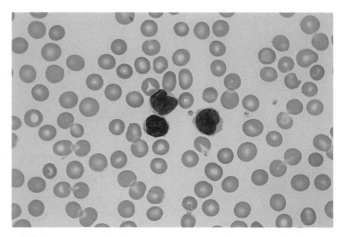

FIGURE 27-11. Peripheral blood smear, mycosis fungoides/Sézary syndrome. Abnormal lymphocytes with deeply cleaved nuclei and condensed chromatin are present.

(33). Other findings include hemophagocytic syndrome and fibrosis, either of which may obscure the underlying malignancy (152,163,167).

Immunophenotyping usually shows expression of CD2, CD3, CD7, TCR γ/δ, granzyme B, and TIA-1. Compared with normal T-cells, expression of pan–T-cell antigens (CD2, CD3, CD5, CD7) may be reduced or absent. CD8, CD16, CD56, and perforin are variably expressed. Occasional cases show expression of TCR α/β rather than TCR γ/δ (150,159). CD1, CD4, CD57, and TdT are not expressed.

Genetic studies often show isochromosome 7q, trisomy 8, and TCR gene rearrangements. Clonal integration of Epstein-Barr virus genome has been reported (153).

The differential diagnosis includes other T-cell neoplasms, especially those expressing TCR γ/δ.

Mycosis Fungoides/Sézary Syndrome

Mycosis fungoides and Sézary syndrome (MF/SS) are the localized and systemic forms, respectively, of CD4+ epidermotropic T-cell lymphoma (168–204) (Fig. 27-11). The clinical course is indolent to progressive. Transformation to large T-cell lymphoma has been reported (175,184, 196,201).

Peripheral blood involvement is frequent and occurs even with minimal skin disease (187,196,199,201). Findings include cytopenias, eosinophilia, and lymphocytosis. The abnormal lymphocytes, or Sézary cells, are variable in size, with irregular to cerebriform nuclei, condensed chromatin, inconspicuous nucleoli, and scant agranular cytoplasm, rarely showing cytoplasmic inclusions or peripheral hairy projections.

Bone marrow aspirate smears show variable numbers of abnormal lymphocytes. Histologic sections of the bone mar-

row show aggregates and infiltrates of abnormal lymphocytes of variable size, usually with smaller cells predominating. Hemophagocytic syndrome may obscure the malignant cells (183). Other findings may include eosinophilia, monocytosis, and storage histiocytosis (185,186,191). Other disorders reported with MF/SS include myeloid diseases, B-cell neoplasms, Hodgkin lymphoma, and plasma cell neoplasms (172,174,182,190,192,194).

Immunophenotyping usually shows expression of CD2, CD3, CD4, CD5, CD7, and TCR α/β. Compared with normal T-cells, expression of pan–T-cell antigens (CD2, CD3, CD5, CD7) may be reduced or absent. Some cases express TCR γ/δ rather than TCR α/β. CD10 and/or CD30 may be expressed. Granzyme B and TIA-1 are not expressed. Rare cases have been reported in which CD8 rather than CD4 is expressed and TIA-1 is coexpressed (170,178); such cases are better classified as peripheral T-cell lymphoma rather than MF/SS.

Genetic studies have shown various clonal karyotypic anomalies, especially del(17p) with *p53* deletion, and TCR gene rearrangements.

The differential diagnosis includes B-cell neoplasms and other T-cell neoplasms, especially those showing Sézary-like morphology (72,189,203).

Peripheral T-Cell Lymphoma

Peripheral T-cell lymphomas (PTCL) are essentially mature T-cell neoplasms that do not fit into other categories (37,205–250) (Figs. 27-12 through 27-16). They have been reported under a variety of names, sometimes according to site of origin or immunophenotype. They arise in lymph nodes, skin, sinuses, nasopharynx, gastrointestinal tract, and other sites. PTCL occurs *de novo* and as a complication of solid organ transplantation and other immunosuppressed states. The course is variable but usually progressive and ultimately fatal.

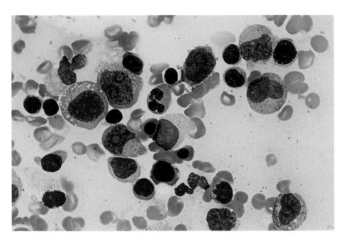

FIGURE 27-12. Bone marrow aspirate, peripheral T-cell lymphoma. Abnormal lymphocytes of varying size are admixed with hematopoietic cells.

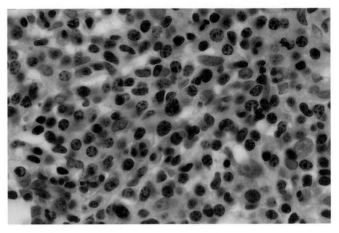

FIGURE 27-15. Bone marrow biopsy specimen, peripheral T-cell lymphoma, CD30+, small cell variant. The hematopoietic tissue is replaced by a diffuse infiltrate of abnormal lymphocytes.

Peripheral blood involvement may occur at any time in the course of the disease. Findings include cytopenias, eosinophilia, and lymphocytosis. The abnormal lymphocytes are typically small to medium-sized, but large cells may also be found. The nuclei are typically irregular, with cleaves and convolutions and condensed chromatin. The cytoplasm is usually agranular, rarely granular.

Bone marrow aspirate smears show variable numbers of abnormal lymphocytes. Histologic sections of the bone marrow show a patchy interstitial or diffuse lymphoid infiltrate. Admixed elements include plasma cells, eosinophils, histiocytes, small blood vessels, and fibrosis. Hemophagocytic syndrome may obscure the underlying malignancy (212,233). Other findings include eosinophilia, pure red cell aplasia, fibrosis, and granulomas (220,230,246). Other disorders reported with peripheral T-cell lymphoma include myeloid diseases, systemic plasmacytosis, B-cell neoplasms, and plasma cell neoplasms (205,209,210,219,221,232,242,247, 248).

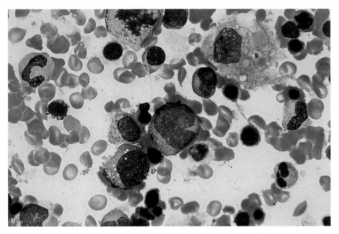

FIGURE 27-13. Bone marrow aspirate smear, peripheral T-cell lymphoma with hemophagocytic syndrome. Abnormal lymphocytes are present as well as a benign-appearing histiocyte with ingested platelets and a red blood cell.

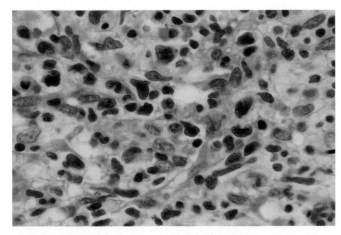

FIGURE 27-14. Bone marrow biopsy specimen, peripheral T-cell lymphoma, CD30+. The hematopoietic tissue is replaced by a pleomorphic infiltrate of abnormal lymphocytes and small blood vessels.

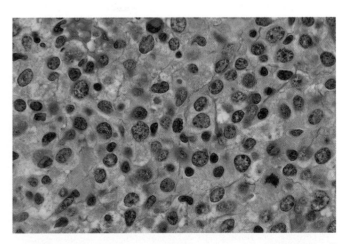

FIGURE 27-16. Bone marrow biopsy specimen, peripheral T-cell lymphoma, CD8+. The hematopoietic tissue is replaced by abnormal lymphocytes with moderately abundant clear cytoplasm.

Immunophenotyping usually shows expression of CD2, CD3, CD5, CD7, either CD4 or CD8, and either TCR α/β or TCR γ/δ. Compared with normal T-cells, expression of pan–T-cell antigens (CD2, CD3, CD5, CD7) may be reduced or absent. CD16, CD30, CD56, granzyme B, perforin, and TIA-1 are variably expressed (128,129,131). CD20 and/or CD79a may be expressed (208,231,249). CD16, CD57, and ALK1 (p80, the NPM/ALK fusion protein) (the NPM/ALK fusion protein)/ALK-1 are not expressed. Cases expressing TCR γ/δ (nonhepatosplenic γ/δ T-cell lymphoma) may express CD4 only, both CD4 and CD8, CD8 only, or neither CD4 nor CD8; they also tend to express the cytotoxic antigens CD16, CD56, granzyme B, and TIA-1. Such cases have been termed nonhepatosplenic γ/δ T-cell lymphoma.

Genetic studies have shown a variety of clonal karyotypic anomalies, TCR gene rearrangements, and, in some cases, clonal integration of Epstein-Barr virus genome.

The differential diagnosis includes reactive T-cell lymphocytosis (which may be clonal although clinically nonmalignant), other T-cell neoplasms, Hodgkin lymphoma (213), and malignant histiocytosis (234).

Anaplastic Large T-Cell Lymphoma

Anaplastic large cell lymphoma (ALCL) may be of the B-cell, T-cell, or null-cell phenotype; the latter two are discussed in this chapter (Fig. 27-17). ALCL tends to presents with either lymph node or skin involvement (33,37,39,223,225,250–291). Cases characterized by nodal disease tend to have an aggressive course, with peripheral blood and bone marrow disease. Cases characterized by localized skin disease have a more favorable course, without systemic manifestations. ALCL arises *de novo*, as a complication of immunosuppression, and as a transformation of MF/SS and TPLL.

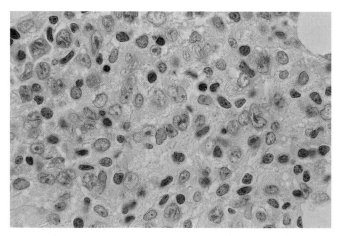

FIGURE 27-17. Bone marrow biopsy specimen, anaplastic T-cell lymphoma. The hematopoietic tissue is replaced by a population of large, abnormal lymphocytes with clear cytoplasm and prominent nucleoli.

The peripheral blood may show anemia and either neutropenia or neutrophilia with absolute lymphocytosis. A leukemic phase is particularly prominent in the small cell variant of ALCL. The abnormal lymphocytes vary in size, ranging from small, relatively nondescript tumor cells to large anaplastic cells with irregular to convoluted nuclei and prominent nucleoli. Either small cells or large cells may predominate. Smaller cells may show small, relatively bland nuclei and scanty cytoplasm. Larger cells show anaplastic features such as large, folded, lobated, bean-shaped, and embryo-shaped nuclei; wreath-shaped arrangements of multiple nuclei; and abundant vacuolated cytoplasm.

Bone marrow aspirate smears show variable numbers of abnormal lymphocytes, which may be difficult to identify among the hematopoietic cells. Myelodysplasia may be present, apparently the result of abnormal cytokine secretion (284). Hematophagocytic syndrome may be present, and may obscure the underlying malignancy (289). Histologic sections of the bone marrow show an intrasinusoidal, interstitial, or diffuse pattern of infiltration. The abnormal lymphocytes are often admixed with inflammatory cells and fibrous tissue and may be difficult to identify among hematopoietic cells. Morphologic variants have been described, consisting predominantly of small cells, large nonanaplastic cells, and neoplastic cells admixed with numerous neutrophils, eosinophils, or histiocytes.

Immunophenotyping usually shows expression of CD2, CD3, either CD4 or CD8, CD5, CD7, CD30, CD45, S100 protein, ALK-1, epithelial membrane antigen, granzyme B, perforin, and TIA-1. Compared with normal T-cells, expression of pan–T-cell antigens (CD2, CD3, CD5, CD7) may be reduced or absent. Some cases express CD8 rather than CD4. CD11c, CD13, CD14, CD15, CD25, CD33, CD56, and CD68 may be expressed. Cases expressing no recognizable T-cell or B-cell antigens are immunophenotypically null and diagnosed as anaplastic null-cell large cell lymphoma.

Genetic studies show, in some cases, t(2;5)(p23;q35) involving *ALK* (anaplastic lymphoma kinase gene) at chromosome 2p23 and *NPM* at chromosome 5q35. Genetic variants involving *ALK* have been described (273,276,282). *TCR* and *IgH* gene rearrangements may also be present.

The differential diagnosis includes drug reaction (290), anaplastic large B-cell lymphoma, Hodgkin lymphoma, acute leukemia, histiocytic neoplasms (274), and nonhematopoietic malignancies.

REFERENCES

Precursor T-Cell Neoplasm

1. Bohlander SK, Muschinsky V, Schrader K, et al. Molecular analysis of the CALM/AF10 fusion: identical rearrangements in acute myeloid leukemia, acute lymphoblastic leukemia and malignant lymphoma patients. *Leukemia* 2000;14:93–99.

2. Chan JK, Sin VC, Wong KF, et al. Nonnasal lymphoma expressing the natural killer cell marker CD56: a clinicopathologic study of 49 cases of an uncommon aggressive neoplasm. *Blood* 1997;89: 4501–4513.

3. Chimenti S, Fink-Puches R, Peris K, et al. Cutaneous involvement in lymphoblastic lymphoma. *J Cutan Pathol* 1999;26: 379–385.

4. Conde-Sterling DA, Aguilera NS, Nandedkar MA, et al. Immunoperoxidase detection of CD10 in precursor T-lymphoblastic lymphoma/leukemia: a clinicopathologic study of 24 cases. *Arch Pathol Lab Med* 2000;124:704–708.

5. Dawson L, Slater R, Hagemeijer A, et al. Secondary T-acute lymphoblastic leukaemia mimicking blast crisis in chronic myeloid leukaemia. *Br J Haematol* 1999;106:104–106.

6. Dorfman DM, Longtine JA, Fox EA, et al. T-cell blast crisis in chronic myelogenous leukemia. Immunophenotypic and molecular biologic findings. *Am J Clin Pathol* 1997;107:168–176.

7. Ginaldi L, Matutes E, Farahat N, et al. Differential expression of CD3 and CD7 in T-cell malignancies: a quantitative study by flow cytometry. *Br J Haematol* 1996;93:921–927.

8. Gloeckner-Hofmann K, Ottesen K, Schmidt S, et al. T-cell/natural killer cell lymphoblastic lymphoma with an unusual coexpression of B-cell antigens. *Ann Hematol* 2000;79:635–639.

9. Hashimoto M, Yamashita Y, Mori N. Immunohistochemical detection of CD79a expression in precursor T cell lymphoblastic lymphoma/leukaemias. *J Pathol* 2002;197:341–347.

10. Hyjek E, Chadburn A, Liu YF, et al. BCL-6 protein is expressed in precursor T-cell lymphoblastic lymphoma and in prenatal and postnatal thymus. *Blood* 2001;97:270–276.

11. Kawakami K, Miyanishi S, Amakawa R, et al. A case of T-lineage lymphoblastic lymphoma/leukemia with t(4;11)(q21;p15) that switched to myelomonocytic leukemia at relapse. *Int J Hematol* 1999;69:196–199.

12. Kell J, Booth M, Jones B, et al. Extramedullary T lymphoblastic transformation of chronic myeloid leukaemia occurring after double allogeneic transplantation. *Bone Marrow Transplant* 1998;22:813–816.

13. Li S, Borowitz MJ. CD79a(+) T-cell lymphoblastic lymphoma with coexisting Langerhans cell histiocytosis. *Arch Pathol Lab Med* 2001;125:958–960.

14. Lim EJ, Peh SC. Bone marrow and peripheral blood changes in non-Hodgkin's lymphoma. *Singapore Med J* 2000;41:279–285.

15. Nah EH, King DE, Craig FE. CD4 and CD8 antigen coexpression: a flow cytometric study of peripheral blood, bone marrow, body fluid, and solid lymphoreticular specimens. *Arch Pathol Lab Med* 1997;121:381–384.

16. Nosaka T, Ohno H, Doi S, et al. Phenotypic conversion of T lymphoblastic lymphoma to acute biphenotypic leukemia composed of lymphoblasts and myeloblasts. Molecular genetic evidence of the same clonal origin. *J Clin Invest* 1988;81:1824–1828.

17. Pilozzi E, Muller-Hermelink HK, Falini B, et al. Gene rearrangements in T-cell lymphoblastic lymphoma. *J Pathol* 1999;188: 267–270.

18. Pilozzi E, Pulford K, Jones M, et al. Co-expression of CD79a (JCB117) and CD3 by lymphoblastic lymphoma. *J Pathol* 1998; 186:140–143.

19. Rosenquist R, Lindh J, Roos G, et al. Immunoglobulin VH gene replacements in a T-cell lymphoblastic lymphoma. *Mol Immunol* 1997;34:305–313.

20. Saito T, Matsuno Y, Tanosaki R, et al. Gamma delta T-cell neoplasms: a clinicopathological study of 11 cases. *Ann Oncol* 2002; 13:1792–1798.

21. Sano K, Goji J, Kosaka Y, et al. Translocation (10;12)(q24;q15) in a T-cell lymphoblastic lymphoma with myeloid hyperplasia. *Cancer Genet Cytogenet* 1998;105:168–171.

22. Soslow RA, Bhargava V, Warnke RA. MIC2, TdT, bcl-2, and

23. Subira M, Domingo A, Santamaria A, et al. Bone marrow involvement in lymphoblastic lymphoma and small non-cleaved cell lymphoma: the role of trephine biopsy. *Haematologica* 1997; 82:594–595.

24. Suzumiya J, Ohshima K, Kikuchi M, et al. Terminal deoxynucleotidyl transferase staining of malignant lymphomas in paraffin sections: a useful method for the diagnosis of lymphoblastic lymphoma. *J Pathol* 1997;182:86–91.

25. Thandla S, Alashari M, Green DM, et al. Therapy-related T-cell lymphoblastic lymphoma with t(11;19)(q23;p13) and MLL gene rearrangement. *Leukemia* 1999;13:2116–2118.

26. Tsutsumi Y, Inada K, Morita K, et al. T-cell lymphomas diffusely involving the intestine: report of two rare cases. *Jpn J Clin Oncol* 1996;26:264–272.

27. van der Kwast TH, van Dongen JJ, Michiels JJ, et al. T-lymphoblastic lymphoma terminating as malignant histiocytosis with rearrangement of immunoglobulin heavy chain gene. *Leukemia* 1991;5:78–82.

28. Velankar MM, Nathwani BN, Schlutz MJ, et al. Indolent T-lymphoblastic proliferation: report of a case with a 16-year course without cytotoxic therapy. *Am J Surg Pathol* 1999;23: 977–981.

29. Wan TS, Ma SK, Chan GC, et al. Complex cytogenetic abnormalities in T-lymphoblastic lymphoma: resolution by spectral karyotyping. *Cancer Genet Cytogenet* 2000;118:24–27.

30. Wolvius EB, van der Valk P, Baart JA, et al. T-cell lymphoblastic lymphoma of the lower jaw in a young child: a case report. *Oral Surg Oral Med Oral Pathol Oral Radiol Endod* 1996;82:434–436.

31. Yeh KH, Cheng AL, Su IJ, et al. Prognostic significance of immunophenotypes in adult lymphoblastic lymphomas. *Anticancer Res* 1997;17:2269–2272.

Mature T-Cell Neoplasms

1. Bartlett NL, Longo DL. T-small lymphocyte disorders. *Semin Hematol* 1999;36:164–170.

2. Baer R, Heppell A, Taylor AM, et al. The breakpoint of an inversion of chromosome 14 in a T-cell leukemia: sequences downstream of the immunoglobulin heavy chain locus are implicated in tumorigenesis. *Proc Natl Acad Sci U S A* 1987;84:9069–9073.

3. Cuneo A, Lanza F, Spanedda R, et al. Alpha interferon in T helper phenotype chronic lymphocytic leukemia: a report of three cases. *J Biol Regul Homeost Agents* 1988;2:31–34.

4. Davey MP, Bertness V, Nakahara K, et al. Juxtaposition of the T-cell receptor alpha-chain locus (14q11) and a region (14q32) of potential importance in leukemogenesis by a 14;14 translocation in a patient with T-cell chronic lymphocytic leukemia and ataxiatelangiectasia. *Proc Natl Acad Sci U S A* 1988;85:9287–9291.

5. Duhrsen U, Uppenkamp M, Uppenkamp I, et al. Chronic T cell leukemia with unusual cellular characteristics in ataxia telangiectasia. *Blood* 1986;68:577–585.

6. Gold JE, Louis-Charles A, Ghali V, et al. T-cell chronic lymphocytic leukemia. Unusual morphologic, phenotypic, and karyotypic features in association with light chain amyloidosis. *Cancer* 1992;70:86–93.

7. Hoyer JD, Ross CW, Li CY, et al. True T-cell chronic lymphocytic leukemia: a morphologic and immunophenotypic study of 25 cases. *Blood* 1995;86:1163–1169.

8. Imamura N, Abe K, Kuramoto A. CD4+, CD45RA+, CD29- T-cell lymphocytic leukemia functioning as T suppressor inducer for B-cell immunoglobulin synthesis. *Leuk Lymphoma* 1993;11:135–139.

9. Kingreen D, Siegert W. Chronic lymphatic leukemias of T and NK cell type. *Leukemia* 1997;11[Suppl 2]:S46–S49.

10. Laneuville P. Cyclosporin A induced remission of CD4+ T-CLL associated with eosinophilia and fasciitis. *Br J Haematol* 1992;80:252–254.

11. Larramendy ML, Peltomaki P, Salonen E, et al. Chromosomal abnormality limited to T4 lymphocytes in a patient with T-cell chronic lymphocytic leukaemia. *Eur J Haematol* 1990;45:52–59.

12. Lutz CT, Galles ME, Kemp JD, et al. Kappa immunoglobulin light chain gene rearrangement in a T-lineage chronic lymphocytic leukemia. *Am J Clin Pathol* 1990;93:702–705.

13. Macey MG, Hou L, Milne T, et al. A CD4+ proliferation of large granular lymphocytes expresses the protease activated receptor-1. *Br J Haematol* 1998;101:78–81.

14. Metzger R, Melmer G, Schondelmaier S, et al. Leukaemic T cells from patients with chronic lymphocytic leukaemia of T-cell origin respond to *Staphylococcus aureus* enterotoxin superantigens. *Scand J Immunol* 1993;37:245–250.

15. Mizuki M, Tagawa S, Machii T, et al. Phenotypical heterogeneity of CD4+CD8+ double-positive chronic T lymphoid leukemia. *Leukemia* 1998;12:499–504.

16. Mori N, Murakami S, Oda S, et al. An HTLV-I carrier who developed CD4+ T-LL expressed the IL-2 receptor beta chain alone without expressing the alpha chain. *Br J Haematol* 1993;85:185–187.

17. Murakami K, Taketazu F, Ida M, et al. True small lymphocytic T-cell chronic lymphocytic leukemia lacking the CD3 molecule and TCR-alpha beta on its cell surface. *Int J Hematol* 1999;70:169–173.

18. Nousari HC, Kimyai-Asadi A, Huang CH, et al. T-cell chronic lymphocytic leukemia mimicking dermatomyositis. *Int J Dermatol* 2000;39:144–146.

19. Raziuddin S, Sheikha A, Latif AA. T-cell chronic lymphocytic leukemia. T-cell function and lymphokine secretion. *Cancer* 1992;69:1146–1152.

20. Russo G, Isobe M, Gatti R, et al. Molecular analysis of a t(14;14) translocation in leukemic T-cells of an ataxia telangiectasia patient. *Proc Natl Acad Sci U S A* 1989;86:602–606.

21. Schmidt HH, Pirc-Danoewinata H, Panzer-Grumayer ER, et al. Translocation (3;5)(p26;q13) in a patient with chronic T-cell lymphoproliferative disorder. *Cancer Genet Cytogenet* 1998;104:82–85.

22. Simpkins H, Kiprov DD, Davis JL, et al. T cell chronic lymphocytic leukemia with lymphocytes of unusual immunologic phenotype and function. *Blood* 1985;65:127–133.

23. Sugimoto K, Tamayose K, Sasaki M, et al. More than 13 years of hypereosinophilia associated with clonal CD3-CD4+ lymphocytosis of TH2/TH0 type. *Int J Hematol* 2002;75:281–284.

24. Uppenkamp M, Dresen IG, Becher R, et al. Molecular analysis of an ataxia telangiectasia T-cell clone with a chromosomal translocation t(14;18)—evidence for a breakpoint in the T-cell receptor delta-chain gene. *Leuk Res* 1992;16:681–691.

25. Watanabe M, Shimamoto Y, Sano M, et al. Unique T-helper leukaemia with cytoplasmic granules and convoluted nuclei. *Leuk Lymphoma* 1993;9:165–167.

26. Witzig TE, Phyliky RL, Li CY, et al. T-cell chronic lymphocytic leukemia with a helper/inducer membrane phenotype: a distinct clinicopathologic subtype with a poor prognosis. *Am J Hematol* 1986;21:139–155.

27. Wong KF, Chan JK, Sin VC. T-cell form of chronic lymphocytic leukaemia: a reaffirmation of its existence. *Br J Haematol* 1996;93:157–159.

28. Zech L, Hammarstrom L, Smith CI. Chromosomal aberrations in a case of T-cell CLL with concomitant IgA myeloma. *Int J Cancer* 1983;32:431–435.

29. Airo P, Rossi G, Facchetti F, et al. Monoclonal expansion of large granular lymphocytes with a CD4+ CD8dim+/− phenotype associated with hairy cell leukemia. *Haematologica* 1995;80:146–149.

30. Amparo E, Kaplan L, Rosenbloom B, et al. T-gamma-lymphoproliferative disorder arising in a background of autoimmune disease and terminating in plasma cell dyscrasia with primary amyloidosis. *Arch Pathol Lab Med* 1991;115:74–77.

31. Bassan R, Rambaldi A, Allavena P, et al. Association of large granular lymphocyte/natural killer cell proliferative disease and second hematologic malignancy. *Am J Hematol* 1988;29:85–93.

32. Blanchong CA, Olshefski R, Kahwash S. Large granular lymphocyte leukemia: case report of chronic neutropenia and rheumatoid arthritis-like symptoms in a child. *Pediatr Dev Pathol* 2001;4:94–99.

33. Costes V, Duchayne E, Taib J, et al. Intrasinusoidal bone marrow infiltration: a common growth pattern for different lymphoma subtypes. *Br J Haematol* 2002;119:916–922.

34. Demeter J, Paloczi K, Foldi J, et al. Immunological and molecular biological identification of a true case of T-hairy cell leukaemia. *Eur J Haematol* 1989;43:339–345.

35. Ergas D, Resnitzky P, Berrebi A. Pure red blood cell aplasia associated with Parvovirus B19 infection in large granular lymphocyte leukemia. *Blood* 1996;87:3523–3524.

36. Evans HL, Burks E, Viswanatha D, et al. Utility of immunohistochemistry in bone marrow evaluation of T-lineage large granular lymphocyte leukemia. *Hum Pathol* 2000;31:1266–1273.

37. Felgar RE, Macon WR, Kinney MC, et al. TIA-1 expression in lymphoid neoplasms. Identification of subsets with cytotoxic T lymphocyte or natural killer cell differentiation. *Am J Pathol* 1997;150:1893–1900.

38. Gentile TC, Uner AH, Hutchison RE, et al. CD3+, CD56+ aggressive variant of large granular lymphocyte leukemia. *Blood* 1994;84:2315–2321.

39. Ginaldi L, Matutes E, Farahat N, et al. Differential expression of CD3 and CD7 in T-cell malignancies: a quantitative study by flow cytometry. *Br J Haematol* 1996;93:921–927.

40. Karakantza M, Matutes E, MacLennan K, et al. Association between sarcoidosis and lymphoma revisited. *J Clin Pathol* 1996;49:208–212.

41. Kishimoto H, Mamada A, Katayama I, et al. Leukaemia cutis in chronic CD8+ T lymphocytic leukaemia. *Dermatology* 1996;192:134–135.

42. Kluin-Nelemans JC, Kester MG, Melenhorst JJ, et al. Persistent clonal excess and skewed T-cell repertoire in T cells from patients with hairy cell leukemia. *Blood* 1996;87:3795–3802.

43. Kondo H, Uematsu M, Watanabe J, et al. CD3+, CD4−, CD8−, TCR alpha beta−, TCR gamma delta+ granular lymphocyte proliferative disorder without lymphocytosis and clinical symptoms. *Acta Haematol* 2000;104:54–56.

44. Kondo H, Watanabe J, Iwasaki H. T-large granular lymphocyte leukemia accompanied by an increase of natural killer cells (CD3−) and associated with ulcerative colitis and autoimmune hepatitis. *Leuk Lymphoma* 2001;41:207–212.

45. Kwong YL, Wong KF. Association of pure red cell aplasia with T large granular lymphocyte leukaemia. *J Clin Pathol* 1998;51:672–675.

46. Kwong YL, Wong KF, Chan LC, et al. Large granular lymphocyte leukemia. A study of nine cases in a Chinese population. *Am J Clin Pathol* 1995;103:76–81.

47. Lamy T, Loughran TP Jr. Current concepts: large granular lymphocyte leukemia. *Blood Rev* 1999;13:230–240.

48. Marolleau JP, Henni T, Gaulard P, et al. Hairy cell leukemia associated with large granular lymphocyte leukemia: immunologic

and genomic study, effect of interferon treatment. *Blood* 1988; 72:655–660.

49. Martin MP, Biggar RJ, Hamlin-Green G, et al. Large granular lymphocytosis in a patient infected with HTLV-II. *AIDS Res Hum Retroviruses* 1993;9:715–719.

50. Matutes E, Coelho E, Aguado MJ, et al. Expression of TIA-1 and TIA-2 in T cell malignancies and T cell lymphocytosis. *J Clin Pathol* 1996;49:154–158.

51. Matutes E, Wotherspoon AC, Parker NE, et al. Transformation of T-cell large granular lymphocyte leukaemia into a high-grade large T-cell lymphoma. *Br J Haematol* 2001;115:801–806.

52. Miyata A, Kojima K, Yoshino T, et al. Concurrent Hodgkin's disease (mixed cellularity type) and T-cell chronic lymphocytic leukemia/prolymphocytic leukemia. *Int J Hematol* 2001;73: 230–235.

53. Mori S, Suzushima H, Nishikawa K, et al. Smoldering gamma delta T-cell granular lymphocytic leukemia associated with pure red cell aplasia. *Acta Haematol* 1995;94:32–35.

54. Morice WG, Kurtin PJ, Leibson PJ, et al. Demonstration of aberrant T-cell and natural killer-cell antigen expression in all cases of granular lymphocytic leukaemia. *Br J Haematol* 2003;120:1026–1036.

55. Morice WG, Kurtin PJ, Tefferi A, et al. Distinct bone marrow findings in T-cell granular lymphocytic leukemia revealed by paraffin section immunoperoxidase stains for CD8, TIA-1, and granzyme B. *Blood* 2002;99:268–274.

56. Moss PA, Gillespie G. Clonal populations of T-cells in patients with B-cell malignancies. *Leuk Lymphoma* 1997;27:231–238.

57. Newland AC, Catovsky D, Linch D, et al. Chronic T cell lymphocytosis: a review of 21 cases. *Br J Haematol* 1984;58: 433–446.

58. Palumbo AP, Corradini P, Battaglio S, et al. Dual rearrangement of immunoglobulin and T-cell receptor gene in a case of T-cell hairy-cell leukemia. *Eur J Haematol* 1991;46:71–76.

59. Rosenblatt JD, Giorgi JV, Golde DW, et al. Integrated human T-cell leukemia virus II genome in CD8+ T cells from a patient with "atypical" hairy cell leukemia: evidence for distinct T-cell and B-cell lymphoproliferative disorders. *Blood* 1988;71: 363–369.

60. Semenzato G, Zambello R, Starkebaum G, et al. The lymphoproliferative disease of granular lymphocytes: updated criteria for diagnosis. *Blood* 1997;89:256–260.

61. Smith JL, Oscier DG, Haegert DG, et al. CD3+ CD8+ T cell lymphocytosis masking B cell leukaemia. *J Clin Pathol* 1988;41: 746–752.

62. Stanworth SJ, Green L, Pumphrey RS, et al. An unusual association of Felty syndrome and TCR gamma delta lymphocytosis. *J Clin Pathol* 1996;49:351–353.

63. Sun T, Cohen NS, Marino J, et al. CD3+, CD4−, CD8− large granular T-cell lymphoproliferative disorder. *Am J Hematol* 1991;37:173–178.

64. Sun T, Susin M, Brody J, et al. T-cell lymphoma associated with natural killer-like T-cell reaction. *Am J Hematol* 1998;57: 331–337.

65. Takami A, Saito M, Nakao S, et al. CD20-positive T-cell chronic lymphocytic leukemia. *Br J Haematol* 1998;102:1327–1329.

66. Tamura K, Sagawa K, Kimura N, et al. A patient of CD4−/ CD8+ chronic T-cell leukemia associated with hypercalcemia. *Leuk Res* 1991;15:43–49.

67. Warzynski MJ, Rosen MH, Golightly MG, et al. An acute form of T gamma lymphoproliferative disease presenting with massive splenomegaly—importance of immunophenotyping for diagnosis. *Clin Immunol Immunopathol* 1993;67:100–108.

68. Wong KF, Chan JC, Liu HS, et al. Chromosomal abnormalities in T-cell large granular lymphocyte leukaemia: report of

two cases and review of the literature. *Br J Haematol* 2002;116: 598–600.

69. Arima N, Matsushita K, Suruga Y, et al. IL-2-induced growth of CD8+ T cell prolymphocytic leukemia cells mediated by NF-kappaB induction and IL-2 receptor alpha expression. *Leuk Res* 1998;22:265–273.

70. Ascani S, Leoni P, Fraternali Orcioni G, et al. T-cell prolymphocytic leukaemia: does the expression of CD8+ phenotype justify the identification of a new subtype? Description of two cases and review of the literature. *Ann Oncol* 1999;10:649–653.

71. Brito-Babapulle V, Hamoudi R, Matutes E, et al. p53 allele deletion and protein accumulation occurs in the absence of p53 gene mutation in T-prolymphocytic leukaemia and Sezary syndrome. *Br J Haematol* 2000;110:180–187.

72. Brito-Babapulle V, Maljaie SH, Matutes E, et al. Relationship of T leukaemias with cerebriform nuclei to T-prolymphocytic leukaemia: a cytogenetic analysis with *in situ* hybridization. *Br J Haematol* 1997;96:724–732.

73. Chan JK, Ng CS, Cheung WC. T-prolymphocytic leukemia with circulating carrot-like cells. *Pathology* 1988;20:64–66.

74. Chan JK, Sin VC, Wong KF, et al. Nonnasal lymphoma expressing the natural killer cell marker CD56: a clinicopathologic study of 49 cases of an uncommon aggressive neoplasm. *Blood* 1997;89:4501–4513.

75. Corwin DJ, Kadin ME, Andres TL. T cell prolymphocytic leukemia. 2 cases having a postthymic helper phenotype with complement receptors and 14q+ chromosome abnormality. *Acta Haematol* 1983;70:43–49.

76. De Schouwer PJ, Dyer MJ, Brito-Babapulle VB, et al. T-cell prolymphocytic leukaemia: antigen receptor gene rearrangement and a novel mode of MTCP1 B1 activation. *Br J Haematol* 2000;110:831–838.

77. Dybjer A, Hellquist L, Johansson B, et al. Seropositive polyarthritis and skin manifestations in T-prolymphocytic leukemia/Sezary cell leukemia variant. *Leuk Lymphoma* 2000;37:437–440.

78. Espinet B, Sole F, Salido M, et al. Application of cross-species color banding (RxFISH) in the study of T-prolymphocytic leukemia. *Haematologica* 2000;85:607–612.

79. Forman SJ, Nathwani BN, Woda BA, et al. Clonal evolution of T-cell prolymphocytic leukemia to a T-large-cell lymphoma. A morphologic and immunologic study. *Arch Pathol Lab Med* 1985;109:1081–1084.

80. Garand R, Goasguen J, Brizard A, et al. Indolent course as a relatively frequent presentation in T-prolymphocytic leukaemia. Groupe Francais d'Hematologie Cellulaire. *Br J Haematol* 1998; 103:488–494.

81. Heinonen K, Mahlamaki E, Hamalainen E, et al. Multiple karyotypic abnormalities in three cases of small cell variant of T-cell prolymphocytic leukemia. *Cancer Genet Cytogenet* 1994;78:28–35.

82. Jehn U, Grunewald R, Goldel N, et al. Prolymphocytic leukemia with suppressor T-cell phenotype: report of two cases. *Anticancer Res* 1989;9:115–118.

83. Kluin-Nelemans HC, Gmelig-Meyling FH, Kootte AM, et al. T-cell prolymphocytic leukemia with an unusual phenotype CD4+ CD8+. *Cancer* 1987;60:794–803.

84. Kojima K, Hara M, Sawada T, et al. Human T-lymphotropic virus type I provirus and T-cell prolymphocytic leukemia. *Leuk Lymphoma* 2000;38:381–386.

85. Laine J, Kunstle G, Obata T, et al. Differential regulation of Akt kinase isoforms by the members of the TCL1 oncogene family. *J Biol Chem* 2002;277:3743–3751.

86. Lauria F, Foa R, Raspadori D, et al. T-cell prolymphocytic leukaemia: a clinical and immunological study. *Scand J Haematol* 1985;35:319–324.

87. Lima M, Coutinho J, Orfao A, et al. Chronic prolymphocytoid leukaemia with an unusual immature immunophenotype. *J Clin Pathol* 1994;47:461–463.

88. Maljaei SH, Brito-Babapulle V, Hiorns LR, et al. Abnormalities of chromosomes 8, 11, 14, and X in T-prolymphocytic leukemia studied by fluorescence *in situ* hybridization. *Cancer Genet Cytogenet* 1998;103:11–116.

89. Matutes E, Brito-Babapulle V, Swansbury J, et al. Clinical and laboratory features of 78 cases of T-prolymphocytic leukemia. *Blood* 1991;78:3269–3274.

90. Matutes E, Catovsky D. Similarities between T-cell chronic lymphocytic leukemia and the small-cell variant of T-prolymphocytic leukemia. *Blood* 1996;87:3520R–3521R.

91. Miyata A, Yoshino T, Kojima K, et al. T-cell prolymphocytic leukemia complicated by diffuse large B-cell lymphoma of the stomach. *Rinsho Ketsueki* 2001;42:47–50.

92. Mossafa H, Brizard A, Huret JL, et al. Trisomy 8q due to i(8q) or der(8) t(8;8) is a frequent lesion in T-prolymphocytic leukaemia: four new cases and a review of the literature. *Br J Haematol* 1994;86:780–785.

93. Nieto LH, Lampert IA, Catovsky D. Bone marrow histological patterns in B-cell and T-cell prolymphocytic leukemia. *Hematol Pathol* 1989;3:79–84.

94. Obara N, Ohkoshi Y, Mukai HY, et al. T-cell prolymphocytic leukemia with CD4+8+25+ phenotype in a patient presenting with venous thrombosis in the lower leg. *Rinsho Ketsueki* 1999;40:1187–1192.

95. Perez-Vila Mf, Espinet B, Sole F, et al. A new case of Sezary cell leukemia: a morphological variant of prolymphocytic leukemia. *Haematologica* 2000;85:775–776.

96. Sakai R, Maruta A, Tomita N, et al. Improvement of quality of life after splenectomy in an HTLV-I carrier with T-cell prolymphocytic leukemia. *Leuk Lymphoma* 1999;35:607–611.

97. Salomon-Nguyen F, Brizard F, Le Coniat M, et al. Abnormalities of the short arm of chromosome 12 in T cell prolymphocytic leukemia. *Leukemia* 1998;12:972–975.

98. Seko Y, Azuma M, Yagita H, et al. Perforin-positive leukemic cell infiltration in the heart of a patient with T-cell prolymphocytic leukemia. *Intern Med* 1995;34:782–784.

99. Serra A, Estrach MT, Marti R, et al. Cutaneous involvement as the first manifestation in a case of T-cell prolymphocytic leukaemia. *Acta Derm Venereol* 1998;78:198–200.

100. Shichishima T, Kawaguchi M, MacHii T, et al. T-prolymphocytic leukaemia with spontaneous remission. *Br J Haematol* 2000;108:397–399.

101. Sohn CC, Blayney DW, Misset JL, et al. Leukopenic chronic T cell leukemia mimicking hairy cell leukemia: association with human retroviruses. *Blood* 1986;67:949–956.

102. Sohn SK, Ahn T, Kim DH, et al. Hepatosplenic T-cell lymphoma: prolymphocytic transformation 18 months after splenectomy. *Int J Hematol* 1997;66:227–232.

103. Sorour A, Brito-Babapulle V, Smedley D, et al. Unusual breakpoint distribution of 8p abnormalities in T-prolymphocytic leukemia. A study with YACS mapping to 8p11-p12. *Cancer Genet Cytogenet* 2000;121:128–132.

104. Stilgenbauer S, Schaffner C, Litterst A, et al. Biallelic mutations in the ATM gene in T-prolymphocytic leukemia. *Nat Med* 1997;3:1155–1159.

105. Stoppa-Lyonnet D, Soulier J, Lauge A, et al. Inactivation of the ATM gene in T-cell prolymphocytic leukemias. *Blood* 1998;91:3920–3926.

106. Sugimoto T, Imoto S, Matsuo Y, et al. T-cell receptor gammadelta T-cell leukemia with the morphology of T-cell prolymphocytic leukemia and a postthymic immunophenotype. *Ann Hematol* 2001;80:749–751.

107. Tamayose K, Sato N, Ando J, et al. CD3-negative, CD20-positive T-cell prolymphocytic leukemia: case report and review of the literature. *Am J Hematol* 2002;71:331–335.

108. Toyota S, Nakamura N, Dan K. T-cell prolymphocytic leukemia with hemorrhagic gastrointestinal involvement and a new chromosomal abnormality. *Int J Hematol* 2002;75:314–317.

109. Wong KF, Chan JK, Sin VC. T-cell prolymphocytic leukemia with a novel translocation (6;11)(q21;q23). *Cancer Genet Cytogenet* 1999;111:149–151.

110. Yuille MA, Coignet LJ, Abraham SM, et al. ATM is usually rearranged in T-cell prolymphocytic leukaemia. *Oncogene* 1998;16:789–796.

111. Dahmoush L, Hijazi Y, Barnes E, et al. Adult T-cell leukemia/lymphoma: a cytopathologic, immunocytochemical, and flow cytometric study. *Cancer* 2002;96:110–116.

112. Hasui K, Sato E, Sakae K, et al. Immunohistological quantitative analysis of S100 protein-positive cells in T-cell malignant lymphomas, especially in adult T-cell leukemia/lymphomas. *Pathol Res Pract* 1992;188:484–489.

113. Hatta Y, Yamada Y, Tomonaga M, et al. Detailed deletion mapping of the long arm of chromosome 6 in adult T-cell leukemia. *Blood* 1999;93:613–616.

114. Inoue Y, Johno M, Matuoka M, et al. A case of adult T-cell lymphoma leukemia with hemophagocytic syndrome. *J Dermatol* 2000;27:280–283.

115. Itoyama T, Chaganti RSK, Yamada Y, et al. Cytogenetic analysis and clinical significance in adult T-cell leukemia/lymphoma: a study of 50 cases from the human T-cell leukemia virus type-1 endemic area, Nagasaki. *Blood* 2001;97:3612–3620.

116. Karlic H, Mostl M, Mucke H, et al. Association of human T-cell leukemia virus and myelodysplastic syndrome in a central European population. *Cancer Res* 1997;57:4718–4721.

117. Kawachi Y, Watanabe A, Sakamoto Y, et al. Acute myeloblastic leukemia associated with an intermediate state between the healthy carrier state and adult T-cell leukemia. *Leuk Lymphoma* 1995;16:505–509.

118. Kawada H, Fukuda R, Suzuki M, et al. Unusual relapse of adult T-cell leukemia/lymphoma after spontaneous remission. *Leuk Res* 1998;22:197–199.

119. Kodama M, Matsuoka H, Maeda K, et al. Smoldering adult T-cell leukemia with B-cell lymphoma and early gastric cancer. *Intern Med* 1995;34:118–121.

120. Lee SN, Nam E, Cha JH, et al. Adult T-cell leukemia/lymphoma with features of CD30-positive anaplastic large cell lymphoma—a case report. *J Korean Med Sci* 1997;12:364–368.

121. Matsushita K, Arima N, Fujiwara H, et al. Spontaneous regression associated with apoptosis in a patient with acute-type adult T-cell leukemia. *Am J Hematol* 1999;61:144–148.

122. Matutes E, Keeling DM, Newland AC, et al. Sezary cell-like leukemia: a distinct type of mature T cell malignancy. *Leukemia* 1990;4:262–266.

123. Mori N, Murakami S, Oda S, et al. An HTLV-I carrier who developed CD4+ T-CLL expressed the IL-2 receptor beta chain alone without expressing the alpha chain. *Br J Haematol* 1993;85:185–187.

124. Mortreux F, Gabet AS, Wattel E. Molecular and cellular aspects of HTLV-1 associated leukemogenesis *in vivo*. *Leukemia* 2003;17:26–38.

125. Ohata J, Matsuoka M, Yamashita T, et al. CD4/CD8 double-positive adult T cell leukemia with preceding cytomegaloviral gastroenterocolitis. *Int J Hematol* 1999;69:92–95.

126. Ohshima K, Haraoka S, Suzumiya J, et al. Absence of cytotoxic molecules in CD8− and/or CD56-positive adult T-cell leukaemia/lymphoma. *Virchows Arch* 1999;435:101–104.

127. Pombo De Oliveira MS, Loureiro P, Bittencourt A, et al.

Geographic diversity of adult T-cell leukemia/lymphoma in Brazil. The Brazilian ATLL Study Group. *Int J Cancer* 1999;83: 291–298.

128. Setoyama M, Katahira Y, Kanzaki T. Clinicopathologic analysis of 124 cases of adult T-cell leukemia/lymphoma with cutaneous manifestations: the smouldering type with skin manifestations has a poorer prognosis than previously thought. *J Dermatol* 1999;26:785–790.

129. Shimamoto Y, Matsunaga C, Suga K, et al. A human T-cell lymphotropic virus type I carrier with temporal arteritis terminating in acute myelogenous leukemia. *Scand J Rheumatol* 1994;23:151–153.

130. Shimamoto Y, Matsuzaki M, Yamaguchi M. Vacuolated Burkitt-like cells in adult T-cell leukaemia/lymphoma. *Clin Lab Haematol* 1992;14:155–157.

131. Siegel RS, Gartenhaus RB, Kuzel TM. Human T-cell lymphotropic-I-associated leukemia/lymphoma. *Curr Treat Options Oncol* 2001;2:291–300.

132. Suzushima H, Asou N, Nishimura S, et al. Double-negative (CD4− CD8−) T cells from adult T-cell leukemia patients also have poor expression of the T-cell receptor alpha beta/CD3 complex. *Blood* 1993;81:1032–1039.

133. Takahara T, Masutani K, Kajiwara E, et al. Adult T-cell leukemia/lymphoma in which the pathohistological diagnosis was identical to that of Ki-1 positive anaplastic large cell lymphoma. *Intern Med* 1999;38:824–828.

134. Takemori N, Hirai K, Onodera R, et al. Vacuolated glycogen-laden leukemic cells in a case of crisis type chronic adult T-cell leukemia. *Leuk Lymphoma* 1993;11:309–314.

135. Takeshita M, Akamatsu M, Ohshima K, et al. CD30 (Ki-1) expression in adult T-cell leukaemia/lymphoma is associated with distinctive immunohistological and clinical characteristics. *Histopathology* 1995;26:539–546.

136. Takeshita M, Ohshima K, Akamatsu M, et al. CD30-positive anaplastic large cell lymphoma in a human T-cell lymphotropic virus-I endemic area. *Hum Pathol* 1995;26:614–619.

137. Takezako Y, Kanda Y, Arai C, et al. Spontaneous remission in acute type adult T-cell leukemia/lymphoma. *Leuk Lymphoma* 2000;39:217–222.

138. Taniguchi S, Yamasaki K, Shibuya T, et al. Spontaneous remission of acute adult T-cell leukaemia with chromosomal abnormality infiltrating to skin and liver. *Br J Haematol* 1993;85:413–414.

139. Tokioka T, Shimamoto Y, Funai N, et al. Coexistence of acute monoblastic leukemia and adult T-cell leukemia: possible association with HTLV-I infection in both cases? *Leuk Lymphoma* 1992;8:147–155.

140. Tsukasaki K, Imaizumi Y, Tawara M, et al. Diversity of leukaemic cell morphology in ATL correlates with prognostic factors, aberrant immunophenotype and defective HTLV-1 genotype. *Br J Haematol* 1999;105:369–375.

141. Tsukasaki K, Koba T, Iwanaga M, et al. Possible association between adult T-cell leukemia/lymphoma and acute myeloid leukemia. *Cancer* 1998;82:488–494.

142. Yamaguchi T, Hirano T, Kumagai K, et al. Osteitis fibrosa cystica generalizata with adult T-cell leukemia: a case report. *Br J Haematol* 1999;107:892–894.

143. Yasukawa M, Arai J, Kakimoto M, et al. CD20-positive adult T-cell leukemia. *Am J Hematol* 2001;66:39–41.

144. Yeh SP, Yu MT, Chow KC, et al. Novel clonal der(8)t(8;14)(p11;q11),del(9)(q13q22) and t(14;22)(q13;q13) in a patient with fulminant adult T-cell leukemia/lymphoma. *Cancer Genet Cytogenet* 2002;139:34–37.

145. Cooke CB, Krenacs L, Stetler-Stevenson M, et al. Hepatosplenic T-cell lymphoma: a distinct clinicopathologic entity of cytotoxic gamma delta T-cell origin. *Blood* 1996;88:4265–4274.

146. Coventry S, Punnett HH, Tomczak EZ, et al. Consistency of isochromosome 7q and trisomy 8 in hepatosplenic gammadelta T-cell lymphoma: detection by fluorescence *in situ* hybridization of a splenic touch-preparation from a pediatric patient. *Pediatr Dev Pathol* 1999;2:478–483.

147. Francois A, Lesesve JF, Stamatoullas A, et al. Hepatosplenic gamma/delta T-cell lymphoma: a report of two cases in immunocompromised patients, associated with isochromosome 7q. *Am J Surg Pathol* 1997;21:781–790.

148. Jonveaux P, Daniel MT, Martel V, et al. Isochromosome 7q and trisomy 8 are consistent primary, non-random chromosomal abnormalities associated with hepatosplenic T gamma/delta lymphoma. *Leukemia* 1996;10:1453–1455.

149. Khan WA, Yu L, Eisenbrey AB, et al. Hepatosplenic gamma/delta T-cell lymphoma in immunocompromised patients. Report of two cases and review of literature. *Am J Clin Pathol* 2001;116:41–50.

150. Macon WR, Levy NB, Kurtin PJ, et al. Hepatosplenic alphabeta T-cell lymphomas: a report of 14 cases and comparison with hepatosplenic gammadelta T-cell lymphomas. *Am J Surg Pathol* 2001;25:285–296.

151. Mastovich S, Ratech H, Ware RE, et al. Hepatosplenic T-cell lymphoma: an unusual case of a gamma delta T-cell lymphoma with a blast-like terminal transformation. *Hum Pathol* 1994;25:102–108.

152. Nosari A, Oreste PL, Biondi A, et al. Hepatosplenic gammadelta T-cell lymphoma: a rare entity mimicking the hemophagocytic syndrome. *Am J Hematol* 1999;60:61–65.

153. Ohshima K, Haraoka S, Harada N, et al. Hepatosplenic gammadelta T-cell lymphoma: relation to Epstein-Barr virus and activated cytotoxic molecules. *Histopathology* 2000;36:127–135.

154. Rossbach HC, Chamizo W, Dumont DP, et al. Hepatosplenic gamma/delta T-cell lymphoma with isochromosome 7q, translocation t(7;21), and tetrasomy 8 in a 9-year-old girl. *J Pediatr Hematol Oncol* 2002;24:154–157.

155. Salhany KE, Feldman M, Kahn MJ, et al. Hepatosplenic gammadelta T-cell lymphoma: ultrastructural, immunophenotypic, and functional evidence for cytotoxic T lymphocyte differentiation. *Hum Pathol* 1997;28:674–685.

156. Sallah S, Smith SV, Lony LC, et al. Gamma/delta T-cell hepatosplenic lymphoma: review of the literature, diagnosis by flow cytometry and concomitant autoimmune hemolytic anemia. *Ann Hematol* 1997;74:139–142.

157. Sohn SK, Ahn T, Kim DH, et al. Hepatosplenic T-cell lymphoma: prolymphocytic transformation 18 months after splenectomy. *Int J Hematol* 1997;66:227–232.

158. Steurer M, Stauder R, Grunewald K, et al. Hepatosplenic gammadelta-T-cell lymphoma with leukemic course after renal transplantation. *Hum Pathol* 2002;33:253–258.

159. Suarez F, Wlodarska I, Rigal-Huguet F, et al. Hepatosplenic alphabeta T-cell lymphoma: an unusual case with clinical, histologic, and cytogenetic features of gammadelta hepatosplenic T-cell lymphoma. *Am J Sur Pathol* 2000;24:1027–1032.

160. Vega F, Medeiros LJ, Bueso-Ramos C, et al. Hepatosplenic gamma/delta T-cell lymphoma in bone marrow. A sinusoidal neoplasm with blastic cytologic features. *Am J Clin Pathol* 2001;116:410–419.

161. Wang CC, Tien HF, Lin MT, et al. Consistent presence of isochromosome 7q in hepatosplenic T gamma/delta lymphoma: a new cytogenetic-clinicopathologic entity. *Genes Chromosomes Cancer* 1995;12:161–164.

162. Weidmann E. Hepatosplenic T cell lymphoma. A review on 45 cases since the first report describing the disease as a distinct lymphoma entity in 1990. *Leukemia* 2000;14:991–997.

163. Weirich G, Sandherr M, Fellbaum C, et al. Molecular evidence of bone marrow involvement in advanced case of Tgammadelta lymphoma with secondary myelofibrosis. *Hum Pathol* 1998;29: 761–765.

164. Wong KF, Chan JK, Matutes E, et al. Hepatosplenic gamma delta T-cell lymphoma. A distinctive aggressive lymphoma type. *Am J Surg Pathol* 1995;19:718–726.

165. Wu H, Wasik MA, Przybylski G, et al. Hepatosplenic gamma-delta T-cell lymphoma as a late-onset posttransplant lymphoproliferative disorder in renal transplant recipients. *Am J Clin Pathol* 2000;113:487–496.

166. Yamaguchi M, Ohno T, Nakamine H, et al. Gamma delta T-cell lymphoma: a clinicopathologic study of 6 cases including extrahepatosplenic type. *Int J Hematol* 1999;69:186–195.

167. Zabernigg A, Fend F, Thaler J, et al. An unusual case of a splenic gamma/delta T-cell lymphoma with angiocentric tendency and haemophagocytic syndrome. *Leuk Lymphoma* 1996;23: 631–634.

168. Bernengo MG, Novelli M, Quaglino P, et al. The relevance of the CD4+ CD26− subset in the identification of circulating Sezary cells. *Br J Dermatol* 2001;144:125–135.

169. Bernengo MG, Quaglino P, Novelli M, et al. Prognostic factors in Sezary syndrome: a multivariate analysis of clinical, haematological and immunological features. *Ann Oncol* 1998;9:857–863.

170. Berti E, Tomasini D, Vermeer MH, et al. Primary cutaneous CD8-positive epidermotropic cytotoxic T cell lymphomas. A distinct clinicopathological entity with an aggressive clinical behavior. *Am J Pathol* 1999;155:483–492.

171. Brito-Babapulle V, Hamoudi R, Matutes E, et al. p53 allele deletion and protein accumulation occurs in the absence of p53 gene mutation in T-prolymphocytic leukaemia and Sezary syndrome. *Br J Haematol* 2000;110:180–187.

172. Cartron G, Roingeard P, Benboubker L, et al. Sezary syndrome in a patient with multiple myeloma: demonstration of a clonally distinct second malignancy. *Eur J Haematol* 1999;63:354–357.

173. Chubachi A, Ishino T, Satoh N, et al. Common acute lymphoblastic leukemia antigen (CD10)-positive Sezary's syndrome. *Am J Hematol* 1994;45:271–272.

174. Crump M, Sutton DM, Pantalony D. Sezary syndrome in a patient with hairy cell leukemia in remission. *Cancer* 1991;68:829–833.

175. Diamandidou E, Colome-Grimmer M, Fayad L, et al. Transformation of mycosis fungoides/Sezary syndrome: clinical characteristics and prognosis. *Blood* 1998;92:1150–1159.

176. Dummer R, Nestle FO, Niederer E, et al. Genotypic, phenotypic and functional analysis of CD4+CD7+ and CD4+CD7− T lymphocyte subsets in Sezary syndrome. *Arch Dermatol Res* 1999;291:307–311.

177. Edelman J, Meyerson H. Diminished CD3 expression is useful for detecting and enumerating Sezary cells. *Am J Clin Pathol* 2000;114:467–477.

178. Goerdt S, Ramaker J, Sonner U, et al. 2 unusual cutaneous T-cell lymphomas with extracutaneous involvement. *Hautarzt* 1996;47:218–224.

179. Karenko L, Kahkonen M, Hyytinen ER, et al. Notable losses at specific regions of chromosomes 10q and 13q in the Sezary syndrome detected by comparative genomic hybridization. *J Invest Dermatol* 1999;112:392–395.

180. Karenko L, Nevala H, Raatikainen M, et al. Communication: chromosomally clonal T cells in the skin, blood, or lymph nodes of two Sezary syndrome patients express CD45RA, CD45RO, CDw150, and interleukin-4, but no interleukin-2 or interferon-gamma. *J Invest Dermatol* 2001;116:188–193.

181. Kim YH, Hoppe RT. Mycosis fungoides and the Sezary syndrome. *Semin Oncol* 1999;26:276–289.

182. Konstantopoulos K, Kapsimalis V, Vaiopoulos G, et al. Simultaneous appearance of mycosis fungoides and chronic lymphocytic leukemia in the same patient. *Haematologia (Budap)* 2000;30:41–43.

183. Lipsker D, Marquart-Elbaz C, Kurtz JE, et al. Macrophage activation syndrome disclosing leukemic transformation of mycosis fungoides. *Ann Dermatol Venereol* 1997;124:544–546.

184. Matutes E, Schulz T, Dyer M, et al. Immunoblastic transformation of a Sezary syndrome in a black Caribbean patient without evidence of HTLV-I. *Leuk Lymphoma* 1995;18:521–527.

185. Meuret G, Schmitt E, Hagedorn M. Monocytopoiesis in chronic eczematous diseases, psoriasis vulgaris, and mycosis fungoides. *J Invest Dermatol* 1976;66:22–28.

186. Miyayama H, Takemiya M, Takahashi K, et al. Massive IgE-hyperimmunoglobulinemia and storage histiocytosis in Sezary syndrome. A postmortem study. *Cancer* 1984;53:1869–1877.

187. Muche JM, Lukowsky A, Asadullah K, et al. Demonstration of frequent occurrence of clonal T cells in the peripheral blood of patients with primary cutaneous T-cell lymphoma. *Blood* 1997;90:1636–1642.

188. Nair CN, Shinde S, Kumar A, et al. Sezary cells with hairy projections. *Leuk Res* 1999;23:195–197.

189. Orero M, Miguel-Sosa A, Miguel-Garcia A, et al. Sezary cell-like leukemia with atypical immunophenotype. *Leukemia* 1997;11: 1383–1385.

190. Paolini R, Poletti A, Ramazzina E, et al. Co-existence of cutaneous T-cell lymphoma and B hairy cell leukemia. *Am J Hematol* 2000;64:197–202.

191. Robinowitz B, Roenigk HH, Smith MM. Sea-blue histiocytes in mycosis fungoides. *Arch Dermatol* 1975;111:1165–1167.

192. Rostoker G, Raphael M, Boisnick S, et al. Coexistence of Sezary syndrome and dysmyelopoiesis with an excess of myeloblasts. *J Am Acad Dermatol* 1986;15:1296–1298.

193. Salhany KE, Greer JP, Cousar JB, et al. Marrow involvement in cutaneous T-cell lymphoma. A clinicopathologic study of 60 cases. *Am J Clin Pathol* 1989;92:747–754.

194. Sano S, Matsui Y, Itami S, et al. Immunological study on CD3 defective cutaneous T cell lymphoma cells from a patient with Sezary syndrome. *Clin Exp Immunol* 1998;113: 190–197.

195. Scarisbrick JJ, Child F, Spittle M, et al. Systemic Hodgkin's lymphoma in a patient with Sezary syndrome. *Br J Dermatol* 2000;142:771–775.

196. Scarisbrick JJ, Whittaker S, Evans AV, et al. Prognostic significance of tumor burden in the blood of patients with erythrodermic primary cutaneous T-cell lymphoma. *Blood* 2001;97: 624–630.

197. So CC, Wong KF, Siu LL, et al. Large cell transformation of Sezary syndrome. A conventional and molecular cytogenetic study. *Am J Clin Pathol* 2000;113:792–797.

198. Suchin KR, Cassin M, Gottlieb SL, et al. Increased interleukin 5 production in eosinophilic Sezary syndrome: regulation by interferon alfa and interleukin 12. *J Am Acad Dermatol* 2001;44: 28–32.

199. Thangavelu M, Finn WG, Yelavarthi KK, et al. Recurring structural chromosome abnormalities in peripheral blood lymphocytes of patients with mycosis fungoides/Sezary syndrome. *Blood* 1997;89:3371–3377.

200. Tokura Y, Yagi H, Seo N, et al. Nonerythrodermic, leukemic variant of cutaneous T-cell lymphoma with indolent clinical course: Th2-type tumor cells lacking T-cell receptor/CD3 expression and coinfiltrating tumoricidal CD8 T cells. *J Am Acad Dermatol* 2000;43:946–954.

201. Trotter MJ, Whittaker SJ, Orchard GE, et al. Cutaneous histopathology of Sezary syndrome: a study of 41 cases with

a proven circulating T-cell clone. *J Cutan Pathol* 1997;24: 286–291.

202. Vergier B, de Muret A, Beylot-Barry M, et al. Transformation of mycosis fungoides: clinicopathological and prognostic features of 45 cases. French Study Group of Cutaneous Lymphomas. *Blood* 2000;95:2212–2218.

203. Whittaker SJ, Smith NP, Jones RR, et al. Analysis of beta, gamma, and delta T-cell receptor genes in mycosis fungoides and Sezary syndrome. *Cancer* 1991;68:1572–1582.

204. Woessner S, Domingo A, Guma J, et al. Lymphocytes with cerebriform nuclei in chronic B-cell lymphoproliferative diseases. *Leuk Res* 1997;21:893–895.

205. Abruzzo LV, Griffith LM, Nandedkar M, et al. Histologically discordant lymphomas with B-cell and T-cell components. *Am J Clin Pathol* 1997;108:316–323.

206. Arnulf B, Copie-Bergman C, Delfau-Larue MH, et al. Non-hepatosplenic gammadelta T-cell lymphoma: a subset of cytotoxic lymphomas with mucosal or skin localization. *Blood* 1998;91:1723–1731.

207. Barth TF, Leithauser F, Dohner H, et al. Primary gastric apoptosis-rich T-cell lymphoma co-expressing CD4, CD8, and cytotoxic molecules. *Virchows Arch* 2000;436:357–364.

208. Blakolmer K, Vesely M, Kummer JA, et al. Immunoreactivity of B-cell markers (CD79a, L26) in rare cases of extranodal cytotoxic peripheral T- (NK/T-) cell lymphomas. *Mod Pathol* 2000;13:766–772.

209. Breccia M, Petti MC, D'Elia GM, et al. Cutaneous pleomorphic T-cell lymphoma coexisting with myelodysplastic syndrome transforming into acute myeloid leukemia: successful treatment with a fludarabine-containing regimen. *Eur J Haematol* 2002;68:1–3.

210. Brumana N, Scheidler D, Bonato M, et al. Peripheral T-cell lymphoma associated with multiple myeloma. *Haematologica* 1993;78:335–337.

211. Charton-Bain MC, Brousset P, Bouabdallah R, et al. Variation in the histological pattern of nodal involvement by gamma/delta T cell lymphoma. *Histopathology* 2000;36:233–239.

212. Ciaudo M, Chauvenet L, Audouin J, et al. Peripheral-T-cell lymphoma with hemophagocytic histiocytosis localised to the bone marrow associated with inappropriate secretion of antidiuretic hormone. *Leuk Lymphoma* 1995;19:511–514.

213. Colon-Otero G, McClure SP, Phyliky RL, et al. Peripheral T-cell lymphoma simulating Hodgkin's disease with initial bone marrow involvement. *Mayo Clin Proc* 1986;61:68–71.

214. Donadieu J, Canioni D, Cuenod B, et al. A familial T-cell lymphoma with gamma delta phenotype and an original location. Possible role of chronic Epstein-Barr virus infection. *Cancer* 1996;77:1571–1577.

215. Gaal K, Sun NC, Hernandez AM, et al. Sinonasal NK/T-cell lymphomas in the United States. *Am J Surg Pathol* 2000;24:1511–1517.

216. Gaulard P, Kanavaros P, Farcet JP, et al. Bone marrow histologic and immunohistochemical findings in peripheral. T-cell lymphoma: a study of 38 cases. *Hum Pathol* 1991;22:331–338.

217. Hanamura A, Kinoshita T, Kurokawa T, et al. Molecular evaluation of bone marrow involvement in peripheral T-cell lymphoma with a PCR-mediated RNase protection assay. *Int J Hematol* 1999;70:283–289.

218. Hanson CA, Brunning RD, Gajl-Peczalska KJ, et al. Bone marrow manifestations of peripheral T-cell lymphoma. A study of 30 cases. *Am J Clin Pathol* 1986;86:449–460.

219. Higuchi T, Tada J, Mori H, et al. Immunoblastic lymphadenopathy-like T cell lymphoma evolving into a massive plasma cell proliferation with biclonal paraproteinemia. *Acta Haematol* 1998;100:151–155.

220. Hung IJ, Kuo TT, Sun CF. Subcutaneous panniculitic T-cell lymphoma developing in a child with idiopathic myelofibrosis. *J Pediatr Hematol Oncol* 1999;21:38–41.

221. Ichinohasama R, Miura I, Takahashi N, et al. Ph-negative non-Hodgkin's lymphoma occurring in chronic phase of Ph-positive chronic myelogenous leukemia is defined as a genetically different neoplasm from extramedullary localized blast crisis: report of two cases and review of the literature. *Leukemia* 2000;14:169–182.

222. Kagami Y, Nakamura S, Suzuki R, et al. A nodal gamma/delta T-cell lymphoma with an association of Epstein-Barr virus. *Am J Surg Pathol* 1997;21:729–736.

223. Kanavaros P, Boulland ML, Petit B, et al. Expression of cytotoxic proteins in peripheral T-cell and natural killer-cell (NK) lymphomas: association with extranodal site, NK or Tgammadelta phenotype, anaplastic morphology and CD30 expression. *Leuk Lymphoma* 2000;38:317–326.

224. Katoh A, Ohshima K, Kanda M, et al. Gastrointestinal T-cell lymphoma: predominant cytotoxic phenotypes, including alpha/beta, gamma/delta T cell and natural killer cells. *Leuk Lymphoma* 2000;39:97–111.

225. Kluin PM, Feller A, Gaulard P, et al. Peripheral T/NK-cell lymphoma: a report of the IXth Workshop of the European Association for Haematopathology. *Histopathology* 2001;38: 250–270.

226. Lavergne A, Brocheriou I, Delfau MH, et al. Primary intestinal gamma-delta T-cell lymphoma with evidence of Epstein-Barr virus. *Histopathology* 1998;32:271–276.

227. Lepretre S, Buchonnet G, Stamatoullas A, et al. Chromosome abnormalities in peripheral T-cell lymphoma. *Cancer Genet Cytogenet* 2000;117:71–79.

228. Lopez-Guillermo A, Cid J, Salar A, et al. Peripheral T-cell lymphomas: initial features, natural history, and prognostic factors in a series of 174 patients diagnosed according to the R.E.A.L. classification. *Ann Oncol* 1998;9:849–855.

229. Marzano AV, Berti E, Paulli M, et al. Cytophagic histiocytic panniculitis and subcutaneous panniculitis-like T-cell lymphoma: report of 7 cases. *Arch Dermatol* 2000;136:889–896.

230. Mitarnun W. Granulomatous reaction in peripheral T-cell proliferative disease: a case report. *J Med Assoc Thai* 1997;80: 795–798.

231. Mohrmann RL, Arber DA. CD20-positive peripheral T-cell lymphoma: report of a case after nodular sclerosis Hodgkin's disease and review of the literature. *Mod Pathol* 2000;13:1244–1252.

232. Nitta Y. Case of malignant lymphoma associated with primary systemic plasmacytosis with polyclonal hypergammaglobulinemia. *Am J Dermatopathol* 1997;19:289–293.

233. Noguchi M, Kawano Y, Sato N, et al. T-cell lymphoma of CD3+CD4+CD56+ granular lymphocytes with hemophagocytic syndrome. *Leuk Lymphoma* 1997;26:349–358.

234. Ohshima K, Kikuchi M, Mizuno S, et al. Hepatosinusoidal leukaemia/lymphoma consisting of Epstein-Barr virus-containing natural killer cell leukaemia/lymphoma and T-cell lymphoma; mimicking malignant histiocytosis. *Hematol Oncol* 1995; 13:83–97.

235. Ohshima K, Suzumiya J, Sugihara M, et al. Clinical, immunohistochemical and phenotypic features of aggressive nodal cytotoxic lymphomas, including alpha/beta, gamma/delta T-cell and natural killer cell types. *Virchows Arch* 1999;435:92–100.

236. Ott MM, Ott G, Klinker H, et al. Abdominal T-cell non-Hodgkin's lymphoma of the gamma/delta type in a patient with selective immunoglobulin A deficiency. *Am J Surg Pathol* 1998;22:500–506.

237. Saito T, Matsuno Y, Tanosaki R, et al. Gamma delta T-cell neoplasms: a clinicopathological study of 11 cases. *Ann Oncol* 2002;13:1792–1798.

238. Salhany KE, Macon WR, Choi JK, et al. Subcutaneous panniculitis-like T-cell lymphoma: clinicopathologic, immunophenotypic, and genotypic analysis of alpha/beta and gamma/delta subtypes. *Am J Surg Pathol* 1998;22:881–893.

239. Scolnik MP, Burgos RA, Paz A, et al. Nonhepatosplenic gamma delta T-cell lymphoma with initial testicular compromise. *Am J Hematol* 2000;65:260–262.

240. Serke S, van Lessen A, Hummel M, et al. Circulating CD4+ T lymphocytes with intracellular but no surface CD3 antigen in five of seven patients consecutively diagnosed with angioimmunoblastic T-cell lymphoma. *Cytometry* 2000;42:180–187.

241. Shapira MY, Caspi O, Amir G, et al. Gastric-mucocutaneous gammadelta T cell lymphoma: possible association with Epstein-Barr virus? *Leuk Lymphoma* 1999;35:397–401.

242. Strickler JG, Amsden TW, Kurtin PJ. Small B-cell lymphoid neoplasms with coexisting T-cell lymphomas. *Am J Clin Pathol* 1992;98:424–429.

243. Takimoto Y, Imanaka F, Sasaki N, et al. Gamma/delta T-cell lymphoma presenting in the subcutaneous tissue and small intestine in a patient with capillary leak syndrome. *Int J Hematol* 1998;68:183–191.

244. Toro JR, Beaty M, Sorbara L, et al. gamma delta T-cell lymphoma of the skin: a clinical, microscopic, and molecular study. *Arch Dermatol* 2000;136:1024–1032.

245. Tsujikawa T, Itoh A, Bamba M, et al. Aggressive jejunal gamma deltaT-cell lymphoma derived from intraepithelial lymphocytes: an autopsy case report. *J Gastroenterol* 1998;33: 280–284.

246. Tsujimura H, Sakai C, Takagi T. Pure red cell aplasia complicated by angioimmunoblastic T-cell lymphoma: humoral factor plays a main role in the inhibition of erythropoiesis from CD34(+) progenitor cells. *Am J Hematol* 1999;62:259–260.

247. Weidmann E, Hinz T, Klein S, et al. Cytotoxic hepatosplenic gd T-cell lymphoma following acute myeloid leukemia bearing two distinct g chains of the T-cell receptor. Biologic and clinical features. *Haematologica* 2000;85:1024–1031.

248. Wickenhauser C, Borchmann P, Diehl V, et al. Development of IgG lambda multiple myeloma in a patient with cutaneous CD30+ anaplastic T-cell lymphoma. *Leuk Lymphoma* 1999;35: 201–206.

249. Yao X, Teruya-Feldstein J, Raffeld M, et al. Peripheral T-cell lymphoma with aberrant expression of CD79a and CD20: a diagnostic pitfall. *Mod Pathol* 2001;14:105–110.

250. Arrowsmith ER, Macon WR, Kinney MC, et al. Peripheral T-cell lymphomas: clinical features and prognostic factors of 92 cases defined by the revised European American lymphoma classification. *Leuk Lymphoma* 2003;44:241–249.

251. Anderson MM, Ross CW, Singleton TP, et al. Ki-1 anaplastic large cell lymphoma with a prominent leukemic phase. *Hum Pathol* 1996;27:1093–1095.

252. Arrowsmith ER, Macon WR, Kinney MC, et al. Peripheral T-cell lymphomas: clinical features and prognostic factors of 92 cases defined by the revised European American lymphoma classification. *Leuk Lymphoma* 2003;44:241–249.

253. Assaf C, Hummel M, Dippel E, et al. Common clonal T-cell origin in a patient with T-prolymphocytic leukaemia and associated cutaneous T-cell lymphomas. *Br J Haematol* 2003;120: 488–491.

254. Bayle C, Charpentier A, Duchayne E, et al. Leukaemic presentation of small cell variant anaplastic large cell lymphoma: report of four cases. *Br J Haematol* 1999;104:680–688.

255. Benharroch D, Meguerian-Bedoyan Z, Lamant L, et al. ALK-positive lymphoma: a single disease with a broad spectrum of morphology. *Blood* 1998;91:2076–2084.

256. Chhanabhai M, Britten C, Klasa R, et al. t(2;5) positive lym-

257. Creager AJ, Geisinger KR, Bergman S. Neutrophil-rich Ki-1-positive anaplastic large cell lymphoma: a study by fine-needle aspiration biopsy. *Am J Clin Pathol* 2002;117:709–715.

258. Dereure O, Portales P, Balavoine M, et al. Rare occurrence of CD30+ circulating cells in patients with cutaneous CD30+ anaplastic large cell lymphoma: a study of nine patients. *Br J Dermatol* 2003;148:246–251.

259. Drexler HG, Gignac SM, von Wasielewski R, et al. Pathobiology of NPM-ALK and variant fusion genes in anaplastic large cell lymphoma and other lymphomas. *Leukemia* 2000;14:1533–1559.

260. Foss HD, Demel G, Anagnostopoulos I, et al. Uniform expression of cytotoxic molecules in anaplastic large cell lymphoma of null/T cell phenotype and in cell lines derived from anaplastic large cell lymphoma. *Pathobiology* 1997;65:83–90.

261. Fraga M, Brousset P, Schlaifer D, et al. Bone marrow involvement in anaplastic large cell lymphoma. Immunohistochemical detection of minimal disease and its prognostic significance. *Am J Clin Pathol* 1995;103:82–89.

262. George DH, Scheithauer BW, Aker FV, et al. Primary anaplastic large cell lymphoma of the central nervous system: prognostic effect of ALK-1 expression. *Am J Surg Pathol* 2003;27: 487–493.

263. Gorczyca W, Tsang P, Liu Z, et al. CD30-positive T-cell lymphomas co-expressing CD15: An immunohistochemical analysis. *Int J Oncol* 2003;22:319–324.

264. Gujral S, Prasad R, Naresh KN. Systemic anaplastic large cell lymphoma in a child presenting with bone marrow involvement and clinical features of acute leukaemia. *Am J Hematol* 2002;69:150–151.

265. Hodges KB, Collins RD, Greer JP, et al. Transformation of the small cell variant Ki-1+ lymphoma to anaplastic large cell lymphoma: pathologic and clinical features. *Am J Surg Pathol* 1999;23:49–58.

266. Jhala DN, Medeiros LJ, Lopez-Terrada D, et al. Neutrophil-rich anaplastic large cell lymphoma of T-cell lineage. A report of two cases arising in HIV-positive patients. *Am J Clin Pathol* 2000;114:478–482.

267. Juco J, Holden JT, Mann KP, et al. Immunophenotypic analysis of anaplastic large cell lymphoma by flow cytometry. *Am J Clin Pathol* 2003;119:205–212.

268. Kadin ME, Morris SW. The t(2;5) in human lymphomas. *Leuk Lymphoma* 1998;29:249–256.

269. Kang SK, Chang SE, Choi JH, et al. Coexistence of CD30-positive anaplastic large cell lymphoma and mycosis fungoides. *Clin Exp Dermatol* 2002;27:212–215.

270. Kasai K, Kon S, Kikuchi K, et al. Expression of carbohydrate antigens, p80NPM/ALK, cytotoxic cell-associated antigens, and Epstein-Barr virus gene products in anaplastic large cell lymphomas. *Pathol Int* 1998;48:171–178.

271. Kato N, Mizuno O, Ito K, et al. Neutrophil-rich anaplastic large cell lymphoma presenting in the skin. *Am J Dermatopathol* 2003;25:142–147.

272. Kutok JL, Aster JC. Molecular biology of anaplastic lymphoma kinase-positive anaplastic large-cell lymphoma. *J Clin Oncol* 2002;20:3691–3702.

273. Lamant L, Dastugue N, Pulford K, et al. A new fusion gene TPM3-ALK in anaplastic large cell lymphoma created by a (1;2)(q25;p23) translocation. *Blood* 1999;93:3088–3095.

274. Lemes A, De La Iglesia S, Santana C, et al. t(2;5) associated with a histiocytic-monocytic neoplasm. *Leuk Lymphoma* 2001;41: 429–433.

275. McCluggage WG, Walsh MY, Bharucha H. Anaplastic large cell

malignant lymphoma with extensive eosinophilic or neutrophilic infiltration. *Histopathology* 1998;32:110–115.

276. Mitev L, Christova S, Hadjiev E, et al. A new variant chromosomal translocation t(2;2)(p23;q23) in CD30+/Ki-1+ anaplastic large cell lymphoma. *Leuk Lymphoma* 1998;28: 613–616.

277. Nakamura S, Shiota M, Nakagawa A, et al. Anaplastic large cell lymphoma: a distinct molecular pathologic entity: a reappraisal with special reference to p80(NPM/ALK) expression. *Am J Surg Pathol* 1997;21:1420–1432.

278. Ng WK, Ip P, Choy C, et al. Cytologic and immunocytochemical findings of anaplastic large cell lymphoma: analysis of ten fine-needle aspiration specimens over a 9-year period. *Cancer* 2003;99:33–43.

279. Paulli M, Vallisa D, Viglio A, et al. ALK positive lymphohistiocytic variant of anaplastic large cell lymphoma in an adult. *Haematologica* 2001;86:260–265.

280. Pileri SA, Pulford K, Mori S, et al. Frequent expression of the NPM-ALK chimeric fusion protein in anaplastic large-cell lymphoma, lympho-histiocytic type. *Am J Pathol* 1997;150:1207–1211.

281. Popnikolov NK, Payne DA, Hudnall SD, et al. CD13-positive anaplastic large cell lymphoma of T-cell origin—a diagnostic and histogenetic problem. *Arch Pathol Lab Med* 2000;124:1804–1808.

282. Rosenwald A, Ott G, Pulford K, et al. t(1;2)(q21;p23) and t(2;3)(p23;q21): two novel variant translocations of the t(2;5) (p23;q35) in anaplastic large cell lymphoma. *Blood* 1999;94: 362–364.

283. Sadahira Y, Hata S, Sugihara T, et al. Bone marrow involvement in NPM-ALK-positive lymphoma: report of two cases. *Pathol Res Pract* 1999;195:657–661.

284. Shimamoto T, Hayashi S, Ando K, et al. Anaplastic large-cell lymphoma which showed severe inflammatory status and myelodysplasia with increased VEGF and IL-6 serum levels after long-term immunosuppressive therapy. *Am J Hematol* 2001;66:49–52.

285. Suzukawa K, Kojima H, Mori N, et al. Anaplastic large-cell lymphoma of null-cell type with multiple bone involvement. *Ann Hematol* 1998;77:287–290.

286. Suzuki R, Kagami Y, Takeuchi K, et al. Prognostic significance of CD56 expression for ALK-positive and ALK-negative anaplastic large-cell lymphoma of T/null cell phenotype. *Blood* 2000;96:2993–3000.

287. ten Berge RL, Oudejans JJ, Ossenkoppele GJ, et al. ALK-negative systemic anaplastic large cell lymphoma: differential diagnostic and prognostic aspects—a review. *J Pathol* 2003;200:4–15.

288. Villamor N, Rozman M, Esteve J, et al. Anaplastic large-cell lymphoma with rapid evolution to leukemic phase. *Ann Hematol* 1999;78:478–482.

289. Wong KF, Chan JK, Ng CS, et al. Anaplastic large cell Ki-1 lymphoma involving bone marrow: marrow findings and association with reactive hemophagocytosis. *Am J Hematol* 1991;37: 112–119.

290. Yeo W, Chow J, Wong N, et al. Carbamazepine-induced lymphadenopathy mimicking Ki-1 (CD30+) T-cell lymphoma. *Pathology* 1997;29:64–66.

291. Yeo W, Wong N, Chow J, et al. Small cell variant of Ki-1 lymphoma associated with myelofibrosis and a novel constitutional chromosomal translocation t(3;4) (q13;q12). *J Clin Pathol* 1996;49:259–262.

NATURAL KILLER CELL NEOPLASMS

Clonal natural killer (NK) cell disorders are the least common of the hematolymphoid malignancies. Their classification has been hampered by their rarity, their similarities to cytotoxic T-cell tumors, and the difficulty of establishing clonality in NK cells (Tables 28-1 and 28-2). Differentiating characteristics of these neoplasms include clinical aggressiveness, morphology, immunophenotype, and relationship to Epstein-Barr virus (EBV) infection (Table 28-3).

PRECURSOR NATURAL KILLER CELL NEOPLASM

Natural Killer Cell Lymphoblastic Lymphoma/Leukemia

NK cell lymphoblastic lymphoma/leukemia has also been reported as blastoid NK cell lymphoma, blastic NK cell lymphoma/leukemia, and monomorphic agranular natural killer cell lymphoma/leukemia (1–17). NK lymphoblastic lymphoma/leukemia usually presents in the skin but may also occur in lymph nodes, mediastinum, and other sites. The clinical course is typically rapid, with development of disseminated disease, a leukemic phase, and death. NK lymphoblastic lymphoma/leukemia occurs *de novo* and as a blast crisis of a myeloproliferative disorder.

The peripheral blood shows one or more cytopenias and/or leukoerythroblastosis. The leukemic phase may be present initially or develop over time. Bone marrow aspirate smears and sections show diffuse infiltration in approximately 50% of cases. The malignant cells are variably sized with oval to irregular nuclei, dispersed chromatin, nucleoli, and variable amounts of agranular cytoplasm. Granules are not visible with light microscopy, but minute granules may

TABLE 28-1. CLASSIFICATION OF NATURAL KILLER CELL NEOPLASMS ACCORDING TO THE WORLD HEALTH ORGANIZATION

Mature NK cell neoplasms
 Aggressive NK cell leukemia
 Extranodal NK/T-cell lymphoma, nasal type
 Blastic NK cell lymphoma

NK, natural killer.

TABLE 28-2. ORGANIZATION OF NATURAL KILLER CELL NEOPLASMS IN THIS CHAPTER

Precursor NK cell neoplasm
 NK cell lymphoblastic lymphoma/leukemia

Mature NK cell neoplasms
 NK cell chronic lymphocytic leukemia
 Aggressive NK cell leukemia/lymphoma
 Other NK cell lymphomas

NK, natural killer.

be identified by electron microscopy. Cohesive cell aggregates and pseudorosettes have been described.

Flow cytometry typically shows expression of CD4, CD45, CD56, and HLA-DR. Cytoplasmic CD3 ε, CD7 and/or terminal deoxynucleotidyl transferase may also be expressed. Surface CD3, CD5, CD16, CD34, and CD57 are typically not expressed. Exceptional cases show expression of CD5 or CD16 or lack expression of CD3 or CD7. Immunostains show positivity for CD43 and CD45 but not TIA-1. Biphenotypic cases showing both myeloid and NK cell differentiation have been reported (see Chapter 19).

Genetic studies show no recurrent karyotypic anomalies. Clonal immunoglobulin and T-cell receptor gene rearrangements are absent. EBV DNA is not found in tumor cells.

The differential diagnosis includes other types of lymphoblastic lymphoma and leukemia and nonhematopoietic small round cell tumors.

TABLE 28-3. DIFFERENTIAL FEATURES OF NATURAL KILLER CELL NEOPLASMS

	ANKL	NK CLL	NK LBL	NKL
Course	Acute	Chronic	Acute	Variable
Leukemia	+	+	+	−
Blasts	−	−	+	−
Granules	+	+	−	+
TdT	−	−	+	−
EBV	+	−	−	+

ANKL, aggressive natural killer cell leukemia/lymphoma; EBV, evidence of Epstein-Barr virus infection; NK CLL, natural killer cell chronic lymphocytic leukemia; NKL, other natural killer cell lymphomas; NK LBL, natural killer cell lymphoblastic lymphoma/leukemia; TdT, terminal deoxynucleotidyl transferase; +, positive; −, negative.

MATURE NATURAL KILLER CELL NEOPLASMS

Natural Killer Cell Chronic Lymphocytic Leukemia

NK cell chronic lymphocytic leukemia, also termed chronic NK cell lymphocytosis and NK cell large granular lymphocytic leukemia, occurs predominantly in male patients (Figs. 28-1 and 28-2). These cases comprise a subset of large granular lymphocytosis (1–11). Hepatomegaly, splenomegaly, and lymphadenopathy are almost always absent. The clinical course is usually indolent, although transformation to aggressive NK cell leukemia/lymphoma has been reported.

The peripheral blood shows an increased number of large granular lymphocytes, with absolute counts ranging from fewer than 2 to more than 50×10^9 cells/L. Other findings include hemolytic anemia, neutropenia, and thrombocytopenia. Bone marrow aspirate smears show similar cells, comprising as much as 50% of cells seen. Histologic sections of the bone marrow show a diffuse lymphoid infiltrate composed of round cells with moderately abundant cytoplasm. Other reported findings include granulomas, pure red cell aplasia, and aplastic anemia.

Flow cytometry shows expression of cytoplasmic CD3 ϵ, CD11c, CD16, and CD56 but not surface CD3 or CD4. CD8, CD57, and HLA-DR are variably expressed. Exceptional cases fail to express CD11b or CD16.

Genetic studies have demonstrated clonal karyotypic anomalies involving chromosomes 5, 6, and 10 and a clonal pattern of X chromosome inactivation. T-cell receptor and immunoglobulin gene rearrangements are absent. Clonal integration of EBV DNA in tumor cells is rarely found.

The differential diagnosis includes other NK cell and cytotoxic T-cell disorders. NK cell lymphocytosis has been reported in several clonal hematolymphoid diseases; in at

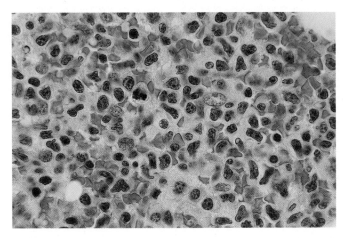

FIGURE 28-2. Bone marrow biopsy specimen, natural killer cell chronic lymphocytic leukemia. The hematopoietic tissue is replaced by a diffuse infiltrate of natural killer cells, showing some nuclear pleomorphism and abundant pale-staining cytoplasm. This disease is morphologically indistinguishable from T-cell large granulocytic leukemia.

least some of these cases, the NK cell proliferation was polyclonal. Immunophenotypic and genetic analysis is required for firm diagnosis of NK chronic lymphocytic leukemia.

Aggressive Natural Killer Cell Leukemia/Lymphoma

Aggressive NK cell leukemia/lymphoma occurs more often in male than female patients and presents with fever, coagulopathy, hepatomegaly, peripheral blood and bone marrow involvement, and variable infiltration of spleen, lymph nodes, skin, and other organs (12–27) (Figs. 28-3 through 28-5). The clinical course is acute and typically fatal. Aggressive NK cell leukemia/lymphoma occurs as a *de novo* malignancy; as a complication of organ transplantation, human immunodeficiency virus infection, and chronic EBV

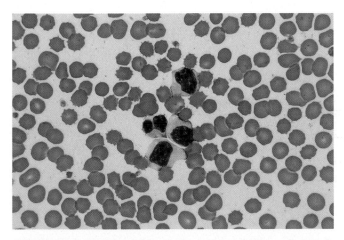

FIGURE 28-1. Peripheral blood smear, natural killer cell chronic lymphocytic leukemia. Natural killer cells show modest nuclear pleomorphism. These cells are morphologically indistinguishable from T-cell large granular lymphocytes.

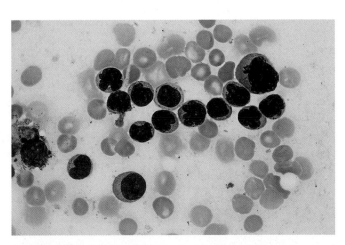

FIGURE 28-3. Bone marrow aspirate smear, aggressive natural killer cell leukemia/lymphoma. Numerous natural killer cells are present, showing marked variability in nuclear size and shape.

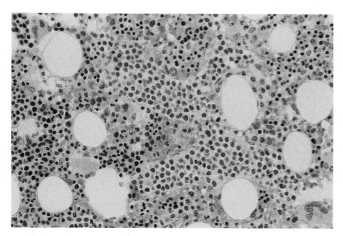

FIGURE 28-4. Bone marrow biopsy specimen, aggressive natural killer cell leukemia/lymphoma. The abnormal natural killer cells fill and distend the sinusoids.

infection; and as a transformation of chronic NK cell lymphocytosis and other NK cell proliferations. Disorders closely associated with aggressive NK cell leukemia/lymphoma include mosquito bite hypersensitivity, hereditary cold urticaria, and hemophagocytic syndrome.

The peripheral blood shows large granular lymphocytosis, with absolute counts as high as 100×10^9 cells/L. The malignant cells show intermediate-sized to large, round to irregular nuclei and pale-staining cytoplasm containing azurophilic granules. Occasional cases show pleomorphic nuclei, prominent nucleoli, and abundant basophilic cytoplasm. Other findings include one or more cytopenias. Bone marrow aspirate smears and histologic sections show similar cells.

Flow cytometry shows expression of CD2, cytoplasmic CD3 ϵ, CD7 (variable), CD38, CD45, CD56 (variable), and HLA-DR. CD16 is rarely expressed. Surface CD3, CD5, immunoglobulin heavy and light chains, T-cell receptor, and terminal deoxynucleotidyl transferase are not expressed. Im-

munostains confirm the above findings and show positivity for granzyme, perforin, TIA-1, and, in some cases, CD30.

Genetic studies show clonal karyotypic anomalies, especially gain and loss of X, and deletions and translocations involving chromosomes 6q, 13q, and 17q. Clonal immunoglobulin and T-cell receptor gene rearrangements are absent. Clonal integration of EBV DNA in tumor cells and other signs of EBV infection are consistently found.

The differential diagnosis includes other NK cell and cytotoxic T-cell proliferations. Immunophenotypic and genetic analysis are required for firm diagnosis of aggressive NK cell leukemia/lymphoma.

Other Natural Killer Cell Lymphomas

Other NK cell lymphomas usually affect male patients, presenting as tumors of the skin and subcutaneous tissue, upper aerodigestive tract, gastrointestinal tract, and other sites (28-42). The clinical course is typically short and aggressive. NK cell lymphoma occurs *de novo;* as a complication of organ transplantation, human immunodeficiency virus infection, and ulcerative colitis; and as a transformation of chronic NK cell lymphocytosis. Complications include hemophagocytic syndrome.

The peripheral blood is typically uninvolved. Cases showing overt leukemia at presentation are probably better considered as aggressive NK cell leukemia/lymphoma. Bone marrow aspirate smears and histologic sections show involvement in less than 10% of cases at diagnosis. The tumor cells are pleomorphic, with irregular nuclei, condensed chromatin, and granular cytoplasm.

Flow cytometry shows expression of CD2, cytoplasmic CD3 ϵ, CD4, CD7, CD16, CD45, and CD56 (variable). Surface CD3, CD5, and T-cell receptor are not expressed. Immunostains may show positivity for CD2 (variable), cytoplasmic CD3 ϵ, CD16, CD56, HLA-DR, granzyme B, perforin, and TIA-1 but not surface CD3 or CD57.

Genetic studies show numerous clonal karyotypic anomalies, especially gain and loss of X and Y, trisomy 7, translocations involving chromosome 11q23, and deletions involving chromosomes 6q, 13q, and 17p. Clonal immunoglobulin and T-cell receptor gene rearrangements are absent. Clonal integration of EBV DNA in tumor cells and other signs of EBV infection are often, although not invariably, found.

The differential diagnosis includes other NK cell and cytotoxic T-cell proliferations. Immunophenotypic and genetic analysis is required for firm diagnosis.

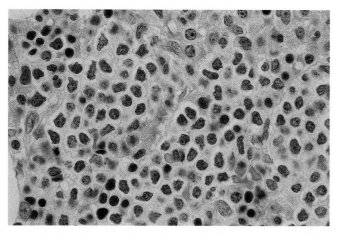

FIGURE 28-5. Bone marrow biopsy specimen, aggressive natural killer cell leukemia/lymphoma. The abnormal natural killer cells show markedly irregular nuclei and moderately abundant clear cytoplasm.

REFERENCES

Precursor Natural Killer Cell Neoplasm

1. Alvarez-Larran A, Villamor N, Hernandez-Boluda JC, et al. Blastic natural killer cell leukemia/lymphoma presenting as overt leukemia. *Clin Lymphoma* 2001;2:178–182.

2. Aoyama Y, Yamane T, Hino M, et al. Blastic NK-cell lymphoma/leukemia with T-cell receptor gamma rearrangement. *Ann Hematol* 2001;80:752–754.

3. Bower CP, Standen GR, Pawade J, et al. Cutaneous presentation of steroid responsive blastoid natural killer cell lymphoma. *Br J Dermatol* 2000;142:1017–1020.

4. DuBois SG, Etzell JE, Matthay KK, et al. Pediatric acute blastic natural killer cell leukemia. *Leuk Lymphoma* 2002;43:901–906.

5. Ginarte M, Abalde MT, Peteiro C, et al. Blastoid NK cell leukemia/lymphoma with cutaneous involvement. *Dermatology* 2000;201:268–271.

6. Gloeckner-Hofmann K, Ottesen K, Schmidt S, et al. T-cell/natural killer cell lymphoblastic lymphoma with an unusual coexpression of B-cell antigens. *Ann Hematol* 2000;79:635–639.

7. Isobe K, Tamaru JI, Nakamura S, et al. Blastic natural killer cell lymphoma arising from the mediastinum with terminal deoxynucleotidyl transferase expression. *Pathol Int* 2001;51:55–59.

8. Khoury JD, Medeiros LJ, Manning JT, et al. CD56(+) TdT(+) blastic natural killer cell tumor of the skin: a primitive systemic malignancy related to myelomonocytic leukemia. *Cancer* 2002;94:2401–2408.

9. Kimura S, Kakazu N, Kuroda J, et al. Agranular CD4+CD56+ blastic natural killer leukemia/lymphoma. *Ann Hematol* 2001;80:228–231.

10. Knudsen H, Gronbaek K, thor Straten P, et al. A case of lymphoblastoid natural killer (NK)-cell lymphoma: association with the NK-cell receptor complex CD94/NKG2 and TP53 intragenic deletion. *Br J Dermatol* 2002;146:148–153.

11. Ko YH, Kim SH, Ree HJ. Blastic NK-cell lymphoma expressing terminal deoxynucleotidyl transferase with Homer-Wright type pseudorosettes formation. *Histopathology* 1998;33:547–553.

12. Liu Q, Ohshima K, Sumie A, et al. Nasal CD56 positive small round cell tumors. Differential diagnosis of hematological, neurogenic, and myogenic neoplasms. *Virchows Arch* 2001;438:271–279.

13. Nagai M, Bandoh S, Tasaka T, et al. Secondary myeloid/natural killer cell precursor acute leukemia following essential thrombocythemia. *Hum Pathol* 1999;30:868–871.

14. Nagatani T, Okazawa H, Kambara T, et al. Cutaneous monomorphous CD4- and CD56-positive large-cell lymphoma. *Dermatology* 2000;200:202–208.

15. Shinoda K, Muraki T, Yano M, et al. Infant leukemia suggestive of natural killer cell precursor origin followed an unusual clinical course. *Acta Haematol* 2000;104:202–206.

16. Tamura H, Ogata K, Mori S, et al. Lymphoblastic lymphoma of natural killer cell origin, presenting as pancreatic tumour. *Histopathology* 1998;32:508–511.

17. Yamada O, Ichikawa M, Okamoto T, et al. Killer T-cell induction in patients with blastic natural killer cell lymphoma/leukaemia: implications for successful treatment and possible therapeutic strategies. *Br J Haematol* 2001;113:153–160.

Mature Natural Killer Cell Neoplasms

1. Dekoninck A, Cartuyvels R, Magerman K, et al. Natural killer (NK) cell leukaemia in a patient with a B cell non-Hodgkin's lymphoma. *Clin Lab Haematol* 2000;22:115–117.

2. De Lord C, Mercieca J, Ashton-Key M, et al. Aggressive NK cell lymphoma preceded by a ten year history of neutropenia associated with large granular lymphocyte lymphocytosis. *Leuk Lymphoma* 1998;31:417–421.

3. Gilsanz F, De La Serna J, Molto L, et al. Hemolytic anemia in chronic large granular lymphocytic leukemia of natural killer cells: cytotoxicity of natural killer cells against autologous red cells is associated with hemolysis. *Transfusion* 1996;36:463–466.

4. Morice WG, Kurtin PJ, Leibson PJ, et al. Demonstration of aberrant T-cell and natural killer-cell antigen expression in all cases of granular lymphocytic leukaemia. *Br J Haematol* 2003;120:1026–1036.

5. Okuno SH, Tefferi A, Hanson CA, et al. Spectrum of diseases associated with increased proportions or absolute numbers of peripheral blood natural killer cells. *Br J Haematol* 1996;93:810–812.

6. Rabbani GR, Phyliky RL, Tefferi A. A long-term study of patients with chronic natural killer cell lymphocytosis. *Br J Haematol* 1999;106:960–966.

7. Semenzato G, Zambello R, Starkebaum G, et al. The lymphoproliferative disease of granular lymphocytes: updated criteria for diagnosis. *Blood* 1997;89:256–260.

8. Sun T, Susin M, Brody J, et al. T-cell lymphoma associated with natural killer-like T-cell reaction. *Am J Hematol* 1998;57:331–337.

9. Tefferi A, Li CY. Bone marrow granulomas associated with chronic natural killer cell lymphocytosis. *Am J Hematol* 1997;54:258–262.

10. Tefferi A, Morice WG, Leibson PJ. Natural killer cells and the syndrome of chronic natural killer cell lymphocytosis. *Leuk Lymphoma* 2001;41:277–284.

11. Vanness ER, Davis MD, Tefferi A. Cutaneous findings associated with chronic natural killer cell lymphocytosis. *Int J Dermatol* 2002;41:852–857.

12. Alvarez-Larran A, Villamor N, Hernandez-Boluda JC, et al. Blastic natural killer cell leukemia/lymphoma presenting as overt leukemia. *Clin Lymphoma* 2001;2:178–182.

13. Camera A, Pezzullo L, Villa MR, et al. Coexistence of two distinct cell populations (CD56(+)TcRgammadelta(+) and CD56(+)TcRgammadelta(−)) in a case of aggressive CD56(+) lymphoma/leukemia. *Haematologica* 2000;85:496–501.

14. De Lord C, Mercieca J, Ashton-Key M, et al. Aggressive NK cell lymphoma preceded by a ten year history of neutropenia associated with large granular lymphocyte lymphocytosis. *Leuk Lymphoma* 1998;31:417–421.

15. Hamaguchi H, Yamaguchi M, Nagata K, et al. Aggressive NK cell lymphoma/leukemia with clonal der(3)t(1;3) (q12;p25), del(6)(q13) and del(13)(q12q14). *Cancer Genet Cytogenet* 2001;130:150–154.

16. Ishihara S, Yabuta R, Tokura Y, et al. Hypersensitivity to mosquito bites is not an allergic disease, but an Epstein-Barr virus-associated lymphoproliferative disease. *Int J Hematol* 2000;72:223–228.

17. Kuroda J, Kimura S, Akaogi T, et al. Aggressive natural killer cell leukemia/lymphoma: a comprehensive cytogenetic study by spectral karyotyping. *Ann Hematol* 2000;79:519–522.

18. Kwong YL, Lam CC, Chan TM. Post-transplantation lymphoproliferative disease of natural killer cell lineage: a clinicopathological and molecular analysis. *Br J Haematol* 2000;110:197–202.

19. Mori N, Yamashita Y, Tsuzuki T, et al. Lymphomatous features of aggressive NK cell leukaemia/lymphoma with massive necrosis, haemophagocytosis and EB virus infection. *Histopathology* 2000;37:363–371.

20. Ohshima K, Suzumiya J, Sugihara M, et al. Clinical, immunohistochemical and phenotypic features of aggressive nodal cytotoxic lymphomas, including alpha/beta, gamma/delta T-cell and natural killer cell types. *Virchows Arch* 1999;435:92–100.

21. Radonich MA, Lazova R, Bolognia J. Cutaneous natural killer/T-cell lymphoma. *J Am Acad Dermatol* 2002;46:451–456.

22. Siu LL, Chan JK, Kwong YL. Natural killer cell malignancies: clinicopathologic and molecular features. *Histol Histopathol* 2002;17:539–554.

23. Siu LL, Chan V, Chan JK, et al. Consistent patterns of allelic loss in natural killer cell lymphoma. *Am J Pathol* 2000;157:1803–1809.

24. Song SY, Kim WS, Ko YH, et al. Aggressive natural killer cell leukemia; clinical features and treatment outcome. *Haematologica* 2002;87:1343–1345.

25. Tao J, Savargaonkar P, Vallejo C, et al. Aggressive natural killer cell lymphoma presenting as an anterior mediastinal mass in a patient with acquired immunodeficiency syndrome. *Arch Pathol Lab Med* 2000;124:304–309.

26. Tokura Y, Ishihara S, Ohshima K, et al. Severe mosquito bite hypersensitivity, natural killer cell leukaemia, latent or chronic active Epstein-Barr virus infection and hydroa vacciniforme-like eruption. *Br J Dermatol* 1998;138:905–906.

27. Wong N, Wong KF, Chan JK, et al. Chromosomal translocations are common in natural killer-cell lymphoma/leukemia as shown by spectral karyotyping. *Hum Pathol* 2000;31:771–774.

28. Abe Y, Muta K, Ohshima K, et al. Subcutaneous panniculitis by Epstein-Barr virus-infected natural killer (NK) cell proliferation terminating in aggressive subcutaneous NK cell lymphoma. *Am J Hematol* 2000;64:221–225.

29. Canioni D, Arnulf B, Asso-Bonnet M, et al. Nasal natural killer lymphoma associated with Epstein-Barr virus in a patient infected with human immunodeficiency virus. *Arch Pathol Lab Med* 2001;125:660–662.

30. Dunphy CH. Natural killer cell lymphoma of the small intestine: diagnosis by flow cytometric immunophenotyping of paracentesis fluid. *Diagn Cytopathol* 1999;20:246–248.

31. Kanavaros P, Boulland ML, Petit B, et al. Expression of cytotoxic proteins in peripheral T-cell and natural killer-cell (NK) lymphomas: association with extranodal site, NK or Tgammadelta phenotype, anaplastic morphology and CD30 expression. *Leuk Lymphoma* 2000;38:317–326.

32. Kato N, Yasukawa K, Onozuka T, et al. Nasal and nasal-type T/NK-cell lymphoma with cutaneous involvement. *J Am Acad Dermatol* 1999;40:850–856.

33. Katoh A, Ohshima K, Kanda M, et al. Gastrointestinal T cell lymphoma: predominant cytotoxic phenotypes, including alpha/beta, gamma/delta T cell and natural killer cells. *Leuk Lymphoma* 2000;39:97–111.

34. Kluin PM, Feller A, Gaulard P, et al. Peripheral T/NK-cell lymphoma: a report of the IXth Workshop of the European Association for Haematopathology. *Histopathology* 2001;38:250–270.

35. Ko YH, Ree HJ, Kim WS, et al. Clinicopathologic and genotypic study of extranodal nasal-type natural killer/T-cell lymphoma and natural killer precursor lymphoma among Koreans. *Cancer* 2000;89:2106–2116.

36. Mhawech P, Medeiros LJ, Bueso-Ramos C, et al. Natural killer-cell lymphoma involving the gynecologic tract. *Arch Pathol Lab Med* 2000;124:1510–1513.

37. Mukai HY, Kojima H, Suzukawa K, et al. Nasal natural killer cell lymphoma in a post-renal transplant patient. *Transplantation* 2000;69:1501–1503.

38. Rodriguez J, Romaguera JE, Manning J, et al. Nasal-type T/NK lymphomas: a clinicopathologic study of 13 cases. *Leuk Lymphoma* 2000;39:139–144.

39. Sadahira Y, Akisada K, Sugihara T, et al. Comparative ultrastructural study of cytotoxic granules in nasal natural killer cell lymphoma, intestinal T-cell lymphoma, and anaplastic large cell lymphoma. *Virchows Arch* 2001;438:280–288.

40. Seiberras S, Hilbert G, Gruson D, et al. Reactive hemaphagocytic syndrome in a patient with midline NK-cell lymphoma. *Ann Med Interne (Paris)* 2000;151:594–596.

41. Wong KF, Chan JK, Cheung MM, et al. Bone marrow involvement by nasal NK cell lymphoma at diagnosis is uncommon. *Am J Clin Pathol* 2001;115:266–270.

42. Yamazaki M, Kakuta M, Takimoto R, et al. Nasal natural killer cell lymphoma presenting as lethal midline granuloma. *Int J Dermatol* 2000;39:931–934.

NONHEMATOLYMPHOID NEOPLASMS

NONHEMATOLYMPHOID NEOPLASMS IN THE BONE MARROW

Nonhematolymphoid tumors in the bone marrow are occasionally primary but more often represent metastatic disease (Table 29-1).

Primary nonhematolymphoid tumors reported in the bone marrow include fibromyxoma, fibrosarcoma, and Kaposi sarcoma (1–3). It is possible that embryonal rhabdomyosarcoma may arise in the bone marrow, although this has not been proven.

Secondary (metastatic) nonhematolymphoid tumors are found with variable frequency, depending on the type of tumor and diagnostic method employed (4–14). Metastatic carcinoma is detected in approximately 20% of bone marrow specimens obtained for staging and stained with hematoxylin and eosin; its presence is a poor prognostic sign. Tumor cells are detected in more than 50% of peripheral blood and bone marrow specimens obtained for staging and studied by immunologic and molecular methods; their presence is of uncertain prognostic import.

A wide variety of tumors metastasize to the bone marrow, including carcinomas, sarcomas, neuroendocrine neoplasms, and malignant melanoma (15–34). Common primary sites of carcinoma metastatic to the bone marrow include the breast, lung, prostate, and stomach; less common sites include the kidney, thyroid, skin, pharynx, gonad, central nervous system, and soft tissue.

Metastatic tumor of unknown primary site is occasionally found in the bone marrow. In adults, most of these are carcinomas, eventually shown to originate in the lung, breast, gastrointestinal tract, or prostate. In children and young adults, most are small round cell tumors, especially embryonal and alveolar rhabdomyosarcoma. Despite exhaustive pre- and postmortem examination, the primary site of embryonal rhabdomyosarcoma remains unidentified in approximately 50% of patients presenting with bone marrow disease. This fact suggests the possibility of bone marrow origin in some cases.

The peripheral blood may show cytopenias and leukoerythroblastosis (signs of marrow replacement or myelophthisis) or microangiopathic hemolytic anemia (35–40). In malignant melanoma, neutrophils and monocytes may contain melanin particles (41). Tumor cell leukemia rarely occurs (see later).

Bone marrow aspirate smears show tumor cells admixed with hematopoietic precursors (Figs. 29-1 through 29-12). Poorly cellular specimens (dry tap) result from bone marrow replacement by tumor, fibrosis, or necrosis. Touch imprints

TABLE 29-1. NONHEMATOLYMPHOID NEOPLASMS IN THE BONE MARROW

Primary neoplasms
  Fibromyxoma
  Fibrosarcoma
  Kaposi sarcoma

Metastatic neoplasms
  Adenocarcinoma
  Embryonal rhabdomyosarcoma
  Hemangiosarcoma
  Malignant melanoma
  Central nervous system neoplasms
  Squamous cell carcinoma
  Undifferentiated carcinoma
  Other sarcomas

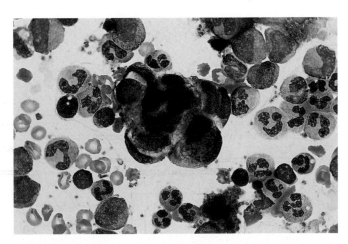

FIGURE 29-1. Bone marrow aspirate, metastatic ductal carcinoma of the breast. A cohesive, three-dimensional group of tumor cells shows nuclei of varying size, displaced by intracellular clear vacuoles.

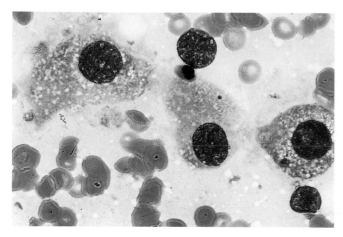

FIGURE 29-2. Bone marrow aspirate, metastatic ductal carcinoma of the breast. Single, large tumor cells show abundant vacuolated cytoplasm.

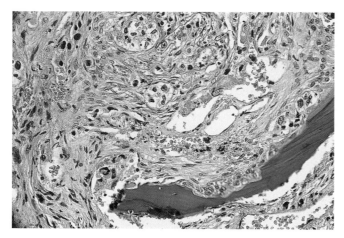

FIGURE 29-3. Bone marrow biopsy specimen, metastatic ductal carcinoma of the breast. Glandlike formations of tumor cells widely infiltrate the bone marrow, surrounded by fibrous stroma and eroded trabecular bone.

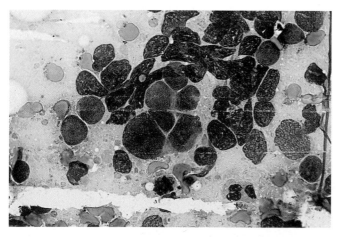

FIGURE 29-4. Bone marrow aspirate, metastatic small cell undifferentiated carcinoma of the lung. Tumor cells with barely discernible cytoplasm are difficult to distinguish from hematolymphoid malignancy; variability in nuclear size, nuclear molding, and absence of nucleoli are helpful clues to the epithelial origin of this tumor.

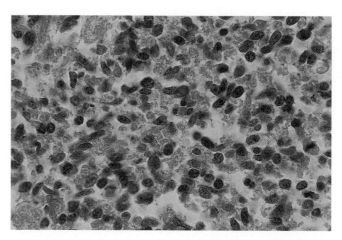

FIGURE 29-5. Bone marrow biopsy specimen, metastatic small cell undifferentiated carcinoma of the lung. Tumor cells with tapered nuclei (oat cells) replace hematopoietic tissue.

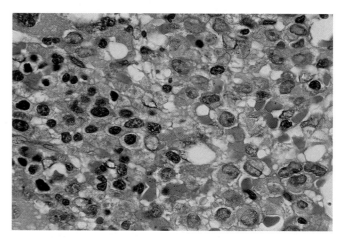

FIGURE 29-6. Bone marrow biopsy specimen, metastatic lobular carcinoma of the breast. The interface between tumor cells and hematopoietic tissue is shown. The tumor cells are similar in size to hematopoietic cells but show abundant cytoplasm with clear vacuoles (signet-ring morphology).

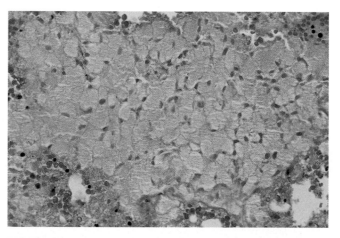

FIGURE 29-7. Bone marrow biopsy specimen, metastatic colon carcinoma. Necrotic tumor cells show abundant cytoplasm and resemble Gaucher cells or other storage histiocytes.

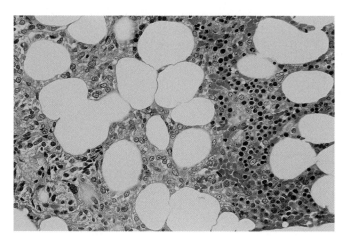

FIGURE 29-8. Bone marrow biopsy specimen, metastatic liposarcoma. The interface between tumor cells and hematopoietic tissue is shown. Adipose cells, either residual or tumor derived, are apparent in both the neoplastic and normal tissue.

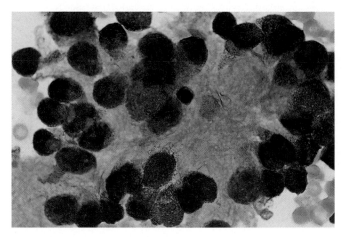

FIGURE 29-11. Bone marrow aspirate, metastatic neuroblastoma. A tumor rosette is seen, with a central accumulation of fibrillary neuropil.

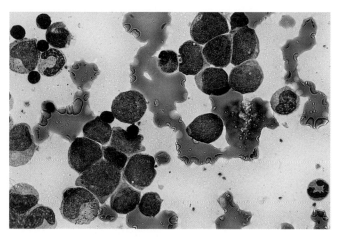

FIGURE 29-9. Bone marrow aspirate, metastatic neuroblastoma. Tumor cells occur singly and in groups and are difficult to distinguish from acute leukemia and malignant lymphoma. The presence of nuclear molding is a helpful clue to the correct diagnosis.

of the core biopsy specimen are particularly helpful in such cases. Isolated tumor cells are often difficult to distinguish from hematopoietic precursors; therefore, definite aggregates of intact tumor cells should be sought before rendering a diagnosis of metastatic tumor.

Tumor cells often show cohesiveness, nuclear molding, and clumped chromatin. They may contain phagocytosed blood cells or tumor cells (42–44). Other morphologic features include acinus formation and intracellular vacuoles in adenocarcinoma and pseudorosette formation in neuroblastoma (Figs. 29-9 through 29-12). Osteoblasts and osteoclasts may be present and are clues to the abnormal bony remodeling often seen in metastatic malignancy.

Histologic sections of the bone marrow show patchy to complete replacement of the marrow by tumor. Residual hematopoietic tissue may be hyperplastic. Most tumors cause architectural distortion of the bone marrow by infiltration,

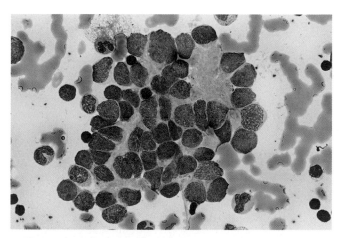

FIGURE 29-10. Bone marrow aspirate, metastatic neuroblastoma. Tumor cells are readily identifiable when they form cohesive clusters and rosettes, as in this specimen.

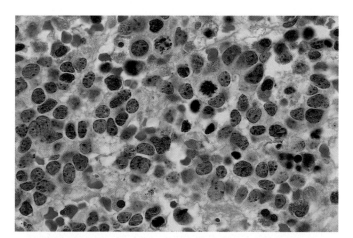

FIGURE 29-12. Bone marrow biopsy specimen, metastatic neuroblastoma. The tumor cells show a high nuclear:cytoplasmic ratio and brisk mitotic activity, often higher than that seen in acute leukemia.

fibrosis, and secondary bony changes. An exception is metastatic lobular breast carcinoma, which may infiltrate the bone marrow with a subtle infiltrate of bland, myelocyte-like cells without notable architectural changes (45). Other findings include nonspecific granulomas and necrosis, which may obscure the underlying diagnosis.

The differential diagnosis includes normal marrow cells and hematolymphoid neoplasms.

Normal cells most likely to be mistaken for tumor cells are erythroid precursors, which are sometimes seen in bone marrow aspirate smears as clumps of smudged nuclei, stripped of their cytoplasm (46). This is a particularly common problem in cases of erythroid hyperplasia. Myeloid precursors may also be mistaken for metastatic tumor, especially in smears made from heparin-anticoagulated bone marrow because heparin causes cell clumping and nuclear smudging. Leukoerythroblastosis with marrow fibrosis owing to metastatic tumor may be misinterpreted as a myeloproliferative disorder (47).

Some nonhematolymphoid tumors may be mistaken for hematolymphoid neoplasms, especially when presenting with a leukemic phase, diffuse marrow involvement, and no apparent primary site (48–51). Conversely, hematolymphoid neoplasms may be mistaken for metastatic tumors (52–55).

Other pitfalls are created by the use of cytochemical and immunologic stains. Peripheral blood and bone marrow samples from patients without malignancies may contain cytokeratin-positive cells (18). Gastric carcinoma cells may produce lysozyme (56). Small cell undifferentiated carcinoma of the lung may express CD15 (57). Neuroblastoma cells express CD56 and, in some cases, CD117 but not CD45 (58,59). Ewing sarcoma and related tumors express CD99 but not CD45 (60).

Most of these potential errors are avoidable by being careful to interpret only intact, well-preserved cells with clearly identifiable nuclear and cytoplasmic membranes and correlating pathologic findings with clinical features.

NONHEMATOLYMPHOID NEOPLASMS IN THE PERIPHERAL BLOOD

Nonhematolymphoid tumors occasionally present with overt peripheral blood disease resembling acute leukemia (Table 29-2). Although often used, the terms "carcinoma cell leukemia" and "carcinocythemia" are not always appropriate because not all cases are attributable to carcinoma.

A leukemic phase has been reported in alveolar and embryonal rhabdomyosarcoma, breast carcinoma, small cell undifferentiated carcinoma of the lung, urothelial carcinoma, malignant melanoma, neuroblastoma, retinoblastoma, and malignant germ cell tumor (1–9). Leukemia may be the first sign of malignancy but is more often a terminal event, presaging death within days.

TABLE 29-2. NONHEMATOLYMPHOID NEOPLASMS IN THE PERIPHERAL BLOOD

Carcinomas
  Breast carcinoma
  Small cell undifferentiated carcinoma of the lung
  Urothelial carcinoma

Other tumors
  Malignant germ cell tumor
  Malignant melanoma
  Neuroblastoma
  Retinoblastoma
  Rhabdomyosarcoma

The peripheral blood shows numerous bizarre cells, often showing coarse chromatin, prominent nucleoli, and basophilic cytoplasm. Auer rods and myelodysplastic changes are absent. The bone marrow aspirate and core biopsy sections typically show massive replacement by malignant cells. Flow cytometry shows no expression of myeloid or lymphoid antigens, with rare exception. Ewing sarcoma and related tumors express CD99 but not CD45 (10). Neuroblastoma expresses CD56 and, in some cases, CD117 but not CD45 (11,12).

The differential diagnosis includes acute leukemia and the leukemic phase of malignant lymphoma (13). Leukemic rhabdomyosarcoma can be particularly difficult to diagnose correctly because many cases show no evidence of a primary site but only peripheral blood and marrow disease. Immunostains, immunophenotyping by flow cytometry, electron microscopy, and/or genetic studies may be both useful and misleading. The correct diagnosis has often made only at autopsy.

It should be kept in mind that, rarely, acute leukemia and leukemic dissemination of a nonhematopoietic tumor may occur simultaneously (14).

REFERENCES

Nonhematolymphoid Neoplasms in the Bone Marrow

1. Kuhne A, Engelhorn T, Homann M, et al. Fibromyxoma of the iliac wing. *Skeletal Radiol* 2003;32:170–173.
2. Ninomiya H, Hato T, Yamada T, et al. Multiple diffuse fibrosarcoma of bone associated with extramedullary hematopoiesis. *Intern Med* 1998;37:480–483.
3. Teh BS, Lu HH, Lynch GR, et al. AIDS-related Kaposi's sarcoma involving bone and bone marrow. *South Med J* 1999;92:61–64.
4. Athale UH, Shurtleff SA, Jenkins JJ, et al. Use of reverse transcriptase polymerase chain reaction for diagnosis and staging of alveolar rhabdomyosarcoma, Ewing sarcoma family of tumors, and desmoplastic small round cell tumor. *J Pediatr Hematol Oncol* 2001;23:99–104.
5. Blaheta HJ, Paul T, Sotlar K, et al. Detection of melanoma cells in sentinel lymph nodes, bone marrow and peripheral blood by a reverse transcription-polymerase chain reaction assay in patients

with primary cutaneous melanoma: association with Breslow's tumour thickness. *Br J Dermatol* 2001;145:195–202.

6. Fukuda M, Miyajima Y, Miyashita Y, et al. Disease outcome may be predicted by molecular detection of minimal residual disease in bone marrow in advanced neuroblastoma: a pilot study. *J Pediatr Hematol Oncol* 2001;23:10–13.

7. Horibe K, Fukuda M, Miyajima Y, et al. Outcome prediction by molecular detection of minimal residual disease in bone marrow for advanced neuroblastoma. *Med Pediatr Oncol* 2001;36:203–204.

8. Marth C, Kisic J, Kaern J, et al. Circulating tumor cells in the peripheral blood and bone marrow of patients with ovarian carcinoma do not predict prognosis. *Cancer* 2002;94:707–712.

9. Naume B, Borgen E, Kvalheim G, et al. Detection of isolated tumor cells in bone marrow in early-stage breast carcinoma patients: comparison with preoperative clinical parameters and primary tumor characteristics. *Clin Cancer Res* 2001;7:4122–4129.

10. Perey L, Benhattar J, Peters R, et al. High tumour contamination of leukaphereses in patients with small cell carcinoma of the lung: a comparison of immunocytochemistry and RT-PCR. *Br J Cancer* 2001;85:1713–1721.

11. Seeger RC, Reynolds CP, Gallego R, et al. Quantitative tumor cell content of bone marrow and blood as a predictor of outcome in stage IV neuroblastoma: a Children's Cancer Group Study. *J Clin Oncol* 2000;18:4067–4076.

12. Thorban S, Rosenberg R, Busch R, et al. Epithelial cells in bone marrow of oesophageal cancer patients: a significant prognostic factor in multivariate analysis. *Br J Cancer* 2000;83:35–39.

13. Weckermann D, Muller P, Wawroschek F, et al. Disseminated cytokeratin positive tumor cells in the bone marrow of patients with prostate cancer: detection and prognostic value. *J Urol* 2001;166:699–703.

14. Z'graggen K, Centeno BA, Fernandez-del Castillo C, et al. Biological implications of tumor cells in blood and bone marrow of pancreatic cancer patients. *Surgery* 2001;129:537–546.

15. Darvishian F, Brody JP, Hajdu SI. Liposarcoma in the bone marrow: a terminal event. *Ann Clin Lab Sci* 2001;31:402–404.

16. de Bono JS, Fraser JA, Lee F, et al. Metastatic extragonadal seminoma associated with cardiac transplantation. *Ann Oncol* 2000;11:749–752.

17. Dunkel IJ, Aledo A, Kernan NA, et al. Successful treatment of metastatic retinoblastoma. *Cancer* 2000;89:2117–2121.

18. Elhasid R, Vlodavsky E, Nachtigal A, et al. Bone marrow involvement in osteosarcoma. *J Clin Oncol* 2001;19:276–278.

19. Hardingham JE, Hewett PJ, Sage RE, et al. Molecular detection of blood-borne epithelial cells in colorectal cancer patients and in patients with benign bowel disease. *Int J Cancer* 2000;89:8–13.

20. Hsu E, Keene D, Ventureyra E, et al. Bone marrow metastasis in astrocytic gliomata. *J Neurooncol* 1998;37:285–293.

21. Koka VN, Julieron M, Bourhis J, et al. Aesthesioneuroblastoma. *J Laryngol Otol* 1998;112:628–633.

22. Kunschner LJ, Kuttesch J, Hess K, et al. Survival and recurrence factors in adult medulloblastoma: the M.D. Anderson Cancer Center experience from 1978 to 1998. *Neurooncology* 2001;3:167–173.

23. Ljungberg B, Abramsson L, Roos G. Diagnosis of renal cell carcinoma by bone marrow aspiration biopsy. *Scand J Urol Nephrol* 2001;35:334–336.

24. Sajedi M, Wolff JE, Egeler RM, et al. Congenital extrarenal non-central nervous system malignant rhabdoid tumor. *J Pediatr Hematol Oncol* 2002;24:316–320.

25. So CC, Wong KF. Bone marrow involvement by angiosarcoma. *Br J Haematol* 2001;115:1.

26. Wong KF, So CC, Wong N, et al. Sinonasal angiosarcoma with marrow involvement at presentation mimicking malignant lymphoma: cytogenetic analysis using multiple techniques. *Cancer Genet Cytogenet* 2001;129:64–68.

27. Greco FA, Burris HA 3rd, Litchy S, et al. Gemcitabine, carboplatin, and paclitaxel for patients with carcinoma of unknown primary site: a Minnie Pearl Cancer Research Network study. *J Clin Oncol* 2002;20:1651–1656.

28. Ise Y, Yanagawa H, Hirose T, et al. An autopsy case of cytokeratin 7-positive minute adenocarcinoma of the lung with systemic metastases. *Intern Med* 1998;37:766–769.

29. Lassen U, Daugaard G, Eigtved A, et al. 18F-FDG whole body positron emission tomography (PET) in patients with unknown primary tumours (UPT). *Eur J Cancer* 1999;35:1076–1082.

30. Torne A, Martinez-Roman S, Pahisa J, et al. Massive metastases from a lobular breast carcinoma from an unknown primary during pregnancy. A case report. *J Reprod Med* 1995;40:676–680.

31. Ambrosiani L, Bellone S, Betto FS, et al. Rhabdomyosarcoma presenting as acute hematologic malignancy: case report and review of the literature. *Tumori* 1996;82:408–412.

32. Kahn DG. Rhabdomyosarcoma mimicking acute leukemia in an adult: report of a case with histologic, flow cytometric, cytogenetic, immunohistochemical, and ultrastructural studies. *Arch Pathol Lab Med* 1998;122:375–378.

33. Morandi S, Manna A, Sabattini E, et al. Rhabdomyosarcoma presenting as acute leukemia. *J Pediatr Hematol Oncol* 1996;18:305–307.

34. Sandberg AA, Stone JF, Czarnecki L, et al. Hematologic masquerade of rhabdomyosarcoma. *Am J Hematol* 2001;68:51–57.

35. Campbell LJ, Van der Weyden MB. Hematological, biochemical and bone scan findings in patients with marrow carcinoma. *Pathology* 1991;23:198–201.

36. Shamdas GJ, Ahmann FR, Matzner MB, et al. Leukoerythroblastic anemia in metastatic prostate cancer. Clinical and prognostic significance in patients with hormone-refractory disease. *Cancer* 1993;71:3594–3600.

37. Mathew P, Fleming D, Adegboyega PA. Myelophthisis as a solitary manifestation of failure from rectal carcinoma. A Batson phenomenon? *Arch Pathol Lab Med* 2000;124:1228–1230.

38. Bhagwati N, Seno R, Dutcher JP, et al. Fulminant metastatic melanoma complicated by a microangiopathic hemolytic anemia. *Hematopathol Mol Hematol* 1998;11:101–108.

39. Lin YC, Chang HK, Sun CF, et al. Microangiopathic hemolytic anemia as an initial presentation of metastatic cancer of unknown primary origin. *South Med J* 1995;88:683–687.

40. Polukhin E, Balla A, Chary K, et al. Microangiopathic hemolytic anemia as the first manifestation of lung adenocarcinoma. *South Med J* 2001;94:550–551.

41. Weil SC, Holt S, Hrisinko MA, et al. Melanin inclusions in the peripheral blood leukocytes of a patient with malignant melanoma. *Am J Clin Pathol* 1985;84:679–681.

42. Caruso RA, Muda AO, Bersiga A, et al. Morphological evidence of neutrophil-tumor cell phagocytosis (cannibalism) in human gastric adenocarcinomas. *Ultrastruct Pathol* 2002;26:315–321.

43. Falini B, Bucciarelli E, Grignani F, et al. Erythrophagocytosis by undifferentiated lung carcinoma cells. *Cancer* 1980;46:1140–1145.

44. Youness E, Barlogie B, Ahearn M, et al. Tumor cell phagocytosis. Its occurrence in a patient with medulloblastoma. *Arch Pathol Lab Med* 1980;104:651–653.

45. Bitter MA, Fiorito D, Corkill ME, et al. Bone marrow involvement by lobular carcinoma of the breast cannot be identified reliably by routine histological examination alone. *Hum Pathol* 1994;25:781–788.

46. Vernon SE. Clumping of erythroblasts simulating a metastatic neoplasm. *Arch Pathol Lab Med* 1985;109:569–570.
47. Yablonski-Peretz T, Sulkes A, Polliack A, et al. Secondary myelofibrosis with metastatic breast cancer simulating agnogenic myeloid metaplasia: report of a case and review of the literature. *Med Pediatr Oncol* 1985;13:92–96.
48. Castella A, Davey FR, Kurec AS, et al. The presence of Burkitt-like cells in non-Burkitt's neoplasms. *Cancer* 1982;50:1764–1770.
49. Cerrotta A, Galante E. A metastatic breast cancer with an unusual lymphoma-like presentation. *Tumori* 1990;76:296–298.
50. Lugassy G, Vorst EJ, Varon D, et al. Carcinocythemia. Report of two cases, one simulating a Burkitt lymphoma. *Acta Cytol* 1990; 34:265–268.
51. Wong KF, So CC, Wong N, et al. Sinonasal angiosarcoma with marrow involvement at presentation mimicking malignant lymphoma: cytogenetic analysis using multiple techniques. *Cancer Genet Cytogenet* 2001;129:64–68.
52. Exner M, Thalhammer-Scherrer R, Kudlacek S, et al. Suspect cell convolutes in the bone marrow of a patient with renal cell carcinoma unmasked as atypical convolutes of hairy cells. *Leuk Lymphoma* 2001;42:239–241.
53. Oyen WJ, Raemaekers JM, Corstens FH. Acute myelofibrosis mimicking multiple bone metastases on Tc-99m MDP bone imaging. *Clin Nucl Med* 1998;23:1–2.
54. Penchansky L, Taylor SR, Krause JR. Three infants with acute megakaryoblastic leukemia simulating metastatic tumor. *Cancer* 1989;64:1366–1371.
55. Pui CH, Rivera G, Mirro J, et al. Acute megakaryoblastic leukemia. Blast cell aggregates simulating metastatic tumor. *Arch Pathol Lab Med* 1985;109:1033–1035.
56. Takahashi T, Akihama T, Yamaguchi A, et al. Lysozyme secreting tumor: a case of gastric cancer associated with myelofibrosis due to disseminated bone marrow metastasis. *Jpn J Med* 1987;26: 58–64.
57. Hyder DM, Beals TF, Schnitzer B. Leu-M1-positive small cell carcinoma. *Hum Pathol* 1986;17:314–316.
58. Beck D, Gross N, Brognara CB, et al. Expression of stem cell factor and its receptor by human neuroblastoma cells and tumors. *Blood* 1995;86:3132–3138.
59. Komada Y, Zhang XL, Zhou YW, et al. Flow cytometric analysis of peripheral blood and bone marrow for tumor cells in patients with neuroblastoma. *Cancer* 1998;82:591–599.
60. Lucas DR, Bentley G, Dan ME, et al. Ewing sarcoma vs lymphoblastic lymphoma. A comparative immunohistochemical study. *Am J Clin Pathol* 2001;115:11–17.

Nonhematolymphoid Neoplasms in the Peripheral Blood

1. Kahn DG. Rhabdomyosarcoma mimicking acute leukemia in an adult: report of a case with histologic, flow cytometric, cytogenetic, immunohistochemical, and ultrastructural studies. *Arch Pathol Lab Med* 1998;122:375–378.
2. Sandberg AA, Stone JF, Czarnecki L, et al. Hematologic masquerade of rhabdomyosarcoma. *Am J Hematol* 2001;68:51–57.
3. Rodriguez-Salas N, Jimenez-Gordo AM, Gonzalez E, et al. Circulating cancer cells in peripheral blood. A case report. *Acta Cytol* 2000;44:237–241.
4. Seronie-Vivien S, Mery E, Delord JP, et al. Carcinocythemia as the single extension of breast cancer: report of a case and review of the literature. *Ann Oncol* 2001;12:1019–1022.
5. Sile CC, Perry DJ, Nam L. Small cell carcinocythemia. *Arch Pathol Lab Med* 1999;123:426–428.
6. Gallivan MV, Lokich JJ. Carcinocythemia (carcinoma cell leukemia). Report of two cases with English literature review. *Cancer* 1984;53:1100–1102.
7. Boyd JE, Parmley RT, Langevin AM, et al. Neuroblastoma presenting as acute monoblastic leukemia. *J Pediatr Hematol Oncol* 1996;18:206–212.
8. Zubizarreta P, Chantada G. Circulating retinoblastoma cells in a patient with metastatic disease. *Ophthalmic Genet* 1999;20: 189–191.
9. Irie J, Kawai K, Ueno Y, et al. Malignant germ cell tumor of the anterior mediastinum with leukemia-like infiltration. *Acta Pathol Jpn* 1985;35:1561–1570.
10. Lucas DR, Bentley G, Dan ME, et al. Ewing sarcoma vs lymphoblastic lymphoma. A comparative immunohistochemical study. *Am J Clin Pathol* 2001;115:11–17.
11. Beck D, Gross N, Brognara CB, et al. Expression of stem cell factor and its receptor by human neuroblastoma cells and tumors. *Blood* 1995;86:3132–3138.
12. Komada Y, Zhang XL, Zhou YW, et al. Flow cytometric analysis of peripheral blood and bone marrow for tumor cells in patients with neuroblastoma. *Cancer* 1998;82:591–599.
13. Gujral S, Prasad R, Naresh KN. Systemic anaplastic large cell lymphoma in a child presenting with bone marrow involvement and clinical features of acute leukaemia. *Am J Hematol* 2002;69: 150–155.
14. Santos-Machado TM, Zerbini MC, Cristofani LM, et al. Simultaneous occurrence of advanced neuroblastoma and acute myeloid leukemia. *Pediatr Hematol Oncol* 2001;18:129–135.